Bioengineering and Biophysical Aspects of Electromagnetic Fields

Fourth Edition

Biological Effects of Electromagnetics Series

Series Editors
Frank Barnes
University of Colorado Boulder, Colorado, U.S.A.

Ben Greenebaum
University of Wisconsin–Parkside Somers, Wisconsin, U.S.A.

Electromagnetic Fields in Biological Systems
Edited by James C. Lin

Epidemiology of Electromagnetic Fields
Edited by Martin Röösli

Advanced Electroporation Techniques in Biology and Medicine
Edited by Andrei G. Pakhomov, Damijan Miklavčič, and Marko S. Markov

The Physiology of Bioelectricity in Development, Tissue Regeneration, and Cancer
Edited by Christine E. Pullar

Handbook of Biological Effects of Electromagnetic Fields, Fourth Edition – Two Volume Set
Edited by Ben Greenebaum and Frank Barnes

For more information about this series, please visit: https://www.crcpress.com/Biological-Effects-of-Electromagnetics/book-series/CRCBIOEFFOFELE

Bioengineering and Biophysical Aspects of Electromagnetic Fields

Fourth Edition

Edited by
Ben Greenebaum and Frank Barnes

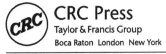

CRC Press is an imprint of the
Taylor & Francis Group, an **Informa** business

CRC Press
Taylor & Francis Group
6000 Broken Sound Parkway NW, Suite 300
Boca Raton, FL 33487-2742

© 2019 by Taylor & Francis Group, LLC
CRC Press is an imprint of Taylor & Francis Group, an Informa business

No claim to original U.S. Government works

Printed on acid-free paper

International Standard Book Number-13: 978-1-138-73530-9 (Hardback)

This book contains information obtained from authentic and highly regarded sources. Reasonable efforts have been made to publish reliable data and information, but the author and publisher cannot assume responsibility for the validity of all materials or the consequences of their use. The authors and publishers have attempted to trace the copyright holders of all material reproduced in this publication and apologize to copyright holders if permission to publish in this form has not been obtained. If any copyright material has not been acknowledged, please write and let us know so we may rectify in any future reprint.

Except as permitted under U.S. Copyright Law, no part of this book may be reprinted, reproduced, transmitted, or utilized in any form by any electronic, mechanical, or other means, now known or hereafter invented, including photocopying, microfilming, and recording, or in any information storage or retrieval system, without written permission from the publishers.

For permission to photocopy or use material electronically from this work, please access www.copyright.com (http://www.copyright.com/) or contact the Copyright Clearance Center, Inc. (CCC), 222 Rosewood Drive, Danvers, MA 01923, 978-750-8400. CCC is a not-for-profit organization that provides licenses and registration for a variety of users. For organizations that have been granted a photocopy license by the CCC, a separate system of payment has been arranged.

Trademark Notice: Product or corporate names may be trademarks or registered trademarks, and are used only for identification and explanation without intent to infringe.

Library of Congress Cataloging-in-Publication Data

Names: Greenebaum, Ben, editor. | Barnes, Frank, 1932- editor.
Title: Handbook of biological effects of electromagnetic fields / [edited by] Ben Greenebaum and Frank Barnes.
Description: Fourth edition. | Boca Raton: Taylor & Francis, 2018. |
Series: Biological effects of electromagnetics series | Includes bibliographical references.
Contents: Volume 1: Bioengineering and biophysical aspects of electromagnetic fields — Volume 2: Biological and medical aspects of electromagnetic fields.
Identifiers: LCCN 2018038369| ISBN 9781138735309 (volume 1: alk. paper) |
ISBN 9781315186580 (volume 1: ebook)
Subjects: LCSH: Electromagnetism—Physiological effect—Handbooks, manuals, etc.
Classification: LCC QP82.2.E43 C73 2018 | DDC 612/.01442—dc23
LC record available at https://lccn.loc.gov/2018038369

Visit the Taylor & Francis Web site at
http://www.taylorandfrancis.com

and the CRC Press Web site at
http://www.crcpress.com

Contents

Preface..vii
Editors..ix
List of Contributors..xi

0. **Introduction to Electromagnetic Fields**..1
   Frank Barnes, Charles Polk, and Ben Greenebaum

1. **Environmental and Occupational DC and Low Frequency Electromagnetic Fields**..29
   Ben Greenebaum and Kjell Hansson Mild

2. **Intermediate and Radiofrequency Sources and Exposures in Everyday Environments**...55
   Javier Vila

3. **Endogenous Bioelectric Phenomena and Interfaces for Exogenous Effects**............73
   Richard H. W. Funk

4. **Electric and Magnetic Properties of Biological Materials**.........................101
   Camelia Gabriel and Azadeh Peyman

5. **Interaction of Static and Extremely Low-Frequency Electric Fields with Biological Materials and Systems**..161
   Frank Barnes

6. **Magnetic Field Interactions with Biological Materials**..........................219
   Frank Barnes

7. **Mechanisms of Action in Bioelectromagnetics**.......................................233
   Ben Greenebaum

8. **Signals, Noise, and Thresholds**...261
   Martin Bier and James C. Weaver

9. **Computational Methods for Predicting Electromagnetic Fields and Temperature Increase in Biological Bodies**...299
   James C. Lin

10. **Experimental Dosimetry**..399
    Rodolfo Bruzon and Hakki Gurhan

v

11. Overcoming the Irreproducibility Barrier: Considerations to Improve the Quality of Experimental Practice When Investigating the Effects of Low-Level Electric and Magnetic Fields on In Vitro Biological Systems 435
Lucas Portelli

12. Radio Frequency Exposure Standards 463
K. R. Foster, C.-K. Chou, and R. C. Petersen

Index 513

Preface

We are honored to have been asked to follow the 2007 3rd Edition of the *Handbook* with this 4th Edition and to carry on the tradition established in the first two editions by Dr. Postow and the late Dr. Polk. In this edition of the *Handbook of Biological Effects of Electromagnetic Fields*, we have added new and newly relevant material on a number of aspects of basic science and on diagnostic and therapeutic applications. While we had to reduce or drop coverage of a few topics that now seem less immediately important, we refer the reader to the material on these in the previous editions. New additions include expanded coverage of brain stimulation, characterization and modeling of epithelial tissue wounds, theoretical models of proposed basic mechanisms giving rise to bioelectromagnetic effects, and dosimetric measurement methods and instrumentation. For the first time in this series we have added coverage of electromagnetic effects in the terahertz region, field effects on plants, and applying electrical engineering concepts of systems engineering and operational amplifiers with feedback to the analysis of biological electromagnetic effects. At the same time, all chapters have been updated in view of what has been learned in the past decade, some receiving relatively minor changes and others being completely revamped.

Research in bioelectromagnetics stems from three sources, all of which are important: Bioelectromagnetics first emerged as a separate scientific subject because of interest in studying possible hazards from exposure to electromagnetic fields and setting human exposure limits. A second interest is in the beneficial use of fields to advance health, both in diagnostics and in treatment, an interest that is as old as the discovery of electricity itself. Finally, the observed interactions between electromagnetic fields and biological systems raise some fundamental, unanswered scientific questions as to how they occur, the answers to which may lead to fields being used as tools to probe basic biology and biophysics. Various chapters treat both basic physical science and engineering aspects and biological and medical aspects of these three. Answering basic bioelectromagnetic questions will not only lead to answers about potential electromagnetic hazards and to better beneficial applications, but they should also contribute significantly to our basic understanding of biological processes. Both strong fields and those on the order of the fields spontaneously generated within biological systems may become tools to perturb the systems, either for experiments seeking to understand how the systems operate or simply to change the systems, such as by injecting a plasmid containing genes whose effects are to be investigated. These three threads are intertwined throughout bioelectromagnetics. Although any specific chapter in this work will emphasize one or another of these threads, the reader should be aware that each aspect of the research is relevant to a greater or lesser extent to all three.

As in previous editions, the authors of the individual chapters were charged with providing the reader, whom we imagine is moderately familiar with one or more of the sciences underlying bioelectromagnetics, though perhaps not in the others or in the interdisciplinary subject of bioelectromagnetics itself, with both an introduction to their topic and a basis for further reading. We asked the chapter authors to imagine and write what they would like to be the first thing they would ask a new graduate student in their laboratory to read. Like its predecessors, this edition is intended to be useful as a reference book but also as a text for introducing the reader to bioelectromagnetics or some of its aspects. For these students and other readers who are not familiar with the basic physical science

vii

behind electromagnetic fields, the Introduction ("Chapter 0") and Chapters 5 and 6 are intended to be helpful.

As a "handbook" and not an encyclopedia, this work does not intend to cover all aspects of bioelectromagnetics. Nevertheless, considering the breadth of topics and growth of research, some ideas are unavoidably duplicated in various chapters, sometimes from different viewpoints that could be instructive to the reader and sometimes presenting different aspects or implications. While the amount of material has led to the publication of the handbook as two separate, but interrelated volumes: Biological and Medical Aspects of Electromagnetic Fields (BMA) and Bioengineering and Biophysical Aspects of Electromagnetic Fields (BBA), there is no sharp dividing line, and some topics are dealt with in parts of both volumes. The reader is urged to go beyond a single chapter is researching a specific topic.

The reader should note that the chapter authors have a wide variety of interests and backgrounds. Their work and interests range from safety standards and possible health effects of low-level fields to therapy through applications in biology and medicine to the fundamental physics and chemistry underlying the biology and bioelectromagnetic interactions. It is therefore not surprising that the authors may have different and sometimes conflicting points of view on the significance of various results and their potential applications. Thus authors should only be held responsible for the viewpoints expressed in their chapters and not in others. We have tried to select the authors and topics so as to cover the scientific results to date that are likely to serve as a starting point for future work that will lead to the further development of the field. Each chapter's extensive reference section should be helpful for those needing to obtain a more extensive background than is possible from a book of this type.

Some of the material, as well as various authors' viewpoints, are controversial, and their importance is likely to change as the field develops and our understanding of the underlying science improves. We hope that this volume will serve as a starting point for both students and practitioners to understand the various parts of the field of bioelectromagnetics, as of mid-to-late 2017, when authors contributing to this volume finished their literature reviews.

The editors would like to express their appreciation to all the authors for the extensive time and effort they have put into preparing this edition. It is our wish that it will prove to be of value to the readers and lead to advancing our understanding of this challenging field.

Ben Greenebaum

Frank Barnes

Editors

Ben Greenebaum retired as professor of physics at the University of Wisconsin—Parkside, Kenosha, WI, in May 2001, but was appointed as emeritus professor and adjunct professor to continue research, journal editing, and university outreach projects. He received his PhD in physics from Harvard University in 1965. He joined the faculty of UW—Parkside as assistant professor in 1970 following postdoctoral positions at Harvard and Princeton Universities. He was promoted to associate professor in 1972 and to professor in 1980. Greenebaum is author or coauthor of more than 50 scientific papers. Since 1992, he has been editor in chief of Bioelectromagnetics, an international peer-reviewed scientific journal, and the most cited specialized journal in this field. He spent 1997–1998 as consultant in the World Health Organization's International EMF Project in Geneva, Switzerland. Between 1971 and 2000, he was part of an interdisciplinary research team investigating the biological effects of electromagnetic fields on biological cell cultures. From his graduate student days through 1975, his research studied the spins and moments of radioactive nuclei. In 1977, he became a special assistant to the chancellor and in 1978, associate dean of faculty (equivalent to the present associate vice chancellor position). He served 2 years as acting vice chancellor (1984–1985 and 1986–1987). In 1989, he was appointed as dean of the School of Science and Technology, serving until the school was abolished in 1996, after which he chaired the physics department through 2001. On the personal side, he was born in Chicago and has lived in Racine, WI, since 1970. Married since 1965, he and his wife have three adult sons and two grandchildren.

Frank Barnes received his BS in electrical engineering in 1954 from Princeton University and his MS, engineering, and PhD degrees from Stanford University in 1955, 1956, and 1958, respectively. He was a Fulbright scholar in Baghdad, Iraq, in 1958 and joined the University of Colorado in 1959, where he is currently a distinguished professor emeritus. He has served as chairman of the Department of Electrical Engineering, acting dean of the College of Engineering, and in 1971 as cofounder/director with Professor George Codding of the Political Science Department of the Interdisciplinary Telecommunications Program (ITP). He has served as chair of the IEEE Electron Device Society, president of the Electrical Engineering Department Heads Association, vice president of IEEE for Publications, editor of the IEEE Student Journal, and the IEEE Transactions on Education, as well as president of the Bioelectromagnetics Society and U.S. Chair of Commission K—International Union of Radio Science (URSI). He is a fellow of the AAAS, IEEE, International Engineering Consortium, and a member of the National Academy of Engineering. Dr. Barnes has been awarded the Curtis McGraw Research Award from ASEE, the Leon Montgomery Award from the International Communications Association, the 2003 IEEE Education Society Achievement Award, Distinguished Lecturer for IEEE Electron Device Society, the 2002 ECE Distinguished Educator Award from ASEE, The Colorado Institute of Technology Catalyst Award 2004, and the Bernard M. Gordon Prize from National Academy of Engineering for Innovations in Engineering Education 2004. He was born in Pasadena, CA, in 1932 and attended numerous elementary schools throughout the country. He and his wife, Gay, have two children and two grandchildren.

List of Contributors

Frank Barnes
University of Colorado Boulder
Boulder, Colorado

Martin Bier
East Carolina University
Greenville, North Carolina

Rodolfo Bruzon
University of Colorado Boulder
Boulder, Colorado

C.-K. Chou
C-K. Chou Consulting
Dublin, California

K. R. Foster
University of Pennsylvania
Philadelphia, Pennsylvania

Richard H. W. Funk
TU-Dresden
Dresden, Germany

Camelia Gabriel
C. Gabriel Consultants
San Diego, California

Ben Greenebaum
University of Wisconsin-Parkside
Kenosha, Wisconsin

Hakki Gurhan
University of Colorado Boulder
Boulder, Colorado

James C. Lin
University of Illinois
Chicago, Illinois

Kjell Hansson Mild
Umeå University
Umeå, Sweden

R. C. Petersen (Deceased)
R. C. Petersen Associates, LLC
Bedminster, New Jersey

Azadeh Peyman
Public Health England
London, United Kingdom

Charles Polk (Deceased)
Deceased. University of Rhode Island
South Kingstown, Rhode Island

Lucas Portelli
Kirsus Institute
Zürich, Switzerland

Javier Vila
Instituto de Salud Global
Barcelona, Spain

James C. Weaver
Massachusetts Institute of Technology
Cambridge, Massachusetts

0

Introduction to Electromagnetic Fields

Frank Barnes
University of Colorado Boulder

Charles Polk*
University of Rhode Island

Ben Greenebaum
University of Wisconsin-Parkside

CONTENTS

0.1 Background 1
0.2 Review of Basic Electromagnetic Theory 2
0.3 Near Fields and Radiation Fields 5
0.4 Penetration of Direct Current and Low-Frequency Electric Fields into Tissue 8
0.5 Direct Current and Low-Frequency Magnetic Fields 10
0.6 RF Fields 15
0.7 Biophysical Interactions of Fields: Ionization, Ionizing Radiation,
Chemical Bonds, and Excitation 22
References 27

0.1 Background

Much has been learned since this handbook's 3rd edition, but a full understanding of biological effects of electromagnetic fields is still to be achieved. The broad range of disciplines that must be studied has to be a factor in the apparent slow progress toward this ultimate end. Understanding how electric and magnetic fields can affect biological systems requires understanding of disciplines that include basic biology, medical science and clinical practice, biological and electrical engineering, basic chemistry and biochemistry, and fundamental physics and biophysics. The subject matter ranges over characteristic lengths and timescales, at one extreme with static fields and low frequencies with wavelengths of tens of kilometers to other extreme with sub-millimeter wavelength fields with periods below 10^{-12} s. Biological systems have response times that range from 10^{-15} s for electronic state transitions in molecules or atoms to many years for generations for humans and other organisms. This chapter is intended to provide a basic review of electric and magnetic fields and the relations between these fields and to define the terms used throughout the

---

* Deceased.

rest of these volumes. Maxwell's equations defining these relations have been known for a long time, however, the solutions to these equations are often complex, as the biological materials can be inhomogeneous, nonlinear, time varying and anisotropic. Additionally, the geometric shapes involved may not lead to simple descriptions. Therefore, a number of approximations which depend on the ratio of the wavelength of the electromagnetic waves to the dimensions of the body being exposed are presented that simplify the calculations of the field strengths at a given location.

0.2 Review of Basic Electromagnetic Theory

The basic force equation for defining electric and magnetic fields is the Lorentz equation.

$$\vec{F} = q(\vec{E} + \vec{v}x\vec{B}) \tag{0.1}$$

where $\vec{F}$ is the force on a charge q. Note $\vec{F}$ is a vector quantity as are the other symbols with arrows over them. $\vec{E}$ is the electric field. $\vec{v}$ is the velocity of the charge and $\vec{B}$ is the magnetic flux density. Thus, $\vec{E}$ is defined as the force on the charge q at a given location due to one or more charges at other locations or

$$\vec{E} = \vec{F}/q \tag{0.2}$$

$\vec{B}$ is similarly defined in the second term of Equation 0.1. In the term $\vec{F} = q(\vec{v}x\vec{B})$, note that $\vec{v}x\vec{B}$ is a vector cross-product so that the force is at right angles to both the velocity of the charge and the magnetic field. The magnetic flux density may also be defined by the incremental force $\vec{F}$ on a current I or charge flowing in an incremental length of a current carrying wire $d\vec{l}$

$$\vec{F} = Id\vec{l}x\vec{B} \text{ and } |\vec{F}| = I|d\vec{l}||\vec{B}|\sin\theta \tag{0.3}$$

where θ is the angle between $d\vec{l}$ and $\vec{B}$

It is to be noted that the magnetic flux density is related to the magnetic field $\vec{H}$ by the magnetic permeability μ at any given point in space so that $\vec{B} = \mu\vec{H}$ or $\vec{B} = \mu_0\vec{H} + \vec{M}_B$. $\vec{M}_B$ is the magnetic polarization per unit volume and μ_o is the magnetic permeability of free space ($\mu_o = 4\pi \times 10^{-7}$ H/m or $4\pi \times 10^{-7}$ kg m/A²s²). For many cases the magnetic field $\vec{H}$ is given by

$$\oint \vec{H} \bullet d\vec{l} = \oiint \vec{J} \bullet d\vec{s} = i \tag{0.4}$$

Where $\vec{H}$ is given by the line integral around the current i or integral of the current density $\vec{J}$ over the surface of the conductor. Thus, we have the electric field defined by the force between charges and the magnetic field defined by the forces associated with the rate of change of charge or charge flow.

Time-changing electrical and magnetic fields lead to radiation and they are associated with the acceleration of charges. The power, P_R, emitted by an accelerated charge is given by

$$P_R = \frac{2q^2a^2}{4\pi\varepsilon_0 3c^3} \tag{0.5}$$

where a is the acceleration, ε_o is the electric permittivity of free space ($\varepsilon_o = 8.845 \times 10^{-12}$ F/m), and c is the velocity of light. The radiation is at right angles to the motion of the accelerated

Introduction to Electromagnetic Fields

charge. Electromagnetic waves are also radiated from atoms and molecules undergoing transitions between energy levels. The radiations occurs at frequency, f, such that $hf = \Delta W$ where h is Planck's constant [$h = 6.63 \times 10^{-34}$ J s] and ΔW is the energy difference between energy levels. Transitions between electronic energy states typically lead to radiation at optical wavelengths. Transitions between vibrational levels are often in the infrared and far infrared and rotational transitions in the millimeter and microwave regions. Hyperfine transitions changing the orientation of electron spins in the earth's magnetic field may yield radiations at radio frequencies (RF).

The general relationship between the electric $\vec{E}$ and magnetic fields $\vec{H}$ are given by Maxwell's equations:

$$\vec{\nabla} x \vec{H} = \vec{J} + \frac{\partial \vec{D}}{\partial t} \tag{0.6}$$

$$\vec{\nabla} x \vec{E} = -\frac{\partial \vec{B}}{\partial t} \tag{0.7}$$

$$\vec{D} = \varepsilon_0 \vec{E} + \vec{P} \tag{0.8}$$

$$\vec{B} = \mu_0 \vec{H} + \vec{M}_B \tag{0.9}$$

where $\vec{D}$ is the displacement vector, related to $\vec{E}$ by the electrical permittivity or dielectric constant ε at a given point in space in Equation 0.8 and ε_o is the dielectric constant of free space, $\vec{p}$ is the electrical polarlization per unit volume, t is time, $\vec{\nabla}$ is the partial differential operator del, μ_o is the magnetic permiability of free space and $\vec{M}_B$ is the magnetic polarization per unit volume. $\vec{p}$ and $\vec{M}_B$ are properties of the material and will be discussed in Chapter 4.

Sources of electric and magnetic fields come in a variety of shapes and sizes and different approximations appropriate for describing them are dependent on the distance from the source to the biological systems of interest and the frequency at which these sources are varying in time. For electrical fields common sources include point sources, parallel plates long wires and dipoles; for magnetic fields, long wires, dipoles and coils

See Figure 0.1 for some common electric and magnetic field distributions.

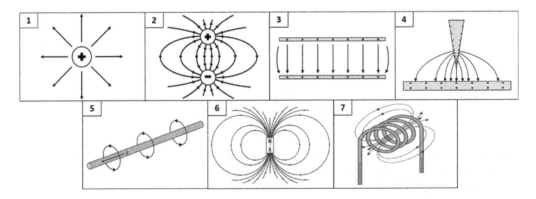

FIGURE 0.1
(1). Electric field of a point charge. (2) Electric field of an electric dipole. (3) Electric field of charge parallel plates. (4) Electric field of a charged probe above a plate. (5) Magnetic field of current carrying wire. (6) Magnetic field of a magnetic dipole. (7) Magnetic field of a current carrying coil.

For point charges the force between two charges is given by Coulomb's Equation

$$\vec{F} = \frac{q_1 q_2}{4\pi \varepsilon \vec{r}^2} \tag{0.10}$$

where q_1 and q_2 are the two charges, ε is the dielectric constant and $\vec{r}$ is the distance between the two charges.

For a large number of cases the distance from the source to the biological object is much larger than the size of the source of the fields, and the source can be approximated by a dipole, a closely spaced pair of equal positive and negative charges or currents. This particularly true at RF, and it can be a first approximation for the fields generated by current-carrying wires.

Another common approximation is that for many cases we can decompose the signal that is being applied into a sum of sine waves using Fourier analysis. In the case of time-changing fields, different terms in Maxwell's equations dominate when distance from the source to the object is large or small compared to the size of the source; these are the far-field and near-field situations. For the case of a single sine wave driving a dipole source, Maxwell's equations are given by Equations 0.11–0.13 [1].

$$H_\vartheta = \frac{I_o L}{4\pi} e^{-jkr} \left(\frac{jk}{r} + \frac{1}{r^2} \right) \sin\theta \tag{0.11}$$

Radiated Field   Near H Field

$$E_r = \frac{I_o L}{4\pi} e^{-jkr} \left(\frac{2\eta}{r^2} + \frac{2}{j\omega\varepsilon r^3} \right) \cos\theta \tag{0.12}$$

Induced E Field   Near E Field

$$E_\theta = \frac{I_o L}{4\pi} e^{-jkr} \left(\frac{j\omega\mu}{r} + \frac{1}{j\omega\mu r^3} + \frac{\eta}{r^2} \right) \sin\theta \tag{0.13}$$

Radiated Field

At radio and microwave frequencies, terms that are important are functions of the ratio L/r of the length of the radiating dipole L and the distance from it, r. Thus, near typical transmitter antennas or close to the antenna of a cell phone, both the near-field and far-field terms of Maxwell's equations often need to be taken into account as ω is a large number. At large distances such as are typical for radio, TV, cell phone base stations, and radars, it is the radiated fields that are important.

0.3 Near Fields and Radiation Fields

At low frequencies such as 50 or 60 Hz, we often are interested in the electric and magnetic fields that are generated by two long parallel wires. In this case, it is the near-field terms in Maxwell's equations that are of interest and it is to be noted that the radiation terms are so small that they are usually unimportant. In general radiation from power lines often does not contribute fields that are most likely to be important in affecting biological materials and one only talks about the near fields or the fields induced in the materials by them. In free space, the electromagnetic wavelength $\lambda = c/f$, where c is the velocity of light and f is the frequency in hertz (cycles/s). In vacuum $c = 3 \times 10^8$ m/s. Therefore, the wave length at the power distribution frequency of 60 Hz is approximately 5000 km, and most available human-made structures are much smaller than one wavelength.

The poor radiation efficiency of electrically small structures, that is, structures whose largest linear dimensions l is small compared to λ, can be illustrated easily for linear antennas. In free space the radiation resistance, R_r of a current element, i.e., an electrically short wire of length l carrying uniform current along its length l [2], is given by (Figure 0.2)

$$R_r = 80\pi^2 \left(\frac{l}{\lambda}\right)^2 \tag{0.14}$$

Thus, the R_r of a 0.01 λ antenna, 50 km long at 60 Hz, would be 0.0197 Ω. The radiated power $P_r = I^2 R_r$ where I is the antenna terminal current, whereas the power dissipated as heat in the antenna wire is $I^2 R_d$ where R_d is the resistance of the wire. When I is uniform, the P_r will be very much less than the power used to heat the antenna, given that the ohmic resistance R_d of any practical wire at room temperature will be very much larger than R_r. For example, the resistance of a 50-km long 2-in. diameter solid copper wire could be 6.65 Ω. At DC, of course, no radiation of any sort takes place, as acceleration of charges is a condition for radiation of electromagnetic waves. A second set of circumstances, which guarantees that any object subjected to low frequency E and H fields usually does not experience effects of radiation, is that any configuration that carries electric currents, sets up E and H field components which store energy without contributing to radiation. A short, linear antenna in free space (short electric dipole) generates, in addition to the radiation field E_r, an electrostatic field E_s and an induced field E_i. Neither E_s nor E_i contribute to the P_r [3,4]. Whereas E_r varies as $1/r$, where r is the distance from the antenna, E_i varies as $1/r^2$, and E_s as $1/r^3$. At a distance from the antenna of approximately one-sixth of the wavelength

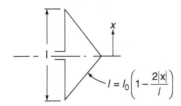

FIGURE 0.2
Current distribution on short, thin, center-fed antenna. $I = I_0\left(1 - \frac{2|x|}{\ell}\right)$.

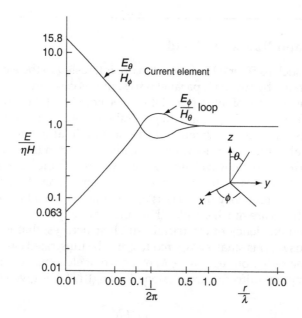

FIGURE 0.3
Ratio of E to H field (divided by wave impedance of free space $\eta = 377\,\Omega$ at $\theta = 90°$; for electric current element at origin along z-axis and for electrically small loop centered at the origin in x–y plane.

($r = \lambda/2\pi$), the E_i equals the E_r, and when $r \ll \lambda/6$ the E_r quickly becomes negligible in comparison with E_i and E_s. Similar results are obtained for other antenna configurations [5]. At 60 Hz the distance $\lambda/2\pi$ corresponds to about 800 km and objects at distances of a few kilometers or less from a 60-Hz system are exposed to low frequency near-field components, which are orders of magnitude larger than the part of the field that contributes to radiation.

A living organism exposed to a static (DC) field or to a low frequency near field may extract energy from it, but the quantitative description of the mechanism by which this extraction takes place is very different than at higher frequencies, where energy is transferred by radiation:

1. In the near field, the relative magnitudes of E and H are a function of the current or charge configuration and the distance from the electric system. The E field may be much larger than the H field or vice versa.

2. In the radiation field, the ratio of the E to H is fixed and equal to 377 Ω in free space, if E is given in volts per meter and H in amperes per meter.

3. In the vicinity of most presently available human-made devices or systems carrying static electric charges, DC, or low-frequency (<1000 Hz) currents, the E and H fields will only under very exceptional circumstances be large enough to produce heating effects inside a living object, as illustrated by Figure 0.4.

(This statement assumes that the living object does not form part of a conducting path that permits direct entrance of current from a wire or conducting ground.) However, effects that are not described by changes in the average temperature are possible; thus, an E field of sufficient magnitude may orient dipoles or translate ions or polarizable neutral particles (see Chapter 4 in this volume)

Introduction to Electromagnetic Fields

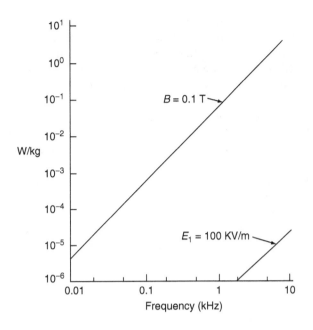

FIGURE 0.4
Top line: Eddy current loss produced in cylinder by sinusoidally time-varying axial *H* field. Cylinder parameters are conductivity $\sigma = 0.1$ S/m, radius 0.1 m, density $D = 1100$ kg/m³, RMS magnetic flux density 0.1 $T = 1000$ G. Watt per kilogram $= \sigma B^2 r^2 w^2/8D$; see Equation 0.29 and use power per volume $= J^2/\sigma$, *Lower line:* Loss produced by 60-Hz E_1 field in Watts per kilogram $= \sigma E_{int}^2/D$, where external field E_1 is related to E_{int} by Equation 0.23 with $\varepsilon_2 = \varepsilon_0 \times 10^5$ at 1 kHz and $\varepsilon_0 = 8 \times 10^4$ at 10 kHz.

The power carried by an electromagnetic wave through space can be calculated by taking the real part of the Poynting vector.

$$\vec{P}_y = \vec{E} \times \vec{H} \quad (0.15)$$

The power emitted through the containing surface of a volume containing a current or accelerated charge can be calculated from.

$$\int_v \left(\vec{H} \cdot \frac{\partial \vec{B}}{\partial t} + \vec{E} \cdot \frac{\partial \vec{D}}{\partial t} + \vec{E} \cdot \vec{J} \right) dV = -\oint_s \left(\vec{E} \cdot \vec{H} \right) \cdot dS \quad (0.16)$$

With radiated power it is relatively easy to produce heating effects in living objects with presently available human-made devices (see Chapter 9 in BMA). This does not imply, of course, that all biological effects of radiated RF power necessarily arise from temperature changes.

The problems we often have are those where a source of electric or magnetic field is specified along with its position with respect to the biological system and we wish to calculate values for $\vec{E}$, $\vec{B}$ or the power density and energy being depoisted in the biological material. Because of the complex geometries and biological material properties, solutions to Equations 0.6–0.9 are often complex. Thus, a large fraction of the time approximations are made to be able to calculate these values and to get insight into how things change with variations in the parameters.

At large distances, the size of a human or other biological system of interest is often small compared to the radius of curvature of the electromagnetic fields and we can approximate the incident fields as plane waves. This greatly simplifies the calculations of the fields interacting with the biological system. Carrying these approximations one step farther in order to get a first approximation to the fields that penetrate or are reflected from the complex shape of a typical biological subject such as a human, we assume that we can approximate the body or biological system with a simple geometric shape. The simplest of these interfaces is the plane sheet of biological material that is infinite in extent.

The results of experiments involving exposure of organic materials and entire living organisms to static E and extremely low frequency (ELF, generally <1 to ~3000 Hz) E fields are described in *BMA*, Chapters 1, 3, and 4.Various mechanisms for the interaction of such fields with living tissue are also discussed there and in *BBA*, Chapter 7. In the present introduction, we shall only point out that one salient feature of static (DC) and ELF E field interaction with living organisms is that the external or applied E field is always larger by several orders of magnitude than the resultant average internal E field [6,7]. This is a direct consequence of the conditions derived from Maxwell's equations (Equations 0.11–0.13).

0.4 Penetration of Direct Current and Low-Frequency Electric Fields into Tissue

Assuming that the two materials illustrated schematically in Figure 0.5 are characterized, respectively, by conductivities σ_1 and σ_2 and dielectric permittivities ε_1 and ε_2, we write E-field components parallel to the boundary as E_P and components perpendicular to the boundary as $E_\perp$. For both static and time-varying fields

$$E_{P1} = E_{P2} \tag{0.17}$$

and for static (DC) fields

$$\sigma_1 E_{\perp 1} = \sigma_2 E_{\perp 2} \tag{0.18}$$

as a consequence of the continuity of current (or conservation of charge). The orientations of the total E fields in media 1 and 2 can be represented by the tangents of the angles between the total fields and the boundary line

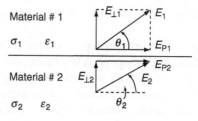

FIGURE 0.5
Symbols used in description of boundary conditions for E-field components.

Introduction to Electromagnetic Fields

$$\tan\theta_1 = \frac{E_{\perp 1}}{E_{P1}}, \quad \tan\theta_2 = \frac{E_{\perp 2}}{E_{P2}} \tag{0.19}$$

From these equations it follows that

$$\tan\theta_1 = \frac{\sigma_2}{\sigma_1}\frac{E_{\perp 1}}{E_{P1}} = \frac{\sigma_2}{\sigma_1}\frac{E_{\perp 2}}{E_{P2}} = \frac{\sigma_2}{\sigma_1}\tan\theta_2 \tag{0.20}$$

If material 1 is air with conductivity [8] $\sigma_1 = 10^{-13}$ S/m and material 2 a typical living tissue with $\sigma_2 \approx 10^{-1}$ S/m (compare Chapter 4 in BBA), $\tan\theta_1 = 10^{12} \tan\theta_2$, and therefore even if the field in material 2 (the inside field) is almost parallel to the boundary so that $\theta_2 \cong 0.5°$ or $\tan\theta_2 \approx (1/100)$, $\tan\theta_1 = 10^{10}$ or $\theta_1 = (\pi/2 - 10)^{-10}$ rad. Thus, an electrostatic field in air, at the boundary between air and living tissue, must be practically perpendicular to the boundary (See Figure 0.6). The situation is virtually the same at ELF although Equation 0.18 must be replaced by

$$\sigma_1 E_{\perp 1} - \sigma_2 E_{\perp 2} = -j\omega\rho_s \tag{0.21}$$

and

$$\varepsilon_1 E_{\perp 1} - \varepsilon_2 E_{\perp 2} = \rho_s \tag{0.22}$$

where $j = \sqrt{-1}$, ω is the radian frequency (= $2\pi \times$ frequency), and ρ_s is the surface charge density. In Chapter 4 in BBA it is shown that at ELF the relative dielectric permittivity of living tissue may be as high as 10^6 so that $\varepsilon_2 = 10^6\,\varepsilon_0$, where ε_0 is the dielectric permittivity of free space $(1/36\,\pi)\,10^{-9}$ F/m; however, it is still valid to assume that $\varepsilon_2 \le 0^{-5}$. Then, from Equations 0.21 and 0.22

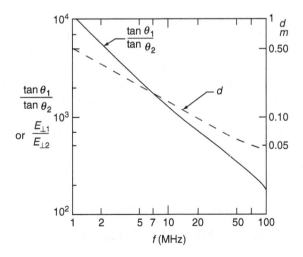

FIGURE 0.6
Orientation of E-field components at air–muscle boundary (or ratio of fields perpendicular to boundary); depth (d) at which field component parallel to boundary surface decreases by approximately 50% (d = 0.6938).

$$E_{\perp 1} = \frac{\sigma_2 + j\omega\varepsilon_2}{\sigma_1 + j\omega\varepsilon_1} E_{\perp 2} \tag{0.23}$$

which gives at 60 Hz with $\sigma_2 = 10^1$ S/m, $\sigma_1 = 10^{-13}$ S/m, $\varepsilon_2 \approx 10^{-5}$ F/m, and $\varepsilon_1 \approx 10^{-11}$ F/m

$$E_{\perp 1} = \frac{10^{-1} + j_4 10^{-3}}{10^{-13} + j_4 10^{-9}} E_{\perp 2} \approx \frac{\sigma_2}{j\omega\varepsilon_1} = -j(2.5 \times 10^7) E_{\perp 2} \tag{0.24}$$

This result, together with Equations 0.17 and 0.19, shows that for the given material properties, the field in air must still be practically perpendicular to the boundary of a living organism: $\tan \theta_1 : 2.5(10^7) \tan \theta_2$.

Knowing now that the living organism will distort the E field in its vicinity in such a way that the external field will be nearly perpendicular to the boundary surface, we can calculate the internal field by substituting the total field for the perpendicular field in Equations 0.18 (DC) and 0.23 (ELF). For the assumed typical material parameters we find that in the static (DC) case

$$\frac{E_{\text{internal}}}{E_{\text{external}}} \approx 10^{-12} \tag{0.25}$$

$$\rho_f = \frac{3(\sigma_2\varepsilon_1 - \sigma_1\varepsilon_2)E_0}{2\sigma_1 + \sigma_2} \cos\vartheta \, \text{C/m}^2$$

and for 60 Hz

$$\frac{E_{\text{internal}}}{E_{\text{external}}} \approx 4(10^{-8}) \tag{0.26}$$

Thus, a 60-Hz external field of 100 kV/m will produce an average E_{internal} field of the order of 4 mV/m.

If the boundary between air and the organic material consists of curved surfaces instead of infinite planes, the results will be modified only slightly. Thus, for a finite sphere (with ε and σ^- as assumed here) embedded in air, the ratios of the internal field to the undisturbed external field will vary with the angle θ and distance r as indicated in Figure 0.6, but will not deviate from the results indicated by Equations 0.21 and 0.22 by more than a factor of 3 [4,9]. Long cylinders ($L \ll r$) aligned parallel to the external field will have interior fields essentially equal to the unperturbed external field, except near the ends where the field component perpendicular to the membrane surface will be intensified approximately as above (see Chapter 5 in this volume).

0.5 Direct Current and Low-Frequency Magnetic Fields

Direct current and ELF H fields are considered in more detail in Chapters 5 and 6 in this volume. As the magnetic permeability μ of most biological materials is practically equal to

Introduction to Electromagnetic Fields 11

the magnetic permeability μ_0 of free space, $4\pi(10^{-7})$ H/m, the DC, or ELF H field "inside" will be practically equal to the H field "outside." The only exceptions are organisms such as the magnetotactic bacteria, which synthesize ferromagnetic material, discussed in Chapter 7 of *BBA*. The known and suggested mechanisms of interaction of DC H fields with living matter are:

1. Orientation of ferromagnetic particles, including biologically synthesized particles of magnetite.

2. Orientation of diamagnetic or paramagnetic anisotropic molecules and cellular elements [11].

3. Generation of potential differences at right angles to a stream of moving ions (Hall effect, also sometimes called a magneto hydrodynamic effect) as a result of the magnetic force $F_m = qvB \sin \theta$, where q is the electric charge, v is the velocity of the charge, B is the magnetic flux density, and $\sin \theta$ is the sine of the angle θ between the directions v and B. One well-documented result of this mechanism is a "spike" in the electrocardiograms of vertebrates subjected to large DC H fields.

4. Changes in intermediate products or structural arrangements in the course of light-induced chemical (electron transfer) reactions, brought about by Zeeman splitting of molecular energy levels or effects upon hyperfine structure. (The Zeeman effect is the splitting of spectral lines, characteristic of electronic transitions, under the influence of an external H field. Hyperfine splitting of electronic transition lines in the absence of an external H field is due to the magnetic moment of the nucleus; such hyperfine splitting can be modified by an externally applied H field.) The magnetic flux densities involved depend upon the particular system and can be as high as 0.2 T (2000 G) but also as low as <0.01 mT (0.1 G). Bacterial photosynthesis and effects upon the visual system are prime candidates for this mechanism [10,12].

5. Induction of E fields with resulting electrical potential differences and currents within an organism by rapid motion through a large static H field. Some magnetic phosphenes are due to such motions [13].

Relatively slow time-varying H fields, which are discussed Chapters 6 and 7 in *BBA*, among others, may interact with living organisms through the same mechanisms that can be triggered by static H fields, provided the variation with time is slow enough to allow particles of finite size and mass, located in a viscous medium, to change orientation or position where required (mechanism 1 and 2) and provided the field intensity is sufficient to produce the particular effect. However, time-varying H fields, including ELF H fields, can also induce electric currents into stationary conducting objects. Thus, all modes of interaction of time-varying E fields with living matter may be triggered by time-varying, but not by static, H fields.

In view of Faraday's law, a time-varying magnetic flux will induce E fields with resulting electrical potential differences and "eddy" currents through available conducting paths. As very large external ELF E fields are required (as indicated by Equations 0.23–0.26) to generate even small internal E fields, many human-made devices and systems generating both ELF E and H fields are more likely to produce physiologically significant internal E fields through the mechanism of magnetic induction.

The induced voltage V around some closed path is given by

$$V = \oint E \cdot dl = -\iint \frac{\partial B}{\partial t} \cdot ds \qquad (0.27)$$

where E is the induced E field. The integration $\oint E \cdot dl$ is over the appropriate conducting path, $\partial B/\partial t$ is the time derivative of the magnetic flux density, and the "dot" product with the surface element, ds, indicates that only the component of $\partial B/\partial t$ perpendicular to the surface, i.e., parallel to the direction of the vector ds, enclosed by the conducting path, induces an E field. To obtain an order-of-magnitude indication of the induced current that can be expected as a result of an ELF H field, we consider the circular path of radius r, illustrated by Figure 0.7. Equation 0.28 then gives the magnitude of the E field as

$$E = \frac{\omega B r}{2} \qquad (0.28)$$

where ω is the $2\pi f$ and f is the frequency. The magnitude of the resulting electric current density J in ampere per square meter is*

$$J = \sigma E = \frac{\sigma \omega B r}{2} \qquad (0.29)$$

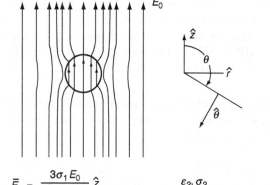

$$r < R \quad \bar{E} = \frac{3\sigma_1 E_0}{2\sigma_1 + \sigma_2} \hat{z}$$

$$r < R \quad \bar{E} = E_0 \cos\theta \left[1 + \frac{2R^3(\sigma_2 - \sigma_1)}{r^3(2\sigma_1 + \sigma_2)}\right]\hat{r} - E\sin\theta \left[1 - \frac{2R^3(\sigma_2 - \sigma_1)}{r^3(2\sigma_1 + \sigma_2)}\right]\hat{r}$$

FIGURE 0.7
E field when sphere of radius R, conductivity σ, and dielectric permittivity ε_2 is placed into an initially uniform static field ($E = 2E_0$) within a medium with conductivity σ_1 and permittivity ε_1. The surface charge density is $\rho_r = \frac{3(\sigma_2 \varepsilon_1 - \sigma_1 \varepsilon_2) E_0}{2\sigma_1 + \sigma_2} \cos\theta \ C/m^2.$

---

* Equation 0.29 neglects the H field generated by the induced eddy currents. If this field is taken into account, it can be shown that the induced current density in a cylindrical shell of radius r and thickness Δ is given by $\Delta r < 0.01 \ m^2/[1 + j\Delta r/\delta_2]$, where $H_0 = B_0/\mu_0$ and δ is the skin depth defined by Equation 0.28 below. However, for conductivities of biological materials ($\sigma < 5$ s/m) one obtains at audio frequencies $\delta > 1$ m and as for most dimensions of interest $\Delta r < 0.01 \ m^2$ the term $j\Delta r/\delta_2$ becomes negligible. The result $-jrH_0/\delta_2$ is then identical with Equation 0.29.

Introduction to Electromagnetic Fields

where σ is the conductivity along the path in Siemens per meter. In the SI (System International) units used throughout this book, B is measured in tesla ($1T = 10^4$ G) and r in meters. Choosing for illustration a circular path of 0.1 m radius, a frequency of 60 Hz, and a conductivity of 0.1 S/m, Equations 0.28 and 0.29 give $E = 18.85\ B$ and $I = 1.885\ B$. The magnetic flux density required to obtain a current density of 1 mA/m² is 0.53 mT or about 5 G. The E field induced by that flux density along the circular path is 10 mV/m. To produce this same 10 mV/m $E_{internal}$ field by an external 60 Hz $E_{external}$ field would require, by Equation 0.24, a field intensity of 250 kV/m.

As the induced voltage is proportional to the time rate of change of the H field (Equation 0.27), implying a linear increase with frequency (Equation 0.28), one would expect that the ability of a time-varying H field to induce currents deep inside a conductive object would increase indefinitely as the frequency increases or conversely, that the magnetic flux density required to induce a specified E field would decrease linearly with frequency, as indicated in Figure 0.8. This is not true, however, because the displacement current density

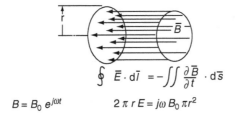

FIGURE 0.8
Circular path (loop) of radius r enclosing uniform magnetic flux density perpendicular to the plane of the loop. For sinusoidal time variation $B = B_0 e^{j\omega t}$.

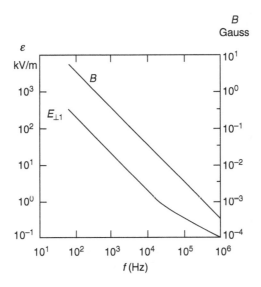

FIGURE 0.9
External E and H field required to obtain an internal E field of 10 mV/m (conductivity and dielectric permittivity for skeletal muscle (From Foster, K.R., Schepps, J.L., and Schwan, H.P. 1980. *Biophys. J.*, 29, 271–281. H-field calculation assumes a circular path of 0.1-m radius perpendicular to magnetic flux).

$\partial D/\partial t$, where $D = \varepsilon E$, must also be considered as the frequency increases. This leads to the wave behavior discussed in Part 3, implying that at sufficiently high frequencies the effects of both external E and H fields are limited by reflection losses (Figures 0.9–0.11) as well as by skin effect [14], i.e., limited depth of penetration d in Figure 0.6.

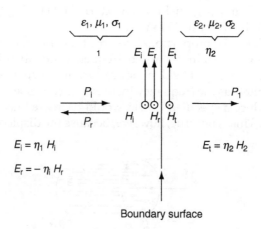

FIGURE 0.10
Reflection and transmission of an electromagnetic wave at the boundary between two different media, perpendicular incidence; P_i = incident power, P_r = reflected power, P_t = transmitted power.

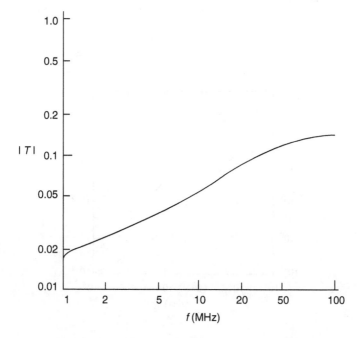

FIGURE 0.11
Magnitude of transmission coefficient T for incident E field parallel to boundary surface. $T = E_t/E_i$: reflection coefficient $r = E_r/E_i = T - 1$. Γ and T are complex numbers; ε_r and σ for skeletal muscle from Chapter 4 in *BBA*.

0.6 RF Fields

At frequencies well below those where most animals and many field-generating systems have dimensions on the order of one free-space wavelength, e.g., at 10 MHz where $\lambda = 30$ m, the skin effect limits penetration of the external field. This phenomenon is fundamentally different from the small ratio of internal to external E fields described in Equation 0.18 (applicable to DC) and Equation 0.23.

Equation 0.23 expresses a "boundary condition" applicable at all frequencies, but as the angular frequency ω increases and in view of the rapid decrease with frequency of the dielectric permittivity ε_2 in biological materials (see Chapter 4 of *BBA*), the ratio of the normal component of the external to the internal E field at the boundary decreases with increasing frequency. This is illustrated by Figure 0.6 where $\tan \theta_1/\tan \theta_2$ is also equal to $E_{\perp_1}/E_{\perp_2}$ in view of Equations 0.17, 0.19, and 0.23. However, at low frequencies the total field inside the boundary can be somewhat larger than the perpendicular field at the boundary; and any field variation with distance from the boundary is not primarily due to energy dissipation, but in a homogeneous body it is a consequence of shape. At RF, on the other hand, the E and H fields of the incoming electromagnetic wave, after reflection at the boundary, are further decreased due to energy dissipation. Both E and H fields decrease exponentially with distance from the boundary

$$g(z) = Ae^{-\frac{z}{\delta}} \tag{0.30}$$

where $g(z)$ is the field at the distance z and A is the magnitude of the field just *inside* the boundary. As defined by Equation 0.30 the skin depth δ is the distance over which the field decreases to $1/e$ ($= 0.368$) of its value just *inside* the boundary. (Due to reflection, the field A just inside the boundary can already be very much smaller than the incident external field; see Figures 0.9 and 0.10.)

Expressions for δ given below were derived [3,4,14,15] for plane boundaries between infinite media. They are reasonably accurate for cylindrical structures if the ratio of radius of curvature to skin depth (r_0/δ) is larger than about five [14]. For a good conductor

$$\delta = \frac{1}{\sqrt{\pi f \mu \sigma}} \tag{0.31}$$

where a good conductor is one for which the ratio p of conduction current, $J = \sigma E$, to displacement current, $\partial D/\partial t = \varepsilon(\partial E/\partial t) = j\omega\varepsilon E$ is large:

$$p = \frac{\sigma}{\omega\varepsilon} \gg 1 \tag{0.32}$$

Since for most biological materials p is of the order of one ($0.1 < p < 10$) over a very wide frequency range (see Chapter 4 of *BBA*), it is frequently necessary to use the more general expression [14]

$$\delta = \frac{1}{\omega\left[\frac{\mu\varepsilon}{2}(\sqrt{1+p^2}-1)\right]^{1/2}} \tag{0.33}$$

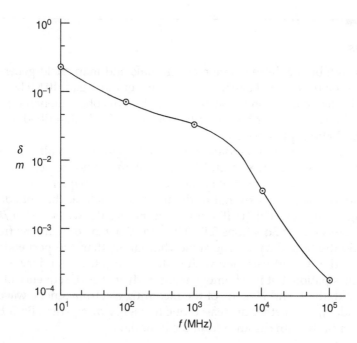

FIGURE 0.12
Electromagnetic skin depth in muscle tissue from plane wave expression (Equation 0.33, Table 0.1).

The decrease in field intensity with distance from the boundary surface indicated by Equation 0.30 becomes significant for many biological objects at frequencies where $r_0/\delta \geq 5$ is not satisfied. However, the error resulting from the use of Equations 0.30 and 0.31 or Equation 0.33 with curved objects is less when $z < \delta$. Thus, at $z = 0.693\,\delta$, where $g(z) = 0.5$ A from Equations 0.30 and 0.31, the correct values of $g(z)$, obtained by solving the wave equation in cylindrical coordinates, differs only by 20% (it is 0.6 A) even when r_0/δ is as small as 2.39 [15]. Therefore, Figure 0.12 shows the distance $d = 0.693\,\delta$, at which the field decreases to half of its value just inside the boundary surface, using Equation 0.33 with typical values for σ and ε for muscle. It is apparent that the skin effect becomes significant for humans and larger vertebrates at frequencies >10 MHz.

Directly related to skin depth, which is defined for fields varying sinusoidally with time, is the fact that a rapid transient variation of an applied magnetic flux density constitutes an exception to the statement that the DC H field inside the boundary is equal to the H field outside. Thus, from one viewpoint one may consider the rapid application or removal of a DC H field as equivalent to applying a high-frequency field during the switching period, with the highest frequencies present of the order of $1/\tau$, where τ is the rise time of the applied step function. Thus, if $\tau < 10^{-8}$ s, the skin effect will be important during the transient period, as d in Figure 0.6 is <5 cm above 100 MHz. It is also possible to calculate directly the magnetic flux density inside a conducting cylinder as a function of radial position r and time t when a magnetic pulse is applied in the axial direction [16,17]. Assuming zero rise time of the applied field B_0, i.e., a true step function, one finds that the field inside a cylinder of radius a is

$$B = B_0 \left[1 - \sum_{k=1}^{\infty} J_0\left(r\frac{v_k}{a}\right) e^{-t/T_k} \right] \tag{0.34}$$

Introduction to Electromagnetic Fields

where $J_0 (r\, v_k/a)$ is the zero-order Bessel function of argument $r\, v_k/a$ and the summation is over the nulls of J_0 designated v_k (the first four values of v_k are 2.405, 5.520, 8.654, and 11.792).* T_k is the rise time of the kth term in the series and is given by

$$T_k = \frac{\mu_0 \sigma a^2}{v_k} \tag{0.35}$$

As v_k increases, the rise time decreases and therefore the longest delay is due to the first term in the summation with $k = 1$

$$T_1 = \frac{\mu_0 \sigma a^2}{2.405} \tag{0.36}$$

For a cylinder with 0.1 m radius and a conductivity $\sigma \approx 1$ S/m, which is a typical value for muscle between 100 and 1000 MHz, Equation 0.36 gives $T_1 = 2.6 \times 10^{-8}$ s. This finite rise time (or decay time in case of field removal) of the internal H field may be of some importance when pulsed H fields are used therapeutically [18]. It might also be used to measure non-invasively the conductivity of biological substances *in vivo* through determination of the final decay rate of the voltage induced into a probe coil by the slowly decaying internal field after the applied field is removed [17].

The properties of biological substances in the intermediate frequency range, above ELF (>300 Hz), and below the higher RFs, where wave behavior and skin effect begin to be important (~20 MHz), are discussed in Chapter 4 of *BBA*. However, many subsequent chapters are concerned with biological effects at DC and ELF frequencies below a few kilohertz, while others deal primarily with the higher RFs >50 MHz. One reason for this limited treatment of the intermediate frequency range is that very little animal data are available for this spectral region in comparison with the large number of experiments performed at ELF and microwave frequencies in recent years.† Another reason is that most electrical processes known to occur naturally in biological systems—action potentials, EKG, EEG, ERG, etc.—occur at DC and ELF frequencies. Therefore, one might expect some physiological effects from external fields of appropriate intensity in the same frequency range, even if the magnitude of such fields is not large enough to produce thermal effects. As illustrated by Figures 0.4 and 0.8, most E fields below 100 kHz set up by currently used human-made devices, and most H fields below 10 kHz except the very strongest, are incapable of producing thermal effects in living organisms, excluding, of course, fields accompanying currents directly introduced into the organism via electrodes. Thus, the frequencies between about 10 and 100 kHz have been of relatively little interest because they have not been seen to be very likely to produce thermal or other biological effects. On the other hand, the higher RFs are frequently generated at power levels where enough energy may be introduced into living organisms to produce local or general heating. In addition, despite skin effect and the reflection loss to be discussed in more detail below, microwaves modulated at an ELF rate may serve as a vehicle for introducing ELF fields into a living organism of at least the same order of magnitude as would be introduced by direct exposure to ELF. Any effect of such ELF-modulated microwaves would, of course, require the existence of some amplitude-dependent demodulation mechanism to extract the ELF from the microwave carrier.

---

* This result is based on solution of $\partial B/\partial t = (1/\mu_0)\nabla^2 B$, which is a consequence of Ampere's and Faraday's laws when displacement is disregarded. Equations 0.20–0.22 are therefore only correct when $p \gg 1$.

† Though this statement was written for the second edition in 1995, it continues to be true.

Among the chapters dealing with RF, Chapters 5, 9, and 10 of *BBA* give the necessary information for establishing the magnitude of the fields present in biological objects: (1) experimental techniques and (2) analytical methods for predicting field intensities without construction of physical models made with "phantom" materials, i.e., dielectric materials with properties similar to those of living objects which are to be exposed. As thermal effects at microwave frequencies are certainly important, although one cannot assume *a priori* that they are the only biological effects of this part of the spectrum, and as some (but not all) thermal effects occur at levels where the thermoregulatory system of animals is activated. Thermoregulation in the presence of microwave fields is discussed in Chapters 9 and 11 of *BMA*, as well as in Chapter 9 of *BBA*. Not only are most therapeutic applications of microwaves based upon their thermal effects, but also it is now experimentally established that there are biological effects for exposure levels that are below the levels where significant changes expected to occur as a result of heating and changes in temperature. See Chapters 7 and 11 in *BBA* and many in *BMA*. Effects at the threshold of large-scale tissue heating in particular living systems also requires thorough understanding of thermoregulatory mechanisms. The vast amount of experimental data obtained on animal systems exposed to microwave is discussed in Chapter 5 in *BMA*. Both non-modulated fields and modulated fields, where the type of modulation had no apparent effect other than modification of the average power level, are considered. These chapters and the Chapters 6 and 7 in *BMA* consider very new extensions of experiments into exposures to ultra-short and to ultra-high-power pulses.

At the higher RF frequencies, the external E field is not necessarily perpendicular to the boundary of biological materials (see Figures 0.5 and 0.11), and the ratio of the total external E field to the total internal field is not given by Equation 0.23. However, the skin effect (Equations 0.30–0.33) and reflection losses still reduce the E field within any biological object below the value of the external field. As pointed out in Chapter 4, dielectric permittivity and electrical conductivity of organic substances both vary with frequency. At RF, most biological substances are neither very good electrical conductors nor very good insulators, with the exception of cell membranes, which are good dielectrics at RF but at ELF can act as intermittent conductors or as dielectrics and are ion-selective [19–21]. The ratio p (Equation 0.32) is neither much smaller nor very much larger than values shown for typical muscle tissue [22,23] in Table 0.1.

Reflection loss at the surface of an organism is a consequence of the difference between its electrical properties and those of air. Whenever an electromagnetic wave travels from one material to another with different electrical properties, the boundary conditions

TABLE 0.1

Ratio p of Conduction Current to Displacement as a Function of Frequency For Typical Muscle Tissue

f (MHz)	σ	ε_r	$p = \dfrac{\sigma}{\omega \varepsilon_0 \varepsilon_r}$
1	0.40	2000	3.6
10	0.63	160	7.1
100	0.89	72	2.2
10^3	1.65	50	0.59
10^4	10.3	40	0.46
10^5	80	6	2.4

Introduction to Electromagnetic Fields 19

(Equations 0.17 and 0.22) and similar relations for the H field require the existence of a reflected wave. The expressions for the reflection coefficient

$$\Gamma = \frac{E_r}{E_i} \tag{0.37}$$

and the transmission coefficient

$$T = \frac{E_t}{E_i} \tag{0.38}$$

becomes rather simple for loss-free dielectrics ($p \ll 1$) and for good conductors ($p \gg 1$). As biological substances are neither the most general expressions for Γ and T, applicable at plane boundaries, are needed [4,14]. For perpendicular incidence, illustrated by Figure 0.9,

$$\Gamma = \frac{\eta_2 - \eta_1}{\eta_2 + \eta_1} \tag{0.39}$$

$$T = \frac{2\eta_2}{\eta_2 + \eta_1} = 1 + \Gamma \tag{0.40}$$

where η_1 and η_2 are the wave impedances, respectively, of mediums 1 and 2. The wave impedance of a medium is the ratio of the E to the H field in a plane wave traveling through that medium; it is given by [14]

$$\eta = \left(\frac{j\omega\mu}{\sigma + j\omega\varepsilon} \right)^{1/2} \tag{0.41}$$

Clearly, Γ and T are in general complex numbers, even when medium 1 is air for which Equation 0.41 reduces to the real quantity $\eta_0 = \sqrt{\mu_0 / \varepsilon_0}$, because medium 2, which here is living matter, usually has a complex wave impedance at RFs.

The incident, reflected, and transmitted powers are given by [14]

$$P_i = R_1 |E_i|^2 \frac{1}{\eta_1^*} = \frac{|E_i|^2}{|\eta_1|^2} R_1 \tag{0.42}$$

$$P_r = R_1 |E_r|^2 \frac{1}{\eta_1^*} = \frac{|E_r|^2}{|\eta_1|^2} R_1 \tag{0.43}$$

$$P_t = R_1 |E_t|^2 \frac{1}{\eta_2^*} = \frac{|E_t|^2}{|\eta_2|^2} R_2 \tag{0.44}$$

where the E fields are effective values ($E_{eff} = E_{peak}/\sqrt{2}$) of sinusoidal quantities, R_1 signifies "real part of," η^*. It is the complex conjugate of η, and R_1 and R_2 are the real parts of η_1 and η_2. If medium 1 is air, $\eta_1 = R_1 = 377 \ \Omega$, it follows from Equations 0.37, 0.38, and 0.42–0.44 and conservation of energy that the ratio of the transmitted to the incident real power is given by

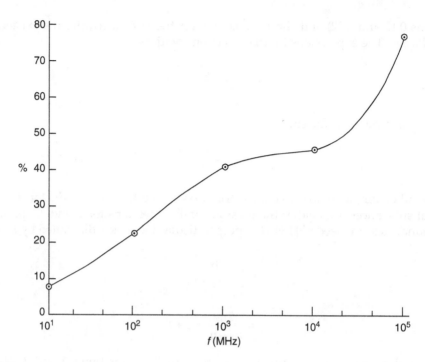

FIGURE 0.13
Ratio of transmitted to incident power expressed as percent of incident power. Air–muscle interface, perpendicular incidence (Equation 0.45, Table 0.1).

$$\frac{P}{P_1} = |T|^2 \frac{\eta_1 \eta_2^* + \eta_1^* \eta_2}{2|\eta_2|^2} = 1 - \frac{P_r}{P_i} = 1 - |\Gamma|^2 \tag{0.45}$$

The magnitude of the transmission coefficient T for the air–muscle interface over the 1- to 100-MHz frequency range is plotted in Figure 0.10, which shows that the magnitude of the transmitted E field in muscle tissue is considerably smaller than the E field in air. The fraction of the total incident power that is transmitted (Equation 0.45) is shown in Figure 0.13, indicating clearly that reflection loss at the interface decreases with frequency. However, for deeper lying tissue this effect is offset by the fact that the skin depth δ (Equation 0.33) also decreases with frequency (Figure 0.12) so that the total power penetrating beyond the surface decreases rapidly.

In addition to reflection at the air–tissue boundary, further reflections take place at each boundary between dissimilar materials. For example, the magnitude of the reflection coefficient at the boundary surface between muscle and organic materials with low-water content, such as fat or bone, is shown in Table 0.2.

The situation is actually more complicated than indicated by Figures 0.10 and 0.12, because the wave front of the incident electromagnetic wave may not be parallel to the air–tissue boundary. Two situations are possible: the incident E field may be polarized perpendicular to the plane of incidence defined in Figure 0.14 (perpendicular polarization, Figure 0.14a) or parallel to the plane of incidence (parallel polarization, Figure 0.14b). The transmission and reflection coefficients [9] are different for the two types of polarization and also become functions of the angle of incidence α_1:

Introduction to Electromagnetic Fields

TABLE 0.2

Reflection Coefficient "Capital Gamma" for Low–Water-Content Materials

	Fat or Bone		
f (MHz)	σ (S/m)	ε_r	Muscle[a]–Fat (Γ)
10^2	0.048	7.5	0.65
10^3	0.101	5.6	0.52
10^4	0.437	4.5	0.52

[a] σ and ε_r for muscle from Table 0.1.

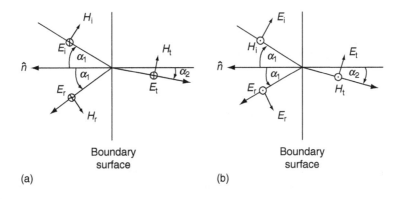

FIGURE 0.14
Oblique incidence of an electromagnetic wave at the boundary between two different media. (a) Perpendicular polarization (E vector perpendicular to plane of incidence); (b) parallel polarization (E vector parallel to plane of incidence). The plane of incidence is the plane formed by the surface normal (unit vector n and the direction of the incident wave); ⊗ indicates a vector into the plane of the paper; ⊙ indicates a vector out of the plane of the paper. The orientation of the field vectors in the transmitted field is shown for loss-free dielectrics. For illustration of the transmitted wave into a medium with finite conductivity, where the wave impedance η_2 becomes a complex number, see Stratton, J.A., *Electromagnetic Theory*, McGraw-Hill, New York, 1941, p. 435.

Perpendicular polarization
$$\begin{cases} T_\perp = \dfrac{2\eta_2 \cos\alpha_1}{\eta_2 \cos\alpha_1 + \eta_1 \cos\alpha_2} \\[2ex] \Gamma_\perp = \dfrac{\eta_2 \cos\alpha_1 - \eta_1 \cos\alpha_2}{\eta_2 \cos\alpha_1 + \eta_1 \cos\alpha_2} \end{cases}$$
(0.46 and 0.47)

Parallel polarization
$$\begin{cases} T_p = \dfrac{2\eta_2 \cos\alpha_1}{\eta_2 \cos\alpha_2 + \eta_1 \cos\alpha_1} \\[2ex] \Gamma_p = \dfrac{\eta_1 \cos\alpha_1 - \eta_2 \cos\alpha_2}{\eta_2 \cos\alpha_2 + \eta_1 \cos\alpha_1} \end{cases}$$
(0.48 and 0.49)

where α_2 is given by the generalized Snell's law (when both the media have the magnetic permeability of free space) by [a]σ and ε_r for muscle from Table 0.1.

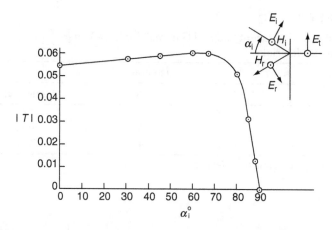

FIGURE 0.15
Magnitude of complex transmission coefficient for parallel polarization versus angle of incidence α_1 at 10 MHz (E field in plane of incidence, H field parallel to boundary plane; $\sigma_2 = 0.7$ S/m, $\varepsilon_{r2} = 150$, $T = E_t/E_r$).

$$\sin \alpha_2 = \frac{\sqrt{\varepsilon_1}}{\sqrt{\varepsilon_2 - j\frac{\sigma_2}{\omega}}} \qquad (0.50)$$

so that $\alpha_2 = \sqrt{1 - \sin^2 \alpha_2}$ is a complex number unless $p_2 = (\sigma_2/\omega\varepsilon_2) = 1$.

As illustration, the variation with angle of incidence of the transmission coefficient for parallel polarization at the air–muscle interface at 10 MHz, is shown in Figure 0.15. It is apparent that the transmitted field is not necessarily maximized by perpendicular incidence in the case of parallel polarization. Furthermore, whenever $p \approx 1$ or $p > 1$ (see Table 0.1, above), α_2 is complex, which causes the waves entering the tissue to be inhomogeneous—they are not simple plane waves, but waves where surfaces of constant phase and constant amplitude do not coincide [4,24]; only the planes of constant amplitude are parallel to the boundary surface.

Analytical solutions for non-planar structures taking into account size and shape of entire animals have been given [25] and are also described in the RF modeling Chapter 9 of *BBA*.

0.7 Biophysical Interactions of Fields: Ionization, Ionizing Radiation, Chemical Bonds, and Excitation

RF fields can be characterized as nonionizing radiation. By this, we mean that there is not enough energy in a single quantum of RF energy, hf, to ionize an atom or a molecule, where h is Planck's constant and f is the frequency. By comparison radiation in the UV or x-ray regions often lead to ionization. It is desirable to begin by reviewing the differences between ionizing and nonionizing radiations, to explain ionization phenomena and also to discuss related excitation phenomena, which require less energy than ionization; a number of proposed models concerning atomic or molecular-level interactions of fields will be

Introduction to Electromagnetic Fields

introduced. A number of these theories will be discussed and their predictions compared with experimental results in many later chapters. Heating, cell excitation, electroporation, and other results of high-intensity fields have been accepted as explanations for many bioelectromagnetic phenomena. For low-intensity exposure, however, no theory is widely accepted as a general explanation for bioelectromagnetic phenomena, and few specific phenomena have accepted explanations. It is quite possible that no general explanation exists and that more than one mechanism of interaction between fields will be found to be operating, depending on the situation. Chapter 7 of BBA has a summary of many proposed mechanisms, including discussion of the possible role of radicals' and other molecular structures' rotational, electronic, and nuclear angular momenta in explaining a number of types of biological effects. Binhi's book [26] contains a good summary of many theoretical proposals, including comparisons with data and critiques of their strong and weak points, as well as his own theory.

We note first that the energy of electromagnetic waves is quantized with the quantum of energy (in joules) being equal to Planck's constant ($h = 6.63 \times 10^{-34}$ J s) times the frequency. This energy can also be expressed in electron volts, i.e., in multiples of the kinetic energy acquired by an electron accelerated through a potential difference of 1 V (1 eV $\approx 1.6 \times 10^{-19}$ J). Energy quanta for a few frequencies are listed in Table 0.3.

Quantized energy can "excite" molecules; appropriate frequencies can couple to vibrational and rotational oscillation; and if the incident energy quantum has sufficient magnitude it can excite other changes in the electron configuration, such as changing an electron to another (unoccupied) energy level or tearing an electron away from one of the constituent atoms. The latter process called as ionization. The energy required to remove one electron from the highest energy orbit of a particular chemical element is called its "ionization potential." Typical ionization potentials are of the order 10 eV; for example, for the hydrogen atom it is 13.6 eV and for gaseous sodium, 5.1 eV. As chemical binding forces are essentially electrostatic, ionization implies profound chemical changes. Therefore, ionization by any outside agent of the complex compounds that make up a living system leads to profound and often irreversible changes in the operation of that system.

Table 0.3 shows that even the highest RF (millimeter waves) has quantum energies well below the ionization potential of any known substance; thus, one speaks of nonionizing radiation when referring to electromagnetic waves below UV light frequencies. Ionizing radiation includes UV and higher frequency electromagnetic waves (x-rays, γ-rays).

This explanation of the difference between ionizing and nonionizing radiation should not imply that nonionizing electromagnetic radiation cannot have profound effects upon

TABLE 0.3

Wave and Quantum Characteristics of Various Types of Radiation

Name of Radiation or Application	Frequency (Hz)	Wavelength (m)	Energy of 1 Quantum of Radiation (eV)
UHF TV	7×10^8	0.43	2.88×10^{-6}
Microwave radar	10^{10}	3×10^{-2}	4.12×10^{-5}
Millimeter wave	3×10^{11}	1×10^{-3}	1.24×10^{-3}
Visible light	6×10^{14}	5×10^{-7}	2.47
Ionizing UV	10^{16}	3×10^{-4}	41.2
Soft x-ray	10^{18}	3×10^{-10}	4120
Penetrating x-ray	10^{20}	3×10^{-12}	4.12×10^5

inorganic and organic substances. As excitation of coherent vibrational and rotational modes requires considerably less energy than ionization, it could occur at RF; this will be discussed in later chapters. In addition, many other possible biological effects require energies well below the level of ionizing potentials. Examples are tissue heating, dielectrophoresis, depolarization of cell membranes, mechanical stress due to piezoelectric transduction, or dielectric saturation, resulting in the orientation of the polar side chains of macromolecules and leading to the breaking of hydrogen bonds. These and other mechanisms will be discussed by the authors of several chapters (see especially Chapter 7 of *BBA*). Returning to the discussion of ionization, it is important to note that ionization of a chemical element can be brought about not only by absorption of electromagnetic energy, but also by collision either with foreign (injected) atoms, molecules, or subatomic particles of the requisite energy, or by sufficiently violent collision among its own atoms. The latter process constitutes ionization by heating, or thermal breakdown of a substance, which will occur when the kinetic energy of the colliding particles exceeds the ionization potential. As the average thermal kinetic energy of particles is related to temperature [27] by $W = kT$ where k is Boltzmann's constant ($= 1.38 \times 10^{-23}$ J/K), we find that the required temperature is

$$1.38(10^{-23})\,T \approx 5\,\text{eV} \approx (5)1.6(10^{-19})\,\text{J}$$

$$T \approx 5(10^4)\,\text{K}$$

which is about twice the temperature inside a lightning stroke [28] and orders of magnitude higher than any temperature obtainable from electromagnetic waves traveling through air.

Actually, initiation of lightning strokes is an example of ionization by collision with injected energetic particles. The few free electrons and ions always present in the air due to ionization by cosmic rays are accelerated by the E fields generated within clouds to velocities corresponding to the required ionization energy. Only when the field is large enough to impart this energy over distances shorter than the mean free path of the free electrons or ions at atmospheric pressure can an avalanche process take place: an accelerated electron separates a low-energy electron from the molecule with which it collides and in the process loses most of its own energy; thus, one high-energy free electron is exchanged for two free low-energy electrons and one positive ion. Both the electrons are in turn accelerated again by the field, giving them high kinetic energy before they collide with neutral molecules; their collision produces four free electrons and the multiplication process continues. The breakdown field strength for air at atmospheric pressure is approximately 3×10^6 V/m, implying a mean free path of electrons

$$\Delta \ell \approx \left[5\text{eV} \, / \, 3 \times 10^6 \text{V/m}\right] \approx 10^{-6}\text{m}$$

However, this model is not entirely accurate because the actual mean free path corresponds to energies of the order of 0.1 eV, which is only sufficient to excite vibrational modes in the target molecule. Apparently such excitation is sufficient to cause ionization if the collision process lasts long enough [29].

Except for some laboratory conditions where a sufficiently high potential difference can be applied directly across a biological membrane to bring about its destruction, collisional ionization is generally not a factor in the interaction of electromagnetic waves

Introduction to Electromagnetic Fields 25

with tissue: The potential difference required for membrane destruction [30] is between 100 nV and 300 mV, corresponding to a field strength of the order of 2×10^7 V/m, assuming a membrane thickness ($d = 100$ Å; $E = V/d$). However, there is a third mechanism of ionization that is particularly important in biological systems. When a chemical compound of the type wherein positive and negative ions are held together by their electrostatic attraction, such as the ionic crystal NaCl, is placed in a suitable solvent, such as H_2O, it is separated into its ionic components. The resulting solution becomes an electrolyte, i.e., an electrically conducting medium in which the only charge carriers are ions.

In this process of chemical ionization, the Na^+ cations and Cl^- anions are separated from the original NaCl crystal lattice and individually surrounded by a sheet of solvent molecules, the "hydration sheath." If the solvent is H_2O, this process is called "hydration," or more generally, for any solvent, "solvation."

A dilute solution of NaCl crystals in H_2O is slightly cooler than the original constituents before the solvation process, indicating that some internal energy of the system was consumed. Actually energy is consumed in breaking up the original NaCl bonds and some, but less, is liberated in the interaction between the dipole moment of the solvent molecule (H_2O in our example) and the electric charges on the ions. Thus, solvents with higher relative dielectric constant ε_r, indicating higher inherent electric dipole moment per unit volume (P), solvate ions more strongly ($\varepsilon_r = 1 + P/[\varepsilon_o E]$, where E is the electric field applied during the measurement of ε_r). For example, H_2O with $\varepsilon_r \approx 80$ solvates more strongly than methanol with $\varepsilon_r \approx 33$. For biological applications, it is worth noting that solvation may affect not only ionic substances, but also polar groups, i.e., molecular components which have an inherent dipole moment, such as $-C=O$, $-NH$, or $-NO_2$. Details of the process are discussed in texts on electrochemistry [31,32].

In biological processes not only chemical ionization and solvation of ionic compounds, but also all kinds of chemical reactions take place. One of the central questions in the study of biological effects of E and H fields is therefore not only whether they can cause or influence ionization, but also whether they can affect—speed up, slow down, or modify—any naturally occurring biologically important chemical reaction.

In Table 0.4 typical energies for various types of chemical bonds are listed. For comparison, the thermal energy per elementary particle at 310 K is also shown. Complementing the numbers in Table 0.4 one should also point out that:

1. The large spread in the statistical distribution of energies of thermal motion guarantees that at physiological temperatures some molecules always have sufficient energy to break the strongest weak bonds [33].

2. The average lifetime of a weak bond is only a fraction of a second.

3. The weak binding forces (Van der Waals) are effective only between the surfaces in close proximity and usually require complementary structures such as a (microscopic) plug and hole, such as are thought to exist, between antigen and antibody, for instance [34].

4. Most molecules in aqueous solution form secondary bonds.

5. The metabolism of biological systems continuously transforms molecules and therefore also changes the secondary bonds that are formed.

Comparison of the last columns in Tables 0.3 and 0.4 shows that millimeter waves have quantum energies which are only about one order of magnitude below typical Van der Waals energies (waves at a frequency of 10^{12} Hz with a quantum energy of 0.004 eV

TABLE 0.4

Bond and Thermal Energies

Type of Bond	Change in Free Energy (Binding Energy) kcal/mol	eV/ Molecule
Covalent	50–100	2.2–4.8
Van der Waals	1–2	0.04–0.08
Hydrogen	3–7	0.13–0.30
Ionic[a]	5	0.2
Avg. thermal energy at 310K	0.62	0.027

[a] For ionic groups of organic molecules such as COO–, $NH3_3^-$ in aqueous solution.

have a wavelength of 0.3 mm and can still be classified as millimeter waves). One might expect therefore that such waves could initiate chemically important events, such as configurational changes, e.g., multiple transitions between closely spaced vibrational states at successively high-energy levels [47].

Energies associated with transition from one to another mode of rotation of a diatomic molecule are given by $W = \ell(\ell + 1)A$ [26,33], where $\ell = 0, 1, 2, 3 \ldots$ and $A = 6 \times 10^{-5}$ eV; thus, an electromagnetic wave with a frequency as low as 29 GHz—still in the microwave region—can excite a rotational mode. Vibrational modes of diatomic molecules [27,34] correspond to energies of the order of 0.04 eV, requiring excitation in the IR region. Vibrational frequencies in a typical H-bonded system [35] are of the order of 3000 GHz; however, attenuation at this frequency by omnipresent free H_2O may prevent any substantial effect [35].

Kohli et al. [36] predict that longitudinal and torsional modes of double helical DNA should not be critically damped at frequencies >1 GHz, although relaxation times are of the order of picoseconds, and Kondepudi [37] suggests the possibility of an influence of millimeter waves at approximately 5×10^{11} Hz upon oxygen affinity of hemoglobin due to the resonant excitation of heme plane oscillations. Although Furia et al. [38] did not find resonance absorption at millimeter waves in yeast, such was reported by Grundler et al. [39,48]. The latter experiment has been interpreted [40,41] as supporting Fröhlich's theory of cooperative phenomena in biological systems. That theory postulates "electric polarization waves" in biological membranes which are polarized by strong biologically generated [19] fields (10^7 V/m). Fröhlich [42,43] suggests that metabolically supplied energy initiates mechanical vibrations of cell membranes. The frequency of such vibrations is determined by the dimensions and the elastic constants of the membranes; based on an estimate of the sound velocity in the membrane of 10^3 m/s and a membrane thickness of 100 Å (equal to one half wavelength) one obtains a frequency of $5(10^{10})$ Hz. Individual molecules within and outside the membrane may also oscillate, and frequency estimates vary between 10^9 Hz for helical RNA [44] and 5×10^{13} Hz for hydrogen-bonded amide structures [45]. As the membranes and molecules involved are strongly polarized, the mechanically oscillating dipole electromagnetic fields those are able to transmit energy, at least in some situations, over distances much larger than the distance to the next adjacent molecule.

Electromagnetic coupling of this type may produce long-range cooperative phenomena. In particular, Fröhlich [46] has shown that two molecular systems may exert strong forces upon each other when their respective oscillation frequencies are nearly equal, provided the dielectric permittivity of the medium between them is strongly dispersive or excitation is supplied by pumping, i.e., by excitation at the correct frequency from an external source. The mechanism is nonlinear in the sense that it displays a step-like dependence

Introduction to Electromagnetic Fields 27

on excitation intensity. Possible long-range effects may be, for example, attraction between enzyme and substrate [43]. These and related topics have been discussed in detail by Illinger [35] and are reviewed in Chapters 5 and 7 in this volume.

References

1. Ramo, S., Whinnery, J.R., and Van Duzer, T., *Fields and Waves in Communication Electronics*, John Wiley & Sons, New York, 1965, p. 644.
2. Jordan, E.C., *Electromagnetic Waves and Radiating Systems*. Prentice-Hall, Englewood Cliffs, NJ, 1950.
3. Schelkunoff, S.A., *Electromagnetic Waves*, D Van Nostrand, New York, 1943, p. 133.
4. Stratton, J.A., *Electromagnetic Theory*, McGraw-Hill, New York, 1941, p. 435.
5. Van Bladel, J., *Electromagnetic Fields*, McGraw-Hill, New York, 1964, p. 274.
6. Kaune, W.T. and Gillis, M.F., General properties of the interaction between animals and ELF electric fields, *Bioelectromagnetics*, 2, 1, 1981.
7. Bridges, J.E. and Preache, M., Biological influences of power frequency electric fields—a tutorial review from a physical and experimental viewpoint, *Proc. IEEE*, 69, 1092, 1981.
8. Iribarne, J.V. and Cho, H.R., *Atmospheric Physics*, D. Reidel, Boston, MA, 1980, p. 134.
9. Zahn, M., *Electromagnetic Field Theory, A Problem Solving Approach*, John Wiley & Sons, New York, 1979.
10. Raybourn, M.S., The effects of direct-current magnetic fields on turtle retina in vitro, *Science*, 220, 715, 1983.
11. Schulten, K., Magnetic field effects in chemistry and biology, in *Festkörperprobleme/Advances in Solid State Physics*, Vol. 22, Heyden, Philadelphia, 1982, p. 61.
12. Blankenship, R.E., Schaafsma, T.J., and Parson, W.W., Magnetic field effects on radical pair intermediates in bacterial photosynthesis, *Biochim. Biophys. Acta*, 461, 297, 1977.
13. Sheppard, A.R., Magnetic field interactions in man and other mammals: An overview, in *Magnetic Field Effect on Biological Systems*, Tenforde, T.S., Ed., Plenum Press, New York, 1979, p. 33.
14. Jordan, E.C., *Electromagnetic Waves and Radiating Systems*, Prentice-Hall, Englewood Cliffs, NJ, 1950, p. 132.
15. Ramo, S., Whinnery, J.R., and Van Duzer, T., *Fields and Waves in Communication Electronics*, John Wiley & Sons, New York, 1965, p. 293.
16. Smyth, C.P., *Static and Dynamic Electricity*, McGraw-Hill, New York, 1939
17. Bean, C.P., DeBlois, R.W., and Nesbitt, L.B., Eddy-current method for measuring the resistivity of metals, *J. Appl. Phys.*, 30(12), 1959, 1976.
18. Bassett, C.A.L., Pawluk, R.J., and Pilla, A.A., Augmentation of bone repair by inductively coupled electromagnetic fields, *Science*, 184, 575, 1974.
19. Plonsey, R. and Fleming, D., *Bioelectric Phenomena*, McGraw-Hill, New York, 1969, p. 115.
20. Houslay, M.D. and Stanley, K.K., *Dynamics of Biological Membranes*, John Wiley & Sons, New York, 1982, p. 296.
21. Wilson, D.F., Energy transduction in biological membranes, in *Membrane Structure and Function*, Bittar, E.D., Ed., John Wiley & Sons, New York, 1980, p. 182.
22. Johnson, C.C. and Guy, A.W., Nonionizing electromagnetic wave effects in biological materials and systems, *Proc. IEEE*, 60, 692, 1972.
23. Schwan, H.P., Field interaction with biological matter, *Ann. NY Acad. Sci.*, 303, 198, 1977.
24. Kraichman, M.B., *Handbook of Electromagnetic Propagation in Conducting Media*, NAVMAT P-2302, U.S. Superintendent of Documents, U.S. Government Printing Office, Washington, DC, 1970.

25. Massoudi, H., Durney, C.H., Barber, P.W., and Iskander, M.F., Postresonance electromagnetic absorption by man and animals, *Bioelectromagnetics*, 3, 333, 1982.
26. Binhi, V.N., *Magnetobiology: Understanding Physical Problems*, Academic Press, London, 473 pp.
27. Sears, F.W., Zemansky, M.W., and Young, H.D., *University Physics*, 5th ed., Addison-Wesley, Reading, MA, 1976, p. 360.
28. Uman, M.A., *Lightning*, McGraw-Hill, New York, 1969, p. 162.
29. Coelho, R., *Physics of Dielectrics for the Engineer*, Elsevier, Amsterdam, 1979, p. 155.
30. Schwan, H.P., Dielectric properties of biological tissue and biophysical mechanisms of electromagnetic field interaction, in *Biological Effects of Nonionizing Radiation*, Illinger, K.H., Ed., ACS Symposium Series 157, American Chemical Society, Washington, DC, 1981, p. 121.
31. Koryta, J., *Ions, Electrodes and Membranes*, John Wiley & Sons, New York, 1982.
32. Rosenbaum, E.J., *Physical Chemistry*, Appleton-Century-Crofts, Education Division, Meredith Corporation, New York, 1970, p. 595.
33. Watson, J.D., *Molecular Biology of the Gene*, W.A. Benjamin, Menlo Park, CA, 1976, p. 91.
34. Rosenbaum, E.J., *Physical Chemistry*, Appleton-Century-Crofts, Education Division, Meredith Corporation, New York, 1970, p. 595.
35. Illinger, K.H., Electromagnetic-field interaction with biological systems in the microwave and far-infrared region, in *Biological Effects of Nonionizing Radiation*, Illinger, K.H., Ed., ACS Symposium Series 157, American Chemical Society, Washington, DC, 1981, p. 1.
36. Kohli, M., Mei, W.N., Van Zandt, L.L., and Prohofsky, E.W., Calculated microwave absorption by double-helical DNA, in *Biological Effects of Nonionizing Radiation*, Illinger, K.H., Ed., ACS Symposium Series 157, American Chemical Society, Washington, DC, 1981, p. 101.
37. Kondepudi, D.K., Possible effects of 10^{11} Hz radiation on the oxygen affinity of hemoglobin, *Bioelectromagnetics*, 3, 349, 1982.
38. Furia, L., Gandhi, O.P., and Hill, D.W., Further investigations on resonant effects of mm-waves on yeast, Abstr. 5th Annu. Sci. Session, Bioelectromagnetics Society, University of Colorado, Boulder, June 12–17, 1983, p. 13.
39. Grundler, W., Keilman, F., and Fröhlich, H., Resonant growth rate response of yeast cells irradiated by weak microwaves, *Phys. Lett.*, 62A, 463, 1977.
40. Fröhlich, H., Coherent processes in biological systems, in *Biological Effects of Nonionizing Radiation*, Illinger, K.H., Ed., ACS Symposium Series 157, American Chemical Society, Washington, DC, 1981, p. 213.
41. Fröhlich, H., What are non-thermal electric biological effects? *Bioelectromagnetics*, 3, 45, 1982.
42. Fröhlich, H., Coherent electric vibrations in biological systems and the cancer problem, *IEEE Trans. Microwave Theory Tech.*, 26, 613, 1978.
43. Fröhlich, H., The biological effects of microwaves and related questions, in *Advances in Electronics and Electron Physics*, Marton, L. and Marton, C., Eds., Academic Press, New York, 1980, p. 85.
44. Prohofsky, E.W. and Eyster, J.M., Prediction of giant breathing and rocking modes in double helical RNA, *Phys. Lett.*, 50A, 329, 1974.
45. Careri, J., Search for cooperative phenomena in hydrogen-bonded amide structures, in *Cooperative Phenomena*, Haken, H. and Wagner, W., Eds., Springer-Verlag, Basel, 1973, p. 391.
46. Fröhlich, H., Selective long range dispersion forces between large systems, *Phys. Lett.*, 39A, 153, 1972.
47. Barnes, F.S. and Hu, C.-L.J., Nonlinear Interactions of electromagnetic waves with biological materials, in *Nonlinear Electromagnetics*, Uslenghi, P.L.E., Ed., Academic Press, New York, 1980, p. 391.
48. Grundler, W., Keilmann, F., Putterlik, V., Santo, L., Strube, D., and Zimmermann, I., Nonthermal resonant effects of 42 GHz microwaves on the growth of yeast cultures, in *Coherent Excitations of Biological Systems*, Frölich, H. and Kremer, F., Eds., Springer-Verlag, Basel, 1983, p. 21.

1

Environmental and Occupational DC and Low Frequency Electromagnetic Fields

Ben Greenebaum
University of Wisconsin-Parkside

Kjell Hansson Mild
Umeå University

CONTENTS

1.1 Introduction 29
1.2 Naturally Occurring Fields 30
1.3 Artificial DC and Power Frequency EM Fields in the Environment 31
    1.3.1 DC Fields 31
    1.3.2 High-Voltage AC Power Lines 32
    1.3.3 Exposure in Homes 36
    1.3.4 Electrical Appliances 40
    1.3.5 ELF Fields in Transportation 42
    1.3.6 ELF Fields in Occupational Settings 45
    1.3.7 Internal ELF Fields Induced by External and Endogenous Fields 47
1.4 Conclusion 50
Acknowledgments 50
References 50

1.1 Introduction

We encounter electromagnetic (EM) fields, both naturally occurring and man-made, every day. This leads to exposure in our homes as well as outdoors and in our various workplaces, and the intensity of the fields varies substantially with the situation. Quite high exposure can occur in some of our occupations as well as during some personal activities, for instance, in trains, where the extremely low-frequency (ELF) magnetic field can reach rather high levels. The frequency of the fields we are exposed to covers a wide range, from static or slowly changing fields to the gigahertz range. However, measurements of the magnetic field at a particular location or near a particular piece of equipment can often be much higher than an individual's average exposure across a day as measured by a personal monitor, since one moves from one place to another throughout the day, both in occupational and everyday settings (Bowman, 2014).

In this chapter, we give an overview of the fields we encounter in the steady direct current (DC) and low-frequency range (ELF, strictly speaking 30–300 Hz but taken here, as is usual in the bioelectromagnetics literature to extend from 0 to 3000 Hz) and in various situations. Higher frequency fields encountered are reviewed in Chapter 2 of *BBA*. Recent published reviews of common field exposures include Bowman (2014) on both ordinary environmental and occupational exposures and Gajšek et al. (2016), which discusses European exposures. The World Health Organization Environmental Health Criteria on static (WHO, 2006) and ELF fields (WHO, 2007) provide chapters on commonly encountered fields.

1.2 Naturally Occurring Fields

The most obvious naturally occurring field is the Earth's magnetic field, known since ancient times. The total field intensity diminishes from the poles, as high as 67 μT at the south magnetic pole to as low as about 30 μT near the equator. In South Brazil, an area with flux densities as low as about 24 μT can be found. In addition, the angle of the Earth's field to the horizontal (inclination) varies, primarily with latitude, ranging from very small near the equator to almost vertical at high latitudes. More information is available in textbooks (see, e.g., Dubrov, 1978) and in databases available on the Web (see, e.g., the U.S. National Geophysical Data Center, 2017).

However, the geomagnetic field is not constant, but is continuously subject to more or less strong fluctuations. There are diurnal variations, which may be more pronounced during the day and in summer than at night and in winter (see, e.g., Konig et al., 1981). There are also short-term variations associated with ionospheric processes. When the solar wind brings protons and electrons toward the Earth, phenomena like the Northern Lights and rapid fluctuations in the geomagnetic field intensity occur. The variation can be rather large; the magnitude of the changes can sometimes be up to 1 μT on a timescale of several minutes. The variation can also be very different in two fairly widely separated places because of the atmospheric conditions. There is also a naturally occurring DC electric field at the surface of the Earth in the order of 100–300 V/m (Earth's surface negative) in calm weather; it can be 100 kV/m in thunderstorms, caused by atmospheric ions (NRC, 1986).

EM processes associated with lightning discharges are termed as atmospherics or "sferics" for short. They consist mostly of waves in the ELF and very low-frequency (VLF) ranges (3–30 kHz) (see Konig et al., 1981). Each second about 100 lightning discharges occur globally; and in the United States, one cloud-to-ground flash occurs about every second, averaged over the year Konig et al. (1981). The ELF and VLF signals travel efficiently in the waveguide formed by the Earth and the ionosphere and can be detected many thousands of kilometers from the initiating stroke. Since 1994, several experiments studying the effects of short-term exposure to simulated 10-kHz sferics have been performed at the Department of Clinical and Physiological Psychology at the University of Giessen, Germany (Schienle et al., 1996, 1999). In the ELF range, very low-intensity signals, called Schumann resonances, also occur. These are caused by the ionosphere and the Earth's surface acting as a resonant cavity, excited by lightning (Konig et al., 1981; Campbell, 1999). These cover the low-frequency spectrum, with broad peaks of diminishing amplitude at 7.8, 14, 20, and 26 Hz and higher frequencies. Higher-frequency fields, extending into the microwave region, are also present in atmospheric or intergalactic sources. These fields are much weaker, usually by many orders of magnitude than those caused by human activity (compare Figure 1.1 and subsequent tables and figures in this chapter).

Environmental DC and Low Frequency Fields

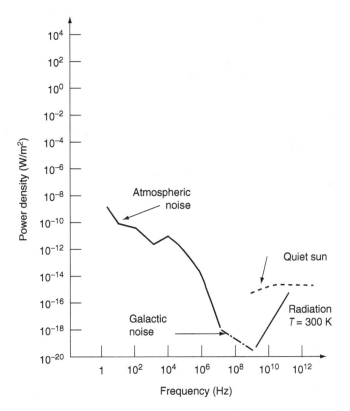

FIGURE 1.1
Power density from natural sources as a function of frequency. (Data from Smith, E. *Proceedings of the IEEE Symposium on Electromagnetic Compatibility*. *Institute of Electrical and Electronic Engineering*, Piscataway, NJ, 1982. Graph adapted from Barnes, F.S. Health Phys. 56, 759–766, 1989. With permission.)

1.3 Artificial DC and Power Frequency EM Fields in the Environment

1.3.1 DC Fields

Although alternate current (AC) power transmission is facilitated by the availability of transformers to change voltages, DC is also useful, especially since high-power, high efficiency solid-state electronic devices have become available. Overland high-voltage DC lines running at up to 1100 kV (circuits at ±550 kV) are found in Europe, North America, and Asia (Hingorani, 1996). Electric and magnetic field intensities near these lines are essentially the same as those for AC lines running at the same voltages and currents, which are discussed below. Because potentials on the cables do not vary in time and there are only two DC conductors (+ and −) instead of the three AC phases, the DC electric fields and space charge clouds of air ions that partially screen them are somewhat different from those near AC transmission lines, though the general features are the same, especially for positions away from the lines. Electric fields, corona, and air ions are discussed further in the AC transmission line section below (Kaune et al., 1983; Fews et al., 2002). For transfer

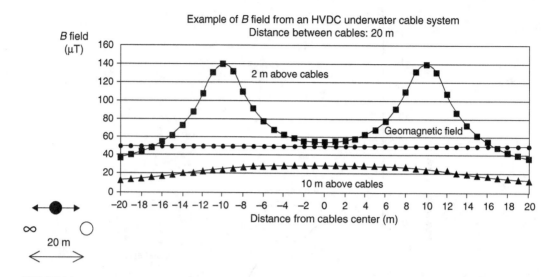

FIGURE 1.2
Predicted DC magnetic field from a high-voltage DC cable with the return cable placed at a distance of 20 m. The current in the cable was assumed to be 1333 A, which is the maximum design current. (From Hansson Mild, K. In Matthes, R., Bernhardt, J.H., and Repacholi, M.H., Eds. *Proceedings from a joint seminar, International Seminar on Effects of Electromagnetic Fields on the Living Environment*, of ICNIRP, WHO, and BfS, Ismaning, Germany, October 4–5, 1999, pp. 21–37. With permission.)

of electric power between countries separated by sea, DC undersea power cables are especially useful, since their higher capacity causes decreased losses than with AC.

Examples are cables between Sweden and Finland, Denmark, Germany, and Gotland, a Swedish island in the Baltic Sea. A 254 km 450 kV 600 MW cable began operation in 2000 from Sweden to Poland (SwePol). In these cables DC is used, and the ELF component of the current is less than a few tenths of a percent. The maximum current in these cables is slightly above 1000 A, and the estimated normal load is about 30% or 400 A. Depending on the location of the return path, the DC magnetic field will range from a maximum disturbance of the geomagnetic field (with a return through water) to a minimal disturbance (with a return through a second cable as close as possible to the feed cable). With a closest distance of 20 m between the cables, the predicted field distribution can be seen in Figure 1.2, immediately above the cables (2 m), practically the same value as that obtained for a single wire. When the distance between cables is increased beyond 20 m, the distortion at a given distance rises above that of Figure 1.2. Since the cables are shielded, no electric field will be generated outside the cable. For a more detailed discussion of the fields associated with this technique, the reader is referred to the paper by Koops (1999).

Few other DC fields from human activity are broadly present in the environment, though very short-range DC fields are found near permanent magnets, usually ranging from a few tenths of a millitesla to a few millitesla at the surface of the magnet and decreasing very rapidly as one moves away. Occupationally encountered DC fields are discussed below.

1.3.2 High-Voltage AC Power Lines

The electric and magnetic fields from high-voltage power lines have been figuring for a long time in the debate on the biological effects of EM fields. Although the AC power systems in the Americas, Japan, the island of Taiwan, Korea, and a few other places are

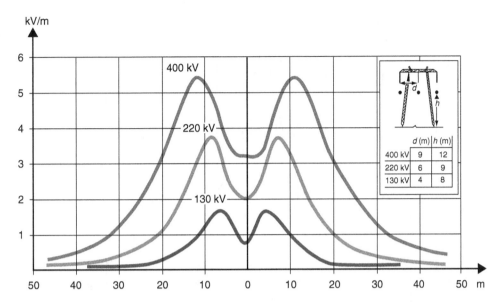

FIGURE 1.3
Electric field from three different high-voltage power lines as a function of the distance from the center of the line. In the inset the distance between the phases as well as the height above ground of the lines are given. (From Hansson Mild, K. In Matthes, R., Bernhardt, J.H., and Repacholi, M.H., Eds. *Proceedings from a joint seminar, International Seminar on Effects of Electromagnetic Fields on the Living Environment, of ICNIRP, WHO, and BfS*, Ismaning, Germany, October 4–5, 1999, pp. 21–37. With permission.)

60 Hz, while most of the rest of the world is 50 Hz, the frequency difference has no effect on high-voltage transmission line fields. In the early days of bioelectromagnetics research, the electric field was considered the most important part, and measurements of field strengths were performed in many places. Figure 1.3 shows an example of such measurements from three different types of lines: 400, 220, and 130 kV lines, respectively. The field strength depends not only on the voltage of the line but also on the distance between the phases and the height of the tower. The strongest field can be found where the lines are closest to the ground, and this usually occurs midway between two towers. Here, field strengths up to a few kilovolts per meter can be found. Since the guidelines of the International Commission on Non-Ionizing Radiation Protection (ICNIRP, 1998) limit public exposure to 5 kV/m and there is no time averaging for low-frequency fields, people walking under high-voltage power lines may on some occasions be exposed in excess of existing international guidelines.

Because electric fields are well shielded by trees, buildings, or other objects, research in the 1970s and 1980s did not turn up any major health effects (see, e.g., Portier and Wolfe, 1998) and because of the epidemiological study by Wertheimer and Leeper (1979) (see also Chapter 13 in *BMA*), attention turned from electric to magnetic fields in the environment. The magnetic field from a transmission line or any other wire depends on the current load carried by the line, as well as the distance from the conductors; in Figure 1.4, calculations of the magnetic flux density from several different types of transmission lines are shown. There is a very good agreement between the theoretical calculation and the measured flux density in most situations. The flux density from two-wire power lines is directly proportional to the electric current, generally inversely proportional to the square of the distance to the power line for distances greater than several times the distance between the phase lines, and directly proportional to the distance between the phase wires. For three and

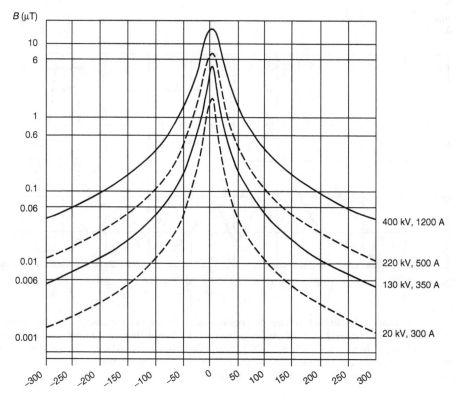

FIGURE 1.4
Magnetic flux density from different high-voltage power lines at a distance (in meters) from the center of the line. The currents in the lines are the maximum values allowed and are given to the right in the figure. (Figure courtesy of Swedish National Institute for Working Life.)

six-wire systems, the fields decrease more rapidly with distance at a rate that is dependent on the phase sequences and the spacing between the wires. For most lower-voltage lines, around 10–20 kV, the distance at which the B field falls below 0.2 µT is generally less than 10 m; this distance still depends on current and the spacing of the wires.

The electric or magnetic field vector from a single AC conductor displays a sinusoidal waveform, oscillating back and forth through zero intensity in a single direction determined by the observation position with respect to the wire, ignoring any small distortions due to harmonics, etc. However, near a three-phase high-voltage transmission line, the electric and magnetic field vectors from the group of conductors, which are at some distance from each other and whose individual sinusoidal variations are out of phase, rotate in space as well as change in magnitude, but their magnitude never decreases exactly to zero (Deno, 1976). This so-called elliptical polarization may or may not have a different biological significance than the single conductor's "plane polarization."

Several approaches have been used for reducing the magnetic field from a line, and in Figure 1.5 some examples are given. Instead of hanging the three phases at the same height and in parallel, the lines can be arranged in a triangular form, thereby reducing the distance between the phases and thus also the flux density. The reduction is of the order of about 1.6. An even greater reduction is obtained if the so-called split phase arrangement is used. Here, five lines are used. One phase is placed in the center, and the other two phases

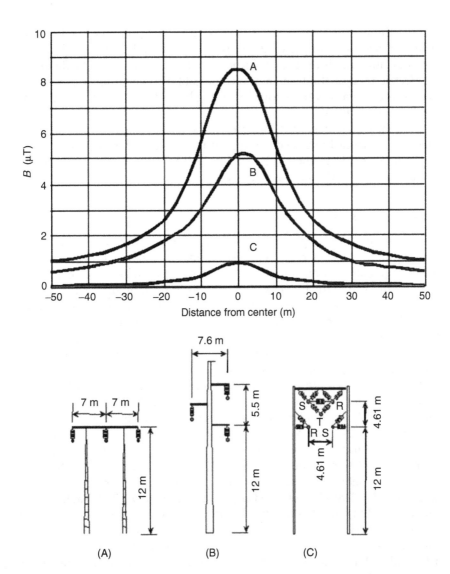

FIGURE 1.5
Examples of reduction of the magnetic flux density from a 220-kV line with a maximum phase current of 500 A. In (A) the normal configuration is used and the maximum flux density is about 8 µT, and in (B) a delta arrangement is used which gives a reduction to about 5 mT maximum under the line. In (C) the split phase arrangement is used leading to a maximum value of only 1 mT. (Figure courtesy of Swedish National Institute for Working Life.)

are split into two lines each, which are placed diagonally (see Figure 1.5). The reduction is almost tenfold.

When high voltage is present, there is a possibility of the insulation breaking down, causing a catastrophic discharge—a spark; lightning is an obvious example. There is also the more common possibility of very minor discharges occurring, in which one or a relatively small number of molecules near the high-voltage element become ionized; this is often called a corona, since in extreme cases a small glow can be seen near parts of the high-voltage system. Corona discharge can also occur at grounded objects near a high voltage and is more likely to occur at more pointed objects; this is the principle of the

36   *Electromagnetic Fields*

lightning rod. Minor corona damage has been observed on pine tree needles very close to a 1200 V transmission line (Rogers et al., 1984). (No other environmental damage to plants or animals from either fields or corona has been found (Lee et al., 1996).) The resulting ions screen the electric field of the transmission line cables to varying extents, because their number depends on a variety of factors, including humidity, dust, rain, and wind (Kaune et al., 1983; Fews et al., 2002).

While a hypothesis has been put forward that ions from power lines make small airborne particles, particularly those carrying naturally occurring radioactive atoms, more likely to enter and remain in the lungs and cause cancer or various other diseases (Fews et al., 1999), it has not found much acceptance.

1.3.3 Exposure in Homes

Although Wertheimer and Leeper (1979) initially used transmission and distribution line sizes and configurations as surrogates for estimating magnetic field exposure from transmission lines, it quickly became apparent that the correlation was not very good and that sources of exposure inside the home were at least as important, unless the home was very close to a transmission line (Portier and Wolfe, 1998). Several studies have explored the exposure to ELF electric and magnetic fields in homes in different countries. Deadman et al. (1999) investigated the exposure of children in Canada. A logging device was used, which recorded the fields during two consecutive 24-h periods. For 382 children up to the age of 15 they found an arithmetic mean (AM) of the magnetic field of 0.121 μT with a range of 0.01–0.8 μT. The corresponding values for the electric field were AM 14.4 V/m, range 0.82–64.7 V/m. Hansson Mild et al. (1996) compared the ELF fields in Swedish and Norwegian residential buildings. The overall mean values were as follows: E fields 54 V/m (SD = 37) and 77 V/m (SD = 58) in Sweden and Norway, respectively; the corresponding values for B fields were 40 nT (SD = 37) and 15 nT (SD = 17). Hamnerius et al. (2011) did a 24-h measurement in 28 apartments and 69 single family homes in three Swedish cities. Apartments averaged 0.17 μT and homes, 0.09 μT, the difference being attributed to wiring in apartment walls leading to other units. A total of 89% had adjusted fields below 0.2 μT. Table 1.1 shows additional comparisons. One should note that European residential power is 220 V while North American power is 110 V, leading to higher currents (and magnetic fields) in North America for the same electric power consumption and distance from the source.

McCurdy et al. (2001) measured women's exposure in the United States by using personal magnetic field exposure meters that were worn during a working day or a day at home. The geometric mean of the time-weighted average for the working day was 0.138 μT with a range of 0.022–3.6 μT, and for the homemakers the corresponding values were 0.113 μT, range 0.022–0.403 μT.

In the meta-analysis by Ahlbom et al. (2000) on childhood cancer and residential magnetic fields, it was stated that 99.2% of the population resided in homes with B < 0.4 μT.

Exposure varies widely in time, according to the time of day and the season. One may be outdoors, far from any field sources at one time, indoors near an operating appliance at another, riding in an electric transit vehicle at some other time, and so forth. Sample exposure values for an individual, recorded as a function of time over a 24-h period in spring and summer, are shown in Figure 1.6.

Since the three-phase systems used for electrical distribution are dimensioned for sinusoidal fields, the harmonic content can create problems. Today we may find large stray currents, usually resulting from unbalanced currents between phases, in water pipes, ventilation systems, concrete reinforcement mesh, etc., and the current flowing also contains

Table 1.1

Selected Residential Exposures to ELF-MFs by Power System Sources, Country, and Area versus Personal Monitoring

	24-hr TWA of ELF-MF (μT)	
Power System Source[a]	GM[b]	P95[c]
Apartment building transformers	0.59	1.30
Transmission lines	0.09	0.49
Overhead primary lines (no neutrals)	0.02	0.60
Overhead secondary lines	0.04	1.58
Underground distribution lines	0.03	0.50
Ground currents	0.01	0.70

			Personal	
Country	Range of GMs	Area	GM	P95
United States	0.06–0.07		0.089	0.389
Canada	0.05–0.11		0.081	0.360
United Kingdom	0.036–0.039			
Germany	0.029–0.047	Europe	0.037	0.311
Norway	0.011–0.015			

Source: Bowman (2014). US Government Copyright.

[a] Random survey of U.S. residences. (Zaffanella L. E., *Survey of Residential Magnetic Field Sources*, Volume 1: Goals, Results, Conclusions, EPRI Report No. TR-102759, Electric Power Research Institute, Palo Alto, CA, 1993.)

[b] GM $\approx$ Median over 24 h and all rooms in the residence.

[c] P95 in the 5% of rooms with the highest MF.

these harmonics. Figure 1.7 gives an example of a measurement of a current flowing in a cable in a large apartment building, and Figure 1.8 shows the corresponding Fourier frequency analysis. The magnetic field in the building thus also has these harmonic components. Often, the largest stray currents, which generate large domestic fields, are due to errors in wiring that violate the building code (Adams et al., 2004) or to a poorly planned wiring layout that has currents flowing in open loops instead of both wires of a circuit being laid next to each other in the same conduit (Moriyama and Yoshitomi, 2005).

From Figures 1.6 through 1.8, as well as the data in the rest of this chapter, it is easy to see that average field strength is far from being the only parameter that is needed to characterize electric or magnetic field exposure. Other parameters include frequency or frequencies present (or the related parameters, the rise and fall times of up-and-down excursions or "transients"), numbers and height of transients, number of times the field exceeds or falls below a certain fraction of its average value, whether both DC and time-varying fields are present, relative directions of multiple fields, etc. As discussed elsewhere (e.g., the Introduction and in Chapters 5 and 6 in this volume and Chapters 13 and 14 in *BMA*), it is not clear, in most cases, which one or group of these parameters is related to a particular biological effect. To date, average field strength is the most commonly used parameter, partly because it is the most easily obtainable summary of exposure over an extended period. For a given frequency range, average field strength is related to some

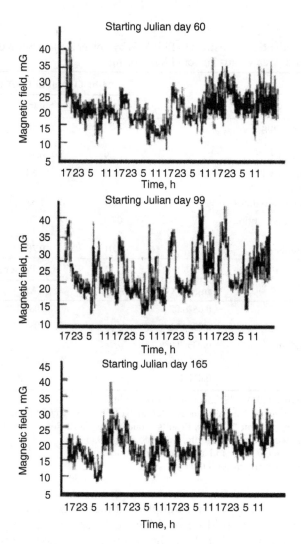

FIGURE 1.6
An individual's measured magnetic field exposure over the course of a day. Note that 1 mG = 0.1 μT. (From Koontz, M.D., Mehegan, L.L., Dietrich, F.M., and Nagda, N.L. Assessment of Children's Long Term Exposure to Magnetic Fields [The Geomet Study]. Final Report TR-101406, Research Project 2966-04, Electric Power Research Institute, Palo Alto, CA, 1992. With permission.)

other parameters, such as fraction of time over a certain threshold, but not to others, such as number of transients per hour. For further discussion of various parameters and their interrelationships, see, for example, Zhang et al. (1997) and Verrier et al. (2005).

Most measurements have been done in detached houses, even though many city dwellers live in apartment buildings. In apartment buildings, the current in the wiring in the ceiling of one unit, for instance, for ceiling lamps, may most strongly affect the magnetic field level of the unit above. Also, some apartment buildings have an electric substation in the basement, where a transformer reduces the medium-voltage distribution line power to 110 or 230 V for domestic use. The low-voltage conductors of the substation may carry substantial currents and create magnetic fields up to several tens of microtesla directly above

Environmental DC and Low Frequency Fields

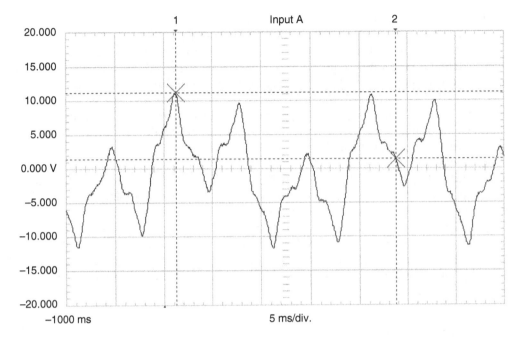

FIGURE 1.7
Stray current wave shape in the 50 Hz power delivery cable in an office building. The peak-to-peak current is of the order 20 A. (Figure courtesy of Swedish National Institute for Working Life.)

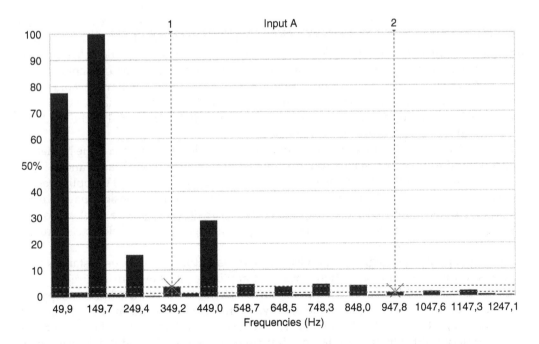

FIGURE 1.8
The Fourier spectrum of the wave shape in Figure 1.5. Note the high 150 Hz (third harmonic) component. (Figure courtesy of Swedish National Institute for Working Life.)

the substation; reduction through placing conductors away from the substation ceiling and shielding with aluminum plates is possible (Forsgren et al., 1994).

In the United States and Canada, though not in other countries, the neutral wire of the AC power distribution system is required to be physically connected to the earth (grounded) at regular intervals to avoid injury from electric shocks; building wiring systems' neutral wires must also be grounded, often by connection to the buried water pipe as it enters the building. Unbalanced loading of the system can produce currents in the ground system, sometimes including currents that leave one residence through the grounding system and return to the power grid through another, which further contributes to the residential magnetic fields (von Winterfeldt and Trauger, 1996; Kaune et al., 2002).

Kavet and colleagues (Kavet and Zaffanella, 2002; Bridges, 2002; Kavet et al., 2004; Kavet, 2005) proposed that effects on leukemia in children, which epidemiology has associated with domestic magnetic fields, are in fact due to small shocks that arise due to potential differences that build up between the water tap and the grounded drain of a tub. Shocks received in the bath were hypothesized to induce in a small child's body current densities of a magnitude known to induce a biological effect. However, subsequent epidemiological studies found no statistical association between these contact currents and childhood leukemia (Does et al., 2011).

1.3.4 Electrical Appliances

The United States, Japan, Canada, and some other countries use 110 V_{rms} AC for basic electrical power, while most of the rest of the world uses 230 V. Since transmission and distribution voltages in the two types of system are about the same, only differences in field exposures due to appliances or building wiring would be expected. For a given power consumption and similar design, 110 V appliances draw twice as much current and create twice as strong a local magnetic field, although their local electric fields are half as strong. However, both types of field fall off rapidly with increasing distance and metal appliance cabinets shield electric fields. Measurements of exposure to magnetic fields have not yielded great differences between the two systems (see Table 1.1). Measurements of magnetic fields from a sample of various appliances show that the fields have a rapid falloff with distance from the device (Kaune et al., 2002). Very close to the appliances or wiring, the values may exceed international guidelines, but at a distance of 0.5–1 m the fields are seldom higher than few tenths of a microtesla.

In general, it can be said that the more power used by a device equipment, the higher the magnetic field. Table 1.2 presents some representative values from 110 V appliances.

Vistnes (2001) recently gave some examples of flux densities near 230 V appliances. Of special interest may be a clock radio, which because of bad electrical design may give rise to exposure of the order of 100 μT nearby. Since people are likely to place a clock radio very close to the pillow, the head may be exposed to quite a large magnetic field, exceeding the normal levels in the house.

The general range of magnetic and electric field magnitudes at various distances from transmission lines, local distribution lines, and appliances is shown in Figure 1.9. Most modern electrical appliances are equipped with an electronically switched power supply in which an electronic circuit replaces the old-style transformer. This means that the current is no longer a pure sinusoidal 50- or 60-Hz signal but contains harmonics. The current used by a low-energy 50-Hz fluorescent lamp is illustrated in Figure 1.10, and the Fourier analysis is shown in Figure 1.11 indicating all the harmonics. Higher harmonics and transients

Environmental DC and Low Frequency Fields

TABLE 1.2

Selected ELF-MF (μT) from Home Appliances at Distances Typical of Personal Exposures

Type	Close (5 cm)		Manual Work Distance (0.5 m)		Far (≥1 m)	
	Median	P95	Median	P95	Median	P95
Light			*Fluorescent lamp*			
			0.10	0.34	0.02	0.08
Heat	*Hair dryer*		*Electric range*		*Baseboard heater*	
	13.01	45.82	0.07	0.22	0.04	0.09
			Electric oven			
			0.82	1.62		
Electronics	*Cell phone[a]*		*Clock radio*		*Stereo*	
	6.00	10.76	0.01	0.06	0.01	0.07
			Microwave			
			0.67	1.15		
Electric motors	*Electric razor*		*Electric can opener*		*Heat pump*	
	164.75	—	1.67	2.15	0.07	0.28
MF-based electronics			*Computer w/CRT[b] monitor*		*TV with CRT*	
			0.13	0.27	0.02	0.06
			Induction range[c]			
			1.00	1.72		

Source: Bowman (2014). US Government Copyright.
[a] 217 Hz pulses converted to rms.
[b] CRT, cathode ray tube.
[c] ELF modulation of 20–50 kHz carrier waves (total MF = 0.4–2 μT at this distance).

(fast spike-like excursions) are also generated by motor-driven appliances and those run by vibrating mechanisms using make-and-break switching contacts, such as older electric shavers or doorbells (Table 1.2).

The magnetic field in different infant incubators used in hospital nurseries varied between 0.23 and 4.4 μT, with an arithmetic average of 1.0 μT (Söderberg et al., 2002). Most of these values are considerably higher than the exposure that can be measured in residential areas close to transmission lines. The technology to reduce the exposure is at hand and can be easily applied.

Occupational exposure from handheld electrical appliances can be quite high. This is mainly equipment that is held close to the body and that uses high power, such as drills and circular saws. These devices usually have adjustable speed, which is done through the switched power supply. Values for the magnetic field of the order 100–200 μT are not uncommon, and in order to show compliance with standards the measurements have to take into account the harmonic contents of the waveform.

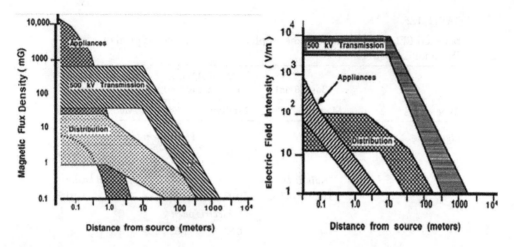

FIGURE 1.9
Magnetic flux density (left, 1 mG = 10 μT) and electric field strength (right) as a function of distance from transmission lines, local distribution lines, and appliances. (From U.S. Office of Technology Assessment. *Biological Effects of Power Frequency Electric and Magnetic Fields.* U.S. Government Printing Office, Washington, DC, Background Paper OTA-BP-E-53, 1989.)

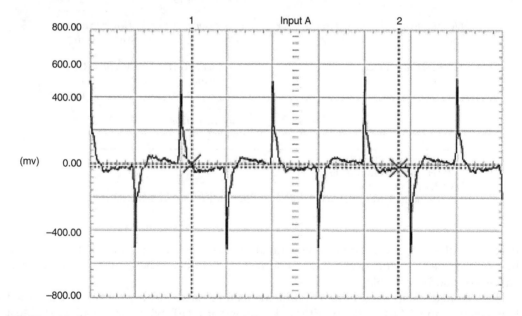

FIGURE 1.10
Wave shape of the current to a low-energy fluorescent lamp. The timescale is 10 ms/div. (Figure courtesy of Swedish National Institute for Working Life.)

1.3.5 ELF Fields in Transportation

Electrified railways and trams have been common for a great many years, both for long distance transportation of freight and passengers and for short trips by city dwellers. Fields are experienced by both train crew members and passengers. Fields are also generated by automobiles, both conventional and electric or hybrid. Fields in both rail systems and electric automobiles are not sinusoidal, but have varying waveforms that contain a variety

Environmental DC and Low Frequency Fields

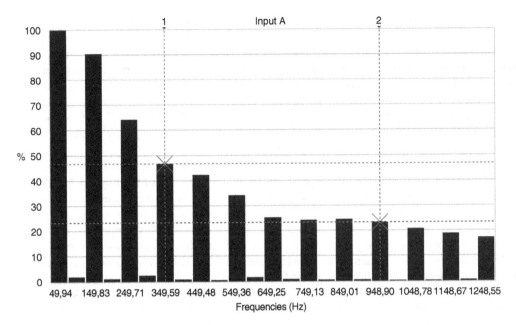

FIGURE 1.11
The Fourier spectrum of the wave shape in Figure 1.7. Note the high 150-Hz component. (Figure courtesy of Swedish National Institute for Working Life.)

of Fourier frequency components. Halgamuge et al. (2010) have summarized principles of operation of electric trains, trams, and automobiles and published results of some studies of field levels in various frequency bands for various AC and DC systems.

In automobiles, electric propulsion systems generate the highest fields. In both electric and conventional cars, the rotation of steel belted tires generates a field, especially near the wheel positions, with frequency depending on road speed. Milham et al. (1999) earlier found AC fields in the rear passenger seat from tires on the order of 2 µT at frequencies below 20 Hz; they also found permanent magnetization in the steel bands of up to 500 µT, measured at the tire surface. Power steering pumps also generate fields.

Intensities inside the passenger cabin from both tire and steering pump fields are much weaker than those from the electrical propulsion components in electric or hybrid (gas-electric) cars. Conventional gasoline engines generate much weaker fields than electric propulsion systems. Vassilev et al. (2015) measured fields in various positions within eight electric or hybrid and three conventional vehicles under various driving conditions using equipment that captured magnetic fields from DC to the MHz region. They quote maximum measured fields from electric propulsion currents of 100–300 µT (0–10 kHz), wheels of 0.2–2 µT (0–20 Hz), steering pumps of about 1 µT (0.5–1 kHz), and internal combustion engines of 50–150 nT (0–200 Hz). Tell et al. (2013) measured fields in 16 electric, hybrid, and gasoline cars driving the same course on a test track, comparing gasoline and hybrids of the same model in four cases, however, their equipment was sensitive only to 40–1,000 Hz. They found geometric means of all measurements for electric and hybrid vehicles of 0.01 µT compared to 0.05 µT for gasoline vehicles, though the 40-Hz low frequency cutoff of the equipment may have removed some drive system fields from electric cars' measurements. Comparing vehicles of the same makes and models, hybrids' geometric mean was 0.06 µT versus 0.05 for gasoline. The highest fields occurred during dynamic braking, when the car's energy of motion is diverted to charging the battery. Using similar equipment, Halgamuge et al. (2010)

found similar levels. These and other authors (Ptitsnaya and Ponzetto, 2012) conclude that electric vehicle fields are comparable to those found elsewhere in the environment.

While electrically powered trains used in long distance service generally are pulled by separate engines, urban transit trains, trams and some very high-speed passenger trains have the electric motors distributed under some or all of the passenger cars. Therefore, exposure to fields of passengers and, to some extent, crews will vary according to the type of vehicle. In general, the waveforms of the magnetic fields from both AC- and DC-powered systems vary significantly and nonuniformly in time, containing many peaks and spikes (Ptitsnaya and Ponzetto, 2012; Ptitsnaya et al., 2003).

Engine drivers of AC electric engines experience rather high magnetic field exposure. The intensity depends of several factors, one of them being the age of the engine. Nordensson et al. (2001) found that drivers of Swedish model RC engines were exposed to flux densities of the order of 10–100 µT (see also Ptitsnaya et al. 1999, 2003). The older models of engines had the higher values. The mean average values for a full workday ranged from 2 to 15 µT. The main input power frequency is 16 2/3 Hz, and this frequency was dominant at idle. But at full power, harmonics up to 150 Hz existed. Wenzl (1997) measured the exposure of rail maintenance workers in the United States and found peak values ranging from 3.4 to 19 µT, and the time-weighted average was in the range 0.3–1.8 mT. Chadwick and Lowes (1998) have examined the exposure of passengers on trains in the United Kingdom, and they found static magnetic flux densities up to several microtesla. The alternating field was also substantial in some locations and reached up to 15 mT at floor level. However, none of the whole-body alternating magnetic flux densities approached the National Radiological Protection Board (NRPB) investigation levels.

Trains operating on DC, such as in the Washington, DC, and San Francisco, CA, municipal transit systems, also produce time-varying fields in the passenger compartments, particularly below 5 Hz (Fraser-Smith and Coates, 1978; Bernardi et al., 1989). Figure 1.12

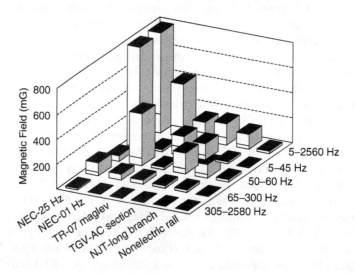

FIGURE 1.12
Maximum (top of bar) and average (horizontal bar) magnetic fields in various frequency bands in the passenger compartment of several intercity rail systems. NEC: U.S. Amtrak Northeast Corridor (Washington, DC, to Boston, MA), which has both 25- and 60-Hz segments; TR-07: German Transrapid maglev system; TGV: French "Train a Grande Vitesse," AC-powered segment of Paris-Tours line; NJT: New Jersey Transit, NJ Coast Line Long Branch section. (From Bernardi, A., Fraser-Smith, A.C., and Villard, O.G., Jr. *IEEE Trans. Electromagn. Compat.* 31, 413–417, 1989.)

shows field intensity in various frequency bands in the passenger compartment of several representative electric rail systems and a nonelectric one. Interestingly, the figure shows that an experimental magnetic levitation (maglev) system does not exhibit substantially different field levels (Dietrich et al., 1993).

1.3.6 ELF Fields in Occupational Settings

Wertheimer and Leeper (1979) were not only the first to publish evidence in support of increased childhood cancer risk with magnetic field exposure, but they also pointed to increased cancer risk in occupations with high magnetic field exposure. Since then, hundreds of studies have looked into this problem, and the assessment of workers' exposure has been debated. There are studies where individual estimates of the exposure have been made for male (Floderus et al., 1996) and females (Deadman and Infante-Rivard, 2002). For workday means, the 25th, 50th, and 75th percentiles were 0.13, 0.17, and 0.27 µT, respectively, for males, and the corresponding values for females were almost similar: 0.14, 0.17, and 0.23 µT. The study on exposure of males investigated the 1,000 most common occupations in Sweden, and the study on female exposure included 61 job categories. Table 1.3 shows additional estimates for various professions.

TABLE 1.3

EMF Exposures in Common Occupational Environments

Personal Measurements of Full-Shift TWA ELF-MF Grouped by Selected Occupational Categories		
Occupation	GM (µT)	P95 (µT)
Teaching professionals	0.11	0.40
Office Occupations		
Library and filing clerks	0.45	0.59
Accounting, bookkeeping, and finance clerks	0.15	0.87
Secretaries and keyboard-operating clerks	0.10	0.51
Manufacturing Occupations		
Ore and metal furnace operators	0.95	9.08
Sewing machine operators	0.83	1.88
Welders and flamecutters	0.80	8.93
Metal moulders and coremakers	0.52	6.08
Electrical and electronic equipment mechanics and fitters	0.23	2.30
Machinery mechanics and fitters	0.20	1.18
Food processing and related trades workers	0.14	0.85
Rubber and plastic products machine operators	0.11	0.39
Transportation Occupations		
Locomotive engine-drivers and related workers	0.13	0.67
Aircraft pilots	0.97	1.87
Ships' engineers	0.55	3.21
Ships' deck officers and pilots	0.22	1.06
Motor vehicle drivers	0.12	0.51
Transport laborers and freight handlers	0.10	0.37
Homemaker	0.06	0.08

Source: Bowman, 2014. US Government copyright.

Sewing machines—Near sewing machines increased magnetic fields can be found and will differ depending on the type of machines used. The mean average value logged during some working hours is of the order of several tenths of a microtesla (Kelsh et al., 2003).

Welders—Among the occupations where quite high exposure exists, electric arc welders are a prominent example. They handle cables carrying hundreds of amperes very close to their bodies. The welder normally grasps the cable, and it sometimes also is in contact with other parts of the body, for instance, it might be draped over the shoulder. Depending on the technique used—DC or AC, type of rectification, etc.—the ELF magnetic field varies, but several studies report values in the range of tens to hundreds of microtesla (Stuchly and Lecuyer, 1989). Skotte and Hjøllund (1997) found a mean of 21 µT for a full-shift average workday of manual metal arc welders. During the actual welding, the B field can be up to several millitesla.

The frequency content of the signal can be rather complex. In one of the most common situations, the welding equipment is connected to a three-phase outlet, and the current for the weld is thus three-phase full-wave rectified. This means that we have first a DC component. To that is added a large AC ripple with main frequency 300 Hz (50 Hz power system), but it is also with harmonics at 600, 900, 1,200 Hz, etc. A newer type of equipment has a pulsed DC (50–200 Hz pulse frequency) as a base frequency with a 53 kHz current applied between the pulses. This leads to frequencies in the current equal to the pulse frequency and its harmonics and also 53 kHz and harmonics. It is a very complex situation to evaluate with respect to compliance with guidelines, because of the complexity of the signal. Since, in many cases, high exposure results from the cables, much can be done to reduce the exposure of the welder by carefully arranging the workstation to keep the cables away from the body. By placing the welding machine on the right hand side of the worker (if right-handed) and seeing that the return cable is as close as possible to the current cable, the exposure can be reduced by one order of magnitude.

Induction heaters—EM induction is used for heating metals for purposes that include surface or deep hardening, welding, melting, soft soldering, brazing, annealing, tempering, and relieving stress. The frequency can be from 50 Hz to the low megahertz range, depending on the desired skin depth and purpose. Since high currents are used, the leakage magnetic field can be substantial. At the operator's position, values of the order of 0.5–8 µT are common, and the maximum field near the coil, where, for instance, the hands can be exposed, can reach several hundreds of microtesla. The field strength is in many cases high compared with recommended limits (ICNIRP, 1998).

Electrochemical plants—In factories producing, for instance, aluminum, copper, or chloride through electrochemical processes, very high DC currents are used, often of the order of tens of kiloamperes. The DC current is obtained through rectification of the incoming three-phase AC power. Often there is still a substantial AC component of the current and hence also an AC magnetic field. Measurements have shown broadband ELF measurements of the order of 10–50 µT, with many different frequencies present that need to be taken into account in the evaluation of the exposure situation. Typically, a 50 Hz component can be present, because of unbalance between the three phases, and the full wave rectification gives 300, 600, and 900 Hz components. The exposure guidelines can often be exceeded in some locations in the plants, and special requirements may be needed to reduce the exposure. DC fields in these smelters are often on the order of several millitesla, with peaks of at least 20–30 mT; up to 70 mT has been reported (NIOSH, 1994; Von Kaenel et al., 1994).

Environmental DC and Low Frequency Fields

1.3.7 Internal ELF Fields Induced by External and Endogenous Fields

Because the bodies of humans, other animals, and even plants contain ionic solutions and because cell cultures, as well as many one-celled and other organisms such as fish or the roots of plants, live in conductive media, external exposure to electric or time-varying magnetic fields can produce internal fields, which can be quite different from the unperturbed external fields.

In an electric field, the conductivity and dielectric constants of tissue are quite different from those of air or vacuum, as discussed in Chapter 4 in this volume. This difference creates a layer of charge due to polarization at the surface of the body, which decreases the internal field, often by many orders of magnitude. For a grounded human standing in the ELF electric field below a high-voltage transmission line, the field inside the body may be only 10^{-6} of the external field. The shape of the body also affects the amount of polarization. Since a standing human's body has more of a "lightning rod" shape than a crouching rat, a rat must be exposed to a much lower external field to achieve an equivalent internal electric field. A squatting human will experience lower and the rearing rat, higher fields. The body shape and foot area also affect the average current densities in various body locations because of the external electric field. Figure 1.13 illustrates these differences (Kaune and Phillips, 1980). As shown in the figure, current densities increase in areas of smaller cross-section, for example, the human neck or leg, and closer to the ground, for example, the upper and lower human torso. When calculated without averaging across a cross-section, current densities are higher near a junction point; for instance, they are higher and more horizontal at the armpit than in the middle of the chest area (Tenforde and Kaune, 1987). However, if the person is insulated from the ground but touching a grounded object, as with for instance an electric substation

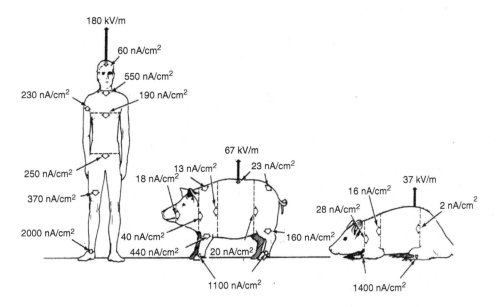

FIGURE 1.13
Estimated external electric field and current densities of a grounded man, pig, and rat exposed to a vertical 0-Hz, 6-kV/m electric field. Calculated internal current densities are averaged over sections through bodies as shown; calculated current densities perpendicular to the body surface are shown for man and pig. (From Figure 4 in Kaune, W.T. and Phillips, R.D. *Bioelectromagnetics* 1, 117–129, 1980; Copyright John Wiley & Sons, reproduced with permission.)

worker with rubber-soled shoes working on some unenergized equipment, the object will offer partial shielding from external fields, and internal fields and currents will be reduced by an amount that depends on how close the person is to the grounded object (Tarao et al., 2013).

It is important to recognize that electric fields and current densities such as those in Figure 1.13 are averages, whether across the whole cross-section of the body or a limb or across a localized region. Fields vary greatly across very small distances when one examines them at dimensions in the order of a cell or a molecule; this is called microdosimetry. Forming a good picture at this level of fields from either endogenous or external sources is an unsolved but very important problem. Chapter 5 in this volume on basic mechanisms discusses this issue further.

An external magnetic field's value is little changed as it enters a biological system, whether the human body or cells in culture, since the average biological magnetic susceptibilities are very close to those of air or vacuum (see Chapter 4 in this). However, the internal electric fields and currents induced in the body according to Faraday's Law are strongly determined by the body (or specimen) shape, electric conductivity, and orientation with respect to the field.

Table 1.4 gives some comparisons between the current induced in a human by the ELF magnetic fields generated in various situations and the external vertical 60 Hz electric field needed to produce the same current densities.

In addition to fields and currents induced in an object by a changing magnetic field, motion of an object in a magnetic field can induce an electric field and current in the object. An example would be an electrical lineman or substation worker (Bowman, 2014). Induction due to motion will occur in either a DC or an AC field, though in the AC case the fields and currents due to the time-changing nature of the field generally would be much stronger than those due to the motion.

A fairly common source of exposure to both strong DC and time-changing fields is the magnetic resonance imaging (MRI) machine, where there is the main DC field, the

TABLE 1.4

Magnetically Induced Total Body Current and Current Densities and Vertical 60-Hz Electric Field Inducing Equivalent Currents

Source	Current (μA)	Current Density (A/m²)	Electric Field (kV/m)
Sinusiodal Waveforms			
Cord-connected household appliance	200–500	0.5–12[a]	1.5–38
Man in 8 kV/m electric field	120	3[a]	8
Electric blanket (not "low field")	7–25	2–40[b]	0.5–1.7
Man in 1.6 kV/m electric field	2.2	0.5[b]	0.16
Nonsinusoidal Waveforms—Medical Devices			
Electric anesthesia device (100 Hz square wave)	10,000	71,000[c]	670
Pacemaker electrode in myocardium[d,e]	6,000	20,000	400
Pacemaker electrode implanted in abdomen[d,f]	6,000	300	400

Source: After Bridges JE and Preache M. 1981. *Proc IEEE* 69: 1092–1120. [a] Through 40 cm² ankle.

[b] 0.63 cm from wire in blanket.

[c] Next to electrode.

[d] Peak pulse current ~1 ms, repeated 0.8 s.

[e] Electrode area 0.3 cm².

[f] Electrode area 20 cm².

Environmental DC and Low Frequency Fields

sinusoidal radiofrequency (RF) resonance field, and the rapidly changing gradient field which effectively changes the position within the patient's body where the imaging resonance occurs. MRI models using 1.5 or 3 T main fields have an RF field for proton imaging of approximately 63.9 or 128 MHz, respectively, at intensities that depend on what is being imaged (Collins and Wang, 2011). MRI DC fields in various models range presently from 1 to 7 T. Gradient fields vary according to model from about 20 to 50 mT/m and change at about 40–200 mT/m/ms (Block Imaging, 2018). Present exposure guidelines limit gradient peak fields to 0.043 mT in any of the three directions, according to Fuentes et al. (2008).

Typical peak field changes on a patient's abdomen upon entering a 3 T MRI were in the range of 0.8 T/s, which induces an electric field of 0.8 V/m; rolling 90° inside the bore produced 1 T/s and 0.15 V/m (Glover and Bowtell, 2008). Medical personnel working in the vicinity of the machines with main fields up to 7 T experienced reduced DC fields that changed at an geometric average rate of 0.3 mT/ms (geometric mean; highest value 131 mT/ms), though for longer periods throughout the workday than a single patient (Bowman, 2014). Fuentes et al. (2008) have measured and calculated field intensities around an MRI machine from the main and gradient coils for 1.5, 2 and 4 T machines. Frankel et al. (2018) have measured the switched gradient field as well as the radiofrequency field in a 3 T machine. The low-frequency field can reach several milliTesla and with a time derivative of the order of some Tesla per second. The radiofrequency (RF) field has a magnitude in the microtesla range giving rise to specific absorption rate values of a few Watts per kilogram.

As discussed further in several chapters in this volume, especially Chapter 3 on endogenous fields, Chapters 5 and 6 on the basic interactions of fields and biological systems, and Chapter 8 on noise, as well as in the various discussions of models of field—biological system interaction, an externally applied field is unlikely to cause a biological effect unless the part of the biological system with which the field interacts is able to distinguish the external field from the internal electric fields and currents that are an integral part of the system. Exactly how to formulate the aspects of the endogenous field or current density that should be compared with the local field or currents in a particular situation is still an open research question; for example, over what region (how many molecules or cells) and over what range of frequencies (very narrow or broad) does the biological system average? These endogenous fields range from the normal 50–100 mV DC transmembrane potentials of most cells (negative in animals, sometimes positive in plants) to the relatively rapid pulses of nerve cell depolarization or repolarization spikes and the less rapid pulses of, for instance, muscle cells (see Figure 1.14 for examples). They also include very large and

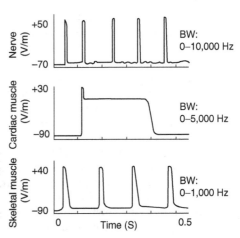

FIGURE 1.14

Typical time course and amplitudes of time-varying membrane potentials (V/m) of various cells. BW is the equivalent frequency bandwidth containing the main Fourier components of each voltage excursion. (From H. Wachtel, University of Colorado, private communication, copyright 1992; reprinted with permission.)

often highly local and hence very nonuniform fields because of local charge densities on some macromolecules or changes in the double-ion layer next to a membrane. The membrane surface and its surrounding layers of ions and molecules can be quite irregular, for instance, because of the inclusion of a protruding structure, such as a channel, at a particular location (see, e.g., diagrams in Chapter 5 in this volume).

1.4 Conclusion

EM fields, both natural and of human origin, are ubiquitous. Fields of human origin are primarily a result of technological developments that did not begin until late in the 19th century. In general, the natural fields in the environment are much smaller than those inside organisms; natural environmental fields are also usually smaller than fields of human origin at the same frequency. Inside an organism, naturally occurring charges, currents, and fields in cells, tissues, and organs are very important physiologically, and electric charges and magnetic moments are crucial factors in determining molecular structure and chemical reaction rates. Since organisms, including humans, evolved in the natural fields alone, it is not clear how their adaptation to artificial ones might affect them. The other chapters of this handbook explore this question.

Acknowledgments

The author wishes to thank his coeditor Prof. Frank Barnes and Dr. Joseph D. Bowman for helpful comments and discussions.

References

Adams, J., Bitler, S., and Riley, K. 2004. Importance of addressing National Electrical Code violations that result in unusual exposure to 60 Hz magnetic fields. *Bioelectromagnetics* 25, 102–106.

Ahlbom, A., Day, N., Feychting, M., Roman, E., Skinner, J., Dockerty, J., Linet, M., McBride, M., Michaelis, J., Olsen, J.H., Tynes, T., and Verkasalo, P.K. 2000. A pooled analysis of magnetic fields and childhood leukemia. *Br. J. Cancer* 83, 692–698.

Bernardi, A., Fraser-Smith, A.C., and Villard Jr, O.G. 1989. Measurement of BART magnetic fields with an automatic geomagnetic pulsation index generator. *IEEE Trans. Electromagn. Compat.* 31, 413–441.

Block Imaging. 2018. https://info.blockimaging.com/bid/98655/1-5t-mri-gradient-slew-rates-compared. (Accessed 1/5/2018).

Bowman J.D. 2014. Exposures to ELF-EMF in everyday environments. In Roosli, M., ed. *Epidemiology of Electromagnetic Fields*. CRC Press, Boca Raton, pp. 94–123.

Bridges, J.E. 2002. Non-perceptible body current ELF effects as defined by electric shock safety data. *Bioelectromagnetics* 23, 542–544.

Campbell, W.C. Geomagnetic pulsations. 1967. In Matsushita, S. and Campbell, W.H., eds. *Physics of Geomagnetic Phenomena*. Academic Press, New York, pp. 822–909.

Chadwick, P. and Lowes, F. 1998. Magnetic fields on British trains. *Ann. Occup. Hyg.* 42, 331–335.

Collins, C.M. and Wang, Z. 2011. Calculation of radiofrequency electromagnetic fields and their effects in MRI of human subjects. *Magn. Reson. Med.* 65, 1470–1482. doi:10.1002/mrm.22845.

Deadman, J.E., Armstrong, B.G., McBride, M.L., Gallagher, R., and Theriault, G. 1999. Exposures of children in Canada to 60 Hz magnetic and electric fields. *Scand. J. Work Environ. Health* 25, 368–375.

Deadman, J.E. and Infante-Rivard, C. 2002. Individual estimation of exposures to extremely low frequency magnetic fields in jobs commonly held by women. *Am. J. Epidemiol.* 155, 368–378. doi:10.1093/aje/155.4.368.

Deno, D.W. 1976. Transmission line fields. *IEEE Trans. Power Appl. Syst.* PAS-95, 1600–1611.

Dietrich, F.M., Feero, W.E., and Jacobs, W.L. 1993. Safety of High Speed Guided Ground Transportation Systems: Final Report to the U.S. Federal Railroad Administration. U.S. Government Printing Office, Washington, DC, DOT-FRA-ORDL-93-07, DOT-VNTSC-TRA-93-13.

Does M., Scélo G, Metayer C., Selvin S., Kavet R., and Buffler P. 2011. Exposure to electrical contact currents and the risk of childhood leukemia. *Radiat. Res.* 175, 390–396.

Dubrov, A.P. 1978. The Geomagnetic Field and Life. In *Geomagnetobiology*. Plenum Press (Springer), New York, p. 318.

Fews, A.P., Henshaw, D.L., Keitch, P.A., Close, J.J., and Wilding, R.J. 1999. Increased exposure to pollutant aerosols under high voltage powerlines. *Int. J. Radiat. Biol.* 75, 1505–1521.

Fews, A.P., Wilding, R.J., Keitch, P.A., Holden, N.K., and Henshaw, D.L. 2002. Modification of atmospheric DC fields by space charge from high-voltage power lines. *Atmos. Res.* 63, 271–289.

Floderus, B., Persson, T., and Stenlund, C. 1996 Magnetic-field exposures in the workplace: Reference distribution and exposures in occupational groups. *Int. J. Occup. Environ. Health* 2, 226–238.

Forsgren, P.G., Berglund, A., and Hansson Mild, K. 1994. Reduktion av lågfrekventa magnetiska fält i nya och befintliga anläggningar för eldistribution. Arbetsmiljöinstitutets undersökningsrapport 35 (in Swedish), 20 pp.

Frankel, J., Wilén, J., and Hansson Mild, K. 2018. Assessing exposures to MRI's complex mixture of magnetic fields for in vivo, in vitro and epidemiologic studies of health effects for staff and patients. *Front. Public Health* 6, 66. doi:10.3389/fpubh.2018.00066.

Fraser-Smith, A.C. and Coates, D.B. 1978.Large amplitude ULF electromagnetic fields from BART. *Radio Sci.* 13, 661–668.

Fuentes, M.A., Trakic, A., Wilson, S.J., and Crozier S. 2008. Analysis and measurements of magnetic field exposures for healthcare workers in selected MR environments. *IEEE Trans. Biomed. Engr.* 55, 1355–1364.

Gajšek, P., Ravazzani, P., Grellier, J., Samaras, T., Bakos, J., and Thuróczy, G. 2016. Review of studies concerning electromagnetic field (EMF) exposure assessment in Europe: Low frequency fields (50 Hz–100 kHz). *Int. J. Environ. Res. Public Health* 13, 875–883. doi:10.3390/ijerph13090875.

Glover, P.M. and Bowtell, R. 2008. Measurement of electric fields induced in a human subject due to natural movements in static magnetic fields or exposure to alternating magnetic field gradients. *Phys. Med. Biol.* 53, 361–373. doi:10.1088/0031-9155/53/2/005.

Halgamuge, M.N., Abeyrathne, C.D., and Mendis, P. 2010. Measurement and analysis of electromagnetic fields from trams, trains and hybrid cars. *Radiat. Protect. Dosimetry* 141, 255–268. doi:10.1093/rpd/ncq168.

Hamnerius, Y., Atefi, S., and Eslami, A. 2011. Distribution of ELF magnetic fields in Swedish dwellings. 30th URSI General Assembly and Scientific Symposium, URSIGASS 2011, Istanbul, 13–20 August 2011.

Hansson Mild, K., Sandstrom, M., and Johnsson, A. 1996. Measured 50 Hz electric and magnetic fields in Swedish and Norwegian residential buildings. *IEEE Trans. Instrum. Meas.* 45, 710–714.

Hingorani, N.G. 1996. High-voltage DC transmission: a power electronics workhorse. *IEEE Spectr.* 33(4), 63–72.

ICNIRP. 1998. Guidelines for limiting exposure to time-varying electric, magnetic, and electromagnetic fields (up to 300 GHz). *Health Phys.* 74(4), 494–522.

Kaune, W.T. and Phillips, R.D. 1980. Comparison of the coupling of grounded humans, swine and and rats to vertical, 60-Hz electric fields. *Bioelectromagnetics* 1, 117–129.

Kaune, W.T., Gilis, M.F., and Weigel, R.J. 1983. Analysis of air ions in biological exposure systems, including HVDC electric power transmission lines, in rooms containing generators, and near exposed humans and animals. *J. Appl. Phys.* 54, 6274–6283.

Kaune, W.T., Miller, M.C., Linet, M.S., Hatch, E.E., Kleinerman, R.A., Wacholder, S., Mohr, A.H., Tarone, R.E., and Haines, C. 2002. Magnetic fields produced by hand held hair dryers, stereo headsets, home sewing machines, and electric clocks. *Bioelectromagnetics* 23, 14–25.

Kaune, W.T., Dovan, T., Kavet, R.I., Savitz, D.A., and Neutra, R.R. 2002. Study of high- and low current-configuration homes from the 1988 Denver childhood cancer study. *Bioelectromagnetics* 23, 177–188.

Kavet, R. 2005. Contact current hypothesis: Summary of results to date. *Bioelectromagnetics* 26, S75–S85.

Kavet, R. and Zaffanella, L.E. 2002. Contact voltage measured in residences: Implications to the association between magnetic fields and childhood leukemia. *Bioelectromagnetics* 23, 464–474.

Kavet, R., Zaffanella, L.E., Pearson, R.L., and Dallapiazza, J. 2004. Association of residential magnetic fields with contact voltage. *Bioelectromagnetics* 25, 530–536.

Kelsh, M.A., Bracken, T.D., Sahl, J.D., Shum, M., and Ebi, K.L. 2003. Occupational magnetic field exposures of garment workers: Results of personal and survey measurements. *Bioelectromagnetics* 24, 316–326.

Konig, H.L., Krueger, A.P., Lang, S., and Sönning, W. 1981. *Biologic Effects of Environmental Electromagnetism.* Springer-Verlag, New York, p. 271.

Koops, F.B.J. 1999. Electric and magnetic fields in consequence of undersea power cables. In Matthes, R., Bernhardt, J., and Repacholi, M., eds. *Effects of Electromagnetic Fields on the Living Environment.* Proceedings from International Seminar, Ismaning, Germany, October. 4–5, ICNIRP 10-2000, pp. 189–210.

Lee, J.M., Pierce, K.S., Spiering, C.A., Stearns, R.D., and VanGinhoven, G. 1996. *Electrical and Biological Effects of Transmission Lines: A Review.* Bonneville Power Administration, Portland, OR, p. 295.

McCurdy, A.L., Wijnberg, L., Loomis, D., Savitz, D., and Nylander-French, L. 2001. Exposure to extremely low frequency magnetic fields among working women and homemakers. *Ann. Occup. Hyg.* 45, 643–650.

Milham, S., Hatfield, J.B., and Tell, R. 1999. Magnetic fields from steel-belted radial tires: Implications for epidemiologic studies. *Bioelectromagnetics* 20, 440–445.

Moriyama, K. and Yoshitomi, K. 2005. Apartment electrical wiring: A cause of extremely low frequency magnetic field exposure in residential areas. *Bioelectromagnetics* 26, 238–241.

NIOSH. 1994. *NIOSH Health Hazard Evaluation Report: Alumax of South Carolina, Centers for Disease Control and Prevention.* National Institute of Occupational Safety and Health, Cincinnati, OH.

Nordensson, I., Hansson Mild, K., Järventaus, H., Hirvonen, A., Sandström, M., Wilén, J., Blix, N., and Norppa, H. 2001. Chromosomal aberrations in peripheral lymphocytes of train engine drivers. *Bioelectromagnetics* 22, 306–315.

NRC. 1986. *The Earth's Electrical Environment.* The National Academies Press, Washington, DC, p. 263. doi:10.17226/898.

Portier, C.J. and Wolfe, M.S., eds. 1998. Assessment of Health Effects from Exposure to Power-Line Frequency Electric and Magnetic Fields. NIH Publication 98–3981, National Institute of Health Sciences, Research Triangle Park, NC, (accessed 19/12/2017, at www.niehs.nih.gov/health/topics/agents/emf/).

Ptitsyna, N.G., Villoresi, G., Kopytenko, Y.A., Tyasto, M.I., Kopytenko, E.A., Iucci, N., Voronov, P.M., and Zaitsev, D.B. 1999. Magnetic field environment in ULF range (0–5 Hz) in urban areas: Manmade and natural fields in St Petersburg (Russia). In Bersani, F., ed. *Electricity and Magnetism in Biology and Medicine.* Kluwer Academic-Plenum Publishers, New York, pp. 279–282.

Ptitsyna, N. and Ponzetto, A. 2012. Magnetic fields encountered in electric transport: rail systems, trolleybus and cars. *IEEE Conference on Electromagnetic Compatibility (EMC EUROPE), International Symposium on Topic(s): Fields, Waves & Electromagnetics* pp. 1–5. doi:10.1109/EMCEurope.2012.6396901.

Ptitsyna, N.G., Kopytenko, Y.A., Villoresi, G., Pfluger, D.H., Ismaguilov, V., Iucci, N., Kopytenko, E.A., Zaitzev, D.B., Voronov, P.M., and Tyasto, M.I. 2003. Waveform magnetic field survey in Russian DC and Swiss AC powered trains: A basis for biologically relevant exposure assessment. *Bioelectromagnetics* 24, 546–556.

Rogers, L.E., Beedlow, P.A., Carlile, D.W., Ganok, K.A., and Lee, J.M. 1984. Environmental Studies of a 1100-kV Prototype Transmission Line: An Annual Report for the 1984 Study Period. Prepared by Battelle Pacific Northwest Laboratories for Bonneville Power Administration, Portland, OR.

Schienle, A., Stark, R., and Vaitl, D. 1999. Electrocortical responses of headache patients to the simulation of 10 kHz sferics. *Int. J. Neurosci.* 97, 211–224.

Schienle, A., Stark, R., Kulzer, R., Klopper, R., and Vaitl, D. 1996. Atmospheric electromagnetism: Individual differences in brain electrical response to simulated sferics. *Int. J. Pschyophysiol.* 21, 177–188.

Skotte, J.H. and Hjøllund, H.I. 1997. Exposure to welders and other metal workers to ELF magnetic fields. *Bioelectromagnetics* 18, 470–477.

Söderberg, K.C., Naumburg, E., Anger, G., Cnattingius, S., Ekbom, A., and Feychting, M. 2002. Childhood leukemia and magnetic fields in infant incubators. *Epidemiology* 13(1), 45–49.

Stuchly, M.A. and Lecuyer, D.W. 1989. Exposure to electromagnetic fields in arc welding. *Health Phys.* 56, 297–302.

Tarao, H., Korpinen, L.H., Kuisti, H.A., Hayashi, N., Elovaara, J.A. and Isaka, K. 2013. Numerical evaluation of currents induced in a worker by ELF non-uniform electric fields in high voltage substations and comparison with experimental results. *Bioelectromagnetics* 34, 61–73.

Tell, R.A., Sias, G., Smith, J., Sahl, J., and Kavet, R. 2013. ELF magnetic fields in electric and gasoline-powered vehicles. *Bioelectromagnetics* 34, 156–161.

Tenforde, T.S. and Kaune, W.T. 1987. Interaction of extremely low frequency electric and magnetic fields with humans. *Health Phys.* 53, 585–606.

U.S. National Geophysical Data Center. 2017. www.ngdc.noaa.gov (accessed 19/12/2017).

Vassilev, A., Ferber, A., Wehrmann, C., Pinaud, O., Schilling, M., and Ruddle, A.R. 2015. Magnetic field exposure assessment in electric vehicles. *IEEE Trans. Electromag. Compat.* 57, 35–43.

Verrier, A., Souques, M., and Wallet, F. 2005. Characterization of exposure to extremely low frequency magnetic fields using multidimensional analysis techniques. *Bioelectromagnetics* 26, 266–274.

Vistnes, A.I. 2001. Electromagnetic fields at home. In Brune, D., Hellborg, R., Persson, B.R.R., and Paakkonen, R., eds. *Radiation at Home, Outdoors and in Workplace*. Scandinavian Science Publisher, Oslo, Norway, ISBN 82-91833-02-8, pp. 286–305.

Von Kaenel, R., Antille J.P., and Steinegger, A.F. 1994. The determination of the exposure to electromagnetic fields in aluminum electrolysis. In Mannweiler, U., ed. *Light Metals*. The Minerals, Metals & Materials Society: Warrendale, PA, pp. 253–260.

von Winterfeldt, D., and Trauger, T. 1996. Managing electromagnetic fields from residential electrode grounding systems: A predecision analysis. *Bioelectromagnetics* 17, 71–84.

Wenzl, T.B. 1997. Estimating magnetic field exposures of rail maintenance workers. *Am. Ind. Hyg. Assoc. J.* 58, 667–671.

Wertheimer, N. and Leeper, E. 1979. Electrical wiring configurations and childhood cancer. *Am. J. Epidemiol.* 109, 273–284.

WHO, 2007. *Extremely Low Frequency Fields (Environmental Health Criteria 238)*. Geneva: World Health Organization, xxiv+519 pp.

WHO. 2006. *Static Fields (Environmental Health Criteria 232)*. Geneva: World Health Organization, xvii + 351 pp.

Zhang, J., Nair, I., and Morgan, M.G. 1997. Effects function simulation of residential appliance field exposures. *Bioelectromagnetics* 18, 116–124.

2

Intermediate and Radiofrequency Sources and Exposures in Everyday Environments

Javier Vila
Instituto de Salud Global, Barcelona, Spain

CONTENTS

2.1 Introduction 55
2.2 Typical IF and RF EMF Sources and Exposures (3 kHz to 300 GHz) 57
    2.2.1 Food Heating Equipment 57
        2.2.1.1 Microwave Ovens 58
        2.2.1.2 Induction Cooking Stoves 58
    2.2.2 Industrial Heating 59
        2.2.2.1 Dielectric Heaters 59
        2.2.2.2 Induction Heaters and Welders 59
    2.2.3 Semiconductor Manufacturing Equipment 60
    2.2.4 Medical Applications 60
        2.2.4.1 Diathermy Devices 60
        2.2.4.2 Electrosurgical Applications 60
        2.2.4.3 Magnetic Resonance Imaging 61
        2.2.4.4 Hyperthermia 61
    2.2.5 Radars 61
        2.2.5.1 Military Radars 62
    2.2.6 Telecommunication Transmitters and Antennas 62
        2.2.6.1 Shortwave Transmission 63
        2.2.6.2 Navigational Transmitters and Antennas 63
        2.2.6.3 FM Radio and TV Transmission 64
        2.2.6.4 Mobile Phone Base Stations and Hand-Held Devices 64
        2.2.6.5 Military Telecommunication Transmitters and Antennas ... 66
        2.2.6.6 Miscellaneous Intermediate and RF Antennas 66
2.3 RF EMF in Everyday Environments 67
2.4 Conclusion 68
References 68

2.1 Introduction

Electromagnetic fields (EMFs) in the intermediate frequency (IF) range (3 kHz–10 MHz) share characteristics with extremely low-frequency (ELF) and radiofrequency (RF) EMF (ICNIRP, 1998a, 2009). Up to 10 MHz, the main effect of the interaction between EMF and the body is nerve electrical stimulation. Above this frequency, the main effect is tissue heating.

55

However, between 100 kHz and 10 MHz both effects occur.[1]* IF EMF have been traditionally considered within the low part of the RF range and very few studies exist until now which focused exclusively on this frequency range (SCENIHR, 2015; Sienkiewicz et al., 2010). IF EMF sources are commonly used for article surveillance (e.g., anti-theft gates) and heating (e.g., induction stoves), although some ELF and RF sources may also emit within this frequency. RF EMF are characterized by their high frequency (10 MHz–300 GHz) and energy which gives them the capacity to heat matter. Sources of RF EMF may also emit in other frequencies, including static, ELF, and/or IF (e.g., mobile phones and other transmitters can emit both RF and ELF EMF), although main emissions are produced within the RF range (Hitchcock, 2015; Hitchcock and Patterson, 1995; Mann, 2011). Microwaves are traditionally considered as the highest extreme of the RF range (300 MHz–300 GHz).

Several physical quantities are used to measure high-frequency EMF, including power density (PD or S, from Specific Power), electric field strength or E-field (in volts per meter, V/m), and magnetic field strength or H-field (in Amperes per meter, A/m). Power density is the power incident on a surface divided by its area. In the International System of units (SI), the unit is Watts per square meter (W/m²). Although E- and H-fields are vector quantities (i.e., they have magnitude and direction), they are generally treated as just magnitudes, since only these are usually measured and reported in safety evaluations. The relationship between these three quantities can be explained by analogy with Ohm's law. Thus, the PD of an EMF is directly proportional to the product of the electric and the magnetic fields (eq. 2.1) (Hitchcock and Patterson, 1995):

$$PD\ (W/m^2) = E\ (V/m) \times H\ (A/m) \qquad (2.1)$$

Other quantities used to characterize RF EMF are specific absorption (SA) and specific absorption rate (SAR). These quantities describe the RF EMF dose and dose rate, respectively, as they refer to the amount of energy absorbed by the body or any other matter. For frequencies up to 10 MHz, dose metrics commonly encountered in the EMF literature are internal electric field and induced current density, which are also related to each other by Ohm's Law (ICNIRP, 1998a). EMF dose metrics are difficult to measure, although measurements performed in phantoms and mathematical models have been developed (Chen et al., 2013; Dimbylow and Mann, 1994; Findlay, 2014) in an effort to estimate internal dose when direct measurements are not feasible.

ELF fields have long wavelengths (~5,000 km at 60 Hz). Thus, exposure to these fields occurs mostly in the near field, where electric and magnetic fields are independent and there is no radiation as such (Hitchcock and Patterson, 1995). However, physical characteristics of high-frequency EMF (i.e., IF and RF fields) differ with distance to the emitting source. In the near field (commonly defined as the space between the source and up to one wavelength), the relationships between electric and magnetic fields are complex and they can be considered independent. In the far field (i.e., the region where the distance from a radiating source exceeds the EMF wavelength), the wave characteristics are more homogeneous (plane-wave model), and the electric and magnetic components of the wave are orthogonal to each other and have a fixed ratio of intensity (Eq. 2.2):

$$E\ [V/m] = H\ [A/m] \times 377\ ohms,$$

$$(2.2)$$

where 377 ohms equals the impedance of free space.

---

* These are the main significant human health effects which are considered scientifically confirmed under current exposure guidelines (ICNIRP, 1998a; IEEE, 2006).

Environmental IF and RF Fields

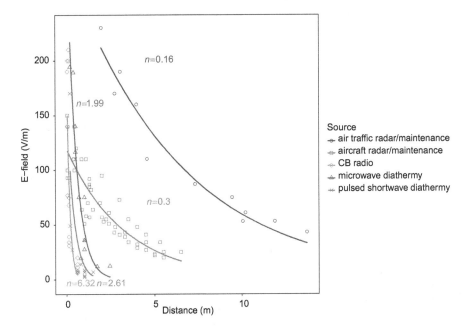

FIGURE 2.1
Electric field strength versus distance for various RF sources. Data collected within the INTEROCC study (Vila et al., 2016). Lines are data fitted by regression to functions of the inverse distance = constant $\times r^{-n}$.

In the far field, the field intensity (e.g., in V/m) decreases inversely with the distance (r) at a rate up to around $1/r^2$, depending on the type of emitting source. Different sources may emit RF EMF with different patterns of propagation. For instance, transmitters, broadcasting, and mobile phone antennas may have a mixture of patterns which vary with distance from the source (Figure 2.1).

The intensity of the electric field may also depend on the frequency of the RF source. Figure 2.2 shows how electric field intensities measured from two RF sources at the same distance may differ depending on their frequency.

In the next section, several RF and IF EMF sources will be described, including information on the levels of exposure to electric and magnetic fields associated with them. These estimates of exposure intensity were obtained by combining information from many literature resources, as part of the INTEROCC project (Vila et al., 2016). The RF and IF EMF sources included here were identified in this study as the most common EMF sources in everyday environments. They have been grouped according to their use/application (e.g., food heating, telecommunication). Thus, both RF and IF EMF sources have been included within each type of application.

2.2 Typical IF and RF EMF Sources and Exposures (3 kHz to 300 GHz)

2.2.1 Food Heating Equipment

Numerous technologies use RF and/or IF EMF to heat, cook, cure, or sterilize foodstuff. Possibly, the most common high-frequency EMF-emitting devices for food heating are microwave ovens and induction cooking stoves.

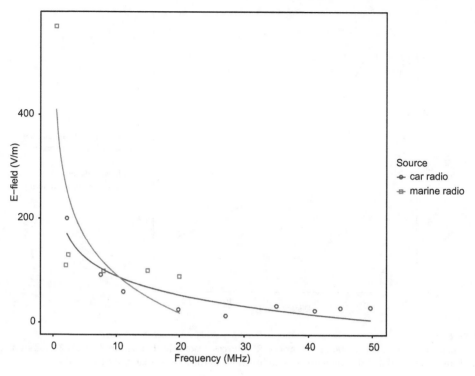

FIGURE 2.2
Electric field strength versus frequency for various RF sources. Data collected within the INTEROCC study (Vila et al., 2016). Curves are modeled regression lines that best fitted the data.

2.2.1.1 Microwave Ovens

Microwave ovens, commonly found in most Western homes nowadays, are one of the most well-known devices for food heating. Domestic ovens use frequencies of 2.45 GHz, while microwave ovens used in industrial and commercial premises often use 915 MHz (21). RF radiation is also used to sterilize food and other materials (e.g., cereals, soils, or wastewater). Average electric fields exposure levels associated with domestic ovens leakage are about 20 V/m (at an average distance of 20 cm) (Mantiply et al., 1997; Plets et al., 2016). Industrial microwave ovens may lead to similar exposures at the operator's eye level (Elder et al., 1974). RF industrial devices are also used for food disinfection. Typical frequencies used are 13.56, 27.12, and 40.68 MHz, in the lower RF range, and 915 or 2,450 MHz, within the MW range (Kim et al., 2012; Lagunas-Solar et al., 2006). To our knowledge, however, information on the operator's exposure to these devices is not available in the literature.

2.2.1.2 Induction Cooking Stoves

In the IF range, induction plates or stoves (22–34 kHz) are commonly found in industrial and commercial premises, as well as in domestic settings. These devices also emit ELF fields and exposure levels depend greatly on the distance to the operator and the number of stoves in use at the time. At distances between 10 and 30 cm from the unit, electric fields mean exposure levels are about 9 V/m, with magnetic fields around 4 A/m (Allen et al., 1994; Stuchly and Lecuyer, 1987).

Environmental IF and RF Fields

2.2.2 Industrial Heating

High-frequency EMF are also used in industrial applications to bond, weld, or seal materials such as metals, plastics, wood, or resins, using induction or dielectric heating equipment.

2.2.2.1 Dielectric Heaters

Dielectric heaters, also called RF sealers, heaters or welders, are used to heat dielectric materials, mainly plastics, fabrics, wood, and paper. These devices can weld, mold or seal plastics or cure glues and resins. The most common frequency of operation is 27 MHz, although lower frequencies such as 13.56 MHz are also common. Some devices can reach frequencies up to 70 MHz and some plastic sealers can work with frequency ranges between 6.5 and 65 MHz (Hitchcock, 2015). High exposure levels, especially to E-fields, have been identified in multiple workplace evaluations (Allen et al., 1994; Bini et al., 1986; Conover et al., 1992; Stuchly et al., 1980; Wilén et al., 2004). RF heaters are considered the most common source of excessive emissions of RF fields (ICNIRP, 1998b), with average E-field levels around 400 V/m and maximum values up to 2,000 V/m (Hitchcock and Patterson, 1995). Magnetic fields of approximately 1 A/m are also present around the sealer. Since exposure occurs in the near-field, the coupling between electric and magnetic fields is complex and levels need to be measured separately.

RF heaters can be named depending on the material being heated and their general appearance. Sealing machines, shuttle trays, turntables, and pressure-sealed applicators are the most common subtypes used for heating plastics (Stuchly et al., 1980). Glue heaters/curers are used to heat, cure and/or dry glue, which is then used for joining wood pieces. Typical frequencies used by these devices range from 4 to 50 MHz. Mean exposure levels range from 30 to 300 V/m for electric fields and 0.1 to 0.7 A/m for magnetic fields (Joyner and Bangay, 1986; Stuchly et al., 1980). Microwave heating (2.45 GHz) can be used to cure optical fiber by using UV lamps which incorporate a source of RF radiation. Near the fiber curing units, electric field mean exposure levels are about 30 V/m, with magnetic fields of approximately 0.1 A/m (Cooper, 2002).

2.2.2.2 Induction Heaters and Welders

Industrial heating equipment in the IF range include induction heaters/furnaces, induction welders, and induction soldering devices used to heat/weld metals, and high-frequency arc welding units used in the production of pipes, tubes and beams for spot welding of metal surfaces. Induction heaters use eddy currents to heat metals or semiconductors by generating a strong alternating magnetic field inside a coil. Frequencies in the RF range can reach 27 MHz although lower frequency units (50 Hz) are also commonly used, which produce stronger magnetic fields with deeper penetration. Magnetic field mean exposure levels associated with RF units are about 0.6 A/m at the operator position, where mean electric field levels are about 50 V/m. Lower frequency units can lead to higher exposure levels around the operator, with magnetic field mean exposures about 5 A/m and electric field mean levels about 300 V/m (Allen et al., 1994; Cooper, 2002; Floderus et al., 2002; Mantiply et al., 1997). High-frequency welders usually operate at 400 to 450 kHz, although operational frequencies can reach 3 MHz. Like with other types of welding equipment, operators can get overexposed in the proximity of the cables, and especially when they encircle an arm or the abdomen with the cable because of the requirements of the specific

60   *Electromagnetic Fields*

task being performed. Power densities near the worker are around 10 W/m² (Hitchcock and Patterson, 1995; Repacholi, 1981).

2.2.3 Semiconductor Manufacturing Equipment

In the chips processing industry, various types of plasma equipment are used with frequencies of 13.56 or 27.12 MHz (e.g., plasma strippers, dry plasma etchers, plasma-enhanced chemical vapor deposition (CVD) and sputtering or metal deposition equipment). Some workplace evaluations have demonstrated that RF leakage can occur even from well-maintained units. Emission levels for E-fields range between 2 and 80 V/m (Cooper, 2002; Ungers et al., 1984).

2.2.4 Medical Applications

Several types of equipment used in the diagnosis and treatment of disease lead to high-frequency EMF exposures. These devices are specifically designed to emit EMF, which are commonly used by physiotherapists to treat specific health problems. Heat is usually applied to patients to achieve muscle relaxation or other purposes. However, unlike patients, therapists and other operators can be exposed to the EMF emitted for longer hours. Therefore, only exposure to operators is considered here.

2.2.4.1 Diathermy Devices

The most common technologies used are continuous or pulsed shortwave (13.56 or 27.12 MHz) and microwave (915 MHz or 2.45 GHz) diathermy. Overexposure of the applicator may occur in the vicinity of the cables, typically unshielded, while the therapist adjusts the equipment during operation. Average electric field levels at about one meter from the source are approximately 60 V/m for pulsed shortwave devices and 300 V/m for continuous shortwave systems. Average magnetic field levels are about 0.20 and 0.70 A/m, respectively. However, maximum exposure levels can reach up to 5,000 V/m for electric fields and 10 A/m for magnetic fields (Allen et al., 1994; Mantiply et al., 1997; Martin et al., 1990; Mild, 1980; Shah and Farrow, 2013; Stuchly et al., 1982).

The antenna design in microwave systems allows directing the beam directly toward the patient, reducing the operator's exposure level. Average exposure levels from microwave devices (2.45 GHz), for distances between 25 and 120 cm from the source, can be approximately 40 V/m for electric fields and 0.3 A/m for magnetic fields (Allen et al., 1994; Martin et al., 1990; Moseley and Davison, 1981). Less common technologies, such as ultrasonic diathermy (0.1–3 MHz), can lead to electric field mean exposure levels of 1 V/m and 0.2 A/m of magnetic fields near the source (Di Nallo et al., 2008).

2.2.4.2 Electrosurgical Applications

Electrosurgical devices are used to cauterize or coagulate tissues. Common frequencies are between 0.5 and 2.4 MHz. Exposure levels may defer depending on the tasks being performed. Surgeons and repairmen typical work distances are between 0.5 and 30 cm from the source. Thus, they can be exposed to mean electric field levels around 740 V/m and mean magnetic fields about 5 A/m. Nurses' mean exposure to electric fields, however, do not commonly exceed 100 V/m in the surroundings of an active equipment (Floderus et al., 2002; Hitchcock, 2015; Liljestrand et al., 2003; Mantiply et al., 1997).

2.2.4.3 Magnetic Resonance Imaging

Magnetic resonance imaging (MRI) and nuclear magnetic resonance (NMR) spectrometers may expose operators and the general public to strong electric and magnetic fields (from static fields to RF fields up to 100 MHz). Average RF electric field levels of repair/maintenance workers can be about 50 V/m, while operators' RF exposure has been typically considered negligible. Static magnetic fields maximum exposure levels of operators near an active device can reach up to 1 T, while mean levels are around 60 mT. Exposure levels of nurses and other technicians are about half the levels associated with operators at distances above one meter from the source. ELF magnetic field mean levels of operators are around 0.6 μT, while nurses and other technicians may be exposed to half this intensity (Bracken, 1994; Smith et al., 1984). Training should be provided to ensure that workers are aware of the tasks associated with the highest levels of exposure (e.g., repair/cleaning or assisting patients near/or inside the magnet's tube, manipulating cables near the magnet) in order to promote exposure reduction.

2.2.4.4 Hyperthermia

Hyperthermia units are used for the treatment of cancer, by applying heat in excess (i.e., above 41°C) to kill cancer cells which tend to be more sensitive to heat than normal cells. Hyperthermia may be used in conjunction with other techniques, such as radio, chemo, and immune therapies, and surgery. Typical frequencies include 13.56, 27.12, 915, and 2450 MHz. Hyperthermia devices are similar to diathermy equipment, although hyperthermia small applicators allow for a more localized treatment. Mean exposure levels to electric fields of operators and other technicians are around 35 V/m between 50 and 200 cm from the source. Mean magnetic fields exposure levels at the same distance range are about 0.2 A/m (Hagmann et al., 1985; Hitchcock and Patterson, 1995; Stuchly et al., 1983).

2.2.5 Radars

Radars are used to detect and monitor moving objects (e.g., aircrafts, ships, or cars). Most radars work in the microwave range of the RF band (300 MHz–15 GHz), using pulse-modulated modes and high transmitting powers (Hitchcock, 2015). Overexposures may occur while performing maintenance tasks in the proximity of commercial radars (e.g., airport traffic control, weather and airport surveillance). Electric field exposure levels associated with these radars differ depending on the activities performed. In the surroundings of the radar, operators can be exposed to an average of 4 V/m at 250–500 m of distance, while repair/maintenance tasks can lead to mean exposure levels around 50 V/m at 1–10 m from the source. Relatively high exposures are also possible inside aircraft cockpits (Tell and Nelson, 1974; Tell et al., 1976), with electric field mean exposures around 80 V/m; near marine/naval radars (Peak, 1975), where mean exposures about 1 V/m are likely to occur at 5–10 m of distance from the source; and police speed devices (Bitran et al., 1992; Bradley, 1991; Fisher, 1993; Lotz et al., 1995). The latter may be hand-held or attached to a vehicle. Exposure of the operator can range from around 6 V/m for fixed radars to 30 V/m for hand-held devices. Security radars are used to detect vehicles and personnel and can lead to mean electric field exposures about 0.5 V/m in the surroundings of the source.

2.2.5.1 Military Radars

Little information exists in the literature about EMF exposure from military radars (mostly pulsed-modulated RF fields at 1–10 GHz with a typical radiated power of 1.5 kW and pulses up to 500 kW). Some available measurements and modeled estimates have shown that exposure levels of most exposed personnel can range from around 30 V/m for acquisition radars to about 300 V/m for illumination radars (Degrave et al., 2009; Szmigielski, 1996). Overall, soldiers in the proximity of directional radars can be exposed to around 10 V/m while the levels associated with non-directional radars can be up to ten times higher. Mean exposure levels inside radar cabins are around 20 V/m (Sobiech et al., 2017).

2.2.6 Telecommunication Transmitters and Antennas

Since the 1930s, the radio section of the International Telecommunications Union (ITU-R), a United Nations specialized agency, has managed the worldwide use of the RF spectrum. Table 2.1 describes the RFs used for telecommunication purposes, as defined by the ITU-R (ITU, 2007).

Telecommunication equipment may be fixed to buildings or built on the ground (e.g., broadcasting antennas). Fixed antennas are typically used for high frequency radio, television, mobile phone, satellite and microwave radio systems, among others. Although, to some extent, we are all exposed to the fields emitted by these antennas, only people living in the proximity of the RF sources or workers involved in repair/maintenance tasks can experiment overexposures.

Transmitters are typically mobile or portable communication devices, either handheld or attached to vehicles. They are frequently used by police, fire, and other emergency services, but also by maintenance staff, security agencies, and other industrial and commercial activities. Portable systems include walkie talkies, cordless telephones, cellular phones, and marine and airplane communication systems. Transmitters commonly attached to vehicles include citizen band (CB) radio and other types of two-way radios. Analogical cordless telephones work with frequencies around 50 MHz, while cellular/mobile phones and modern DECT phones work in the range between 380 up to 3,500 MHz, depending on the technology used. Exposure levels depend on the power of the device and its frequency. Electric field strengths between 20 and 700 V/m have been measured near transmitters attached to vehicles working at 800 MHz. Hand-held transmitters or

TABLE 2.1

ITU Frequency Bands for the Radio Spectrum

ITU Band	Label	Frequency Band	Frequency Range
Extra high frequency	EHF	RF/MW	30–300 GHz
Super high frequency	SHF	RF/MW	3–30 GHz
Ultra high frequency	UHF	RF/MW	300–3,000 MHz
Very high frequency	VHF	RF	30–300 MHz
High frequency	HF	IF-RF	3–30 MHz
Medium frequency	MF	IF	300–3,000 kHz
Low frequency	LF	IF	30–300 kHz
Very low frequency	VLF	IF	3–30 kHz
Ultra low frequency	ULF	IF	300–3,000 Hz
Extremely low frequency	ELF	ELF	30–300 Hz

Note: ELF: Extremely low frequency; IF: Intermediate frequency; MW: Microwave; RF: Radiofrequency.

Environmental IF and RF Fields

TABLE 2.2

Characteristics of Telecommunication Antennas/Transmitters

Source	Frequency Band	Frequency Range
DECT (digital)	UHF-MW	900–2,400 MHz
DECT (analogue)	HF-VHF	50 MHz
Mobile communication – GSM	UHF-MW	380–1,900 MHz
Mobile communication – UMTS	UHF-MW	700–3,500 MHz
Mobile communication – LTE	UHF-MW	450–3,700 MHz
Navigational antennas	VLF-LF	10–70 kHz
Radio broadcasting – FM	HF-VHF	87.5–108 MHz
Radio broadcasting – AM	MF-HF	500–1,700 kHz
Roof-top paging antennas	HF-VHF/UHF-MW	152–929 MHz
Shortwave transmission	HF	3–300 MHz
TV broadcasting	UHF	470–854 MHz
TV broadcasting	VHF	54–216 MHz

Note: FM: Frequency modulated; AM: Amplitude modulated; GSM: Global system for mobile communications; UMTS: Universal mobile telecommunications system; LTE: Long-term evolution; DECT: Digital enhanced cordless telecommunications.

transceivers' emissions occur near the head of the users, so recommended exposure limits can sometimes be exceeded (Hitchcock and Patterson, 1995; Lambdin and EPA, 1979; Ruggera, 1979). Table 2.2 summarizes the characteristics of the antennas and transmitters further described in this section.

2.2.6.1 Shortwave Transmission

Shortwave stations use from a few watts to several hundreds of kilowatts to transmit information worldwide, depending on the type of source (e.g., amateur radio operators, commercial broadcasts by governments and private organizations, military communications). Studies looking at the levels of exposure of the general population (Altpeter et al., 2006; Michelozzi et al., 2002) have shown that average magnetic field exposure levels of those living relatively close to the antennas (i.e., ~500 m) are around 10 mA/m (which in far-field conditions corresponds to an electric field strength of around 4 V/m). Workers performing repair/maintenance tasks near energized antennas can be exposed to about 10 V/m, although maximum values up to 100 V/m have also been recorded (Mantiply et al., 1997). The shortwave or high frequency (HF) band is one of the amplitude modulated (AM) radio bands, which also include the low frequency (LF) and the medium frequency (MF) bands, the latter being the most commonly used AM broadcasting band. Measurements for this frequency band have shown mean exposure levels on the ground near the towers between 50 and 200 V/m. Subjects working on the masts can be exposed to similar average levels, with maximum values up to 400 V/m (Allen et al., 1994; Conover, 1999; Mantiply et al., 1997).

2.2.6.2 Navigational Transmitters and Antennas

Similar high-frequency transmitters and antennas are used for navigational purposes by marine boats, such as Fast Patrol Boats (Baste et al., 2010). Frequencies between 2 and 8 MHz and powers between 10 and 250 W are typically used. Mean exposure levels on the boats can be around 10 V/m, although maximum levels over 100 V/m have been measured (Baste et al., 2010; Skotte, 1984; Tynes et al., 1996).

Ground-based communication antennas using the IF range (16–60 kHz) are sometimes used to communicate with boats or submarines at sea. Mean exposure levels near LF antennas can be around 200 V/m while levels around very low frequency (VLF) towers are even higher, with average exposures about 600 V/m (Cooper et al., 2007).

2.2.6.3 FM Radio and TV Transmission

Although broadcast transmitters have much higher radiated power (i.e., several kilowatts against a few hundred watts) compared to mobile telephone base stations, there are fewer masts with TV and/or radio antennas, these are typically located on very tall masts (i.e., over 100 m in height), and beams are directed toward the horizon leading to small exposure levels on the ground (Mann, 2010).

FM radio broadcasting commonly uses a frequency range, differing by country, within the very-high frequency (VHF) band, from 30 to 300 MHz (ITU, 2007). Antenna towers, which are not part of the transmitting system, are usually high and emissions are directed to reach longer distances. Mean exposure levels of the population are around 0.1 V/m although a small proportion of subjects can be exposed to up to 2 V/m. Workers in the surroundings of a tower can be exposed to up to 800 V/m while in the proximity to the emitting antenna, levels can reach 1,000 V/m and about 5 A/m (Allen et al., 1994; Mantiply et al., 1997; Moss and Conover, 1999).

Television transmission may use the VHF or the ultra-high frequency (UHF) bands. Measurements of the general population have shown that most people are exposed to levels around 0.1 V/m while less than 1% of subjects might be exposed to around 2 V/m. Workers at ground level can be exposed to levels around 10 V/m while those climbing the towers can reach up to 900 V/m (Cooper et al., 2007; Mantiply et al., 1997). The TV signal consists of an amplitude-modulated video signal and a frequency-modulated audio signal. The modulation is similar for both VHF and UHF signals. A common input power for the video in Europe is 30 kW while 5 kW is used for the audio, which combined with the antenna gain gives an effective radiated power of 1,000 kW. The number of towers has not increased in the last years due in part to the introduction of new technologies, such as digital radio and TV which use lower power, but larger frequency bandwidth and may lead to higher exposure levels (Mann, 2010).

UHF-TV signals usually work with transmitting powers around 30 kW, which gives an effective radiating power (i.e. input power times antenna gain) up to 5 MW. Measurement campaigns have shown that around 20% of the population is exposed above 0.1 V/m while less than 1% have exposures above 1 V/m. Near the masts on the ground, exposures range between 1 and 20 V/m, while levels over 600 V/m have been measured beside the antenna element (Mantiply et al., 1997; Tell and Mantiply, 1980).

2.2.6.4 Mobile Phone Base Stations and Hand-Held Devices

Current mobile phone telephony operates with frequencies between 800 and 2,100 MHz although specialized systems used by professionals such as police, firemen, or ambulances, use lower frequencies around 400 MHz. Mobile telephony systems involve communication between hand-sets (uplink) with nearby base stations (downlink) which cover specific areas (cells), achieving the desired coverage. In recent years, the number of technologies has increased enormously, and several networks have been put in place, which make use

Environmental IF and RF Fields 65

of different frequency bands (Table 2.1). The "Groupe Spécial Mobile" or Global system for mobile communications (GSM) networks cover over 90% of the market. This includes the original 1G analogue network, plus the digital networks 2G and 3G (UMTS). The new 4G network is not part of the GSM standard. An important feature of mobile telecommunication systems is adaptive power control, which allows avoiding unnecessarily high power that would lead to interference and reduced capacity. However, for the purpose of exposure assessment it is assumed that the radiated power equals the maximum possible, although this is seldom used (ICNIRP, 1996). Base station transmitting antennas are formed of vertical arrays of collinear dipoles phased to give a narrow beamwidth (typically between 7 and 10 degrees). The antennas are mounted on buildings or on high towers. They are a source of whole-body exposure of people in their proximity. Exposure of the general public typically occurs in the far field zone, where the electric and magnetic fields vary inversely with distance (radiating far field) and there is commonly compliance with basic limits.

Hand-sets are small portable transceivers that are typically held near the head while calls take place although new technologies have led to new behaviors as mobile phones allow more and more capabilities (e.g., email, Internet, music, games). Modern phones contain internal monopole or dipole antennas mounted on a metal box. Phone calls lead to exposure in the near field of the source since the emitted radiation has a wavelength of a few centimeters, which is the typical call distance. Other configurations may lead to different scenarios of exposure. Methods to estimate the exposure levels associated with some of these scenarios have been proposed (Kelsh et al., 2011; Roser et al., 2015) and modeling approaches using personal use data obtained through questionnaires and mobile apps (e.g., XMobiSense) are under development (Schüz et al., 2011). Exposure in the near field, during calls or other activities, leads to localized energy absorption (ICNIRP, 1996). Demonstration of compliance with basic limits, typically in terms of SAR, is obtained through calculations of absorbed energy and measurements using anatomical tissue-equivalent phantoms. Because of the complex patterns of energy absorption, both calculations and experimental studies have revealed that basic limits might be significantly exceeded when using portable units at lower distances than recommended by manufacturers. For instance, iPhone 4 recommends using and transporting the phone at a minimum distance of 10 mm from the body to comply with European and U.S. basic restrictions. However, this recommendation is frequently breached since phones are commonly held touching the head or transported inside the clothes pockets.

Output power is the main factor determining energy absorption (Hillert et al., 2006; Kelsh et al., 2011). Several exposure limits have been proposed by international organizations to avoid well-established adverse health effects due to significant temperature increase above normal body temperature. Both the International Commission on Non-Ionizing Radiation Protection (ICNIRP, 1998a) and the Institute of Electrical and Electronics Engineers (IEEE, 2006) have proposed basic limits for whole-body and localized (peak spatial) average SAR (Table 2.2). Under normal use and typical peak output powers of 1–2 W, commonly used by most devices, recommended exposure limits are not exceeded (ICNIRP, 1996). However, certain circumstances (e.g., small head-phone separation, higher output power due to low coverage) may lead to violation of these limits.

In occupational settings, dosimetric assessments in the form of SAR values are rarely performed and exposures are typically expressed in units of field strength or power density. Overexposures may occur to maintenance workers while climbing or working on energized antennas mounted on towers or buildings, or on the ground. Exposure levels vary depending on the specific source and exposure configuration. Mean electric fields of an operator can range from around 0.5 V/m, while working on the ground near the mast, to around 13 V/m, while working on the mast (Cleveland et al., 1995; Cooper et al., 2004). There is little information in the literature regarding exposure levels from the use of occupational portable hand-held transmitters/transceivers such as walkie-talkies. Some reviews show that mean electric field strength values are around 500 V/m near the antenna, although maximum levels up to 1,000 V/m are possible (Bernhardt and Matthes, 1992; Mantiply et al., 1997). Mean magnetic field strength levels are around 0.2 A/m, but maximum levels can reach up to 1 A/m (Vermeeren et al., 2015).

Commercial development is under way for the so-called 5G communications system that is intended to serve not only telephones, but a wide variety of "smart" devices (ITU, 2017). Many frequencies are being considered within the range 3–100 GHz, with first priority being given to 3.4-3.8 GHz and 24.25-27.5 GHz. The system will use more numerous base stations that transmit at lower power than current telephone systems. Larger, multiple channel antennas using narrow beam-forming technology are also being considered. Little data are currently available on potential environmental exposures from these devices.

2.2.6.5 Military Telecommunication Transmitters and Antennas

As with military radars, there is also little information in the literature about the levels associated with military telecommunication transmitters and antennas. In a review of military naval equipment (Sylvain et al., 2006), mean electric field levels near (i.e., about 1 m) HF and VLF antennas were found around 70 V/m, while almost 1,000 V/m were measured in some locations. Electric fields emitted by portable radios used by the Polish Armed Forces (Sobiech et al., 2017) showed average levels around 50 V/m near the soldier's head. For manpack radio operators, mean levels might be even higher (around 100 V/m), while mean exposure levels inside vehicles with radio transmitters were found to be around 20 V/m.

2.2.6.6 Miscellaneous Intermediate and RF Antennas

The paging communication system, consisting of fixed transmitters and pagers or beepers (i.e., portable receivers/transceivers), was highly used in the 1980s. However, the widespread use of mobile phones since the 2000s has made this type of system almost a rarity nowadays. However, ground or building-based antennas can still be found in some countries. Mean electric field levels about 50 V/m have been recorded (Cleveland et al., 1995) in the vicinity of paging antennas (around 200 m from the source).

Recent years have seen an increase in the number and types of IF EMF emitting sources. Induction heating equipment for both industrial and domestic purposes, as described above, commonly use frequencies between 400 kHz and 2.4 GHz. Other induction technologies include soldering (10–800 kHz) and welding (208–371 kHz). Mean magnetic field levels around 200 A/m are possible at 30 cm from induction soldering devices; while induction welding equipment can lead to average magnetic field exposure levels around 4 A/m (Jonker and Venhuizen). Some newer technologies include security tags and antennas, such as electronic article surveillance (EAS) and RF identification (RF ID) systems. EAS devices use frequencies between 58 kHz and 9.1 MHz and H-field exposures near them can reach around 25 A/m (Joseph et al., 2012a). RF IDs are similar to EAS systems, except that transponder tags respond with a data signal – not only disturbing the signal between the transmitting and receiving antenna panels – which allows the identification of the detected object due to the transmission of coded information. They usually work with slightly higher frequencies, around 13.56 MHz, and may lead to mean electric fields around 20 V/m and mean magnetic field levels around 2 A/m near the antennas (Senić et al., 2010).

2.3 RF EMF in Everyday Environments

Typical exposure to RF EMF of the general public is difficult to characterize due to the complex nature of RF EMF, the variety of telecommunication technologies and the large spatial and temporal variability associated with these physical agents. RF EMF measurement campaigns and/or long-term monitoring networks have been developed in several countries (Breckenkamp et al., 2012; EPA, 1978; Gotsis et al., 2008; Hankin, 1986; Rufo et al., 2011; Troisi et al., 2008). Available measurements in Europe (Gajsek et al., 2013; Joseph et al., 2010; Sagar et al., 2017) have shown that average levels of RF electric fields tend to be up to ten times below the reference levels for residential exposure recommended by international bodies (ICNIRP, 1998b) or European regulations (EC, 1999). Most measurements tend to be below 1 V/m and only around 0.1% is above 20 V/m. The strictest reference level established by this legislation for environmental (residential) exposure is 28 V/m, which corresponds with the limit set for the 10–400 MHz frequency, typically associated with FM radio and VHF TV broadcasting.

Studies on frequencies associated with mobile telecommunications (Gajsek et al., 2013; Hutter et al., 2006) have shown that mean RF exposure levels tend to be slightly higher in rural areas (0.13 V/m) compared to urban areas (0.08 V/m). This could be due to the need to transmit higher powers to reach longer distances but also to the shielding effect of buildings and other physical obstacles in cities compared to more rural open spaces. RF indoor exposure depends on the number and intensity of sources inside households and those outside. A study in Austria (Tomitsch et al., 2010) found that only 15% of the indoor exposure was due to RF sources inside the house (e.g. DECT phones, WiFi), while 85% was attributed to outside sources. In Germany, mean values around 1 V/m were found near public spaces such as schools or hospitals (Bornkessel et al., 2007). Measurements in Belgium, the Netherlands and Sweden (Joseph et al., 2012b), investigating the impact of new technologies of mobile telecommunications, have shown that the contribution to the total RF electric fields was higher for GSM (>60%), followed by UMTS (>3%) and LTE and WiMAX (<1%). Measurements in the United Kingdom near macro and microcell base stations showed higher levels associated with the latter technology, although all measurements were largely below international exposure limits. The highest intensity measured near a base station was around 9% of the corresponding ICNIRP reference level.

Population exposure to RF fields from TV and radio broadcasting tends to be low, since these transmitters are typically located away from heavily populated areas (Hitchcock, 2015). However, relatively high exposures can happen due to radio AM towers, which need high transmitting powers (up to 70 KW). The mean exposure of the general public in Switzerland due to RF fields from AM radio antennas was established around 0.6 V/m (Altpeter et al., 2006). Comparisons between RF field exposures from analogue and digital TV and radio systems have been carried out in Germany (Schubert et al., 2007). Although overall exposure levels were found to be higher for analogue systems, the planned increase of transmitting power for digital systems will likely reduce these differences in the future.

Exposure levels previously described were mostly obtained through fixed monitoring networks or spot measurements in indoor and outdoor environments, and typically refer to exposures due to specific RF EMF sources. Personal measurements, which potentially reflect exposure levels due to emissions from several sources at once, as well as changes of physical location (e.g., home, work, leisure) are, however, scarce (Sagar et al., 2017). This possibly indicates the difficulty of using personal exposimeters due to technical problems such as body shielding, calibration errors, or measurement artifacts, which tend to lead to under or over estimations of the true exposure levels (Bolte et al., 2011; Knafl et al., 2008).

2.4 Conclusion

Recent years have seen an outstanding increase in the availability and use of high-frequency EMF-emitting sources, with applications in medicine, telecommunication, and manufacturing, but also for cooking/heating of foodstuffs. Without any doubt, these RF and IF EMF sources have meant an enormous technological breakthrough, as they provide new tools that make our lives more comfortable, smarter and more productive, and give access to leisure and updated information in a continuously changing society. However, these advances not only entail benefits but also have the drawback of an important increase in the levels of exposure to high-frequency electric and magnetic fields, compared with the levels due to (unavoidable) exposures from natural sources.

Except for occupational activities, such as maintenance and repair tasks, and the use of mobile telecommunications devices (e.g., mobile phones), exposures to most of these sources occur at distances which can go from a few meters to kilometers and, therefore, are typically below the limits established by national and international regulations. However, exposure limits in place in most Western countries have been established to protect the exposed populations from short-term heating effects due to high exposure levels, since the evidence to date for low-level non-thermal chronic health effects is still considered insufficient to be used in the establishment of environmental and occupational reference levels. Therefore, following the precautionary principle, it would be advisable to reduce, to the degree possible, both the intensity and duration of exposure to these and other EMF sources, to avoid or limit potential not yet clearly identified risks.

References

Allen, S.G., Chadwick, P.J., Pearson, A.J., Whillock, M.J., Unsworth, C., Blackwell, R.P., and Driscoll, C.M.H. (1994). *Review of occupational exposure to optical radiation and electric and magnetic fields with regard to the proposed CEC physical agents directive* (Chilton, Didcot, Oxon: National Radiological Protection Board).

Altpeter, E.-S., Röösli, M., Battaglia, M., Pfluger, D., Minder, C.E., and Abelin, T. (2006). Effect of short-wave (6–22 MHz) magnetic fields on sleep quality and melatonin cycle in humans: The Schwarzenburg shut-down study. *Bioelectromagnetics 27*, 142–150.

Baste, V., Mild, K.H., and Moen, B.E. (2010). Radiofrequency exposure on fast patrol boats in the Royal Norwegian Navy—An approach to a dose assessment. *Bioelectromagnetics 31*, 350–360.

Bernhardt, J.H., and Matthes, R. (1992). *ELF and RF electromagnetic sources in proceedings 2nd international non-ionizing radiation workshop* (Vancouver, British Columbia, Canada: Institute of Radiation Hygiene Federal Office for Radiation Protection D 8042 Munich-Neuherberg).

Bini, M., Checcucci, A., Ignesti, A., Millanta, L., Olmi, R., Rubino, N., and Vanni, R. (1986). Exposure of workers to intense RF electric fields that leak from plastic sealers. *J. Microw. Power Electromagn. Energy 21*, 33–40.

Bitran, M.E., Charron, D.E., and Nishio, J.M. (1992). *Microwave emissions and operator exposure from traffic radars used in Ontario* (Ontario, Canada: Non Ionizing Radiation Section Radiation Protection Service Occupational Health & Saety Branch Ontario Ministry of Labour).

Bolte, J.F.B., van der Zande, G., and Kamer, J. (2011). Calibration and uncertainties in personal exposure measurements of radiofrequency electromagnetic fields. *Bioelectromagnetics 32*, 652–663.

Bornkessel, C., Schubert, M., Wuschek, M., and Schmidt, P. (2007). Determination of the general public exposure around GSM and UMTS base stations. *Radiat. Prot. Dosimetry 124*, 40–47.

Bracken, T.D. (1994). *Electric and magnetic fields in a magnetic resonance imaging facility: Measurements and exposure assessment procedures* (Portland, OR: Prepared for National Institute for Occupational Safety and Health Cincinnati, OH).

Bradley, R. (1991). *Traffic RADAR power densities: Summary of findings* (Institute of Police Technology and Management).

Breckenkamp, J., Blettner, M., Schüz, J., Bornkessel, C., Schmiedel, S., Schlehofer, B., and Berg-Beckhoff, G. (2012). Residential characteristics and radiofrequency electromagnetic field exposures from bedroom measurements in Germany. *Radiat. Environ. Biophys. 51*, 85–92.

Chen, X.-L., Benkler, S., Chavannes, N., De Santis, V., Bakker, J., van Rhoon, G., Mosig, J., and Kuster, N. (2013). Analysis of human brain exposure to low-frequency magnetic fields: a numerical assessment of spatially averaged electric fields and exposure limits. *Bioelectromagnetics 34*, 375–384.

Cleveland, R.F., Sylvar, D.M., Ulcek, J.L., and Mantiply, E.D. (1995). *Measurement of radiofrequency fields and potential exposure from land-mobile paging and cellular radio base station antennas* (Boston, MA (USA): Bioelectromagnetics Society).

Conover, D. (1999). *New and existing methods for assessing worker exposure to AM towers: Field survey results* (Bioelectromagnetics Society).

Conover, D.L., Moss, C.E., Murray, W.E., Edwards, R.M., Cox, C., Grajewski, B., Werren, D.M., and Smith, J.M. (1992). Foot currents and ankle SARs induced by dielectric heaters. *Bioelectromagnetics 13*, 103–110.

Cooper, T.G. (2002). *Occupational exposure to electric and magnetic fields in the context of the ICNIRP guidelines* (UK: National Radiological Protection Board. HSE).

Cooper, T., Mann, S., Blackwell, R., and Allen, S. (2007). *Occupational exposure to electromagnetic fields at radio transmitter sites* (Chilton, Didcot, UK: Health Protection Agency, Radiation Protection Division).

Cooper, T.G., Allen, S.G., Blackwell, R.P., Litchfield, I., Mann, S.M., Pope, J.M., and van Tongeren, M.J.A. (2004). Assessment of occupational exposure to radiofrequency fields and radiation. *Radiat. Prot. Dosimetry 111*, 191–203.

Degrave, E., Meeusen, B., Grivegnée, A.-R., Boniol, M., and Autier, P. (2009). Causes of death among Belgian professional military radar operators: A 37-year retrospective cohort study. *Int. J. Cancer 124*, 945–951.

Di Nallo, A.M., Strigari, L., Giliberti, C., Bedini, A., Palomba, R., and Benassi, M. (2008). Monitoring of people and workers exposure to the electric, magnetic and electromagnetic fields in an Italian National Cancer Institute. *J. Exp. Clin. Cancer Res.* 27: 16, 8 pp.

Dimbylow, P.J., and Mann, S.M. (1994). SAR calculations in an anatomically realistic model of the head for mobile communication transceivers at 900 MHz and 1.8 GHz. *Phys. Med. Biol. 39*, 1537–1553.

EC (1999). *Council recommendation on the limitation of exposure of the general public to electromagnetic fields (0 Hz to 300 GHz)* (Brussels, Belgium: Official Journal of the European Communities).

Elder, R.L., Eure, J.A., and Nicolls, J.W. (1974). Radiation leakage control of industrial microwave power devices. *J. Microw. Power 9*, 51–61.

EPA (1978). Nonionizing radiation in the New York metropolitan area (New York).

Findlay, R.P. (2014). Induced electric fields in the MAXWEL surface-based human model from exposure to external low frequency electric fields. *Radiat. Prot. Dosimetry 162*, 244–253.

Fisher, P.D. (1993). Microwave exposure levels encountered by police traffic radar operators. *IEEE Trans. Electromagn. Compat. 35*, 36–45.

Floderus, B., Stenlund, C., and Carlgren, F. (2002). Occupational exposures to high frequency electromagnetic fields in the intermediate range (>300 Hz–10 MHz). *Bioelectromagnetics 23*, 568–577.

Gajsek, P., Ravazzani, P., Wiart, J., Grellier, J., Samaras, T., and Thuróczy, G. (2013). Electromagnetic field (EMF) exposure assessment in Europe - Radio Frequency Fields (10 MHz–6 GHz). *J. Exp. Sci. Env. Epidemiol.* 25(1):37–44.

Gotsis, A., Papanikolaou, N., Komnakos, D., Yalofas, A., and Constantinou, P. (2008). Non-ionizing electromagnetic radiation monitoring in Greece. *Ann. Telecommun. 63*, 109–123.

Hagmann, M.J., Levin, R.L., and Turner, P.F. (1985). A comparison of the annular phased array to helical coil applicators for limb and torso hyperthermia. *IEEE Trans. Biomed. Eng. 32*, 916–927.

Hankin, N.N. (1986). *The radiofrequency radiation environment: Environmental exposure levels and RF radiation emitting sources* (Washinton (USA): Environmental Protection Agency (EPA)).

Hillert, L., Ahlbom, A., Neasham, D., Feychting, M., Järup, L., Navin, R., and Elliott, P. (2006). Call-related factors influencing output power from mobile phones. *J. Expo. Sci. Environ. Epidemiol. 16*, 507–514.

Hitchcock, R. (2015). Radio-frequency radiation. In *Hamilton and Hardy's industrial toxicology* (John Wiley and Sons, Inc.).

Hitchcock, R.T., and Patterson, R.M. (1995). *Radio-frequency and ELF electromagnetic energies: A handbook for health professionals* (New York: Van Nostrand Reinhold).

Hutter, H.-P., Moshammer, H., Wallner, P., and Kundi, M. (2006). Subjective symptoms, sleeping problems, and cognitive performance in subjects living near mobile phone base stations. *Occup. Environ. Med. 63*, 307–313.

ICNIRP (1996). Health issues related to the use of hand-held radiotelephones and base transmitters. International Commission on Non-Ionizing Radiation Protection. *Health Phys. 70*, 587–593.

ICNIRP (1998a). Guidelines for limiting exposure to time-varying electric, magnetic, and electromagnetic fields (up to 300 GHz). International Commission on Non-Ionizing Radiation Protection. *Health Phys. 74*, 494–522.

ICNIRP (1998b). Safety in the use of radiofrequency dielectric heaters and sealers: A practical guide.

ICNIRP (2009). Exposure to high frequency electromagnetic fields, biological effects and health consequences (100 kHz–300 GHz) - Review of the scientific evidence and health consequences.

IEEE (2006). IEEE standard for safety levels with respect to human exposure to radio frequency electromagnetic fields, 3 kHz to 300 GHz. IEEE Std C951-2005 Revis. IEEE Std C951-1991 1–238.

ITU (2007). Frequency and wavelength bands. In *Radio regulations* (Geneve: International Telecommunications Union).

ITU (2017). 5G technology and human exposure to RF EMF. Geneva: International Telecommunications Union, ITU-T Series K, Suppl. 9, 12 pp.

Jonker, H.T., and Venhuizen, R. (2005). Summary of EM field strength measurements KEMA Quality 1995–2005 in relation to public health aspects (KEMA Quality B.V.).

Joseph, W., Frei, P., Roösli, M., Thuróczy, G., Gajsek, P., Trcek, T., Bolte, J., Vermeeren, G., Mohler, E., Juhász, P., et al. (2010). Comparison of personal radio frequency electromagnetic field exposure in different urban areas across Europe. *Environ. Res. 110*, 658–663.

Joseph, W., Goeminne, F., Verloock, L., Vermeeren, G., and Martens, L. (2012a). In situ occupational and general public exposure to VHF/UHF transmission for air traffic communication. *Radiat. Prot. Dosimetry 151*, 411–419.

Joseph, W., Verloock, L., Goeminne, F., Vermeeren, G., and Martens, L. (2012b). Assessment of RF exposures from emerging wireless communication technologies in different environments. *Health Phys. 102*, 161–172.

Joyner, K.H., and Bangay, M.J. (1986). Exposure survey of operators of radiofrequency dielectric heaters in Australia. *Health Phys. 50*, 333–344.

Kelsh, M.A., Shum, M., Sheppard, A.R., McNeely, M., Kuster, N., Lau, E., Weidling, R., Fordyce, T., Kühn, S., and Sulser, C. (2011). Measured radiofrequency exposure during various mobile-phone use scenarios. *J. Expo. Sci. Environ. Epidemiol. 21*, 343–354.

Kim, S.-Y., Sagong, H.-G., Choi, S.H., Ryu, S., and Kang, D.-H. (2012). Radio-frequency heating to inactivate Salmonella Typhimurium and Escherichia coli O157:H7 on black and red pepper spice. *Int. J. Food Microbiol. 153*, 171–175.

Knafl, U., Lehmann, H., and Riederer, M. (2008). Electromagnetic field measurements using personal exposimeters. *Bioelectromagnetics 29*, 160–162.

Lagunas-Solar, M.C., Zeng, N.X., Essert, T.K., Truong, T.D., and Cecilia Piña, U. (2006). Radiofrequency power disinfects and disinfests food, soils and wastewater. *Calif. Agric. 60*, 192–199.

Lambdin, D.L., and EPA, U.S. (1979). *An investigation of energy densities in the vicinity of vehicles with mobile communications equipment and near a hand-held walkie talkie* (Las Vegas, NV (USA): Environmental Protection Agency, Office of Radiation Programs, Electromagnetic Radiation Analysis Branch).

Liljestrand, B., Sandström, M., and Hansson Mild, K. (2003). RF exposure during use of electrosurgical units. *Electromagn. Biol. Med. 22*, 127–132.

Lotz, W.G., Rinsky, R.A., and Edwards, R.D. (1995). *Occupational exposure of police officers to microwave radiation from traffic radar device* (Cincinnati, Ohio (USA): National Institute for Occupational Safety and Health).

Mann, S. (2010). Assessing personal exposures to environmental radiofrequency electromagnetic fields. *Physique 11*, 541–555.

Mann, S. (2011). *Exposure assessment for epidemiological studies* (Brussels, Belgium).

Mantiply, E.D., Pohl, K.R., Poppell, S.W., and Murphy, J.A. (1997). Summary of measured radiofrequency electric and magnetic fields (10 kHz to 30 GHz) in the general and work environment. *Bioelectromagnetics 18*, 563–577.

Martin, C.J., McCallum, H.M., and Heaton, B. (1990). An evaluation of radiofrequency exposure from therapeutic diathermy equipment in the light of current recommendations. *Clin. Phys. Physiol. Meas. 11*, 53–63.

Michelozzi, P., Capon, A., Kirchmayer, U., Forastiere, F., Biggeri, A., Barca, A., and Perucci, C.A. (2002). Adult and childhood leukemia near a high-power radio station in Rome, Italy. *Am. J. Epidemiol. 155*, 1096–1103.

Mild, K.H. (1980). Occupational exposure to radio-frequency electromagnetic fields. *Proc. IEEE 68*, 12–17.

Moseley, H., and Davison, M. (1981). Exposure of physiotherapists to microwave radiation during microwave diathermy treatment. *Clin. Phys. Physiol. Meas. 2*, 217–221.

Moss, C.E., and Conover, D.L. (1999). *John Tyrone, Seminole, Florida* (Cincinnati, Ohio (USA): NIOSH).

Peak, D.W. (1975). *Measurement of power density from marine radar* (Rockville, Md. , Washington: U.S. Dept. of Health, Education, and Welfare, Public Health Service, Food and Drug Administration, Bureau of Radiological Health).

Plets, D., Verloock, L., Van Den Bossche, M., Tanghe, E., Joseph, W., and Martens, L. (2016). Exposure assessment of microwave ovens and impact on total exposure in WLANs. *Radiat. Prot. Dosimetry 168*, 212–222.

Repacholi, M.H. (1981). Sources and applications of radiofrequency (RF) and microwave energy. In *Biological effects and dosimetry of nonionizing radiation*, M. Grandolfo, S.M. Michaelson, and A. Rindi, eds. (Springer US), pp. 19–41.

Roser, K., Schoeni, A., Bürgi, A., and Röösli, M. (2015). Development of an RF-EMF exposure surrogate for epidemiologic research. *Int. J. Environ. Res. Public. Health 12*, 5634–5656.

Rufo, M.M., Paniagua, J.M., Jiménez, A., and Antolín, A. (2011). Exposure to high-frequency electromagnetic fields (100 kHz–2 GHz) in Extremadura (Spain). *Health Phys. 101*, 739–745.

Ruggera, P.S. (1979). Measurements of electromagnetic fields in the close proximity of CB antennas (Rockville, MD (USA): Final Report Bureau of Radiological Health, Div. of Electronic Products).

Sagar, S., Dongus, S., Schoeni, A., Roser, K., Eeftens, M., Struchen, B., Foerster, M., Meier, N., Adem, S., and Röösli, M. (2017). Radiofrequency electromagnetic field exposure in everyday micro-environments in Europe: A systematic literature review. *J. Expo. Sci. Environ. Epidemiol. 28*: 147–160

SCENIHR (2015). *Opinion on: Potential health effects of exposure to electromagnetic fields (EMF)* (Luxembourg: Scientific Committee on Emerging and Newly Identified Health Risks).

Schubert, M., Bornkessel, C., Wuschek, M., and Schmidt, P. (2007). Exposure of the general public to digital broadcast transmitters compared to analogue ones. *Radiat. Prot. Dosimetry 124*, 53–57.

Schüz, J., Elliott, P., Auvinen, A., Kromhout, H., Poulsen, A.H., Johansen, C., Olsen, J.H., Hillert, L., Feychting, M., Fremling, K., et al. (2011). An international prospective cohort study of mobile phone users and health (Cosmos): Design considerations and enrolment. *Cancer Epidemiol. 35*, 37–43.

Senić, D., Poljak, D., and Šarolić, A. (2010). Electromagnetic field exposure of 13.56 MHz RFID loop antenna. In *SoftCOM 2010, 18th International Conference on Software, Telecommunications and Computer Networks*, pp. 121–125.

Shah, S.G.S., and Farrow, A. (2013). Assessment of physiotherapists' occupational exposure to radio-frequency electromagnetic fields from shortwave and microwave diathermy devices: A literature review. *J. Occup. Environ. Hyg. 10*, 312–327.

Sienkiewicz, Z., Schüz, J., and Cardis, E. (2010). Risk analysis of human exposure to electromagnetic fields (revised). Deliverable Report D2 of EHFRAN project.

Skotte, J. (1984). Exposure of radio officers to radio frequency radiation on Danish merchant ships. *Am. Ind. Hyg. Assoc. J. 45*, 791–795.

Smith, M.A., Best, J.J., Douglas, R.H., and Kean, D.M. (1984). The installation of a commercial resistive NMR imager. *Br. Inst. Radiol. 57*, 1145–1148.

Sobiech, J., Kieliszek, J., Puta, R., Bartczak, D., and Stankiewicz, W. (2017). Occupational exposure to electromagnetic fields in the Polish Armed Forces. *Int. J. Occup. Med. Environ. Health 30*, 565–577.

Stuchly, M.A., and Lecuyer, D.W. (1987). Electromagnetic fields around induction heating stoves. *J. Microw. Power 22*, 63–69.

Stuchly, M.A., Repacholi, M.H., Lecuyer, D., and Mann, R. (1980). Radiation survey of dielectric (RF) heaters in Canada. *J. Microw. Power 15*, 113–121.

Stuchly, M.A., Repacholi, M.H., Lecuyer, D.W., and Mann, R.D. (1982). Exposure to the operator and patient during short wave diathermy treatments. *Health Phys. 42*, 341–366.

Stuchly, M.A., Repacholi, M.H., and Lecuyer, D.W. (1983). Operator exposure to radiofrequency fields near a hyperthermia device. *Health Phys. 45*, 101–107.

Sylvain, D.C., Cardarelli, J.J., Lotz, W.G., Conover, D.L., and Feldman, D. (2006). *Niosh health hazard evaluation report naval computer and telecommunications station cutler, Maine* (Cincinnati, Ohio: National Institute for Occupational Safety and Health).

Szmigielski, S. (1996). Cancer morbidity in subjects occupationally exposed to high frequency (radio-frequency and microwave) electromagnetic radiation. *Sci. Total Environ. 180*, 9–17.

Tell, R.A., and Mantiply, E.D. (1980). Population exposure to VHF and UHF broadcast radiation in the united states. *Proc. IEEE 68*, 6–12.

Tell, R.A., and Nelson, J.C. (1974). RF pulse spectral measurements in the vicinity of several air traffic control radars (US Environmental Protection Agency. Office of Radiation Programs).

Tell, R.A., Hankin, N.M., and Janes, D.E. (1976). *Aircraft radar measurements in the near field* (Denver, Colorado).

Tomitsch, J., Dechant, E., and Frank, W. (2010). Survey of electromagnetic field exposure in bedrooms of residences in lower Austria. *Bioelectromagnetics 31*, 200–208.

Troisi, F., Boumis, M., and Grazioso, P. (2008). The Italian national electromagnetic field monitoring network. *Ann. Telecommun. 63*, 97–108.

Tynes, T., Hannevik, M., Andersen, A., Vistnes, A., and Haldorsen, T. (1996). Incidence of breast cancer in Norwegian female radio and telegraph operators. *Cancer Causes Control 7*, 197–204.

Ungers, L.J., Mihlan, G.J., and Jones, J.H. (1984). In-depth survey report: Control technology for micro-electronics industry at Xerox Corporation, Microelectronics Center, El Segundo, California (National Institute for Occupational Safety and Health).

Vermeeren, G., Joseph, W., and Martens, L. (2015). SAR compliance assessment of PMR 446 and FRS walkie-talkies. *Bioelectromagnetics 36*, 517–526.

Vila, J., Bowman, J.D., Richardson, L., Kincl, L., Conover, D.L., McLean, D., Mann, S., Vecchia, P., van Tongeren, M., Cardis, E., et al. (2016). A source-based measurement database for occupational exposure assessment of electromagnetic fields in the INTEROCC study: A literature review approach. *Ann. Occup. Hyg. 60*, 184–204.

Wilén, J., Hörnsten, R., Sandström, M., Bjerle, P., Wiklund, U., Stensson, O., Lyskov, E., and Mild, K.H. (2004). Electromagnetic field exposure and health among RF plastic sealer operators. *Bioelectromagnetics 25*, 5–15.

3

Endogenous Bioelectric Phenomena and Interfaces for Exogenous Effects

Richard H. W. Funk

TU-Dresden

CONTENTS

3.1 Introduction 74
    3.1.1 Overview of the Detection of Endogenous Bioelectrical Phenomena 74
    3.1.2 Cell Membrane 74
    3.1.3 Cell Membrane Potential (Resting Potential) 75
    3.1.4 Situations Were Endogenous EF Can Be Found 77
        3.1.4.1 Endogenous EF during Early Embryogenesis 77
        3.1.4.2 Differentiation of Single Organs 80
        3.1.4.3 Wound Healing 81
        3.1.4.4 Regeneration 81
        3.1.4.5 Polarization 83
        3.1.4.6 Migration 84
        3.1.4.7 Nerve Sprouting and Growth Cones 85
        3.1.4.8 Transporters and Ion Channels Involved in the
                 Bioelectric Processes 86
3.2 Electromagnetic Fields 86
    3.2.1 Endogenous EMF 86
    3.2.2 Effects from Environmental EMF 87
    3.2.3 Pulsed EMFs in Therapy 88
3.3 Coupling EF and EMF Endogenous and Environmental Fields with the
    Biological Interface 89
    3.3.1 Cyclotron Resonance? 89
    3.3.2 EMF Ligand–Receptor Interaction 89
    3.3.3 Larmor Precession 89
    3.3.4 Faraday Coupling 90
    3.3.5 Voltage-Sensitive Receptors 91
3.4 Summary 91
Acknowledgment 92
References 92

3.1 Introduction

In this chapter, results are compiled from authors, who studied "electrical" phenomena in biology from Galvani onwards. This field developed in several phases (see Section 3.1.1) and now is growing very strong in the last decade. This is because now it is possible to link this topic of bioelectricity to modern developmental biology, to molecular and cell biology and even to bioinformatics.

Due to the methods used, most of the findings of modern bioelectricity show more quasi-static to ultra-low frequency electromagnetic fields (EMFs). That is why we focus on this part of the EMF spectrum.

An interface and a counterpart exits in the natural environment for this part of the EMF spectrum, thus some related aspects are presented. Also links to pulsed EMF are given, because this form is mostly used in medicine as therapy. In the outlook, we consider possible coupling phenomena between the environment and the biological interface.

3.1.1 Overview of the Detection of Endogenous Bioelectrical Phenomena

Already in the 16th-century Galvani performed experiments using frog legs regarding "bioelectricity" ("bioelectricity" in contrast to the "vis vitalis," the vital force, discussion of Galvani with B. Franklin). In the 19th century, DuBois Reymond demonstrated electric currents circulating in his own body, e.g., in his wounded forearm. With help of more sophisticated measuring instruments of his time he measured a wounding potential of 70 mV and more (1, 2). Using sensitive voltmeters, the anatomist H.S. Burr began experimenting (1930–1950) on the "life field" by measuring differences in electrical potentials of plants, animals, and patients (3, 4). In humans, Burr found, e.g., a static electric field (EF) between the left and the right forefinger of 2–10 mV. Later on more and more electrode measurements were performed in embryos and adult animals (5–10). With aid of self-calibrating vibrating probes it was possible to measure electrical potentials even in the sub-millivolt range (11–14). For the first time tissue-folding processes going on in very early embryogenesis (like gastrulation) could be recorded electrically and could be compared with the microscopic picture of the folding processes. It could be shown that tissue folds coincide with sharp electric gradients and that the electric gradients even shortly precede the subsequent tissue movements (15–18).

The introduction of new methods like membrane potential- and ion-sensitive *in vivo* dyes as well as other constructs for imaging and molecular tracing enabled us to show that the electrical phenomena are an integral part of cell and tissue behavior (14, 19–22). In this sense, the topic of endogenous ion gradients and electric fields (EFs) is not an alternative or complementary view of cell biology but an intrinsic part of mainstream cell – and molecular biology.

In living organisms electric phenomena are generated endogenously, mostly as direct current (DC) fields or ultra-low frequency electromagnetic fields (ULF-EMF) (20). The fields arise from the segregation of charges by molecular pumps, transporters, and ion channels situated in the plasma membrane (23). Thus, they are not spikes of action potentials like in nerve cells (required field 10–20 V/cm) but smoothly changing—like ULF-EMF. Thus, we have first to look at the plasma membrane with its pumps and transporters.

3.1.2 Cell Membrane

The cell membrane surrounds the cytoplasm of the cell and separates intracellular components from the extracellular environment—like a skin. The arrangement of hydrophilic

Bioelectric Phenomena and Interfaces 75

heads and hydrophobic tails of the *lipid bilayer* can halt polar solutes (e.g., amino acids, nucleic acids, carbohydrates, proteins, and ions) from diffusing across the membrane, but generally allows for the passive diffusion of hydrophobic molecules. This enables the cell to control the movement of these substances via pores and gates (all composed mainly of proteins) for the ion transport—rendering a selective permeability.

Electrically the cell membrane acts like a Faraday cage. This is because of the relative high membrane potential (voltage across the membrane of 0.05–0.1 V); however, the membrane is only 10 nm thick which results in a potential gradient of 10^7 V/m!

This Faraday cage is sheltering the interior of the cell from stochastic EMF from the environment. Furthermore, the cell must be able to discern cell biologically relevant information from the "EMF—noise". As discussed later, at the surface of the cell membrane or in ion channels between neighboring cells (gap junctions—see below) EF rhythms can be detected via charged molecules or other mechanisms. However, the magnetic component of EMF can enter into the cell and induce EF (Faraday's law, see Section 3.2 on EMF).

3.1.3 Cell Membrane Potential (Resting Potential)

All bioelectric phenomena are first generated within the cell membrane. And, interestingly the cell membrane of a living cell is steadily generating a membrane *potential* or *resting potential* itself. This is established by ion gradients which are generated (1) by passive processes due to the semipermeable membrane barrier and thus unequal distribution of ions and (2) by active transporters (see below). This membrane potential is a key characteristic of every living cell. Each cell type—not only neural cells—generates this membrane potential! Interestingly, the height of the membrane potential is specific for each cell type and tissue (see below).

In evolution, this membrane potential was probably the first guided control system through the cell membrane coming up with the more and more oxygenated atmosphere, about 1.5 billions of years ago. Energy-fueled membrane transport systems had to control osmoregulation within the archaic surrounding through ionic separation (24). Later on, ions like Ca^{++} could then develop as first messenger and information transmission systems. This should be relevant for single membrane surrounded ancestors of Archaebacteria and Eubacteria. Here, stretch-activated and electric channels evolved, shifting the membrane potential away from being neutral, thus producing a membrane potential. Much later during development of primitive multicellular systems, ionic channels from one cell to the neighboring cell may represent the ancestor of the hormone and nervous systems (25). In vertebrates, connexins (gap junction components, see below) are first detected at the eight-cell stage (26), and gap junctions themselves contribute to conveying electrical information.

Later during evolution of the nervous system specialized cells (like nerve and muscle cells) are able to "fire" an action potential (often regarded erroneously as the only electrical event in a biological cell). This action potential was then discerned from the state in the "firing pauses," the "resting potential." In the case of the resting membrane potential, potassium (and sodium) gradients are established by specific molecular machines ("ion - pumps") like the Na^+/K^+-ATPase (sodium–potassium pump) which transports two potassium ions inside and three sodium ions outside at the cost of one ATP molecule. In other cases, for example, a membrane potential may be established by acidification of the inside of a membranous compartment or alcalinization of the outside in most cases by proton (NHE) transporters (Figure 3.1).

Normally, quiescent and differentiated cells possess a high membrane potential (–50 mV) with the highest for neurons (–75 mV), glia (–90 mV), and muscle cells. It is very intriguing that, in general, malignant cancer cells (0–10 mV) as well as proliferating cells (CHO, 3T3, etc., –12 to –25 mV) have low-cell membrane potentials. However, to depolarize

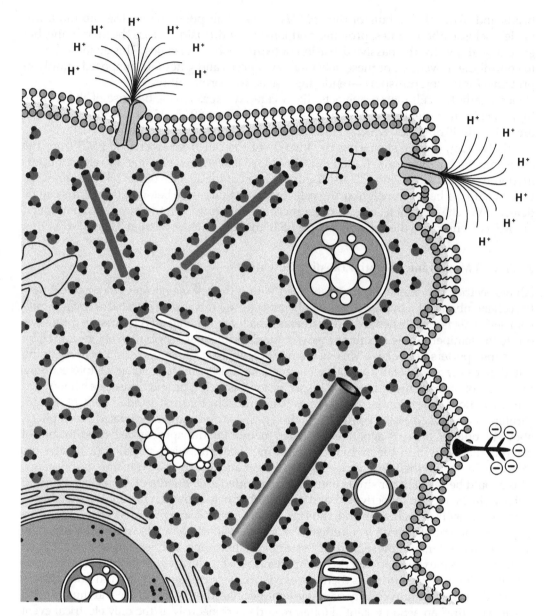

FIGURE 3.1
Part of a cell with cell organelles—e.g., nucleus at the bottom, charged particle with polarized water molecules (bound water) around the cell organelles. At the top and at the right side of the cell proton transporters (pumps like NHE) are integrated within the cell membrane. At the bottom of the right side a receptor protein with a charged moiety is symbolized. The charged, movable lever can be set in resonance by an adequate EMF frequency. Thus, it is possible that a receptor opens up and starts biochemical signaling processes within the cell.

a neuron and fire an action potential using surface electrodes requires field stimulation of 1–2 V/mm. The technique of electroporation for drug or gene delivery into cells uses extremely large pulses of Direct Current (DC) EF stimulation, roughly 100–500 V/mm. The DC EFs that play physiological roles in development and regeneration (see below) are three or four orders of magnitude less than this (1–100 mV/mm) (see (27, 28))!

Bioelectric Phenomena and Interfaces 77

The resting potential of all other non-neural and non-muscle cells, however, can be subjected to great changes (e.g., during injury and wound healing), fluctuations (during embryonic development), and oscillations (by biochemical and metabolic cycles).

In this respect, recent studies imply that the resting potential is a key regulator of the further fate of the cell, the cell cycle as well as of proliferation in tissues. Depolarization of cell membrane potential by external changes in ion concentration inhibits G1/S progression of Schwann cells, astrocytes, fibroblasts, and lymphocytes. This suggests that hyperpolarization should be important for initiating S-phase (29–31). Many proteins are involved in this membrane potential triggered cell cycle control (31). For G2/M transition, depolarization of the plasma membrane should be mandatory. In total a rhythmic change to hyperpolarization before DNA synthesis to longer depolarization during mitosis can be found as general pattern in tissue embryogenesis and regeneration (32).

Cell cycle can also determine cell fate in diseases, depending on outside conditions, and the resting membrane potential level can switch in a flip-flop manner into different states—especially if the order between the cells is perturbed during a diseased state. This may happen also between larger groups of cells; because ion transmitting gap junctions exist as well as other ways to convey information. Nowadays, computer modeling studies arise, showing how groups of cells with altered membrane potential level behave compared to normal cells (33).

3.1.4 Situations Were Endogenous EF Can Be Found

3.1.4.1 Endogenous EF during Early Embryogenesis

During early development of amphibian and chicken embryos, endogenous ionic currents can be measured. Those currents and related fields are actively generated by Na^+ uptake from the environment that leads to a potential difference between inside and outside of the single layers of closely connected cells, which appear in these early stages (transepithelial potential—TEP) (Figure 3.2). TEP in the early embryo are sources of current loops that were detected with non-invasive vibrating electrodes (see above). Here, differences in TEP between various regions form intra-embryonic voltage gradients. The arising endogenous static EF is on the order of 1–5 V/cm—well above the minimum level needed for externally applied voltage gradients to affect morphology and migration of embryonic cells *in vitro* (22, 34, 35).

Domains of distinct membrane potentials can be observed even in single cells (34), beginning in the fertilized egg and also in the electric and then calcium wave-mediated polyspermia block (36), triggering the neighboring cell to build up an EF. EF gradients are detectable already within the subsequent 2, 4, 8, etc. stages. Vandenberg and Levin (37) showed patterns of a changing membrane potential arising within the cell surfaces, reaching from one to the neighboring cell. Later on these fields spread over the early embryo at the epithelial surface and via gap junctions (Figure 3.3). EFs are in general the first information cues that determine domains like anterior/posterior or left/right in the very early embryo, e.g., in the flatworm (*planaria*) (38, 39). Even within the circumference of a plasma membrane in unicellular organisms (*protozoa*), regular and sharply confined patterns could be found that define, e.g., the position of cilia and other features (34).

So *in toto,* a patterned surface of the *morula* and in the later stages appeared. These EM patterns can be followed in smaller animals like the flatworm *planaria* also during later stages, e.g., in front-end and right-left polarization (40–43). Furthermore, organ fields become demarcated like the eye field and others. Levin (44) states: "one mode of membrane potential signaling is as a pre-pattern. Much like Hox genes, whose combinatorial patterns

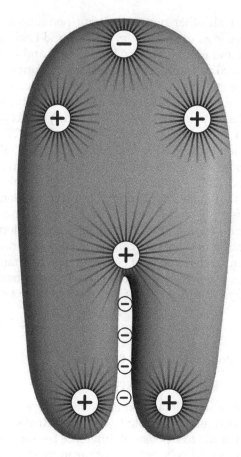

FIGURE 3.2
Local charge domains appearing temporarily within an early embryo (general example) measured at the surface.

of gene expression encode specific body regions during development, it has recently been shown that bioelectric pre-patterns in the developing face of the frog and planarian models regulate the gene expression, size, and shape of craniofacial components" (39, 45). Nogi and Levin (46) suggested that gap junctional communication might be required for long-range anterior/posterior patterning in *planaria*. Oviedo et al. (38) could indeed show in this species that gap junctions are required for signaling long-range information on anterior/posterior body axis to the blastema during regeneration. In this case, information spreads over many hundreds, if not thousands, of cells (see below for further explanation on how this might work). Still, more studies are needed to show how this occurs in larger animals including also mammals, where it is known for local areas, e.g., during craniofacial patterning in *xenopus* embryos (37). Finally, studies that show a possible cooperation between gap junctional signaling and signaling of the nervous system remain to be conducted.

Functionally and especially for time coordination, an absolutely important feature is that the EFs precede mechanical actions of epithelial folding, gastrulation, and other further organ development. It is well documented that vertebrate embryos possess steady voltage gradients, particularly in areas where major developmental events occur in relation to cell movement and cell division (37). Even internal signaling and genetic processes such as

Bioelectric Phenomena and Interfaces

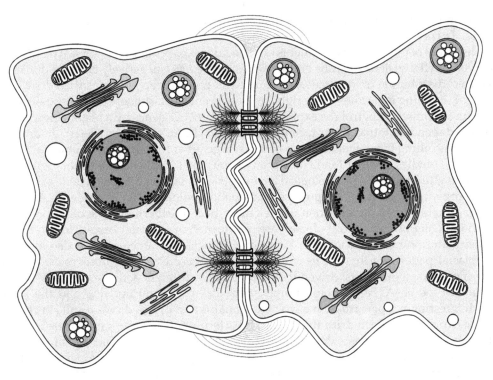

FIGURE 3.3
Two surface (epithelial) cells with their own local charge domains (gray field lines at the bottom and top) and gap junctions (depicted are two groups of connexin molecules) to serve for ion transport.

further cell differentiation and internal cell polarization is preceded by respective EF patterns (25). For example, the position of the eye field in the whole body plan is marked first by the EF. Only after this pre-patterning, typical eye differentiation markers like Pax 6 can be detected (order of appearance of "biomarkers," see below in more detail). Regarding the development of the nervous system—e.g., in axolotl embryos—outward electric currents are found at the lateral edges of the neural ridges and at the blastopore, whereas inward currents are found at the center of neural groove across the wall of neural tube and at lateral skin (27, 47). Across the neural tube a voltage gradient exists and neuroblasts differentiate in this gradient (27). If in axolotl this trans-neural tube potential is eliminated during stages 34–36, major abnormalities in development of the cranial and central nervous system occur (27). Simply by ablation of the trans-neural tube potential, the internal structure of most of these embryos reduces to a formless mass of dedifferentiated cells. Remarkably, the external form of some embryos with collapsed trans-neural tube potential continues to develop, despite the complete absence of concomitant internal histogenesis (48).

Furthermore, electric currents precede and predict the point of emergence of the limb bud by several days in the amphibian embryo pre-limb bud region (27, 49, 50).

As an example of coupling EF signals into well-known pathways in molecular biology, let us look to left-right patterning in more detail, because it directs the position of organs like heart, liver, and organs of the digestive tract asymmetrically to the left-right axis. This example shows, how the subtle field information of the EF is transferred to more fixed biochemical signaling pathways and transferred down to the genome level, finally ending in morphological patterning (51, 52). Distribution of cell membrane components begins already in the fertilized egg and ends in an asymmetric distribution of ion channels and pumps. This can lead to asymmetric ion gradients (51, 53), which subsequently drive the establishment of physiological gradients of molecules (e.g., serotonin) (54, 55). After the first embryonic cell divisions the cells on the right side are more negatively charged due to the polarized distribution of ion gradients. A network of open gap junctions then distributes left-right signaling molecules to the right and most ventral blastomere (34). These signaling molecules ultimately control the expression of asymmetric genes by a histone deacetylase (HDAC)-dependent intracellular receptor (52). Thus, HDAC activity is a left-right determinant in controlling the epigenetic state of defined genes at the early developmental stages. The HDAC binding partner Mad3 may then be the new serotonin-dependent regulator of asymmetry, linking early physiological asymmetries to stable changes in gene expression during organogenesis (52). This process sets the foundations for an asymmetric Anlage of cilia and thereby also the direction of the cilium beat. Furthermore, the other body axes (anterior–posterior and ventral–dorsal) are pre-formed in a similar cascade of events and further patterning of substructures. Electrophysiological parameters were also found for craniofacial patterning in *xenopus* embryos: Vandenberg et al. (37) observed a complex pattern of voltage gradients, driven by the regionally different activities of the V-ATPase (Vacuolar-type H^+-ATPase) proton pump at the primitive oral opening and the neural tube. Interestingly, a perturbation of voltage domains and pH gradients results in changes of gene expression, which drive this orofacial patterning, resulting in malformations.

Regarding early embryonic development and subsequent cell migratory pathways, multiple possibilities of conveying, storing, and transducing information into classical cell and molecular pathways exist: First, they exist by the magnitude of the membrane potential of the cell itself. Second, different domains with distinct resting membrane potentials can exist, as an example, they can be driven by different transporters, exchangers, etc. within dendrites and axons of nerve cells. These different domains arise even in unicellular organisms, e.g., where these membrane potential domains indicate the position of cilia (34). Third, different frequencies of membrane potential fluctuations exist (as outlined above). Fourth, different types of ions and charged biomolecules like histamine convey different streams of information recognized by different transporters, exchangers, and receptors on the cell membrane.

3.1.4.2 Differentiation of Single Organs

The activities of EMF observed in embryos may also apply to differentiation of single organs, e.g., in the vertebrate lens, basolateral membranes of anterior epithelial cells produce a DC EF by Na^+/K^+ pumps (35). Using published values for equatorial and polar lens resistivity (0.5 and 500 kΩ/cm) McCaig et al. (27) have calculated that lens currents give rise to steady DC EF of between 0.02 and 6 V/cm, a normal physiological range. Current flow draws associated water through the avascular lens, and this may flush out metabolites (56). The main current efflux is concentrated at the lens equator, where important aspects of lens physiology, such as growth of new cells, take place. During adult life, lens epithelial cells move toward the equator, probably by active migration, proliferate and trans-differentiate into lens fiber cells (57).

Cao et al. (58) detected that mature, denucleated lens fibers expressed high levels of the $\alpha 1$ and $\beta 1$ subunits of Na^+/K^+-ATPase (ATP1A1 and ATP1B1 of the sodium pump) and had a hyperpolarized membrane potential difference (V mem). In contrast, differentiating, nucleated lens fiber cells had little ATP1A1 and ATP1B1 and a depolarized membrane potential.

Mimicking the natural equatorial epithelial stream with an applied EF induced a striking reorientation of lens epithelial cells to lie perpendicular to the direction of the EF. EF also

Bioelectric Phenomena and Interfaces

promoted the expression of β-crystallin, aquaporin-0, and the Beaded Filament Structural Protein 2 in lens epithelial cells, all of which are hallmarks of differentiation (58).

3.1.4.3 Wound Healing

Again, the McCaig group (27, 47), Pullar (59–62) and others studied in cellular dimensions the electric phenomena near wounded tissues using modern molecular biological techniques (see below).

During the process of wound healing the tissues "fall back" into a kind of embryological state so it is not astonishing that also during wound healing processes such endogenous EF appear. An enhanced TEP is generated immediately upon wounding. A natural cathode arises at the breach in the epithelial layer as wound center. Also here, EF as earliest detectable signal initiates directional migration of cells into the dermal wound bed (63, 64). The wound-induced electrical signal then lasts for many hours (47, 65). It regulates different cell behaviors within 500 μm to 1 mm from the wound edge. After complete covering by the epithelium the signal fades. In corneal epithelial wound healing, the EF lines control even the orientation of the mitotic spindle in the proliferating epithelial cells as well as the orientation of the re-growing nerve sprouts (47). Similarly, in cultured hippocampal neural and glial cells the cleavage planes were oriented perpendicular to the EF field lines (66).

During the subsequent pattern of events, other factors (like growth factors, etc.) take over. Finally, EF-induced gene activation follows. Zhao et al. (67) could show that during wound healing, e.g., phosphatase and tensin (PTEN) homolog enzymes are directly involved. Inhibiting the cystic fibrosis transmembrane conductance regulator (cAMP-regulated chloride channel) significantly reduced wound currents in airway epithelial wounds (68).

And again, all these examples together show that the mentioned small DC EFs are ideally suited to bridge the information gap for short time periods and for the spatial dimensions between the short-range action of molecules, e.g., by local hormones, growth factors, etc. and the far-reaching control from the organism, e.g., via hormones distributed via blood stream and the autonomic nerves.

3.1.4.4 Regeneration

The process of regeneration is also related to wound healing; however, it also includes the natural turnover and replacement of cells within a tissue. Here, also stem cells come into play. Under both situations, we find again a reset into embryologic conditions combined with the origin of endogenous EF.

Regarding regeneration, it has been known for a long time that like in wound healing the cells of the injured tissue dedifferentiate to embryonic stages. This is especially true for the so-called blastema—the regenerating tissue in wound and bone fracture healing. It has been reported in a paper by Adams et al. (51) that H^+ pump (V-ATPases)-dependent changes in membrane voltage are an early mechanism, which is necessary and sufficient, to induce tail (spinal cord, muscle, and vasculature) regeneration in Xenopus. After amputation, the normal regeneration bud depolarizes, but after 24 h it repolarizes due to V-ATPase activity. More recently, our group (69) demonstrated that ion contents in the axolotl tail blastema change dynamically during regeneration and, in most cases, are still fluctuating at 48 h *post amputationem*. After 6 h the membrane potential was depolarized by fivefold in the bud region blastema compared with other regions and the uncut tail. The further time line was investigated by Tseng et al. (70): 6 h after amputation a V-ATPase-dependent proton extrusion occurs (Figure 3.4). Furthermore, the cells in the bud region

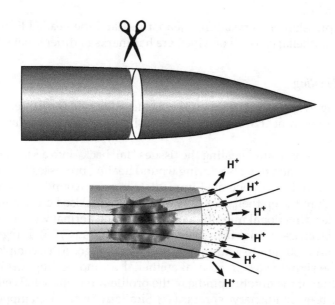

FIGURE 3.4
Tail of a Xenopus laevis larva after cutting. Cells depolarize and form a "blastemal" zone (cells, which fall back into an embryological state; cloudy area). One of the first tissue reactions is a positioning of proton pumps within the cell membrane of the regenerating edge (arrows, H$^+$ is extruding). The subsequent transepithelial potential results in an EF.

have a relatively high pH and they extruded protons (see also (51)). The proton extrusion induces an EF with the negative pole being outwardly directed, which is large enough to induce the directed growth of nerves of the spinal cord. Later on an increased Na$^+$ influx follows in the regeneration bud. After 24 hours an activation of downstream pathways (BMP, Notch, Msx, Wnt, and Fgfs) starts. After 7 days the regeneration is completed.

Experimental models like limb regeneration in salamanders and newts (15, 17, 71) encompass so many facets that it is currently quite difficult to unravel all molecular aspects of ion transporter locations. Especially the epidermal and mesenchymal cells were involved in these early events with both having elevated membrane potentials compared with, e.g., melanophores.

Artificial modulation of wound physiology by addressing the right ion transporters may therefore be a promising approach for augmenting and inducing regeneration in otherwise non-regenerative tissues. Interestingly, serotonin often transmits bioelectric signals into classical signaling pathways, e.g., in left/right patterning (see above).

In a recent paper, Sabin et al. (72) could show that after spinal cord injury in axolotl a prolonged depolarization of ependymoglial cells inhibits proliferation of these cells and subsequent axon regeneration. The authors identified c-Fos as a key voltage sensitive early response gene that is expressed specifically in these cells after injury.

However, especially with regard to stem cells, further EF studies in the context of regeneration are urgently needed. Up to now it is reported in this line that mild electrical stimulation strongly influenced embryonic stem cells to assume a neuronal fate (73). Here, the induction of calcium ion influx is significant, e.g., in embryoid bodies forming ES cells. Because Ca^{++} is one of the most important signaling ions, many downstream pathways may be involved. For example, Ca^{++} is known to be involved in the non-canonical Wnt signaling pathway. Yamada et al. (73) further point out that physical alteration of cell surface membranes may initiate signaling, even though normal signaling molecules take over

Bioelectric Phenomena and Interfaces

later. Again, we see that ionic flux constitutes a novel category of differentiation signals. Regarding Ca^{2+} fluxes, D'Ascenzo et al. (74) could demonstrate that neural stem/progenitor cells differentiation is strongly correlated with the expression of voltage-gated Ca^{2+} channels, especially the Ca(v)1, and that Ca^{2+} influx through these channels plays a key role in promoting neuronal differentiation. Finally, membrane potential, IK(DR) and I(KCa) channels change with cell cycle progression in rat bone marrow-derived mesenchymal stem cells (75). Human mesenchymal stem cells (hMSC) (76), as do many other cell types, possess characteristic Ca^{2+} waves that are involved in intracellular signaling.

These waves come in short and long periods—the longer also operate during transcellular signaling. Sun et al. (76) showed that a DC 0.1 V/cm stimulus (30 min/day for 10 days) facilitated, synergistically with osteoinductive factors, hMSC differentiation into the osteogenic cell lineage by reducing the Ca^{2+} wave frequency, which is typically found in differentiation processes. These naturally occurring fluctuations in Ca^{2+}, or other metabolic or signaling waves (rhythms of the cell), can be accessible to appropriate EMF impulses. However, the coupling devices and mechanisms channeling EMF information into these pathways are now the subjects of detailed investigation.

For regenerative therapy the fact is important, that in normal human mesenchymal stem cells (hMSCs), cell differentiation is accompanied by a progressive hyperpolarization. Artificial depolarization holds these cells in an undifferentiated (stem-like) state, while artificial hyperpolarization accelerates differentiation (77). An increasing Ca^{++} entry into the cell and a positive feedback loop between Ca^{++} entry and Ca^{++}-dependent potassium channels is discussed as the next step after the changes in resting potential (78). In further signaling cascades till gene regulation, e.g. phosphatase and tensin homolog (PTEN) is involved as well as epigenetic regulators like histone decarboxylase (HDAC). Also Feng et al. (79) report that DC EF induces directional migration of neural precursor cells. Whole cell patching revealed that the cell membrane depolarized in the EF, and buffering of extracellular calcium via EGTA prevented cell migration. Immunocytochemical staining indicated that the same electric intensity could also enhance differentiation and increases the percentage of cell differentiation into neurons, but not astrocytes and oligodendrocytes. The results indicate that DC EF is capable of promoting cell directional migration and orchestrating functional differentiation, suggestively mediated by calcium influx during DC field exposure.

Again, endogenous electric phenomena are present in all three situations where fast changes of tissue remodeling are needed: embryology, wound healing, and regeneration. Here, the pre-formative capacity EM field contains the major component of early information and coordination. A comprehensive literature survey of endogenous bioelectricity phenomena is also given by Levin et al. (80, 81).

3.1.4.5 Polarization

At cell-, organelle-, and molecular dimensions, DC-EF can induce changes in position of the Golgi apparatus (GA) and nucleus. Also, cytoskeletal proteins are affected such as the microtubule-organizing center (MTOC), actin and microtubules (MT) proper (82–85). Furthermore, plasma and mitochondrial membrane potentials change (86). Regarding directional migration, MTOC, GA, and actin were reoriented into the direction of the leading edge of the cells, while the MT accumulated in the rear edge of the cells. Also, the nucleus was located at the back of the cells. Saltukoglu et al. (87) found spontaneous and EF-controlled front-rear polarization of human keratinocytes. The EF directionality targeted the plasma membrane molecules. This finding fits well with the notion that the EF

3.1.4.6 Migration

Polarization is the first step in preparing and initiating migration for tissue and organ formation, regeneration, and wound healing. Interestingly, bioelectric factors override most chemical gradients. *In vitro* experiments revealed that many cell types prefer to migrate to the cathode when the externally applied field strengths is around 0.1–10 V/cm (electrotaxis), e.g., neural crest cells, fibroblasts, keratinocytes, chondrocytes, rat prostate cancer cells, and many epithelial cell types (47, 88–92). In contrast, only a few cell types move to the anode, among them corneal endothelial cells, bovine lens epithelium, human granulocytes, and human vascular endothelial cells (20). Both speed and direction of the movement are voltage dependent. Electrotaxis as the movement of cells along an EF gradient is further modulated by species and cell subtype differences. For example, SAOS (an osteosarcoma cell line) migrate in the opposite direction than rat calvaria osteoblasts in primary cell cultures (93).

This opens up the question of what the mechanisms are behind the directed movement of a cell in an EF gradient. First, there should be charges on the cell membrane surface which are either mobile or which are able to translate into a reorientation of the cell (electrophoretic mechanism (94)). Furthermore, if the guidance cue, e.g., a gap in an epithelial layer, is distant, a persistent movement has to be achieved. Finally, all these interactions need to be reapplied periodically until the cell has arrived at the correct site. All molecular components which are needed for persistent directional cell migration are currently analyzed in detail. The simplest signal is the unidirectional signal of a linear breach in an epithelial layer during wound healing (see above). Here, the signal of the wounding gradient must be sensed first at the cell membrane, either by charged molecules which then indirectly leads to grouping of receptors for these molecules at the site of influx of the plasma membrane circumference, or more probably by a reorientation of charged molecules at the cell membrane (electrophoretic redistribution of membrane components (95)), which is directly elicited by the field gradient itself (see (96)).

In *Dictyostelium* cells, Gao et al. (97) could also show that the initial directional sensing mechanisms for electrotaxis sit at the cell membrane. They could also prove that the EF sensors differ from those of chemotaxis. During migration differences in pH between the front and the rear end have been observed in many cell types. Here, Na^+/H^+ exchanger (NHE) are located in the cell membrane and in intracellular organelles of mammals (98). NHE1 regulates intracellular pH and volume, while NHE3 is involved in Na^+ reabsorption and proton secretion (99). In a previous study, we reported on patchy accumulations of physiologically active sodium-hydrogen exchanger (NH3). In addition, H^+ bubbles were seen outside the cell membrane particularly at the leading edge of migrating cells. Furthermore, β-actin accumulated inside the leading edge membrane (93). After NHE3 silencing, cells lost their characteristic polarity and orientation (93). In a previous paper, we found that the directional information of NHE3 is transferred via mechanisms involving PIP2 maintaining electrotaxis (93). Furthermore, we found that pNHE3 forms complexes with both protein kinase C (PKC) isoform η and γ-tubulin at filopodia, suggesting that these molecules may regulate the MTOC. Our data further suggest that PKCη-dependent phosphorylation of NHE3 and the formation of pNHE3/PKCη/γ-tubulin complexes at the leading edge of the cell (87, 93) (Figure 3.5).

Nakajima et al. (100) propose a two-molecule sensing and coupling of EF in directional migration. Weak extracellular EF redistribute positively charged polyamines, which then bind to the potassium channel Kir 4.2 to regulate K^+ fluxes. Polyamines are able to gate and

Bioelectric Phenomena and Interfaces

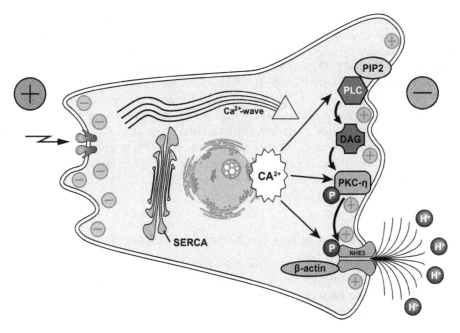

FIGURE 3.5
In the presence of a directional cue (external EF polarity see + and −) there is a depolarization of the rear end of cell movement (arrow at a voltage sensitive receptor), then it starts a Ca^{++} influx and a Ca^{++} wave to the front end. "SERCA" is the calcium store within the smooth endoplasmic reticulum. In addition, the NHE3 proton pump is activated via PKC. Note the aggregation of ß-actin at the front end and of MT (cell adhesion) at the rear end.

rectify K^+ channels by direct plugging the ion channel pore (101). Interestingly, this two-molecule sensing mechanism should be essential for cathode as well as for anode migrating cells (100). Recently, Lin et al. (102) could show that lipid rafts on the cell membrane are drawn into the direction of EF electrodes, in a kind of micro-iontophoresis (40). Notably, this sensing and directional polarization is working also in symmetric alternating currents in a frequency depending manner.

Protrusion is important for the motoric response; here adhesion and retraction represent components, which are driven directly by the actin cytoskeleton. In electrically stimulated cells, the stress fibers became oriented perpendicular to the field and a band of actin became associated with the lamellae at the cathode edge at the end of the cells. However, polarizations usually requires the cooperation of MT. MT sense points of traction between the actin cytoskeleton and the substrate and deliver signals to antagonize adhesion at these sites, in migrating cells. MTs can potentiate retraction in one region of the cell and influence protrusion in another, to induce and maintain polarization, through the spatially selective targeting of adhesion sites. The GA and the MTOC is replaced at the forward end. This is followed by a myosin contraction at the rear end and a nuclear translocation toward the displaced MTOC and GA (66, 85, 103).

3.1.4.7 Nerve Sprouting and Growth Cones

Nerve cells find normally their way with a special elongated process and a groping hand-like triangle, the growth cone. Regarding the instructive—and many other cues overriding—role of EF, Ranjnicek et al. (104) demonstrated the involvement of dynamic microfilaments and MT in EF-directed migration and orientation. The above-mentioned authors studied the dynamics of the growth cone in cultured *Xenopus* embryonic spinal neurons. With the use of specific inhibitors they could reveal an orchestrated interplay of microfilaments and MT. Dynamically, the filopodia of the growth cone turned to the cathode, suggesting an instructive role in EF-induced steering. Lamellipodial asymmetry accompanied this turning. The filopodia and lamellipodia are regulated by the GTPases Cdc42 and Rac, respectively, and peptides that selectively prevented effector binding to Cdc42 or Rac abolished cathodal growth cone turning.

As a promising application of electric migration cues, Feng et al. (79) demonstrated migration of human neural stem cell in the rat brain after implantation of stimulation electrodes. They could show that under stimulation these stem cells migrate along the EF field lines, even against the normal cell migration route.

3.1.4.8 Transporters and Ion Channels Involved in the Bioelectric Processes

Pumps, ion channels, and transporters are essential for most bioelectrical phenomena. We have reported about sensing EF via K^+ channel Kir 4.2 and we have seen pre-formative mapping and indicating sites of subsequent biomechanical events in embryogenesis and organ differentiation. In mature organs the Na^+/K^+ ATPase holds "lens fibers" (in reality they are still lens cells) in a differentiated means hyperpolarized state.

Wound EF and currents are produced by directional flow of ions present within the cytoplasm (105). The same group reported an inward flux of chloride with a smaller component of inward sodium flux (106). In human corneal epithelium special types of chloride channels are getting active (107). In wound healing of amphibian, early embryos chloride and sodium channels are active (108).

Again, the first reaction in regeneration after amputation is that of proton pump (V-ATPase), later Na^+ influx increases. Thus, the above-mentioned bioelectric processes are characterized by shifting ions and by this producing ion gradients and electric currents (80).

Please note the important role of further spreading of the EF and ion gradients via gap junctions, along the cellular and extracellular structures—described in the respective paragraphs of this chapter (Figure 3.2).

3.2 Electromagnetic Fields

3.2.1 Endogenous EMF

As we have seen in the chapter endogenous bioelectric phenomena, there exists a biological counterpart for the influence of electromagnetic waves (mostly ULF-EMF) on cell and cell systems. However, it is clear that amplitude and frequencies must hit the right "window," to get into tune with the endogenous signals.

For the endogenous EMF counterpart within the organism, one should keep in mind that many EMF rhythms are present in the body: in the nervous system, in the musculoskeletal system, and within all connective tissue. Frequencies from 5 to 30 Hz were found during muscle activity during quiet standing and of 10 Hz during walking (109). So everything in living systems is in motion and—clearly—changing magnetic fields are associated with changing EF. Furthermore, mechanical deformation of dry bone causes piezoelectricity—in

Bioelectric Phenomena and Interfaces

the living bone this should be more—or in addition—a streaming potential. This is the electric potential difference between a liquid and a capillary, diaphragm, or porous solid through which it is forced to flow (110). Bending strain also couples to the spatial gradients of permanent dipoles in collagen molecules (111, 112).

At the dimensions of single cells, enzymatic and metabolic activities of cells are mostly processed rhythmically. Thus, every substrate change and every small metabolic cycle has its own up and down in a sine wave with a typical frequency (113). For example, frequencies in the low Hz range are to be found in metabolic situations (biorhythm of cell reactions, e.g., 1–25 Hz, Ca^{++} pulses in combination with 0.5 Hz metabolic oscillations, see Funk et al. (20) and Rosenspire et al. (64, 111). However, the situation within cells and tissues is extremely complex and far from being completely understood. We have more than ten thousands of biochemical reactions happening simultaneously within a single cell (114). For example, during early embryogenesis very low frequency oscillators appear which are responsible for tissue organization (115). The next higher frequencies are caused by the action of cells by motion; it is slow in smooth muscle cells and faster in heart muscle cells (ECG). Neuronal networks fire in faster trains—up to hundreds of Hz in neurons (EEG and cerebellum neurons). Here, it seems that the (also human) organism has internalized the frequencies of the natural environment. For example, the brainstem mainly fires with 10 Hz, which is a frequency near the so-called Schumann resonance. This is a reflection of charges (especially lightning, about 200/s worldwide) between the earth's surface and the ionosphere causing EMF in the range of 7.83–250 Hz (ground frequency and additional harmonics), travelling around the globe as standing waves.

Often, these endogenous rhythms seem to be chaotic but then reveal as "ordered" (deterministic) chaos. For nature, this kind of chaotic dynamics between cells or within cells is easier to control (116). In this respect, Skarda and Freeman (117) found chaotic patterns in spatiotemporal temporal oscillations within the olfactory bulb of the rabbit, which were related to sensing of odor. Also complex dynamics can be revealed in cardiac (118), neural (119) systems. These authors used chaos-control techniques in an attempt to manipulate such complex rhythms, although all mechanisms still are enigmatic.

Regarding frequencies of cellular signals emitted by different organisms (algae, yeast, frog muscle, crab nerve, etc.) Cifra et al. (120) presented a comprehensive compilation and listed frequencies from kHz to MHz and at higher frequencies in wavelengths of mm to visible and UV light. Here, also distant interaction wavelengths of biosystems were listed in wavelengths or frequency tables (compare also with frequencies of external radiation exposures: Blackman (121) and also Leszczynski et al. (122).

Cells and tissues are also sensitive to and also emit at certain circumstances infrared and visible light. Here also a huge amount of studies exist, however, these wavelengths are not in the focus of this chapter—so we have concentrated on EMF in the lower range. As we have seen in the chapters above there exists an endogenous interface for EMF. However, as in many kinds of resonance phenomena, the right window of frequency and signal intensity must be hit.

3.2.2 Effects from Environmental EMF

As a vast amount of literature exist dealing with EMF effect on cells tissues and organ systems only some examples of EMF effects from outside sources should be given. Furthermore, there exists an ample and partly contradictory literature. Many effects can be explained on a more causal (means molecular biological level), because the models of coupling into the bio-interface seem to be relevant.

Effective EMF-stimuli have to be coherent (123), presenting a train of regularly recurring signals. The stimuli must be present for a certain minimum duration (124). "Windows" were found for certain frequencies at cell and molecular levels: for the brain (125–127) and also for non-neural cells (128, 129). In human granulocytes, Sontag and Dertinger (130) investigated the liberation of prostaglandin E2 (PGE2) during application of EMF of different frequencies: here "windows" at 6 and 16 Hz were found, where PGE was 200% above 0 Hz baseline. Beneath these "windows" (e.g. at 10 Hz) PGE was only slightly above the baseline.

3.2.3 Pulsed EMFs in Therapy

On the side of therapy, mainly Pulsed Electromagnetic Fields (PEMFs) are often used, motivated by positive therapeutic results of PEMF treatment. On the other hand, PEMF pulsation frequencies and application profiles have often been "copied" from the above mentioned naturally occurring frequencies in order to give "healing signals" to the body. However, one has to consider that pulsing in near rectangular shape produces a spectrum of multiple frequencies. Although the repetition rate normally falls in the extremely low frequency range (1–100 Hz), the frequency contents (discreet Fourier transform) ranges from 1 Hz to greater than 1 MHz (39, 40).

The cell biological effects described after such therapies reach from general enhancement of viability to an increase of neurotrophic or other growth factors, to influence of cytokines as well as cell protection. Also, activation of the vasodilatative nitrogen oxide (NO) may be of significance (131). A direct enhancement of NO produced by endothelial cells recently has been demonstrated in an *in vitro* study (132). These mechanisms combined with increased blood circulation and the signal cascade of NO might be an important part of the PEMF effect. Magnetic fields at 1 and 60 Hz destabilize rhythmic oscillations in brain hippocampal slices via yet unidentified nitric oxide mechanisms (133). Rhythmic EEG wave bursts in rat brain hippocampal tissue can also change due to exposure to weak (peak amplitudes 0.08 and 0.8 mT) 1 Hz sinusoidal magnetic fields (133). Adey (134) reports that these field effects depend on synthesis of NO in the tissue. They are consistent with reports of altered EEG patterns in man and laboratory animals by extremely low-frequency (ELF) EMF (135, 136).

PEMF can also increase osteoblast activity but significantly reduce osteoclast formation (110, 137, 138). Thus, treatment with PEMF may shift the balance toward osteogenesis. Osteogenic differentiation is enhanced in MSCs by PEMF if the cells are pre-committed (139). Also, MSCs derived from adipocytes differentiate faster and more expressed if they are cultured in a medium favoring osteogenic differentiation. What is more; Zhai et al. could show that PEMF stimulation with 15.38 Hz at 20 Gs (2 mT) for 2 h/day enhanced osteoblastic functions through amelioration of the cytoskeletal organization; increased proliferation-related gene expressions as well as upregulated gene and protein expressions of collagen type 1 of the Runt-related transcription factor 2 and of Wnt/β-catenin signaling at proliferation and differentiation phases (140).

Furthermore, a cell protective effect was found via the activation of the PI3K/Akt/Bad signaling pathway. In nerve crush experiments in rats, peripheral nerve regeneration could be ameliorated by PEMF as well as by addition of Schwann-like cells derived from human dental pulp stem cells (141). In guinea pigs, Veronesi et al. could show that PEMF (75 Hz) dampened all symptoms of knee osteoarthritis (142).

A chondroprotective effect of PEMF is observed on joint cartilage and on spontaneous osteoarthritis in animal models (143–150). At the same time, the catabolic effect of IL-1b

Bioelectric Phenomena and Interfaces

is reduced by PEMF (151, 152). Furthermore increased gene expression in members of the Transforming Growth Factor (TGF) family takes place (153). The local expression of TGF hereby also results in improved bone fracture healing (154), together with an increased proliferation, differentiation, and synthesis of cartilage matrix proteins (145, 155).

3.3 Coupling EF and EMF Endogenous and Environmental Fields with the Biological Interface

With the exception of the gap junction contacts (see above), the cell membrane represents a significant barrier to charged molecules such as peptide hormones and neurotransmitters that may carry signals from one cell type to another. Similarly, due to its high resistance, the cell membrane represents a huge barrier to electric currents that are flowing in the medium outside the cell. Mechanisms developed by living cells to sense the presence of signaling molecules are comparable to those that are required to receive an electrical signal. For example, sensitive detection, amplification, rectification, and transduction can be accomplished by enzyme systems residing in cell membrane. A kind of receptor or antenna at the outside of the membrane is needed, too (see below: microvilli).

3.3.1 Cyclotron Resonance?

Historically, the first phenomenon which was discussed, was the coherent vibration of charged molecules (mostly ions and here Ca^{2+}) with the EMF in phase. This led to the discussion of signal–noise ratio with the thermal noise as background vibration. Then, the cyclotron resonance was discussed for ions (156, 157). However, it could be shown that the force applied by an MF on a charge ("free", means outside a binding site) is too weak compared to the background thermal noise (158, 159).

3.3.2 EMF Ligand–Receptor Interaction

Pilla proposed in 1972 that EMF might affect ion adsorption/binding and possibly alter the related cascade of biological processes. This hypothesis of electrochemical information transfer postulated that the cell membrane is the site of interaction of low-level EMF ligand–receptor interaction. Via this mechanism, signal cascade events inside the cell membrane were mediated by altering the rate of binding of, e.g., calcium ions to enzymes and/or receptor sites. The ligand–receptor interactions play a pivotal role in mediating the following signal cascade events inside the cell membrane (159).

3.3.3 Larmor Precession

Also, Larmor precession is a very strong candidate for EMF coupling. Here, the precession frequency is unaffected by thermal noise while the oscillator is bound. According to Pilla (159) the threshold for the Larmor precession mode is therefore determined only by the bound lifetime of the charged oscillator. Thus, magnetic fields in the 0.1–1 mT can be detected if the oscillator (e.g., protein-bound ion) remains bound in the order of a second. The topography of the binding site can create locally a hydrophobic region from which dipolar molecules (like water) are repelled (159). Thus, in the binding site the bound ion experiences only few collisions in a surrounding which has a significant lower viscosity than the bulk water. This fact accounts for the long bound times reported for the Ca^{2+}–Calmodulin system. Thus, Larmor precession can explain such low intensities as 20 mT in 65 ms bursts of pulsed radio frequencies. Under these circumstances, 600 bursts/s were enough to increase the myosin phosphorylation reaction twofold in a cell-free system (159). In general, time dependence (phase, coherence) and charge to mass ratio are also decisive factors that can lead to linear shifts in the cell membrane, such as electrophoretic mobility in DC EF. Ion channel or receptor clustering can occur in the cell membrane: (96); this is also a special form of micro-iontophoresis (40).

3.3.4 Faraday Coupling

EMF is able to induce movement of surface charges on the cell membrane (160). Further, Coulombic forces at the surface of the cell membrane can couple EF components. These forces are able to distort the shape of the membrane and of the underlying cytoskeleton (161). If such a Coulombic force is large enough then an insertion of actin monomer between the cytoskeleton and cell membrane occurs—then, the cell shape is altered more durably after the polymerization of actin. Such manipulations distort, e.g., transmembrane proteins (ion channels, etc.) and thus lead to intracellular signaling to the cytoskeleton.

Also charged receptors or other kinds of "antennae" on the outside of the cell membrane recognize EMF by their ability to resonate with EMF frequencies because of the appropriate lengths of the moving parts that hold a charge on the free end (Figure 3.3). The resonance frequency thereby depends on the length of this lever and induced surface charge movements on the membrane trigger a signaling pathway (162, 163). This phenomenon is similar to the electrophoretic mobility of charged molecules in the cell membrane exposed to a static EF. The induced charge movement would represent at least a modification of Coulombic forces on the outside of the cell (161). Kindzelskii and Petty (96) found that application of a phase-matched EF in the presence of ion channel clusters caused myeloperoxidase (MPO) to traffic to the cell surface suggesting a link between the signaling apparatus and subsequent metabolic changes. Furthermore, EF effects could be blocked by MPO inhibition or removal while certain EF effects were mimicked by the addition of MPO to untreated cells. Therefore, channel clustering plays an important role in EF detection and downstream responses of morphologically polarized neutrophils. Via the magnetic component of EMF or PEMF also Faraday coupling is possible, as discussed by Schimmelpfeng and Dertinger (164). They found in mouse fibroblasts after treatment with a sinusoidal 2 mT 50 Hz magnetic field that cell growth was only affected by an induced EF above a threshold between 4 and 8 mVpeak/m at 2 mT.

A resonance can also take place in the movement of ions bound to, e.g., linear microfilament or other structures, which pre-determine a preferred direction. In addition there is a kind of molecular ratchet (165). The binding of calcium or other cations is very important to special sides, as ions are not only herded in vesicles or membrane compartments (e.g., in the endoplasmic reticulum), but are also bound to polyanions, such as polyamines. Polyamines have the highest charge/mass ratio of any biomolecule. They "herd and queue" (134) K^+ ions toward, e.g., transmembrane exit (166, 167). Interestingly, polyamines are synthesized from ornithine in response to ELF exposure (128).

The idea of Ca^{2+} storage at the high-affinity polyanionic binding sites of actin filaments will be presented as an alternative hypothesis of Gartzke and Lange (168). Cellular sites of F-actin-based Ca^{2+} storage are located, e.g., in the cortical (submembrane) cytoskeleton,

Bioelectric Phenomena and Interfaces

in the microvilli, and in all cell protrusions (geometric sharp anisotropy, "nonlinearity"). Cho et al. (169) showed that a 1 or 10 Hz field changed microfilament structure from an aligned form to globular patches, whereas higher frequencies (20–120 Hz) had no effect. Possibly, the actin fibers could not follow the changing field at higher frequencies (moment of inertia) thus, the reaction is as if no field would influence. However, at low frequencies the steady distortion inhibited formation of the typical cable-like structures. A drift of conduction charges (electrons, protons, ions) builds up a current, and this current produces new EFs that did not exist before the E-field was applied (170). Thermal excitation causes random motion of the conduction charges, and the force due to the applied fields superimposes a slight movement in the direction of the force on this random movement.

3.3.5 Voltage-Sensitive Receptors

Complex voltage-sensitive receptors, like the voltage-sensitive phosphatase (VSP) were found as direct EF sensors. This is again a special case of coupling by changing of conformation in channel proteins. Here, e.g., a molecular lever is moved by the charges leading to changes of topography), which leads to an ion flux and hence produces new currents and fields by this ion flux. Furthermore, voltage-sensitive phosphatases (VSP) were found to be direct EF sensors and links to relevant signaling cascades (171). VSP is a phosphoinositide phosphatase that converts PtdIns (3,4,5)P3 to PtdIns (4,5) P2, under regulation of a voltage sensor domain (172). Levin (22) reports that the lipid phosphatase PTEN was found to be a component of an intrinsic voltage sensor (171). PTEN negatively regulates the PI3K and Akt pathway by reducing the available amount of PtdIns (3,4,5) P3. Furthermore, genetic abrogation of PTEN enhanced ERK and Akt phosphorylation, and potentiated field-induced keratinocyte migration (22, 67).

The effects of static magnetic fields are not covered in this chapter. Also omitted are the still enigmatic ways of coupling the magnetic force into the various cell biological sites.

Buchachenko (173) found effects of magnetic effects on the radical pair mechanism enhancing ATP synthesis rate. In this chapter, he reflected about the problem, which is also the title "Why Magnetic and Electromagnetic Effects in Biology Are Irreproducible and Contradictory." For biological effects of hypomagnetic fields, very detailed and comprehensive overview is given by Binhi and Prato (174).

3.4 Summary

Regarding the endogenous EFs, we are at the beginning of a new understanding of the "physics of life." These novel findings, however, link very well into the classical cell- and molecular biological pathways. Here, we are able to present a consistent body of findings which adds important aspects to the already accepted understanding of biological phenomena.

In contrast to endogenous DC EF, subtle EMF phenomena produced endogenously by the organism, organs and cells are mostly *"terra incognita"* and now await investigation. This becomes more and more feasible with all this new methods like life cell imaging in highest resolution, molecular detection by high end confocal, cryo-electron microscopy, and the combination with physical methods of spectroscopy, charge distribution, mechanical and electric force measurements, etc.—all combined with cutting-edge informatics and visualization.

Like the endogenous EMF, the same is true for the problem of impact of EMF or PEMF. Here, many questions are still open, regarding linking the information and energetic impact of these exogenous EMF into the organism. Also in this topic our toolbox of new methods and the rapidly growing arsenal of new devices will help us.

Acknowledgment

The author thanks Torsten Schwalm and Kathrin Rienäcker for excellent technical assistance. Many thanks to all PhDs, PostDocs, and Professors of the institute who collaborated with me in this topic, especially N. Ozkucur, T. Monsees, C. Roehlecke, R. Blaesche, S. Bola, W. Kandhavivorn, and H.H. Epperlein.

References

1. P. Ruff: *Emil du Buis-Reymond*. Teubner-Verlag, (1997).
2. J. A. Cox: Interactive properties of calmodulin. *Biochem J*, 249(3), 621–9 (1988).
3. H. Burr: *Blueprint for immortality: Electric patterns of life discovered in scientific break-trougth*. C.W. Daniel Co. Ltd (1972).
4. H. S. Burr and F. S. C. Northrop: The electro-dynamic theory of life. *Q Rev Biol*, 10, 322–33 (1935).
5. G. Marsh and H. W. Beams: Electrical control of growth polarity in regenerating Dugesia tigrina. *Fed Proc*, 6(1 Pt 2), 163 (1947).
6. G. Marsh and H. W. Beams: Electrical control of axial polarity in a regenerating annelid. *Anat Rec*, 105, 513–14 (1949).
7. G. Marsh and H. W. Beams: Electrial control of growth axis in a regenerating annelid. *Anat Rec*, 108, 512 (1950).
8. G. Marsh and H. W. Beams: Electrical control of morphogenesis in regenerating Dugesia tigrina. I. Relation of axial polarity to field strength. *J Cell Comp Physiol*, 39(2), 191–213 (1952).
9. G. Marsh and H. W. Beams: Electrical control of morphogenesis in regenerating Dugesia tigrina. *J Cell Comp Physiol*, 39, 191–211 (1957).
10. E. J. Lund: The electrical polarity of Obelia and frog's skin, and its reversible inhibition by cyanide, ether and chloroform. *J Exp Zool*, 44, 383–96 (1926).
11. L. F. Jaffe and R. Nuccitelli: An ultrasensitive vibrating probe for measuring steady extracellular currents. *J Cell Biol*, 63(2 Pt 1), 614–28 (1974).
12. R. Nuccitelli: Ionic currents in morphogenesis. *Experientia*, 44(8), 657–66 (1988).
13. R. B. Borgens: *Electric fields in vertebrate repair: Natural and applied voltages in vertebrate regeneration and healing*. A.R. Liss (1989).
14. K. B. Hotary and K. R. Robinson: Evidence of a role for endogenous electrical fields in chick embryo development. *Development*, 114(4), 985–96 (1992).
15. R. B. Borgens: Are limb development and limb regeneration both initiated by an integumentary wounding? A hypothesis. *Differentiation*, 28(2), 87–93 (1984).
16. R. B. Borgens and R. Shi: Uncoupling histogenesis from morphogenesis in the vertebrate embryo by collapse of the transneural tube potential. *Dev Dyn*, 203(4), 456–67 (1995) doi:10.1002/aja.1002030408.
17. R. B. Borgens, J. W. Vanable, Jr. and L. F. Jaffe: Bioelectricity and regeneration: large currents leave the stumps of regenerating newt limbs. *Proc Natl Acad Sci U S A*, 74(10), 4528–32 (1977).

18. R. B. Borgens, M. E. McGinnis, J. W. Vanable, Jr. and E. S. Miles: Stump currents in regenerating salamanders and newts. *J Exp Zool*, 231(2), 249–56 (1984) doi:10.1002/jez.1402310209.

19. M. S. Cooper and R. E. Keller: Perpendicular orientation and directional migration of amphibian neural crest cells in dc electrical fields. *Proc Natl Acad Sci U S A*, 81(1), 160–4 (1984).

20. R. H. Funk, T. Monsees and N. Ozkucur: Electromagnetic effects - From cell biology to medicine. *Prog Histochem Cytochem*, 43(4), 177–264 (2009) doi:10.1016/j.proghi.2008.07.001.

21. L. F. Jaffe: Developmental currents, voltages and gradients. In: *Developmental order: Its origin and regulation*. Alan R Liss pp, New York (1982).

22. M. Levin: Large-scale biophysics: ion flows and regeneration. *Trends Cell Biol*, 17(6), 261–70 (2007) doi:10.1016/j.tcb.2007.04.007.

23. D. Simanov, I. Mellaart-Straver, I. Sormacheva and E. Berezikov: The flatworm macrostomum lignano is a powerful model organism for ion channel and stem cell research. *Stem Cells Int*, 2012, 167265 (2012) doi:10.1155/2012/167265.

24. F. Franciolini and A. Petris: Evolution of ionic channels of biological membranes. *Mol Biol Evol*, 6(5), 503–13 (1989).

25. K. G. Sullivan, M. Emmons-Bell and M. Levin: Physiological inputs regulate species-specific anatomy during embryogenesis and regeneration. *Commun Integr Biol*, 9(4), e1192733 (2016) doi :10.1080/19420889.2016.1192733.

26. F. D. Houghton: Role of gap junctions during early embryo development. *Reproduction*, 129(2), 129–35 (2005) doi:10.1530/rep.1.00277.

27. C. D. McCaig, A. M. Rajnicek, B. Song and M. Zhao: Controlling cell behavior electrically: current views and future potential. *Physiol Rev*, 85(3), 943–78 (2005) doi:10.1152/physrev.00020.2004.

28. R. Binggeli and R. C. Weinstein: Membrane potentials and sodium channels: hypotheses for growth regulation and cancer formation based on changes in sodium channels and gap junctions. *J Theor Biol*, 123(4), 377–401 (1986).

29. B. D. Freedman, M. A. Price and C. J. Deutsch: Evidence for voltage modulation of IL-2 production in mitogen-stimulated human peripheral blood lymphocytes. *J Immunol*, 149(12), 3784–94 (1992).

30. G. F. Wilson and S. Y. Chiu: Mitogenic factors regulate ion channels in Schwann cells cultured from newborn rat sciatic nerve. *J Physiol*, 470, 501–20 (1993).

31. D. J. Blackiston, K. A. McLaughlin and M. Levin: Bioelectric controls of cell proliferation: ion channels, membrane voltage and the cell cycle. *Cell Cycle*, 8(21), 3527–36 (2009) doi:10.4161/cc.8.21.9888.

32. P. Bregestovski, I. Medina and E. Goyda: Regulation of potassium conductance in the cellular membrane at early embryogenesis. *J Physiol Paris*, 86(1–3), 109–15 (1992).

33. J. Cervera, S. Meseguer and S. Mafe: The interplay between genetic and bioelectrical signaling permits a spatial regionalisation of membrane potentials in model multicellular ensembles. *Sci Rep*, 6, 35201 (2016) doi:10.1038/srep35201.

34. D. S. Adams and M. Levin: Endogenous voltage gradients as mediators of cell-cell communication: Strategies for investigating bioelectrical signals during pattern formation. *Cell Tissue Res*, 352(1), 95–122 (2013) doi:10.1007/s00441-012-1329-4.

35. E. Wang, M. Zhao, J. V. Forrester and C. D. McCaig: Bi-directional migration of lens epithelial cells in a physiological electrical field. *Exp Eye Res*, 76(1), 29–37 (2003).

36. R. D. Grey, M. J. Bastiani, D. J. Webb and E. R. Schertel: An electrical block is required to prevent polyspermy in eggs fertilized by natural mating of Xenopus laevis. *Dev Biol*, 89(2), 475–84 (1982).

37. L. N. Vandenberg, D. S. Adams and M. Levin: Normalized shape and location of perturbed craniofacial structures in the Xenopus tadpole reveal an innate ability to achieve correct morphology. *Dev Dyn*, 241(5), 863–78 (2012) doi:10.1002/dvdy.23770.

38. N. J. Oviedo, J. Morokuma, P. Walentek, I. P. Kema, M. B. Gu, J. M. Ahn, J. S. Hwang, T. Gojobori and M. Levin: Long-range neural and gap junction protein-mediated cues control polarity during planarian regeneration. *Dev Biol*, 339(1), 188–99 (2010) doi:10.1016/j.ydbio.2009.12.012.

39. W. S. Beane, J. Morokuma, J. M. Lemire and M. Levin: Bioelectric signaling regulates head and organ size during planarian regeneration. *Development*, 140(2), 313–22 (2013) doi:10.1242/dev.086900.

40. M. Poo: In situ electrophoresis of membrane components. *Annu Rev Biophys Bioeng*, 10, 245–76 (1981) doi:10.1146/annurev.bb.10.060181.001333.
41. M. Poo and K. R. Robinson: Electrophoresis of concanavalin A receptors along embryonic muscle cell membrane. *Nature*, 265(5595), 602–5 (1977).
42. A. J. Rosenspire, A. L. Kindzelskii and H. R. Petty: Pulsed DC electric fields couple to natural NAD(P)H oscillations in HT-1080 fibrosarcoma cells. *J Cell Sci*, 114(Pt 8), 1515–20 (2001).
43. A. J. Rosenspire, A. L. Kindzelskii, B. J. Simon and H. R. Petty: Real-time control of neutrophil metabolism by very weak ultra-low frequency pulsed magnetic fields. *Biophys J*, 88(5), 3334–47 (2005) doi:10.1529/biophysj.104.056663.
44. M. Levin, G. A. Buznikov and J. M. Lauder: Of minds and embryos: left-right asymmetry and the serotonergic controls of pre-neural morphogenesis. *Dev Neurosci*, 28(3), 171–85 (2006) doi:10.1159/000091915.
45. L. N. Vandenberg and M. Levin: Polarity proteins are required for left-right axis orientation and twin-twin instruction. *Genesis*, 50(3), 219–34 (2012) doi:10.1002/dvg.20825.
46. T. Nogi and M. Levin: Characterization of innexin gene expression and functional roles of gap-junctional communication in planarian regeneration. *Dev Biol*, 287(2), 314–35 (2005) doi:10.1016/j.ydbio.2005.09.002.
47. C. D. McCaig and M. Zhao: Physiological electrical fields modify cell behaviour. *Bioessays*, 19(9), 819–26 (1997) doi:10.1002/bies.950190912.
48. R. Shi and R. B. Borgens: Three-dimensional gradients of voltage during development of the nervous system as invisible coordinates for the establishment of embryonic pattern. *Dev Dyn*, 202(2), 101–14 (1995) doi:10.1002/aja.1002020202.
49. A. M. Altizer, L. J. Moriarty, S. M. Bell, C. M. Schreiner, W. J. Scott and R. B. Borgens: Endogenous electric current is associated with normal development of the vertebrate limb. *Dev Dyn*, 221(4), 391–401 (2001) doi:10.1002/dvdy.1158.
50. M. Levin: Endogenous bioelectrical networks store non-genetic patterning information during development and regeneration. *J Physiol*, 592(11), 2295–305 (2014) doi:10.1113/jphysiol.2014.271940.
51. D. S. Adams, K. R. Robinson, T. Fukumoto, S. Yuan, R. C. Albertson, P. Yelick, L. Kuo, M. McSweeney and M. Levin: Early, H^+-V-ATPase-dependent proton flux is necessary for consistent left-right patterning of non-mammalian vertebrates. *Development*, 133(9), 1657–71 (2006) doi:10.1242/dev.02341.
52. K. Carneiro, C. Donnet, T. Rejtar, B. L. Karger, G. A. Barisone, E. Diaz, S. Kortagere, J. M. Lemire and M. Levin: Histone deacetylase activity is necessary for left-right patterning during vertebrate development. *BMC Dev Biol*, 11, 29 (2011) doi:10.1186/1471-213X-11-29.
53. M. Levin, T. Thorlin, K. R. Robinson, T. Nogi and M. Mercola: Asymmetries in H^+/K^+-ATPase and cell membrane potentials comprise a very early step in left-right patterning. *Cell*, 111(1), 77–89 (2002).
54. T. Fukumoto, R. Blakely and M. Levin: Serotonin transporter function is an early step in left-right patterning in chick and frog embryos. *Dev Neurosci*, 27(6), 349–63 (2005) doi:10.1159/000088451.
55. T. Fukumoto, I. P. Kema and M. Levin: Serotonin signaling is a very early step in patterning of the left-right axis in chick and frog embryos. *Curr Biol*, 15(9), 794–803 (2005) doi:10.1016/j.cub.2005.03.044.
56. R. T. Mathias, J. L. Rae and G. J. Baldo: Physiological properties of the normal lens. *Physiol Rev*, 77(1), 21–50 (1997).
57. R. H. Funk, D. Apple and G. Naumann: Embryologie, Anatomie und Untersuchungstechnik. In: *Pathologie des Auges*. Ed. G. Naumann. Springer, Berlin (2002).
58. L. Cao, J. Liu, J. Pu, J. M. Collinson, V. J. Forrester. and C.D. McCaig..: Endogenous bioelectric currents promote differentiation of the mammalian lens. *J Cell Physiol* (2017) doi:10.1002/jcp.26074.
59. C. E. Pullar, M. Zhao, B. Song, J. Pu, B. Reid, S. Ghoghawala, C. McCaig and R. R. Isseroff: Beta-adrenergic receptor agonists delay while antagonists accelerate epithelial wound healing: evidence of an endogenous adrenergic network within the corneal epithelium. *J Cell Physiol*, 211(1), 261–72 (2007) doi:10.1002/jcp.20934.

60. C. E. Pullar and R. R. Isseroff: Cyclic AMP mediates keratinocyte directional migration in an electric field. *J Cell Sci*, 118(Pt 9), 2023–34 (2005) doi:10.1242/jcs.02330.

61. F. X. Hart, M. Laird, A. Riding and C. E. Pullar: Keratinocyte galvanotaxis in combined DC and AC electric fields supports an electromechanical transduction sensing mechanism. *Bioelectromagnetics*, 34(2), 85–94 (2013) doi:10.1002/bem.21748.

62. A. Riding and C. E. Pullar: ATP Release and P2 Y Receptor Signaling are Essential for Keratinocyte Galvanotaxis. *J Cell Physiol*, 231(1), 181–91 (2016) doi:10.1002/jcp.25070.

63. R. Nuccitelli: A role for endogenous electric fields in wound healing. *Curr Top Dev Biol*, 58, 1–26 (2003).

64. J. C. Ojingwa and R. R. Isseroff: Electrical stimulation of wound healing. *J Invest Dermatol*, 121(1), 1–12 (2003) doi:10.1046/j.1523-1747.2003.12454.x.

65. B. Song, M. Zhao, J. Forrester and C. McCaig: Nerve regeneration and wound healing are stimulated and directed by an endogenous electrical field in vivo. *J Cell Sci*, 117(Pt 20), 4681–90 (2004) doi:10.1242/jcs.01341.

66. L. Yao, C. D. McCaig and M. Zhao: Electrical signals polarize neuronal organelles, direct neuron migration, and orient cell division. *Hippocampus*, 19(9), 855–68 (2009) doi:10.1002/hipo.20569.

67. M. Zhao, B. Song, J. Pu, T. Wada, B. Reid, G. Tai, F. Wang, A. Guo, P. Walczysko, Y. Gu, T. Sasaki, A. Suzuki, J. V. Forrester, H. R. Bourne, P. N. Devreotes, C. D. McCaig and J. M. Penninger: Electrical signals control wound healing through phosphatidylinositol-3-OH kinase-gamma and PTEN. *Nature*, 442(7101), 457–60 (2006) doi:10.1038/nature04925.

68. Y. H. Sun, B. Reid, J. H. Fontaine, L. A. Miller, D. M. Hyde, A. Mogilner and M. Zhao: Airway epithelial wounds in rhesus monkey generate ionic currents that guide cell migration to promote healing. *J Appl Physiol (1985)*, 111(4), 1031–41 (2011) doi:10.1152/japplphysiol.00915.2010.

69. N. Ozkucur, H. H. Epperlein and R. H. Funk: Ion imaging during axolotl tail regeneration in vivo. *Dev Dyn*, 239(7), 2048–57 (2010) doi:10.1002/dvdy.22323.

70. A. S. Tseng, W. S. Beane, J. M. Lemire, A. Masi and M. Levin: Induction of vertebrate regeneration by a transient sodium current. *J Neurosci*, 30(39), 13192–200 (2010) doi:10.1523/JNEUROSCI.3315-10.2010.

71. A. M. Altizer, S. G. Stewart, B. K. Albertson and R. B. Borgens: Skin flaps inhibit both the current of injury at the amputation surface and regeneration of that limb in newts. *J Exp Zool*, 293(5), 467–77 (2002) doi:10.1002/jez.10141.

72. K. Sabin, T. Santos-Ferreira, J. Essig, S. Rudasill and K. Echeverri: Dynamic membrane depolarization is an early regulator of ependymoglial cell response to spinal cord injury in axolotl. *Dev Biol*, 408(1), 14–25 (2015) doi:10.1016/j.ydbio.2015.10.012.

73. M. Yamada, K. Tanemura, S. Okada, A. Iwanami, M. Nakamura, H. Mizuno, M. Ozawa, R. Ohyama-Goto, N. Kitamura, M. Kawano, K. Tan-Takeuchi, C. Ohtsuka, A. Miyawaki, A. Takashima, M. Ogawa, Y. Toyama, H. Okano and T. Kondo: Electrical stimulation modulates fate determination of differentiating embryonic stem cells. *Stem Cells*, 25(3), 562–70 (2007) doi:10.1634/stemcells.2006-0011.

74. M. D'Ascenzo, R. Piacentini, P. Casalbore, M. Budoni, R. Pallini, G. B. Azzena and C. Grassi: Role of L-type Ca^{2+} channels in neural stem/progenitor cell differentiation. *Eur J Neurosci*, 23(4), 935–44 (2006) doi:10.1111/j.1460-9568.2006.04628.x.

75. X. L. Deng, C. P. Lau, K. Lai, K. F. Cheung, G. K. Lau and G. R. Li: Cell cycle-dependent expression of potassium channels and cell proliferation in rat mesenchymal stem cells from bone marrow. *Cell Prolif*, 40(5), 656–70 (2007) doi:10.1111/j.1365-2184.2007.00458.x.

76. S. Sun, Y. Liu, S. Lipsky and M. Cho: Physical manipulation of calcium oscillations facilitates osteodifferentiation of human mesenchymal stem cells. *FASEB J*, 21(7), 1472–80 (2007) doi:10.1096/fj.06-7153com.

77. S. Sundelacruz, M. Levin and D. L. Kaplan: Membrane potential controls adipogenic and osteogenic differentiation of mesenchymal stem cells. *PLoS One*, 3(11), e3737 (2008) doi:10.1371/journal.pone.0003737.

78. A. E. West, W. G. Chen, M. B. Dalva, R. E. Dolmetsch, J. M. Kornhauser, A. J. Shaywitz, M. A. Takasu, X. Tao and M. E. Greenberg: Calcium regulation of neuronal gene expression. *Proc Natl Acad Sci U S A*, 98(20), 11024–31 (2001) doi:10.1073/pnas.191352298.

79. J. F. Feng, J. Liu, L. Zhang, J. Y. Jiang, M. Russell, B. G. Lyeth, J. A. Nolta and M. Zhao: Electrical Guidance of Human Stem Cells in the Rat Brain. *Stem Cell Reports*, 9(1), 177–189 (2017) doi:10.1016/j.stemcr.2017.05.035.

80. M. Levin: Molecular bioelectricity: how endogenous voltage potentials control cell behavior and instruct pattern regulation in vivo. *Mol Biol Cell*, 25(24), 3835–50 (2014) doi:10.1091/mbc.E13-12-0708.

81. M. Levin, G. Pezzulo and J. M. Finkelstein: Endogenous bioelectric signaling networks: Exploiting voltage gradients for control of growth and form. *Annu Rev Biomed Eng*, 19, 353–87 (2017) doi:10.1146/annurev-bioeng-071114-040647.

82. B. Song, M. Zhao, J. V. Forrester and C. D. McCaig: Electrical cues regulate the orientation and frequency of cell division and the rate of wound healing in vivo. *Proc Natl Acad Sci U S A*, 99(21), 13577–82 (2002) doi:10.1073/pnas.202235299.

83. L. Cao, J. Pu and M. Zhao: GSK-3beta is essential for physiological electric field-directed Golgi polarization and optimal electrotaxis. *Cell Mol Life Sci*, 68(18), 3081–93 (2011) doi:10.1007/s00018-010-0608-z.

84. V. Millarte and H. Farhan: The Golgi in cell migration: regulation by signal transduction and its implications for cancer cell metastasis. *ScientificWorldJournal*, 2012, 498278 (2012) doi:10.1100/2012/498278.

85. E. K. Onuma and S. W. Hui: Electric field-directed cell shape changes, displacement, and cyto-skeletal reorganization are calcium dependent. *J Cell Biol*, 106(6), 2067–75 (1988).

86. N. Ozkucur, B. Song, S. Bola, L. Zhang, B. Reid, G. Fu, R. H. Funk and M. Zhao: NHE3 phosphorylation via PKCeta marks the polarity and orientation of directionally migrating cells. *Cell Mol Life Sci*, 71(23), 4653–63 (2014) doi:10.1007/s00018-014-1632-1.

87. D. Saltukoglu, J. Grunewald, N. Strohmeyer, R. Bensch, M. H. Ulbrich, O. Ronneberger and M. Simons: Spontaneous and electric field-controlled front-rear polarization of human keratinocytes. *Mol Biol Cell*, 26(24), 4373–86 (2015) doi:10.1091/mbc.E14-12-1580.

88. K. R. Robinson: The responses of cells to electrical fields: a review. *J Cell Biol*, 101(6), 2023–7 (1985).

89. K. Y. Nishimura, R. R. Isseroff and R. Nuccitelli: Human keratinocytes migrate to the negative pole in direct current electric fields comparable to those measured in mammalian wounds. *J Cell Sci*, 109(Pt 1), 199–207 (1996).

90. M. Zhao, C. D. McCaig, A. Agius-Fernandez, J. V. Forrester and K. Araki-Sasaki: Human corneal epithelial cells reorient and migrate cathodally in a small applied electric field. *Curr Eye Res*, 16(10), 973–84 (1997).

91. M. B. A. Djamgoz, M. Mycielska, Z. Madeja, S. P. Fraser and W. Korohoda: Directional movement of rat prostate cancer cells in direct-current electric field: Involvement of voltagegated Na+ channel activity. *J Cell Sci*, 114(Pt 14), 2697–705 (2001).

92. C. E. Pullar, B. S. Baier, Y. Kariya, A. J. Russell, B. A. Horst, M. P. Marinkovich and R. R. Isseroff: Beta4 integrin and epidermal growth factor coordinately regulate electric field-mediated directional migration via Rac1. *Mol Biol Cell*, 17(11), 4925–35 (2006) doi:10.1091/mbc.E06-05-0433.

93. N. Ozkucur, S. Perike, P. Sharma and R. H. Funk: Persistent directional cell migration requires ion transport proteins as direction sensors and membrane potential differences in order to maintain directedness. *BMC Cell Biol*, 12, 4 (2011) doi:10.1186/1471-2121-12-4.

94. P. Lammert, J. Prost and R. Bruinsma: Ion drive for vesicles and cells. *Journal of Theoretical Biology*, 4(178), 387–91 (1996).

95. G. M. Allen, A. Mogilner and J. A. Theriot: Electrophoresis of cellular membrane components creates the directional cue guiding keratocyte galvanotaxis. *Curr Biol*, 23(7), 560–8 (2013) doi:10.1016/j.cub.2013.02.047.

96. A. L. Kindzelskii and H. R. Petty: Ion channel clustering enhances weak electric field detection by neutrophils: apparent roles of SKF96365-sensitive cation channels and myeloperoxidase trafficking in cellular responses. *Eur Biophys J*, 35(1), 1–26 (2005) doi:10.1007/s00249-005-0001-2.

97. R. C. Gao, X. D. Zhang, Y. H. Sun, Y. Kamimura, A. Mogilner, P. N. Devreotes and M. Zhao: Different roles of membrane potentials in electrotaxis and chemotaxis of dictyostelium cells. *Eukaryot Cell*, 10(9), 1251–6 (2011) doi:10.1128/EC.05066-11.

98. M. Donowitz and X. Li: Regulatory binding partners and complexes of NHE3. *Physiol Rev*, 87(3), 825–72 (2007) doi:10.1152/physrev.00030.2006.

99. M. G. Wheatly and Y. Gao: Molecular biology of ion motive proteins in comparative models. *J Exp Biol*, 207(Pt 19), 3253–63 (2004) doi:10.1242/jeb.01132.

100. K. Nakajima, K. Zhu, Y. H. Sun, B. Hegyi, Q. Zeng, C. J. Murphy, J. V. Small, Y. Chen-Izu, Y. Izumiya, J. M. Penninger and M. Zhao: KCNJ15/Kir4.2 couples with polyamines to sense weak extracellular electric fields in galvanotaxis. *Nat Commun*, 6, 8532 (2015) doi:10.1038/ncomms9532.

101. K. Igarashi and K. Kashiwagi: Modulation of cellular function by polyamines. *Int J Biochem Cell Biol*, 42(1), 39–51 (2010) doi:10.1016/j.biocel.2009.07.009.

102. B. J. Lin, S. H. Tsao, A. Chen, S. K. Hu, L. Chao and P. G. Chao: Lipid rafts sense and direct electric field-induced migration. *Proc Natl Acad Sci U S A* (2017) doi:10.1073/pnas.1702526114.

103. J. V. Small, T. Stradal, E. Vignal and K. Rottner: The lamellipodium: where motility begins. *Trends Cell Biol*, 12(3), 112–20 (2002).

104. A. M. Rajnicek, L. E. Foubister and C. D. McCaig: Growth cone steering by a physiological electric field requires dynamic microtubules, microfilaments and Rac-mediated filopodial asymmetry. *J Cell Sci*, 119(Pt 9), 1736–45 (2006) doi:10.1242/jcs.02897.

105. B. Reid and M. Zhao: The electrical response to injury: Molecular mechanisms and wound healing. *Adv Wound Care (New Rochelle)*, 3(2), 184–201 (2014) doi:10.1089/wound.2013.0442.

106. A. C. Vieira, B. Reid, L. Cao, M. J. Mannis, I. R. Schwab and M. Zhao: Ionic components of electric current at rat corneal wounds. *PLoS One*, 6(2), e17411 (2011) doi:10.1371/journal.pone.0017411.

107. L. Cao, X. D. Zhang, X. Liu, T. Y. Chen and M. Zhao: Chloride channels and transporters in human corneal epithelium. *Exp Eye Res*, 90(6), 771–9 (2010) doi:10.1016/j.exer.2010.03.013.

108. T. Fuchigami, T. Matsuzaki and S. Ihara: Exposure to external environment of low ion concentrations is the trigger for rapid wound closure in Xenopus laevis embryos. *Zoolog Sci*, 28(9), 633–41 (2011) doi:10.2108/zsj.28.633.

109. E. K. Antonsson and R. W. Mann: The frequency content of gait. *J Biomech*, 18(1), 39–47 (1985).

110. M. W. Otter, K. J. McLeod and C. T. Rubin: Effects of electromagnetic fields in experimental fracture repair. *Clin Orthop Relat Res*, (355 Suppl), S90–104 (1998).

111. R. O. Becker: *The body electric: Electromagnetism and the foundation of life*. William Morrow and Company, New York (1985).

112. G. W. Hastings and F. A. Mahmud: Electrical effects in bone. *J Biomed Eng*, 10(6), 515–21 (1988).

113. R. Bertram, A. Sherman and L. S. Satin: Metabolic and electrical oscillations: partners in controlling pulsatile insulin secretion. *Am J Physiol Endocrinol Metab*, 293(4), E890–900 (2007) doi:10.1152/ajpendo.00359.2007.

114. R. Milo and R. Philips: Cell biology by the numbers. In: *Garland Science*, USA (2015).

115. A. Mara and S. A. Holley: Oscillators and the emergence of tissue organization during zebrafish somitogenesis. *Trends Cell Biol*, 17(12), 593–9 (2007) doi:10.1016/j.tcb.2007.09.005.

116. L. Glass: Synchronization and rhythmic processes in physiology. *Nature*, 410(6825), 277–84 (2001) doi:10.1038/35065745.

117. C. A. Skarda and W. J. Freeman: How brains make chaos in order to make sense of the world. *Behavioral and Brain Sciences*, 10(2), 161–73 (2010) doi: 10.1017/S0140525X00047336.

118. A. Garfinkel, M. L. Spano, W. L. Ditto and J. N. Weiss: Controlling cardiac chaos. *Science*, 257(5074), 1230–5 (1992).

119. S. J. Schiff, K. Jerger, D. H. Duong, T. Chang, M. L. Spano and W. L. Ditto: Controlling chaos in the brain. *Nature*, 370(6491), 615–20 (1994) doi:10.1038/370615a0.

120. M. Cifra, J. Z. Fields and A. Farhadi: Electromagnetic cellular interactions. *Prog Biophys Mol Biol*, 105(3), 223–46 (2011) doi:10.1016/j.pbiomolbio.2010.07.003.

121. C. Blackman: Cell phone radiation: Evidence from ELF and RF studies supporting more inclusive risk identification and assessment. *Pathophysiology*, 16(2–3), 205–16 (2009) doi:10.1016/j.pathophys.2009.02.001.

122. D. Leszczynski, D. de Pomerai, D. Koczan, D. Stoll, H. Franke and J. P. Albar: Five years later: the current status of the use of proteomics and transcriptomics in EMF research. *Proteomics*, 12(15–16), 2493–509 (2012) doi:10.1002/pmic.201200122.

123. W. R. Adey: Electromagnetics in biology and medicine. In: *Modern radio science*. Ed. H. Matsumoto. Oxford University Press, Oxford (1993).

124. T. A. Litovitz, D. Krause, M. Penafiel, E. C. Elson and J. M. Mullins: The role of coherence time in the effect of microwaves on ornithine decarboxylase activity. *Bioelectromagnetics*, 14(5), 395–403 (1993).

125. S. M. Bawin, L. K. Kaczmarek and W. R. Adey: Effects of modulated VHF fields on the central nervous system. *Ann N Y Acad Sci*, 247, 74–81 (1975).

126. C. F. Blackman, S. G. Benane, D. E. House and W. T. Joines: Effects of ELF (1–120 Hz) and modulated (50 Hz) RF fields on the efflux of calcium ions from brain tissue in vitro. *Bioelectromagnetics*, 6(1), 1–11 (1985).

127. O. Kolomytkin, M. Yurinska and S. Zharikov: Response of brain receptor systems to microwave energy. In: *On the nature of electromagnetic field interactions with biological systems*. Ed. A. H. Frey. GR Landes, Austin, TX (1994).

128. C. V. Byus, S. E. Pieper and W. R. Adey: The effects of low-energy 60-Hz environmental electromagnetic fields upon the growth-related enzyme ornithine decarboxylase. *Carcinogenesis*, 8(10), 1385–9 (1987).

129. J. Walleczek: Immune cell interactions with extremely low frequency magnetic fields: experimental verification and free radical machanisms. In: *On the nature of electromagnetic field interactions with biological systems*. Ed. A. H. Frey. RG Landes, Austin, TX (1994).

130. W. Sontag and H. Dertinger: Response of cytosolic calcium, cyclic AMP, and cyclic GMP in dimethylsulfoxide-differentiated HL-60 cells to modulated low frequency electric currents. *Bioelectromagnetics*, 19(8), 452–8 (1998).

131. G. Grohmann, M. Krauß, G. Pöhlmann, H. Bär and H. R. Figulla: Zur Makro- und Mikrozirkulation am Vorfuß unter verschiedenen Kompressionsdrücken bei gesunden Probandinnen. *Phlebologie*, 29(5), 114–18 (2000).

132. R. H. Funk, L. Knels, A. Augstein, R. Marquetant and H. F. Dertinger: Potent stimulation of blood flow in fingers of volunteers after local short-term treatment with low-frequency magnetic fields from a novel device. *Evid Based Complement Alternat Med*, 2014, 543564 (2014) doi:10.1155/2014/543564.

133. S. M. Bawin, W. M. Satmary, R. A. Jones, W. R. Adey and G. Zimmerman: Extremely-low-frequency magnetic fields disrupt rhythmic slow activity in rat hippocampal slices. *Bioelectromagnetics*, 17(5), 388–95 (1996) doi:10.1002/(SICI)1521-186X(1996)17:5<388::AID-BEM6>3.0.CO;2-#.

134. W. R. Adey: Evidence for nonthermal electromagnetic bioeffects: Potential health risks in evolving lowfrequency and microwave environments. In: *Electromagnetic environments and safety in buildings*. Ed. D. Clements-Ccroome., Taylor & Francis, London pp. 35-52.(2003).

135. W. Bell, J. Hollingworth and J. McGillivray: Physicians and the environment. *CMAJ*, 147(12), 1749–50 (1992).

136. E. B. Lyskov, J. Juutilainen, V. Jousmaki, J. Partanen, S. Medvedev and O. Hanninen: Effects of 45-Hz magnetic fields on the functional state of the human brain. *Bioelectromagnetics*, 14(2), 87–95 (1993).

137. M. Hartig, U. Joos and H. P. Wiesmann: Capacitively coupled electric fields accelerate proliferation of osteoblast-like primary cells and increase bone extracellular matrix formation in vitro. *Eur Biophys J*, 29(7), 499–506 (2000).

138. W. H. Chang, L. T. Chen, J. S. Sun and F. H. Lin: Effect of pulse-burst electromagnetic field stimulation on osteoblast cell activities. *Bioelectromagnetics*, 25(6), 457–65 (2004) doi:10.1002/bem.20016.

139. L. Ferroni, I. Tocco, A. De Pieri, M. Menarin, E. Fermi, A. Piattelli, C. Gardin and B. Zavan: Pulsed magnetic therapy increases osteogenic differentiation of mesenchymal stem cells only if they are pre-committed. *Life Sci*, 152, 44–51 (2016) doi:10.1016/j.lfs.2016.03.020.

140. M. Zhai, D. Jing, S. Tong, Y. Wu, P. Wang, Z. Zeng, G. Shen, X. Wang, Q. Xu and E. Luo: Pulsed electromagnetic fields promote in vitro osteoblastogenesis through a Wnt/beta-catenin signaling-associated mechanism. *Bioelectromagnetics* (2016) doi:10.1002/bem.21961.

141. W. H. Hei, S. Kim, J. C. Park, Y. K. Seo, S. M. Kim, J. W. Jahng and J. H. Lee: Schwann-like cells differentiated from human dental pulp stem cells combined with a pulsed electromagnetic field can improve peripheral nerve regeneration. *Bioelectromagnetics* (2016) doi:10.1002/bem.21966.

142. F. Veronesi, P. Torricelli, G. Giavaresi, M. Sartori, F. Cavani, S. Setti, M. Cadossi, A. Ongaro and M. Fini: In vivo effect of two different pulsed electromagnetic field frequencies on osteoarthritis. *J Orthop Res*, 32(5), 677–85 (2014) doi:10.1002/jor.22584.

143. F. Benazzo, M. Cadossi, F. Cavani, M. Fini, G. Giavaresi, S. Setti, R. Cadossi and R. Giardino: Cartilage repair with osteochondral autografts in sheep: effect of biophysical stimulation with pulsed electromagnetic fields. *J Orthop Res*, 26(5), 631–42 (2008) doi:10.1002/jor.20530.

144. D. M. Ciombor, R. K. Aaron, S. Wang and B. Simon: Modification of osteoarthritis by pulsed electromagnetic field--a morphological study. *Osteoarthritis Cartilage*, 11(6), 455–62 (2003).

145. M. De Mattei, A. Caruso, F. Pezzetti, A. Pellati, G. Stabellini, V. Sollazzo and G. C. Traina: Effects of pulsed electromagnetic fields on human articular chondrocyte proliferation. *Connect Tissue Res*, 42(4), 269–79 (2001).

146. M. De Mattei, M. Fini, S. Setti, A. Ongaro, D. Gemmati, G. Stabellini, A. Pellati and A. Caruso: Proteoglycan synthesis in bovine articular cartilage explants exposed to different low-frequency low-energy pulsed electromagnetic fields. *Osteoarthritis Cartilage*, 15(2), 163–8 (2007) doi:10.1016/j.joca.2006.06.019.

147. M. De Mattei, M. Pasello, A. Pellati, G. Stabellini, L. Massari, D. Gemmati and A. Caruso: Effects of electromagnetic fields on proteoglycan metabolism of bovine articular cartilage explants. *Connect Tissue Res*, 44(3–4), 154–9 (2003).

148. M. Fini, G. Giavaresi, P. Torricelli, F. Cavani, S. Setti, V. Cane and R. Giardino: Pulsed electromagnetic fields reduce knee osteoarthritic lesion progression in the aged Dunkin Hartley guinea pig. *J Orthop Res*, 23(4), 899–908 (2005) doi:10.1016/j.orthres.2005.01.008.

149. M. Fini, P. Torricelli, G. Giavaresi, N. N. Aldini, F. Cavani, S. Setti, A. Nicolini, A. Carpi and R. Giardino: Effect of pulsed electromagnetic field stimulation on knee cartilage, subchondral and epyphiseal trabecular bone of aged Dunkin Hartley guinea pigs. *Biomed Pharmacother*, 62(10), 709–15 (2008) doi:10.1016/j.biopha.2007.03.001.

150. V. Nicolin, C. Ponti, G. Baldini, D. Gibellini, R. Bortul, M. Zweyer, B. Martinelli and P. Narducci: In vitro exposure of human chondrocytes to pulsed electromagnetic fields. *Eur J Histochem*, 51(3), 203–12 (2007).

151. A. Ongaro, A. Pellati, F. F. Masieri, A. Caruso, S. Setti, R. Cadossi, R. Biscione, L. Massari, M. Fini and M. De Mattei: Chondroprotective effects of pulsed electromagnetic fields on human cartilage explants. *Bioelectromagnetics*, 32(7), 543–51 (2011) doi:10.1002/bem.20663.

152. P. R. Boopalan, S. Arumugam, A. Livingston, M. Mohanty and S. Chittaranjan: Pulsed electromagnetic field therapy results in healing of full thickness articular cartilage defect. *Int Orthop*, 35(1), 143–8 (2011) doi:10.1007/s00264-010-0994-8.

153. R. K. Aaron and D. M. Ciombor: Pain in osteoarthritis. *Med Health R I*, 87(7), 205–9 (2004).

154. P. R. Boopalan, A. J. Daniel and S. B. Chittaranjan: Managing skin necrosis and prosthesis subluxation after total knee arthroplasty. *J Arthroplasty*, 24(2), 322 e23–7 (2009) doi:10.1016/j.arth.2008.03.001.

155. D. M. Ciombor, G. Lester, R. K. Aaron, P. Neame and B. Caterson: Low frequency EMF regulates chondrocyte differentiation and expression of matrix proteins. *J Orthop Res*, 20(1), 40–50 (2002) doi:10.1016/S0736-0266(01)00071-7.

156. A. R. Liboff: Geomagnetic cyclotron resonance in living cells. *Journal of Biological Physics*, 13(4), 99–102 (1985) doi:10.1007/bf01878387.

157. A. R. Liboff: The 'cyclotron resonance' hypothesis: experimental evidence and theoretical constraints. In: *Interaction mechanisms of low-level electromagnetic fields in living systems*. Ed. B. Norden and K. Ramel. Oxford University Press, New York (1992).

158. B. Bianco and A. Chiabrera: From the Langevin-Lorentz to the Zeeman model of electromagnetic effects on ligand-receptor binding. *Bioelectrochemistry and Bioenergetics*, 28, 355–65 (1992).

159. A. A. Pilla: Mechanisms and therapeutic applications of time-varying and static magnetic fields. In: *Biological and medical aspects of electromagnetic fields; handbook of biological effects of electromagnetic fields*. Ed. F. S. Barnes and B. Greenebaum. CRC Press, Taylor & Francis Group, Boca Raton (2007).

160. K. J. McLeod, C. T. Rubin and H. J. Donahue: Electromagnetic fields in bone repair and adaptation. *Radio Sci*, 30(1), 233–44 (1995).

161. C. S. Peskin, G. M. Odell and G. F. Oster: Cellular motions and thermal fluctuations: The Brownian ratchet. *Biophys J*, 65(1), 316–24 (1993) doi:10.1016/S0006-3495(93)81035-X.

162. R. J. Fitzsimmons, D. D. Strong, S. Mohan and D. J. Baylink: Low-amplitude, low-frequency electric field-stimulated bone cell proliferation may in part be mediated by increased IGF-II release. *J Cell Physiol*, 150(1), 84–9 (1992) doi:10.1002/jcp.1041500112.

163. R. J. Fitzsimmons and D. J. Baylink: Growth factors and electromagnetic fields in bone. *Clin Plast Surg*, 21(3), 401–6 (1994).

164. J. Schimmelpfeng and H. Dertinger: Action of a 50 Hz magnetic field on proliferation of cells in culture. *Bioelectromagnetics*, 18(2), 177–83 (1997).

165. R. D. Astumian: Thermodynamics and kinetics of a Brownian motor. *Science*, 276(5314), 917–22 (1997).

166. M. Nishida and R. MacKinnon: Structural basis of inward rectification: cytoplasmic pore of the G protein-gated inward rectifier GIRK1 at 1.8 A resolution. *Cell*, 111(7), 957–65 (2002).

167. H. Matsuda, K. Oishi and K. Omori: Voltage-dependent gating and block by internal spermine of the murine inwardly rectifying K+ channel, Kir2.1. *J Physiol*, 548(Pt 2), 361–71 (2003) doi:10.1113/jphysiol.2003.038844.

168. J. Gartzke and K. Lange: Cellular target of weak magnetic fields: Ionic conduction along actin filaments of microvilli. *Am J Physiol Cell Physiol*, 283(5), C1333–46 (2002) doi:10.1152/ajpcell.00167.2002.

169. M. R. Cho, H. S. Thatte, R. C. Lee and D. E. Golan: Reorganization of microfilament structure induced by ac electric fields. *FASEB J*, 10(13), 1552–8 (1996).

170. A. A. Pilla, J. J. Kaufmann and J. T. Ryaby: Electrochemical kinetics at the cell membrane: A physicochemical link for electromagnetic bioeffects. In: *Mechanistic approaches to interactions of electric and electromagnetic fields with living systems*. Ed. M. Blank and E. Findl, Premum Press, New York (1987).

171. Y. Murata, H. Iwasaki, M. Sasaki, K. Inaba and Y. Okamura: Phosphoinositide phosphatase activity coupled to an intrinsic voltage sensor. *Nature*, 435(7046), 1239–43 (2005) doi:10.1038/nature03650.

172. M. Iijima, Y. E. Huang, H. R. Luo, F. Vazquez and P. N. Devreotes: Novel mechanism of PTEN regulation by its phosphatidylinositol 4,5-bisphosphate binding motif is critical for chemotaxis. *J Biol Chem*, 279(16), 16606–13 (2004) doi:10.1074/jbc.M312098200.

173. A. Buchachenko: Why magnetic and electromagnetic effects in biology are irreproducible and contradictory? *Bioelectromagnetics*, 37(1), 1–13 (2016) doi:10.1002/bem.21947.

174. V. N. Binhi and F. S. Prato: Biological effects of the hypomagnetic field: An analytical review of experiments and theories. *PLoS One*, 12(6), e0179340 (2017) doi:10.1371/journal.pone.0179340.

4

Electric and Magnetic Properties of Biological Materials

Camelia Gabriel

C. Gabriel Consultants

Azadeh Peyman

Public Health England

CONTENTS

4.1 Introduction 102
4.2 Dielectric Properties—Molecular Origin 104
    4.2.1 Quasi-Static Response 104
    4.2.2 Permittivity of Low Pressure Gases 105
    4.2.3 Permittivity of Liquids and Dense Gases 105
    4.2.4 Time and Frequency Dependence of the Dielectric Response 106
        4.2.4.1 Time-Dependent Polarization – Impulse Response – Kramers–Krönig Relations 106
        4.2.4.2 Permittivity of a Polar Substance—The Debye Equation 108
        4.2.4.3 Nonpolar Molecules 109
4.3 Observed Responses of Real Systems – Multiple Relaxations – the Universal Law 109
    4.3.1 Multiple Relaxation Models – Distribution of Relaxation Times 110
    4.3.2 Universal Law of Dielectric Relaxation 112
4.4 Dielectric Properties of Biological Materials—Main Components 113
    4.4.1 Water 113
    4.4.2 Electrolytes 115
    4.4.3 Carbohydrates 117
    4.4.4 Proteins and Other Macromolecules 118
    4.4.5 Dielectric Dispersions in Tissue 119
        4.4.5.1 α Dispersion 120
        4.4.5.2 β Dispersion 121
        4.4.5.3 γ Dispersion 122
        4.4.5.4 δ Dispersion 123
4.5 Dielectric Properties of Tissue – Effective Permittivity - State-of-Knowledge 124
    4.5.1 Measurement Concepts 124
    4.5.2 Uncertainty in the Measurement of Biological Materials 125
    4.5.3 Review of the Dielectric Properties of Tissues 126
        4.5.3.1 The 1996 Database 126
        4.5.3.2 *In Vivo* versus *In Vitro* Measurements 128
        4.5.3.3 Anisotropy of Tissue Dielectric Properties 129
        4.5.3.4 Variation of Dielectric Properties with Age 130

101

		4.5.3.5 Changes Following Death	132
		4.5.3.6 Healthy versus Pathological Tissue	133
		4.5.3.7 Species Specific Tissue: Skin	134
	4.5.4	Conductivity of Tissue at Low Frequency	137
	4.5.5	Nonlinear Dielectric Properties	138
	4.5.6	Electric Properties Tomography	139
4.6	Magnetic Properties of Matter		140
	4.6.1	Molecular origin	141
	4.6.2	Diamagnetic Materials	141
	4.6.3	Paramagnetic Materials	142
	4.6.4	Ferromagnetic Materials	143
		4.6.4.1 Anti-ferromagnetism	144
		4.6.4.2 Ferrimagnetism	144
	4.6.5	Temperature Dependence of Ferromagnetism	145
4.7	Magnetic Susceptibility of Biological Materials		146
	4.7.1	Factors that Affect the Magnetic Susceptibility of Tissue	147
		4.7.1.1 Iron	147
		4.7.1.2 Structure of Tissue (Magnetic Anisotropy)	149
	4.7.2	MRI Techniques for Magnetic Susceptibility Mapping	149
		4.7.2.1 Quantitative Susceptibility Mapping (QSM)	149
		4.7.2.2 QSM versus SQUID Susceptometry	149
		4.7.2.3 Magnetic Susceptibility in Diagnostic Applications	150
Acknowledgments			150
References			150

4.1 Introduction

The electric and magnetic properties of materials are a measure of their response to stimulation by external electric and magnetic fields, respectively. They are intrinsic properties of matter determined by the extent of interactions with an external electric or magnetic field at all levels of organization within matter including structural, molecular, atomic, and electronic. The electric permittivity and magnetic permeability are the properties used to characterize and quantify these interactions. The electrical properties used to characterize non-metallic materials are commonly referred to as dielectric properties and will be referred to as such throughout this chapter.

Biological matter has an abundance of free and bound charges, an applied electric field will cause them to drift and displace thus inducing conduction and polarization currents that occur over time scales from seconds to pico seconds. Translated to the frequency domain, this amounts to an eventful permittivity spectrum spanning from few Hz to 100s of GHz. Dielectric spectroscopy is the science that relates the permittivity (or dielectric property) and its variation with frequency to the underlying microscopic mechanisms of polarization and conduction.

Today, electromagnetic fields are ever omnipresent in the environment the world over. The development of standards for safe exposure to such fields has necessitated detailed knowledge of the dielectric properties of body tissues in order to quantify the interaction and assess their biological effects. Moreover, electromagnetic fields are increasingly used

Properties of Biological Materials 103

to probe the body for diagnostic or therapeutic purposes. The concept, design, optimization, and safety of such medical devices require good knowledge of the dielectric properties of body tissues. For this reason, a great deal of the dielectric measurement work of the past two decades has been dedicated to providing a credible database of dielectric properties of tissues to provide essential data to such fields of studies. This continues to be an active field of research.

Magnetic fields in matter originate from the movement of charged entities and their associated magnetic moments. The magnetic properties of materials are determined by the alignment of magnetic moments and their interaction with external fields.

For most biological materials, the magnetic permeability is close to that of free space, which implies that there is very little direct interaction with the external magnetic fields at low-field strengths. However, as for dielectric properties, the magnetic properties of tissues are determined by their molecular composition and structure, so different tissues have different magnetic susceptibilities. Recently, it has become possible to determine these properties and use the variation between tissues to great advantage in numerous biological applications (Deistung et al. 2017). Moreover, recent discovery of biogenic ferrimagnetic substances in human tissue including the brain, open new questions regarding possible direct interactions with external field (Dobson and Grassi 1996 and Dobson 2004).

At a fundamental level permittivity and permeability are implicitly defined within the solution to Maxwell's electromagnetic field equations as the electric permittivity and magnetic permeability and inform on the ability of a material to carry an electric or magnetic field compared to free space. In free space, the constitutive relations to Maxwell's equations are:

$$D = \varepsilon_0 E \text{ and } B = \mu_0 H \tag{4.1}$$

where E and D are the electric and displacement fields, H and B the magnetic and induction fields, ε_0 and μ_0 are the permittivity and permeability of free space. In a homogenous and linear system they become:

$$D = \varepsilon\varepsilon_0 E \text{ and } B = \mu\mu_0 H \tag{4.2}$$

where ε and μ are the relative permittivity and permeability of the material. The relative permittivity and permeability are dimensionless factors that relate to the interaction within the material creating additional polarization and magnetization fields, respectively, and will be used throughout this chapter to characterize the dielectric and magnetic properties.

Homogeneity is a relative description of matter, meaning that the microscopic behaviors relate to a bulk property that is reflected in the constitutive relations between the electromagnetic field components. Linearity is observed in most practical situations where weak fields interact with matter. Non-linear behavior occurs in strong electric and magnetic fields and is not the focus of this chapter.

This chapter aims at providing an overview of the fundamental concepts underpinning the dielectric and magnetic properties of matter and a review of the state of knowledge on the subject. In recent years, it has become possible to determine the dielectric and magnetic properties of tissues from data gathered during magnetic resonance imaging (MRI). These developing technologies are the tools of the future; they provide a welcome new approach to a century-old quest and are bound to invigorate research in this field.

4.2 Dielectric Properties—Molecular Origin

This section will start with the fundamental concepts of the interaction of homogenous matter with static fields and proceed, in steps, to heterogenous mixtures and their dynamic response to time-varying fields leading to the dielectric properties of tissues.

4.2.1 Quasi-Static Response

Considering the simple case of a monomolecular material, three main interaction mechanisms are possible: electronic, atomic, and molecular polarization. Electronic polarization is the shift of electrons, in the direction of the field, from their equilibrium position with respect to the positive nuclei. Atomic polarization is the relative displacement of atoms or atom groups relative to each other. The orientation of permanent or induced molecular dipoles, when present, is known as molecular polarization. Materials that possess permanent or induced dipoles are described as polar. The total polarizability α_T is the sum of the contribution of, in this case, all three processes, termed α_e, α_a, and α_d.

In view of the dominance of molecular-orientation processes in defining the total polarization $((\alpha_e + \alpha_a) < \alpha_d)$ and hence the dielectric properties, it is usual to differentiate between polar and nonpolar materials when these properties are considered.

When a dielectric material becomes polarized by the application of an external electric field E, the dipole moment of the constituent molecules is given by

$$\bar{m} = \alpha_T \bar{E}_1 \tag{4.3}$$

where E_1 is the local field acting on the molecules. The dipole moment per unit volume of the material P increases the total displacement flux density D, defined from the relationship $D = \varepsilon_0 E$ in vacuum and $D = \varepsilon_0 \varepsilon E$ in a medium of relative permittivity ε. The latter expression may also be written as:

$$D = \varepsilon_0 E + P \tag{4.4}$$

The dependence of P on E can take several forms, the simplest and most common being a scalar proportionality:

$$P = \varepsilon_0 \chi E \tag{4.5}$$

where $\chi = \varepsilon - 1$ is the relative dielectric susceptibility. This simple relationship is valid for a perfect isotropic dielectric, at low or moderate field intensities and at static or quasi-static field frequencies.

If the material contains N dipoles per unit volume, then

$$P = N\alpha_T E_1 \tag{4.6}$$

and

$$\varepsilon - 1 = \frac{N\alpha_T}{\varepsilon_0} \frac{E_1}{E} \tag{4.7}$$

Properties of Biological Materials 105

The molecular description of the permittivity requires that the relationship between the microscopic and the macroscopic field intensities be known. In most cases, there is no exact solution to this problem, only more or less good approximations that hold within the confines of the assumptions and simplifications made, as will be briefly illustrated for typical classes of materials.

4.2.2 Permittivity of Low Pressure Gases

At low pressures, the molecules are far apart from each other, and their interaction with each other may be assumed to be negligible in comparison with the macroscopic field intensity E. Under these conditions $E_1 \approx E$ and

$$\varepsilon - 1 = \frac{N\alpha_T}{\varepsilon_0} \tag{4.8}$$

The relative permittivity of a nonpolar gas is very close to 1, typically of the order of 1.0001 at atmospheric pressure.

4.2.3 Permittivity of Liquids and Dense Gases

When the intermolecular interactions are such that $E_1 \neq E$, the local field must be estimated. One approach is to consider a spherical region inside the dielectric that is large compared to the size of a molecule and to assume that the field from the molecules inside the cavity average out due to isotropy and do not contribute to the local field. The local field arising from the polarization in the material under the action of the external field is

$$E_1 = \left(\frac{\varepsilon + 2}{3}\right) E \tag{4.9}$$

which yields

$$\frac{3(\varepsilon - 1)}{\varepsilon + 2} = \frac{N}{\varepsilon_0} \alpha_T \tag{4.10}$$

The above expression is known as the Clausius–Mossoti–Lorentz formulation. It is not always valid, such as when the density of the material corresponds to $N = 3\varepsilon_0/\alpha_T$. An alternative formulation, valid when the molecules are polarizable point dipoles of permanent moment μ, was provided by Onsager 1936:

$$\frac{(\varepsilon - n^2)(2\varepsilon + n^2)}{\varepsilon(n^2 + 2)^2} = \frac{N\mu^2}{9kT\varepsilon_0} \tag{4.11}$$

where k is the Boltzman constant and T is the absolute temperature.

Debye separated out the contribution to the total polarization of the permanent dipole from those associated with electronic and atomic displacements and arrived at the following relationship

$$\frac{\varepsilon - 1}{\varepsilon + 2} = \frac{N}{3\varepsilon_0}\left(\alpha + \mu^2/3kT\right) \tag{4.12}$$

While Onsager (1936) and Debye (1929) used semi-statistical techniques to estimate the local field, others like Kirkwood (1936), and later Fröhlich (1955), used statistical methods to obtain a rigorous expression of the permittivity after taking local interactions into consideration and obtained:

$$\frac{(\varepsilon-1)(2\varepsilon+1)}{3\varepsilon} = \frac{N}{\varepsilon_0}\left(\alpha + g\mu^2/3kT\right) \tag{4.13}$$

This is Kirkwood's equation for permittivity in which g is known as the Kirkwood correlation parameter, introduced to account for the effect of local ordering in the material. Fröhlich's theory gives:

$$\frac{\left(\varepsilon-n^2\right)\left(2\varepsilon+n^2\right)}{\varepsilon\left(n^2+2\right)^2} = \frac{Ng\mu^2}{9kT\varepsilon_0} \tag{4.14}$$

which except for the correlation parameter g, is identical to Onsager's equation.

This brief outline of the dielectric theory gives an idea of the nature of the electric field interaction problems and of the various techniques used to partially solve them under static field conditions. The solutions hold for slow time-varying fields as long as there is a quasi-static state. References to the original work by Debye (1929), Kirkwood (1936), Onsager (1936), and Fröhlich (1955) are given in Böttcher and Bordewijk (1978) and other well-known texts (Hill et al. 1969; Hill and Jonscher 1983).

4.2.4 Time and Frequency Dependence of the Dielectric Response

Much of the interest in the dielectric properties of biological materials is concerned with their response to time-varying electric fields. This can be explained by the same macroscopic variables used for the quasi-static state except for the introduction of a time dependence for the excitation and response. The general discussion will assume sinusoidal fields and linear and isotropic responses, nonsinusoidal fields and material anisotropy, and nonlinearity being special cases.

4.2.4.1 Time-Dependent Polarization – Impulse Response – Kramers–Krönig Relations

The following relationship holds irrespective of the polarization mechanism:

$$P(t) = D(t) - \varepsilon_0 E(t) \tag{4.15}$$

For an ideal dielectric material with no free charge, the polarization follows the pulse with a delay determined by the time constant of the polarization mechanism. Assuming a rate process, which is that the rate of polarization is proportional to the constantly decreasing number of unpolarized units, the simplest expression for the polarization is obtained from the solution of the first-order differential rate equation with constant coefficients and time constant τ, giving

$$P(t) = P\left(1 - e^{-t/\tau}\right) \tag{4.16}$$

The decay of polarization is also an exponential function

$$P(t) = e^{-t/\tau} \tag{4.17}$$

Properties of Biological Materials 107

For a linear system, the response to a unit-step electric field is the impulse response $f(t)$ of the system. The response of the system to a time-dependent field can be obtained from summation in a convolution integral of the impulses corresponding to a sequence of elements making up the electric field. For a harmonic field and a causal, time-independent system, the Fourier transform exists and yields

$$P(\omega) = \varepsilon_0 \chi(\omega) E(\omega) \tag{4.18}$$

indicating that the dielectric susceptibility $\chi(\omega)$ is the Fourier transform of $f(t)$. In general, the susceptibility is a complex function reflecting the fact that it informs on the magnitude and phase of the polarization with respect to the polarizing field:

$$\chi(\omega) = \chi' - j\chi'' \tag{4.19}$$

The real and imaginary parts of $\chi(\omega)$ can be obtained from the separate parts of the Fourier transform:

$$\chi'(\omega) = \int_{-\infty}^{+\infty} f(t)\cos(\omega t)\,dt = \int_0^{+\infty} f(t)\cos(\omega t)\,dt$$

$$\chi''(\omega) = \int_{-\infty}^{+\infty} f(t)\sin(\omega t)\,dt = \int_0^{+\infty} f(t)\sin(\omega t)\,dt \tag{4.20}$$

The limit of integration can be changed from $-\infty$ to 0 since $f(t)$ is causal.

The impulse response $f(t)$ defines the dielectric response and, conversely, knowledge of the complex susceptibility allows the determination of the impulse response by carrying out the reverse transformation, which gives $f(t)$ in terms of either $\chi'(\omega)$ or $\chi''(\omega)$

$$f(t) = (2/\pi)\int_0^{+\infty} \chi'(\omega)\cos(\omega t)\,d\omega$$

$$f(t) = (2/\pi)\int_0^{+\infty} \chi''(\omega)\sin(\omega t)\,d\omega \tag{4.21}$$

Eliminating $f(t)$ from the above equations gives an expression of $\chi'(\omega)$ in terms of $\chi''(\omega)$ and vice versa. Thus, there is a relationship between the real and imaginary parts of the complex susceptibility of any material, such that knowledge of either enables the other to be calculated. The expressions of real and imaginary parts of the susceptibility or permittivity in terms of each other are known as the Kramers–Krönig relations and have been derived as:

$$\chi'(\omega) = \chi'(\infty) + \frac{2}{\pi}\int_0^\infty \frac{u\chi''(u) - \omega\chi''(\omega)}{u^2 - \omega^2}\,du$$

$$\chi''(\omega) = \frac{2}{\pi}\int_0^\infty \frac{\chi'(u) - \chi'(\omega)}{u^2 - \omega^2}\,du \tag{4.22}$$

where u is a variable of integration. Recalling the relationship between relative dielectric susceptibility and relative permittivity $\chi = \varepsilon - 1$, the permittivity is a complex function given by

$$\hat{\varepsilon}(\omega) = \varepsilon'(\omega) - j\varepsilon''(\omega) = \left(1 + \chi'(\omega) - j\chi''(\omega)\right) \tag{4.23}$$

108   *Electromagnetic Fields*

Thus, the Kramers–Krönig relations relate ε' to the complete spectrum of ε'' and vice versa. A clear account of their derivation can be found in Jonscher (1983).

4.2.4.2 Permittivity of a Polar Substance—The Debye Equation

When a step field E is applied to a polar dielectric material, the electronic and atomic polarizations are established almost instantaneously compared to the time scale of the molecular orientation; the total polarization reaches a steady state as a first-order process characterized by the time constant of the dipolar rotation. When the field is removed, the process is reversed; electronic and atomic polarizations subside first, followed by a relatively slow decay in dipolar polarization. The time constant τ depends on the physical process, in this case the rotational dynamics of the dipole determined by the size, shape, and intermolecular relations of the molecules. If P_∞ and P_0 are the instantaneous and steady state polarization then the total polarization for a first-order process characterized by a time constant τ is

$$P = P_\infty + (P_0 - P_\infty)\left(1 - e^{-t/\tau}\right) \tag{4.24}$$

In time-varying fields the permittivity is a complex function originating from the magnitude and phase shift of the polarization with respect to the polarizing field:

$$\hat{\varepsilon} = \varepsilon' - j\varepsilon'' = \varepsilon' - j\sigma/\omega\varepsilon_0 \tag{4.25}$$

the real part ε' is a measure of the induced polarization per unit field and the imaginary part ε'' is the out of phase loss factor associated with it. The loss factor can also be represented by a conductivity term $\sigma = \omega\varepsilon_0\varepsilon''$ where ω is the angular frequency. The SI unit of conductivity is siemens per metre (S/m).

The frequency response of the first-order system is obtained from the Laplace transformation which gives the relationship known as the Debye equation:

$$\hat{\varepsilon} = \varepsilon_\infty + \frac{(\varepsilon_0 - \varepsilon_s)}{1 + j\omega\tau} = \varepsilon' - j\varepsilon'' \tag{4.26}$$

The limiting values of the permittivity ε_s and ε_∞ are known as static and infinite permittivity, respectively. The relaxation time τ corresponds to a relaxation frequency $f_r = 1/2\pi\tau$. For a highly associated liquid such as water the static permittivity can be expressed in terms of molecular parameters in accordance with the discussions in the previous section as:

$$\varepsilon_s = \varepsilon_\infty + \frac{Ng\mu^2}{2kT\varepsilon_0} \tag{4.27}$$

The relaxation time may be identified with the time constant of the molecular polarization and expressed in terms of molecular parameters. If η is the viscosity, then for a spherical molecule of radius a

$$\tau = 4\pi a^3 \eta/kT \tag{4.28}$$

For most polar materials, though not for water, ε_∞ corresponds to the optical permittivity and is equal to the square of optical refractive index n of the medium

$$\varepsilon_\infty = n^2 \tag{4.29}$$

Properties of Biological Materials

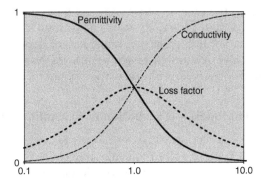

FIGURE 4.1
Normalized permittivity $(\varepsilon' - \varepsilon_\infty)/(\varepsilon_S - \varepsilon_\infty)$, loss factor $\varepsilon''(\varepsilon_S - \varepsilon_\infty)$, and conductivity $\omega\varepsilon_0\varepsilon''(\varepsilon_S - \varepsilon_\infty)$ for a single time constant relaxation plotted against f/f_r.

The dielectric properties of polar molecules vary with temperature, in general, both ε_s and τ decrease with increasing temperature.

As with the charge density and polarization, the time dependence of the current density J and σ the current density per unit field also follows a first-order law such that

$$J/E = \sigma_\infty + (\sigma_s - \sigma_\infty)\left(1 - e^{-t/\tau}\right) \tag{4.30}$$

This transforms into the conductivity equivalent of the Debye equation:

$$\hat{\sigma} = \sigma_\infty + \frac{(\sigma_s - \sigma_\infty)}{1 + j\omega\tau} \tag{4.31}$$

Figure 4.1 shows the variation in the permittivity, loss factor, and conductivity with frequency for a single time constant relaxation, such behavior pertain to an idealized monomolecular polar substance with no residual frequency-independent conductivity, that is $\sigma_s = 0$. An example of such material is pure water as will be discussed later.

At the relaxation frequency, the permittivity is halfway between its limiting values and the loss factor at its highest. In the case of a single time constant as described in Figure 4.1, the conductivity is halfway between its limiting values at the relaxation frequency.

4.2.4.3 Nonpolar Molecules

The permittivity of nonpolar materials is virtually constant throughout the frequency range. In general, the temperature dependence is not significant. The static and optical values of the permittivity are almost identical, hence the Maxwell relation $\varepsilon = n^2$ holds true throughout the frequency and temperature range.

4.3 Observed Responses of Real Systems – Multiple Relaxations – the Universal Law

Although the Debye model was specifically derived to describe the polarization and relaxation of a polar molecule, it was found to apply whenever the decay of polarization is exponential, which is often the case, in more complex biological systems. However, few systems exhibit single relaxation time dispersions as in the Debye model, real materials depart from this ideal behavior to a greater or lesser extent depending on the complexity of the molecular mechanisms. A number of semi-empirical variants of the Debye model were derived to account for observed multi-relaxation phenomena.

4.3.1 Multiple Relaxation Models – Distribution of Relaxation Times

The occurrence of multiple interaction processes or the presence of more than one molecular conformational state or type of polar molecule may cause the dielectric behavior of a substance to exhibit multiple relaxation time dispersions. Deviation from Debye behavior may also indicate a polarization process whose kinetics are not first order or the presence of a complex intermolecular interaction. Models are needed to analyze the dielectric spectra of complex systems to unravel the underlying interaction mechanisms.

The simplest case is that of a dielectric response arising from multiple first-order processes; in this case, the dielectric response will consist of multiple Debye terms to correspond to the polarization processes such that

$$\hat{\varepsilon} = \varepsilon_{\infty} + \frac{\Delta\varepsilon_1}{1 - j\omega\tau_1} + \frac{\Delta\varepsilon_2}{1 - j\omega\tau_2} + \cdots \tag{4.32}$$

Where $\Delta\varepsilon_n$ corresponds to the limits of the dispersion characterized by time constant τ_n. If the relaxation times are well separated such that $\tau_1 \ll \tau_2 \ll \tau_3 \ldots$, a plot of the dielectric properties as a function of frequency will exhibit clearly resolved dispersion regions.

If, as is quite often the case, the relaxation times are not well separated, the material will exhibit a broad dispersion encompassing all the relaxation times. At the limit of a continuous distribution of relaxation times, the multiple Debye expression would be:

$$\hat{\varepsilon} = \varepsilon_{\infty} + \left(\varepsilon_s - \varepsilon_{\infty}\right) \int_0^{\infty} \frac{\rho(\tau)d\tau}{1 - j\omega\tau} \tag{4.33}$$

where

$$\int_0^{\infty} \rho(\tau)d\tau = 1 \tag{4.34}$$

The above equations can be used to represent all dielectric dispersion data, provided an appropriate distribution function $\rho(\tau)$ is available. Conversely, it should also be possible, at least in principle, to invert dielectric relaxation spectra to determine $\rho(\tau)$ directly; however, this is not easily achievable in practice. More commonly, one has to assume a distribution to describe the frequency dependence of the dielectric properties observed experimentally. The choice of distribution function should depend on the cause of the multiple dispersions in the material. For example, one can assume a Gaussian distribution as is known to occur for other physical characteristics $\rho(\tau)$ would be:

$$\rho\left(t/\tau\right) = \frac{b}{\sqrt{\pi}} e^{-b^2\left[\ln(t/\tau)\right]^2} \tag{4.35}$$

where τ is the mean relaxation time. The shape of the Gaussian function depends on the parameter b; it reduces to the delta function when b tends to infinity and becomes very

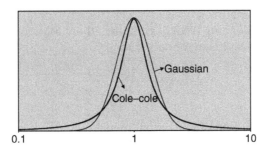

FIGURE 4.2
Gaussian distribution with $b = 2$ and Cole–Cole distribution with $\alpha = 0.09$ as a function of t/τ.

broad when b decreases; the area under the curve remains the same as required by the normalization condition. Incorporated into the expression for complex permittivity, it produces an expression that cannot be solved analytically, which makes it impractical for experimental data analysis.

Numerous empirical distribution functions or models have been proposed to model the experimental data without elaboration of the underlying mechanisms. One of the most commonly used models, a modified version of the Debye expression, was proposed by Cole and Cole (1941) and is widely known as the Cole–Cole model:

$$\hat{\varepsilon} = \varepsilon_\infty + \frac{(\varepsilon_s - \varepsilon_\infty)}{1 - (j\omega\tau)^{1-\alpha}} = \varepsilon' - j\varepsilon'' \qquad (4.36)$$

in which α is a distribution parameter in the range $1 > \alpha \geq 0$ for $\alpha = 0$ the model reverts to the Debye equation.

The distribution function that corresponds to the Cole–Cole model is

$$p(t/\tau) = \frac{1}{2\pi} \frac{\sin(\alpha\pi)}{\cosh[(1-\alpha)\ln(t/\tau) - \cos(\alpha\pi)]} \qquad (4.37)$$

here again, τ is the mean relaxation time. As with the Gaussian, this distribution is logarithmically symmetrical about t/τ (Figure 4.2).

Davidson and Cole (1951) proposed another variant of the Debye equation in which an exponent β is applied to the whole denominator:

$$\hat{\varepsilon} = \varepsilon_\infty + \frac{(\varepsilon_s - \varepsilon_\infty)}{(1 - j\omega\tau)^\beta} \qquad (4.38)$$

The corresponding distribution of relaxation times is

$$p(t/\tau) = \frac{1}{\pi}\left(\frac{t}{\tau - t}\right)^\beta \sin(\pi\beta) \qquad (4.39)$$

When $\beta = 1$, the model reverts to the Debye equation.

Another expression, sometimes used to model dielectric data, is the Havriliak–Negami relation (Havriliak and Negami 1966). It combines the variations introduced in both the Cole–Cole and the Cole–Davidson models, giving

$$\hat{\varepsilon} = \varepsilon_\infty + \frac{(\varepsilon_s - \varepsilon_\infty)}{\left(1 - (j\omega\tau)^{(1-\alpha)}\right)^\beta} \tag{4.40}$$

the corresponding distribution of relaxation times is

$$\rho(t/\tau) = \frac{1}{\pi} \frac{(t/\tau)^{\beta(1-\alpha)} \sin(\beta\theta)}{\left((t/\tau)^{2(1-\alpha)} + 2(t/\tau)^{(1-\alpha)} \cos(\pi(1-\alpha)) + 1\right)^{(\beta/2)}} \tag{4.41}$$

where $\theta = \arctan\{[(\sin(1-\alpha)\pi)/((t/\tau)\cos(1-\alpha)\pi)]\}$.

Havriliak–Negami expressions revert to their Cole–Cole, Cole–Davidson, and Debye equivalents at the limiting values of β, α, and α and β, respectively. In principle, this should be the model of choice for dielectric data analysis. In practice, it is not widely used to describe the dielectric properties of biological material, as will be discussed later. It is important to recall that these empirical distribution functions lack mechanistic justification; however, they do serve a useful purpose in enabling the parameterization of the experimental data, albeit with very limited clarification of the underlying mechanisms.

Another limitation of this type of analysis is the possibility of obscuring multi-relaxation processes, particularly the presence of a small amplitude dispersion following in the high-frequency tail end of a much larger principal one. This point is well illustrated by Wei and Sridhar (1993); they point out that a graphical representation of the parameter $\sigma'' = \omega\varepsilon_0(\varepsilon' - \varepsilon_0)$ versus $\sigma' = \omega\varepsilon_0\varepsilon''$ provides a more sensitive visualization of multi-relaxation processes.

4.3.2 Universal Law of Dielectric Relaxation

The Debye model and its many variations, including those described in this section, have been widely used over more than half a century primarily because they lend themselves to simple curve-fitting procedures. In particular, the Cole–Cole model is used almost as a matter of course in the analysis of the dielectric properties of biological materials. Mathematically, at the limit of high frequencies, the Cole–Cole function simplifies to a fractional power law, that is, both ε' and ε'' are proportional to $(\omega\tau)^{(\alpha-1)}$. This fractional power law behavior is at the basis of what is known as the universal law of dielectric phenomena developed by Jonscher, Hill, and Dissado (Jonscher 1983) for the analysis of the frequency dependence of dielectric data.

A model that combines features from Debye-type and universal dielectric response behavior was proposed by Raicu (1999). In the course of modeling broad dielectric dispersions, as is often observed in the dielectric spectrum of biological materials, Raicu (1999) found that neither approach was good enough over a wide frequency range. He proposed the following very general function

$$\hat{\varepsilon} = \varepsilon_\infty + \frac{\Delta}{\left[(j\omega\tau)^\alpha + (j\omega\tau)^{1-\beta}\right]^\gamma} \tag{4.42}$$

where α, β, and γ are real constants in the range of 0–1, τ is the characteristic relaxation time, and Δ is a dimensional constant, which becomes the dielectric increment ($\varepsilon_s - \varepsilon_\infty$)

Properties of Biological Materials 113

when $\alpha = 0$, and the above expression reverts to the Havriliak–Negami model, which further reduces to the Debye, Cole–Cole, or Cole–Davison models with an appropriate choice of the α, β, and γ parameters. For $\gamma = 1$, it reverts to Jonsher's universal response model; in the special case where $\gamma = 1$ and $\alpha = 1 - \beta$, it becomes

$$\hat{\varepsilon} = \varepsilon_\infty + \left(j \frac{\omega}{s} \right)^{\beta - 1} \qquad (4.43)$$

which is known as the constant phase angle model (Dissado 1990). In this expression S is a scaling factor given by $s = (\Delta/2)^{1/(1 - \beta)} \tau^{-1}$. The above expression was successfully used to model the dielectric spectrum of a biological material over five frequency decades from $10^3\,Hz$ to $10^8\,Hz$.

4.4 Dielectric Properties of Biological Materials—Main Components

Tissue is a heterogenous material containing water, dissolved organic molecules, macromolecules, ions, and insoluble matter. The constituents are highly organized in cellular and subcellular structures forming macroscopic elements and soft and hard tissues. The presence of ions plays an important role in the interaction with an electric field, providing means for ionic conduction and polarization effects. Ionic charge drift creates currents and also initiates polarization mechanisms through charge accumulation at structural interfaces, which occur at various organizational levels. Their dielectric properties will thus reflect contributions to the polarization from both structure and composition. In this section, the contribution of each of the components will be determined individually and then collectively, leading to the formulation of models for the dielectric response of biological tissue.

4.4.1 Water

Water is a constituent of all living things; it is the environment in which body electrolytes and biomolecules reside and interact. Knowledge of its properties must precede the study of the more complex system. Many of the physical properties peculiar to water are due to its molecular asymmetry, polar nature, and ability to hydrogen bond, which are all interrelated. Water is described as an associated liquid because of its intermolecular hydrogen bonding. One practical reason for emphasizing the study of water in this chapter is its increasing use as a reference liquid, that is, a material of well-known dielectric properties. Consequently, it is often used as a standard for the calibration and testing of dielectric measuring procedures. The dielectric properties of water are among the most studied and reported in the literature. Over the past decades, many experimental studies have been carried out to determine the dielectric properties of water over wide frequency and temperature ranges. These include Haggis et al. (1952), Lane and Saxton (1952), Hasted and El Sabeh (1953), Grant et al. (1957), Grant and Shack (1967), Grant and Sheppard (1974), Schwan et al. (1976), Grant et al. (1981), Hasted et al. (1985), Kaatze (1986, 1988), Buckmaster (1990), and Buchner et al. (1998). A comprehensive list of references and a historical overview of the subject can be found in Ellison et al. (1996). Other notable reviews were carried out by Kaatze (1989) and Liebe et al. (1991).

Data up to 100 GHz exhibit a near-perfect Debye dispersion with fairly well-defined parameters. Table 4.1 gives the Debye parameters for water at 20°C from three relatively

TABLE 4.1

Debye Parameters for Pure Water at 20°C

Review	ε_s	τ (ps)	ε_∞
Kaatze (1989)	80.2	9.47	5.2
Liebe et al. (1991)	80.1	9.35–9.39	5.3–5.4
Buchner et al. (1998)	80.2	9.32–9.52	5.9–6.0

Notes: For Liebe et al. (1991), τ and ε_∞ values are those of the single-Debye model (<100 GHz) and of the principal dispersion in the two-Debye model (up to 1 THz). Buchner et al. (1998) provide upper and lower bounds for τ and ε_∞ of the principal relaxation of a two-Debye model.

recent reviews. Kaatze (1989) used a Debye expression to model his own extensive experimental data covering –4°C to 60°C and 1 to 57 GHz in addition to what he considered to be credible data from other sources.

Liebe et al. (1991) gathered extensive static and high-frequency data. For frequencies up to 100 GHz and temperatures from 0°C to 30°C, the data were a very good fit to the Debye function. However, including data at higher frequency somewhat reduced the goodness of the fit, suggesting the possible presence of a much smaller secondary dispersion in the hundreds of gigahertz range. The next logical step was then to use a two-Debye model. This proved a good fit to all experimental data up to 1 THz, thus confirming the presence of a small, high-frequency dispersion, probably due to some subtle molecular mechanism. This secondary dispersion, centered around 670 GHz, brought down the high-frequency permittivity from 5.4 to 3.3 and made practically no impact on the characteristics of the principal dispersion, which were almost unchanged (Table 4.1). Liebe et al. (1991) extended the model to the far infrared (30 THz) by accounting for two near-infrared resonance absorption terms.

The most recent and comprehensive analysis of the dielectric properties of water is provided by Ellison et al. (1996), who critically reviewed the literature spanning the late 19th and most of the 20th centuries. With respect to the static permittivity, they obtained a function $\varepsilon_s = ae^{-b}$ with $a = 87.85306$ and $b = 0.00456992$, which predicts the value of ε_s at a given temperature to well within the limits of experimental accuracy for the range $-35°C < t < 100°C$. All high-frequency data (up to 1 THz) that met their selection criteria are tabulated. They stopped short of formulating models for the frequency dependence of the data; instead, they invited comments from the scientific community prior to the determination of what would probably be the ultimate model and spectral parameters for the dielectric properties of pure water, a finding that will greatly benefit this field of study. Already, other researchers have used this extensive survey. For example, Buchner et al. (1998) reported values for τ and ε_∞ of the principal water dispersion (Table 4.1) by fitting a two-Debye model to combined experimental data from Ellison et al. (1996) and other, more recent, studies (Barthel et al. 1995).

It is evident from Table 4.1 that the static permittivity and the relaxation time are fairly well-defined, less so the infinite permittivity. Fortunately, this parameter has little impact on the dielectric data in the gigahertz range because its value is only a small percentage of the permittivity in that frequency range. This relatively large uncertainty highlights the fact that even this most studied, pure substance is not a perfect reference liquid and that much remains to be done in the characterization of the dielectric properties of water at terahertz frequencies. Figure 4.3 is a plot of the dielectric properties of water at 20° tabulated by Ellison et al. (1996).

In biological materials, water is a solvent for salts, protein, nucleic acids, and smaller molecules. It is, therefore, important to study the effect of solutes on its dielectric response.

Properties of Biological Materials 115

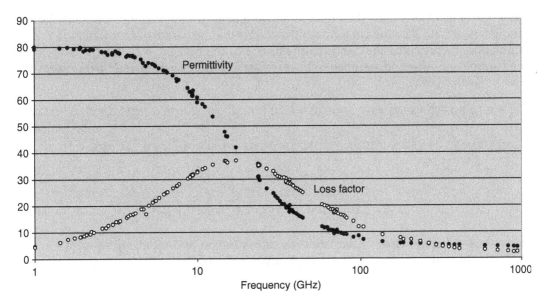

FIGURE 4.3
Experimental data from numerous sources reviewed and tabulated by Ellison et al. (1996).

4.4.2 Electrolytes

Electrolytes in the form of sodium, potassium, calcium, magnesium, chloride, and other ions play an important role in the function of biological systems. Many vital processes depend upon a subtle balance being established between the concentration of electrolytes inside and outside the cell. The cell membrane is, to a great extent, impermeable to the passive exchange of ions but allows directed movement under physiological control. In terms of dielectric properties, electrolytes have two effects. The direct effect is the production of ohmic currents and energy loss in the system. The indirect effect, polarization due to charge accumulation and ionic diffusion is discussed later in this section. Ionic conduction gives the system an additional conductivity term, σ_s, its value is commensurate with the ionic concentration and mobility and is conventionally referred to as static conductivity.

The Debye model for electrolytes in solution is thus:

$$\hat{\varepsilon} = \varepsilon_\infty + \frac{(\varepsilon_s - \varepsilon_\infty)}{1 - j\omega\tau} - \frac{j\sigma_s}{\omega\varepsilon_0} \tag{4.44}$$

The total conductivity σ is given by

$$\sigma = \omega\varepsilon_0\varepsilon'' = \sigma_s + \frac{(\varepsilon_s - \varepsilon_\infty)\varepsilon_0\omega^2\tau}{1 + (\omega\tau)^2} \tag{4.45}$$

It is customary to present the dielectric properties as ε' and σ versus frequency.

The dielectric properties of aqueous solutions of NaCl have been extensively measured and it was shown that the above model is applicable at low salt concentration (<0.5 mol/L). At higher concentrations, the data are better fitted to a Cole–Cole (Peyman et al. 2007a) and more recently Levy et al. (2012).

Peyman et al. (2007a) used their data to derive models for the variation of the dielectric parameters of NaCl solutions in terms of the corresponding parameter for water - (w) - and as function of concentration c and temperature t in the range 0–5 Mol/l and 5°C–30°C. The parameter ε_∞ was and assumed to have the same value as water, water parameters are those of Kaatze (1989).

$$\varepsilon_s = \varepsilon_s(w)\left(0.999 + 8.521 \times 10^{-4} tc + 0.013 c^2 - 0.175 c + 2.344 \times 10^{-4} t - 1.235 \times 10^{-5} t^2\right) \quad (4.46)$$

$$\tau(\sec) = \tau(w)\left(1.03 + 9.387 \times 10^{-5} tc + 0.012 c^2 - 0.091 c - 3.093 \times 10^{-3} t + 4.932 \times 10^{-5} t^2\right) \quad (4.47)$$

$$\sigma_i = 0.096 tc - 0.8 c^2 + 6.554 c \quad (4.48)$$

$$\alpha = 2.474 \times 10^{-4} tc + 2.101 \times 10^{-3} c^2 + 0.021 c \quad (4.49)$$

Figures 4.4–4.5 show effect of variation in concentration and temperature on dielectric properties of sodium chloride solutions (Peyman et al. 2007).

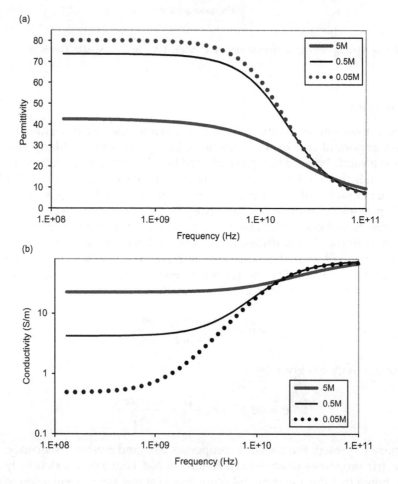

FIGURE 4.4
(a) Permittivity and (b) conductivity of different concentrations of sodium chloride solutions-data taken from Peyman et al. (2007a).

4.4.3 Carbohydrates

In quantitative terms, carbohydrates are not major constituents of animal cells; they are present at the surface of the cell membrane and are known to play a role in cellular communications. They are responsible for the gel consistency that gives certain body fluids such as vitreous humor and synovial fluid cushioning or lubricating properties. They are important constituents of certain tissues such as cartilage, tendon, and ligament. In terms of molecular structure, they vary in complexity and molecular size; they have in common the presence of one or more hydroxyl groups and the ability to hydrogen bond with each other or with water molecules. In aqueous solution, they modify the principal dispersion of water to an extent that depends on the nature and concentration of the organic radical. In general, the dispersion is likely to be broader than a Debye, the static permittivity lower, and the relaxation time longer than for pure water, as observed and reported by Bateman and Gabriel (1987) and more recently Levy et al. (2012).

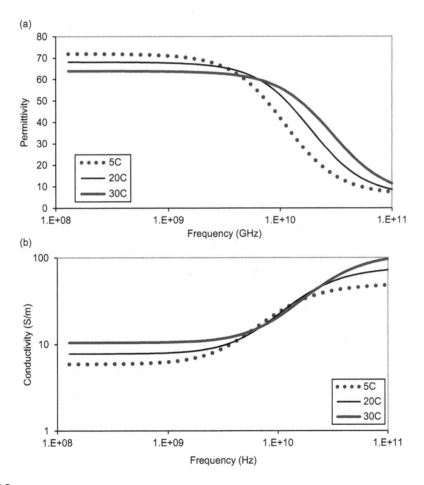

FIGURE 4.5
Effect of temperature on (a) Permittivity and (b) conductivity of 1 Molar sodium chloride solution-data taken from Peyman et al. (2007a).

4.4.4 Proteins and Other Macromolecules

Protein constitutes the bulk of the organic matter in the body. Proteins are described as biopolymers each molecule being a sequence of amino acids folded into a specific three-dimensional structure enclosing its hydrophobic sites within it. The surface has polar, hydrophilic groups with an affinity to bind water molecules from its surrounding aqueous environment. Part of the function of a protein resides in its structure, if the structure unfolds the protein is said to be denatured, and is no longer functional.

A good model for a globular protein in solution is that of a cluster of organic matter surrounded by a layer of strongly bound water, the solvent is referred to as free water to differentiate it from bound water. The size of the cluster depends on the molecular weight of the protein, which is typically of the order of tens or hundreds of thousands, that is, significantly larger than a water molecule. In an aqueous environment, most biological macromolecules including proteins act like polar molecules with permanent or induced dipole moment the magnitude of which depends on the molecular structure, configuration, and size. Dielectric spectroscopy is therefore an important tool in the study of these molecular properties.

Typically, the dielectric dispersion of a protein will be in the megahertz frequency range, corresponding to a time constant of the order of microseconds. The dielectric spectrum of an aqueous globular protein solution will have two dispersion regions corresponding to the polarization of the protein and water molecules, the larger the protein the more clearly defined they will be, conventionally, they are referred to as β and γ dispersion, respectively (Figure 4.6).

Figure 4.6 shows a conceptual spectrum of a binary, protein-water system, in practice, to maintain the conformational stability of the biological molecules inorganic ions, in the form of dissolved salts, must also be present. Table 4.2 has actual data, gathered from the literature, on the magnitude of the dielectric increment and the relaxation time for proteins

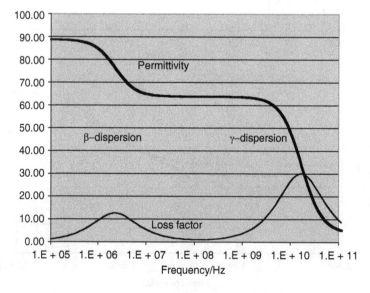

FIGURE 4.6
Conceptual representation of the dielectric spectrum of an aqueous protein solution. In practice, the two dispersions may overlap. The nearest to this picture is the complex permittivity spectrum of an aqueous solution of 1,2-dimyristoyl-L-3-phosphatidycholine reported by Kaatze and Giese (1980).

TABLE 4.2

Dielectric Parameters of Various Protein at 25°C

Protein	Mol wt ($\times 10^{-3}$)	$\Delta\varepsilon$	μD	$\tau - 10^8$ (s)	a/b
Myoglobin	17	0.15	170	2.9	
b-Lactoglobulin (in 0.25 M glycine)	40	1.51	730	15; 5.1	4
Ovalbumin	44	0.10	250	18; 4.7	5
Horse carboxyhemoglobin	67	0.33	480	8.4	1.6
Horse serum albumin	70	0.17	380	36; 7.5	6
Horse serum pseudoglobulin	142	1.08	1100	250; 28	9

Notes: a/b is the axial ratio that determines the shape of the molecule. Where the shape deviates significantly from the spherical, two relaxation times are observed (from Foster and Schwan 1989). The dielectric increment $\Delta\varepsilon$ (per g/l) the dipole moment μ is given in Debye unit (1 D = 3.33×10^{-30} Coulomb meter (Cm)).

of different shape, size, and dipole moment. Many authors have reported the presence of a small dispersion that is attributed to bound water, described as molecules that are more or less strongly bound or otherwise affected by the presence of organic matter. When present, the spectral region of the bound water is termed δ dispersion. The book by Grant et al. (1978) is a good introduction to this topic.

For aqueous solutions of small nucleotides (such as adenosine monophosphate/adenosine-5′-triphosphate) a single relaxation process is observed that reflects the water property and its variations at different solute concentrations (Puzenko et al. 2012).

Larger biopolymers such as DNA, whose molecular weight may be of the order of several million, have more complex dielectric spectra with dispersions extending from kilohertz to megahertz. The elucidation of the polarization mechanisms responsible for the dielectric spectrum of aqueous DNA solution is an area of active research. A good introduction to the subject is the book on biopolymers by Takashima (1989).

There is more than just academic interest in the study of biopolymers, advances in nanotechnology are such that biological macromolecules are being considered as possible nanoscale electronic devices for fast information processing and transfer.

4.4.5 Dielectric Dispersions in Tissue

The dielectric properties of a tissue relate to the bulk of the material, they are determined by its composition and cellular structure. Water, the main component of tissue is a polar molecule and most biological molecules are polar or polarizable; all contribute to the total polarization of a tissue. Other major polarizations originate from the structure of the tissue into cells enclosed by cell membrane and other intracellular membranous structures present in an aqueous ionic medium. The cell membrane is a barrier to the flow of ions. The boundary conditions at and around the interfaces gives rise to interfacial polarization and ionic diffusion effects quite apart from dipolar type dispersions that occur in the surrounding media.

The dielectric spectrum of a biological tissue (spleen at 37°C) is given in Figure 4.7 as an example of the response of a high water content tissue. Three main dispersion regions are immediately obvious and are referred to as α, β, and γ dispersions at low, intermediate and high frequency. The dispersions are broad indicating the possible overlap of discrete relaxations arising from the polarization mechanisms encountered in the complex biological environment. The main β dispersion is often analyzed as having an auxiliary smaller δ dispersion. Ionic conductivity contributes significantly to the loss factor, obliterating its

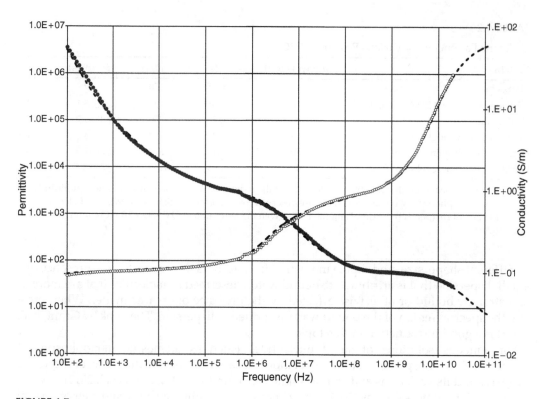

FIGURE 4.7
Dielectric spectrum of a high water content tissue (spleen at 37°C); experimental data from Gabriel et al. (1996b); dotted line is a best fit to a model of four Cole–Cole and a conductivity term.

features and it is more informative to express the dielectric properties of tissues as permittivity and conductivity as in Figure 4.7.

4.4.5.1 α Dispersion

The α or low-frequency dispersion is characterized by very high permittivity values. Such large dispersions are predicted by theories of ionic diffusion in ionic media near charged surfaces leading to the formation of counterions or electric double layers. The distribution of ions in the vicinity of charged interfaces is subject to concentration and electric field gradients. The time constant associated with this mechanism is long compared to other polarization mechanisms. Counterion phenomena are difficult to analyze rigorously; they involve coupled electrodynamic and hydrodynamic mechanisms. The theories are complex, but good reviews are available as an introduction to the subject (Dukhin 1971; Dukhin and Shilov 1974; Fixman, 1980, 1983; Mandel and Odijk, 1984).

While it is not possible to model the complexity of a tissue for counterion relaxation, simpler models predict dielectric increments of the right order of magnitude. One example that provides exact solutions has been proposed (Grosse and Foster 1987; Grosse 1988) where coupled differential equations for the ion concentrations and current densities are obtained for a macroscopic charged sphere in an ionic medium. Their solution yields a broad, asymmetrical, low-frequency dispersion. The time constant of this dispersion is depends on the size of the particle and the diffusion coefficient of ions in the bulk electrolyte.

Properties of Biological Materials   121

Other mechanisms, may also contribute to the α dispersion, many relate to the cell membrane which is a complex, dynamic structure. The main element of the cell membrane is a phospholipid bilayer with the hydrophilic groups covering the inner and outer surface and the hydrophobic lipids forming an inner layer. Embedded in the bilayer are proteins, transport organelles, and ionic channels that operate under physiological control. The ionic balance between the intra- and extra-cellular media maintains a 60–70 mV potential difference between them of about 10 kV/mm across the membrane, assuming a 6–7 nm thickness. Membrane-related mechanisms that are thought to contribute to the α dispersion include the charging of intracellular membrane-bound organelles and a frequency dependence in the impedance of the cell membrane itself. An important reason for the uncertainty in the determination of this dispersion is the paucity of error-free dielectric data in its frequency range. The α dispersion has a very large permittivity increment, the corresponding decrement in conductivity is small, this however, does not contravene the principle of causality and the Kramers–Kronig relations which predict a change in conductivity of about 0.005 S/m for a 10^6 increment in permittivity and relaxation frequency of 100 Hz.

4.4.5.2 β Dispersion

The β dispersion occurs at intermediate frequencies and originates mostly from the capacitive charging of the cellular membranes and those of membrane-bound intracellular bodies. This phenomenon, also known as interfacial polarization, has been studied theoretically and experimentally.

Modeling the electrodynamics of a simplified tissue-like system, for example, a suspension of spherical inclusions in conductive media, has established theoretical grounds for the presence of the β dispersions. It enables the computation of an effective permittivity for the mixture of similar order of magnitude to the β dispersion. The solution for the case of a dilute suspension of spherical inclusions in a continuum is given by the formulation known as the Maxwell–Wagner equation

$$\frac{\hat{\varepsilon} - \hat{\varepsilon}_1}{\hat{\varepsilon} + 2\hat{\varepsilon}_1} = v_2 \frac{\hat{\varepsilon}_2 - \hat{\varepsilon}_1}{\hat{\varepsilon}_2 + 2\hat{\varepsilon}_1} \tag{4.50}$$

where the subscripts 1 and 2 refer to the suspending medium and inclusions, respectively. Interfacial polarization is described as a Maxwell–Wagner effect.

Numerous mixture equations exist for different shape inclusions such as oblate and prolate spheroids. An interesting case is that of ellipsoids with their axes aligned in the same direction. The effective permittivity would be different depending on the direction of the field, the mixture would be electrically anisotropic and the effective permittivity represented by a tensor. The subject has been reviewed by, among others, Hanai (1968), Van Beek (1967), Dukhin (1971), Tinga (1992), Greffe and Grosse (1992), and Sihvola and Lindell (1992).

For a system of concentric shells in conductive media, (Hanai et al. 1988; Irimajiri et al. 1991), mixture theory predicts the presence of dielectric dispersions equal in number to the number of interfaces. These interfacial polarizations are boundary effects that occur in addition to other polarizations that may occur in the components of the system.

Another model of practical interest is that of layered spherical inclusions simulating cellular structures surrounded by a membrane of finite thickness. Solutions for the effective permittivity of this model were provided by, among others, Zhang et al. (1983) and Grosse

122 *Electromagnetic Fields*

(1988). These authors applied two mixture models once to the concentric bodies thus obtaining an effective permittivity for the inclusions and then treating the mixture as a suspension of homogeneous spheres. The parameters of the dispersion could be expressed in terms of the physical dimensions and electrical characteristics of the cell and cell membrane, simplified versions of these expressions are reported by Foster and Schwan (1989). Sihvola (1989), Irimajiri et al. (1991), among others, extended the treatment to several concentric shells by using a recursive technique. These complex models are more relevant to the study of biological system and to the understanding of the interactions at the cellular level, they are not sufficiently developed for the quantitative characterization of the interfacial polarization in biological tissue but do provide an insight into the factors that determine its characteristics.

An example is the modeling of the dielectric response of heart tissue by Schaefer et al. (2002). The model is function of the cell shape, electrical cell coupling, and polarization of cell membranes and intracellular structure. It describes heart cells and subcellular organelles as rotational ellipsoids filled with electrolyte enclosed by an isolating membrane and is capable of reproducing the main features of the dielectric spectrum of heart tissue.

In recent years, statistical methods using probabilistic descriptions of the physical mixture in terms of a spatial density function have been developed to provide realistic bounds for the effective permittivity of mixtures. This approach, developed by, among others, Bergman (1978) and Milton (2002), provides an analytic integral representation of the effective permittivity of an arbitrary binary mixture in terms of a spatial density function $g(x)$:

$$\frac{\hat{\varepsilon} - \hat{\varepsilon}_1}{\hat{\varepsilon}_1} = \int_0^1 \frac{g(x)\mathrm{d}x}{x + \hat{\varepsilon}_1/\hat{\varepsilon}_2 - \hat{\varepsilon}_1} \tag{4.51}$$

where, as before, the subscripts 1 and 2 refer to continuum and dispersed phases, respectively, and the integration is over all possible positions. Depending on the choice of distribution function $g(x)$, it is possible for the above equation to revert to some of the well-known binary mixture equations. Recursive application is possible; modeling biological systems remains challenging.

A new tool for the study of mixtures, including biological materials, has evolved with the development of increasingly powerful numerical modeling packages for the propagation of electromagnetic fields in complex structures from full solutions of Maxwell's equations. With structures being defined at the nanoscale, the characterization of fields within cells and subcellular structures appears to be within reach (Gimsa and Wachner, 1998, 1999, 2001a, 2001b; Bianco et al. 2000; Sebastian et al. 2001; Munoz et al. 2003).

It was established experimentally that damage to the cell membrane changes the features of the β dispersion. Numerous biomedical applications are based on the variation of the parameters of the β dispersion with pathological conditions involving changes in cell physiology and morphology. Tissue with directed, anisotropic cellular structure would, in theory, exhibit an anisotropic dielectric response in the frequency range of the β dispersion.

4.4.5.3 γ Dispersion

The γ dispersion is due to the molecular polarization of tissue water. At frequencies in excess of a few hundred MHz, where the response of tissue water is the dominant mechanism, the

Properties of Biological Materials

TABLE 4.3

Dielectric Parameters of Water Dispersion in Tissues Obtained By Analysis of Experimental Results at 37°C from Gabriel et al. (1996c)

Tissue	ε_s	τ (ps)	α	σ (S/m)
Bone (cortex)	14.9	13.8	0.26	0.092
Bone (section)	22.1	14.4	0.22	0.208
Cartilage	43.6	12.8	0.27	0.58
Cornea	53.0	8.72	0.13	1.05
Lens (cortex)	52.1	9.18	0.11	0.72
Lens (nucleus)	38.1	11.3	0.20	0.33
Retina	67.3	7.25	0.05	1.42
Brain (gray)	55.5	7.76	0.12	1.03
Brain (white)	37.0	8.04	0.24	0.47
Cerebellum	50.2	8.52	0.09	0.89
Dura	49.2	9.63	0.14	0.77
Brain stem	34.6	8.45	0.20	0.47
Tongue (in vivo)	57.7	9.12	0.08	0.63
Aq. humour	74.2	6.81	0.01	1.83
Water	74.1	6.2	0.0	<0.0001

complex permittivity may be expressed as Cole–Cole plus a conductivity term to simulate the dipolar dispersion of water and the contribution of the electrolytes, thus

$$\hat{\varepsilon}(\omega) = \varepsilon_\infty + \frac{\varepsilon_s - \varepsilon_\infty}{1 + (j\omega\tau)^{1-\alpha}} + \frac{\sigma}{j\omega\varepsilon_0} \tag{4.52}$$

where σ is the conductivity due to ionic currents and to the lower frequency polarization mechanisms. Table 4.3 gives the parameters of the γ dispersion of tissues modeled to the above expression. The water content of the tissues considered ranges from >95% for vitreous humor and >85% for retina to <20% for cortical bone. The correlation between ε_s and tissue water content is an obvious and expected result. The value of the distribution parameter α is significant for most tissues and negligible for body fluids (as for aqueous humor, for example). The mean relaxation time τ is generally longer than the value for water indicating a restriction in the rotational ability of at least some of the tissue water molecules. The lengthening of the relaxation time of water in biological material is a well-studied hypothesis, the effect is common to most organic solutes and is known to increases with solute concentration (Grant et al. 1981; Bateman et al. 1990) and has previously been observed in tissues (Gabriel et al. 1983).

4.4.5.4 δ Dispersion

The δ dispersion identified in some protein solution between the β and γ dispersions may also occur in tissue in the hundreds of megahertz range; when present, its magnitude is small compared to the adjacent ones. Possible mechanisms include the dipolar relaxation of bound water, relaxation of small dipolar segments or side chains of biological molecules and counterion diffusion along small regions of charged surface. Under these conditions, it is difficult to isolate and, in view of the multiplicity of possible mechanisms, difficult to interpret. It is often treated as the tail end of the β dispersion or a broadening of the γ dispersion.

4.5 Dielectric Properties of Tissue – Effective Permittivity - State-of-Knowledge

To account for the main dispersion regions and where adequate experimental data are available in the frequency range from Hz to GHz, the complex permittivity of a tissue can be adequately modeled with four Cole–Cole dispersions and a static conductivity term.

$$\hat{\varepsilon}(\omega) = \varepsilon_\infty + \sum_{n=1}^{4} \frac{\Delta\varepsilon_n}{1+\left(j\omega\tau_n\right)^{(1-\alpha_n)}} + \sigma_s/j\omega\varepsilon_0 \qquad (4.53)$$

In practice, the dispersion regions overlap resulting in interdependence of some of the parameters. It is a useful descriptive model, imparting no quantitative information on the polarization mechanisms. The measured dielectric properties represent the bulk response of the tissue.

In the last few decades, the research was driven, above all else, by the need to establish a credible database of dielectric properties of all body tissues for use in electromagnetic dosimetry studies, where the object is to quantify the exposure of people to external electromagnetic fields from knowledge of the effective internal fields and currents induced in them. In these studies, tissues are characterized by their measured dielectric properties.

4.5.1 Measurement Concepts

As with most physical quantities, the measurement of the dielectric properties of tissues is inherently simple in concept but relatively complex and varied in implementation. The choice of experimental procedure depends mostly, but not exclusively, on the frequency and temperature of interest, the nature of the sample, and the purpose of the measurement. At radio and microwave frequencies, the basic elements of a measurement system are: a source, transmission line, detector, and data acquisition instrumentation from which the characteristics of the line are determined. A sample placed within the transmission line will alter its characteristics in a manner depending on its dielectric properties which enable their calculation. For decades, researchers used single or narrow frequency sources and designed elaborate cells to contain the sample to be measured within a coaxial or waveguide line. The determination of a wide frequency spectrum was a tedious enterprise, limited mostly by hardware (for example: Nightingale et al. 1983 and Steel and Sheppard 1988).

At low frequencies, below about 100 MHz, full implementation of transmission line theory is not necessary; it becomes possible to measure the capacitive and conductive properties of the sample directly using impedance measuring circuitry from which the dielectric properties are calculated. In principle, sampling can be achieved with electrodes of any configuration and stray impedances from the circuitry can be calibrated out. However, the determination of the impedance of the sample is not straightforward because of the buildup of charges at the electrodes, a phenomenon known as electrode polarization. Electrode polarization is a naturally occurring phenomenon; it contributes to the measured dielectric properties. Its effects are most prominent at frequencies below about 10 kHz. Compensating for this phenomenon remains a challenge (Gabriel et al. 2009), a review of the subject by Chassagne et al. (2016) includes an assessment of the methods used to correct for its effect.

Properties of Biological Materials 125

Measurement at radio and microwave frequencies benefited from one main development, that is, the use of open-ended coaxial probes as samplers together with swept frequency instrumentation capable of characterizing the network parameters operating in the time or frequency domain (Gabriel et al. 1986; Gabriel et al. 1987; Gabriel et al. 1994). The analysis of the relationship between reflection coefficient and dielectric properties of the sample terminating the line has a much earlier history (Marcuvitz 1951; Galejs 1969; Hodgetts 1989; Nevels et al. 1985; Jenkins et al. 1992). Some early adaptation to the measurement of biological material include Burdette et al. (1980) and Stuchly and Stuchly (1980).

Today, open-ended coaxial probes are most commonly used with vector network analyzers running essentially in the frequency domain but offering some time domain capabilities. Open-ended probes are fairly broadband, the optimal probe size depends on the frequency range, centimeter size probes at frequencies below 100 MHz; millimeter size at higher frequencies. A tissue sample need only be placed in contact with the probe for measurement, no special encasing required. The sample is assumed semi-infinite relative to the size of the probe, isotropic, and homogeneous.

Advantages of this sampling technique are that it is non-destructive, requires minimal handling of the sample and could be used to measure tissue *in vivo*. One main limitation is that its radial geometry does not provide the directionality required for measuring anisotropic material.

The technique has been shown to be suitable for measurement of glossy liquids (Wei and Sridhar 1991 and Peyman et al. 2007a) and fairly robust when adequate conditions are used to measure standard liquids (Gabriel and Peyman 2006). For example, for a 2.98 mm probe in the frequency range of 300 MHz to 10 GHz, the total combined uncertainty, from random and systematic errors, did not exceed 1 percent for permittivity and conductivity across the whole frequency range.

A developing technology described as "electric properties tomography" (EPT) is a novel approach to the determination of the dielectric properties of tissue from data gathered during MRI. A brief description is provided under a separate heading at the end of this section.

4.5.2 Uncertainty in the Measurement of Biological Materials

A certain level of variability in structure and composition is inherent in biological tissue. The extent of variability depends on the tissue type, for instance, fat and bone tissues show greater variability than high water content tissues. For a measurement system free of systematic errors, sample variability, and sample handling are the main contributors to the measurement uncertainty for all tissue types. The standard deviation of the mean has been shown to be by far the largest element in the uncertainty budget for tissue dielectric properties (Gabriel and Peyman 2006). This is a statistical element that can be improved by ensuring the integrity of the sample, maintaining consistency in the sampling technique and increasing the number of samples. This statement applies to temperature-controlled excised tissue, that is, to measurements carried out *in vitro*. For best results, the probe is fixed in position and the sample brought in contact with it.

Measurements carried out on tissue *in vivo* could be subject to additional sources of error. For instance, it is sometimes necessary to reach out to the tissue sample by moving the probe and test cable, the change in position of the test cable introduces phase errors depending on the quality of the cable and the frequency range, these are evaluated experimentally and, when present, added to the total uncertainty. Limited access to and/or limited visibility of the target tissues may lead to poor sampling. Errors from other sources such as contamination of the contact surface by bodily fluid may also happen

4.5.3 Review of the Dielectric Properties of Tissues

The earliest reports of dielectric properties of tissues date from the turn of the 20th century. Some of the early work has been reviewed by Duck (1990) and Gabriel et al. (1996a, b and c) complemented the review with experimental data on 56 tissue types and analyzed the data in terms of Cole–Cole models. The resulting models are referred to as the 1996 database which remains widely used by researchers in the field. For this reason it will be briefly described and discussed.

More recent data will be presented in the context of conditions resulting in systematic variations in tissue properties.

4.5.3.1 The 1996 Database

The backbone of the 1996 database is a large experimental study providing data pertaining, almost exclusively, to excised animal tissue at 37°C. For most tissues, the characterization was over a wide frequency range, 10 Hz to 20 GHz, using three previously established experimental setups with overlapping frequency ranges.

Some examples (Figures 4.8–4.10) were selected to highlight aspects of the state of knowledge of the dielectric properties of tissues that are still current. Note the scarcity of literature data for brain at low frequencies. The data for muscle shows reasonable agreements at radiofrequency (RF) and microwave frequencies and a wide spread at low frequencies.

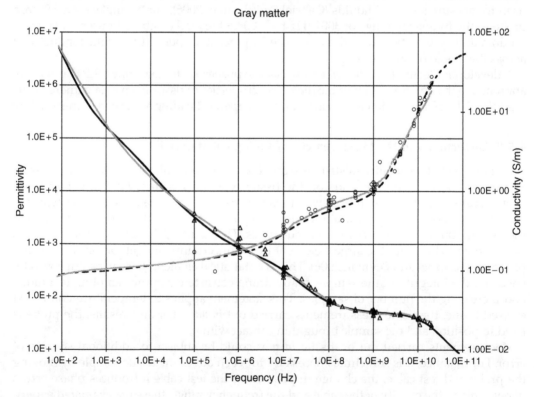

FIGURE 4.8
Permittivity and conductivity of gray matter at 37°C; gray lines are experimental data from Gabriel et al. (1996b), triangles and circles are permittivity and conductivity values from the pre-1996 literature, black solid and dashed lines are the predictions of the model.

Properties of Biological Materials

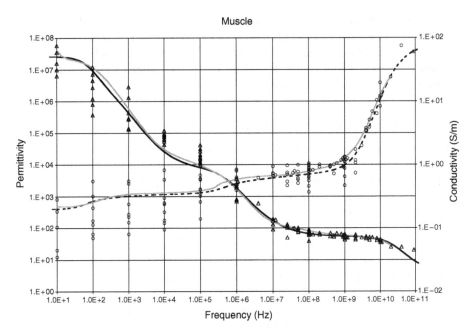

FIGURE 4.9
Permittivity and conductivity of skeletal muscle at 37°C; legend as in Figure 4.15, The very wide spread of data below 1 MHz is, at least partially, due to the anisotropy in the dielectric properties of muscle tissue. The literature data pertain to measurement along and across the muscle fibers and to measurements where the direction was not specified.

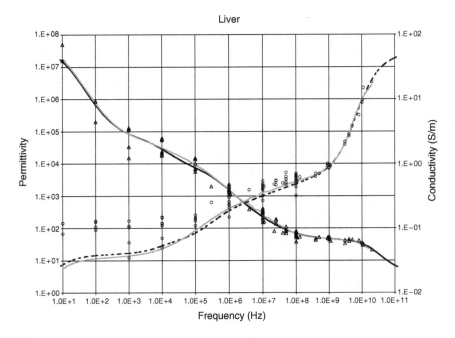

FIGURE 4.10
Permittivity and conductivity of liver tissue at 37°C; legend as in Figure 4.15, Liver tissue exhibit no significant anisotropy in its dielectric properties but as with all tissue, the characteristics of the dispersion and the static conductivity are sensitive the viability and time after death when the measurements were made.

This is attributed to the anisotropy of the tissue; the literature data includes both measurements along and across the muscle fibers. The 1996 measurement was carried out with a coaxial probe that is not designed for directionality. The structure of liver tissue is isotropic, the spread of data at low frequencies highlights the other possible source of differences between *in vivo* versus *in vitro* measurements.

4.5.3.2 In Vivo versus In Vitro Measurements

In an ideal case scenario, *in vivo* measurements would be preferred as more relevant biological applications. If systematic differences exist, between *in vivo* and *in vitro* measurements, they can lead to a better understanding of the underlying mechanisms. One fact, established with reasonable confidence, is that at high frequencies, the site of the γ-dispersion systematic differences have not been observed (Stauffer et al. 2003; Peyman et al. 2005; Farrugia et al. 2016). In this frequency range, tissue water content is the main determinant of the dielectric properties, when care is taken to avoid dehydration of the tissue sample, no systematic differences are observed between measurement carried out *in vivo* and *in vitro* as illustrated in (Figures 4.11 and 4.12) for gray matter, white matter, and spinal cord.

Bao et al. (1997) carried out measurements *in vitro*, with sample immersed in saline. Schmid et al. (2003a and b) measured porcine gray matter (*in vivo*) and human gray matter (*in vitro*). Their porcine gray matter data were obtained under conditions designed for the study of variation with time over a period spanning the time of death and beyond. In their human study, they measured postmortem human brain immediately after excision, in the frequency range of 800–2450 MHz. The measurements were carried out at room temperature in the range 18°C–25°C and extrapolated to 37°C using experimentally determined

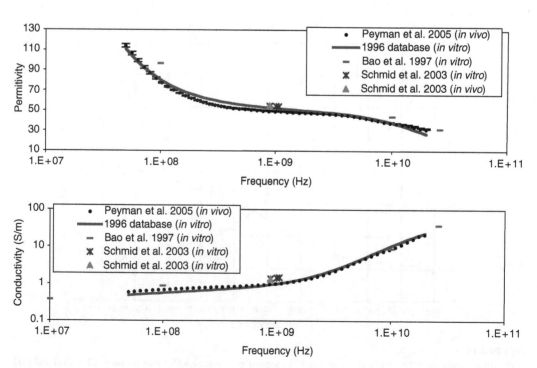

FIGURE 4.11
Reported (a) permittivity and (b) conductivity of skull tissues.

Properties of Biological Materials

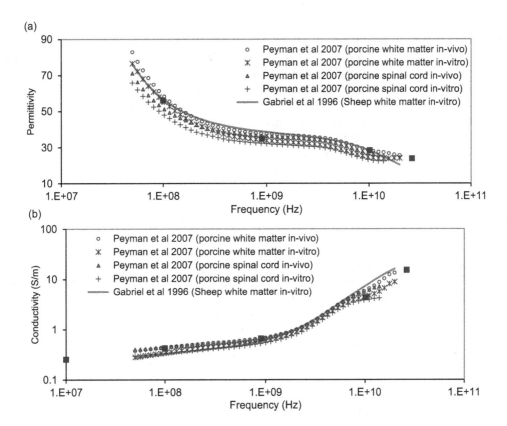

FIGURE 4.12
Dielectric properties (a) permittivity and (b) conductivity of gray matter, at 37°C. Data from recent studies compared to the prediction of the 1996 database.

thermal coefficients, the dielectric properties at 900 MHz were in good agreement with their data for porcine gray matter *in vivo*.

In vivo measurement are more relevant at lower frequencies, in the range of the α and β dispersions in view of the sensitivity of their causal mechanism on the physiological state of the tissue. Latikka et al. (2001) reported conductivity values at 50 kHz for gray matter (0.28 S/m), white matter (0.25 S/m), cerebrospinal fluid (CSF) (1.25 S/m) and tumors (0.1–0.43 S/m). They used a monopolar needle electrode during brain surgery on nine patients who had deep brain tumors. The authors noted that the measured values differ from those given by Schwan and Kay (1957), Geddes and Baker (1967), and Gabriel et al. (1996a). They ascribe the differences to the fact that their measurements were done *in vivo*.

4.5.3.3 Anisotropy of Tissue Dielectric Properties

The theory of interfacial polarization predicts that if the cells are elongated and aligned their dielectric properties would be anisotropic. The longitudinal fiber arrangement of skeletal, myocardial, lingual, and other muscle tissue are examples of anisotropic structures. Epstein and Foster (1983) observed marked differences in the dielectric response along and across the fibers at frequencies below 1 MHz. Notably, the static conductivity along the fiber was 6.6 times higher than across. Other aspects of the dielectric spectrum were also dependent on direction, the α dispersion was more prominent and the

β dispersion is less defined in the longitudinal direction. This is in accordance with the effective permittivity modeling of elongated structures predicted by Semenov et al. (2002) and Peters et al. (2001). The theory predicts an anisotropy ratio of the order of ten for the static conductivity of the muscle tissue model.

Practical difficulties in achieving field-fiber alignment means that anisotropy is not easy to observe experimentally (Fallert et al. 1993; Tsai et al. 2000; Gabriel et al. 2009) some of the problems associated with obtaining good data at frequencies below 1 MHz have been described by Tsai et al. (2000 and 2002) in the context of their *in vivo* measurement of swine myocardial resistivity. They did not observe anisotropy but report changes in the myocardial resistivity as a function of time after death.

Anisotropy has also been observed in tissues of the nervous system. Nicholson and Freeman (1975) used low-frequency current source mapping to determine the conductivity tensor for anuran (frogs and toads) cerebellum *in vivo* ($\sigma_x = 0.118 \pm 0.012$ S/m, $\sigma_y = 0.022 \pm 0.003$ S/m, and $\sigma_z = 0.012 \pm 0.004$ S/m). The conductivity component is highest in the direction parallel to the fibers (σ_x), and the components transverse to the fibers but parallel to the surface are much lower. Nicholson (1965) had previously reported similar anisotropy for white matter (cat, *in vivo*), a factor of 9–10 between the conductivity along and across the fibers. Ranck and BeMent (1965) pulsed low-frequency non-stimulating currents on the surface of the dorsal columns in the cervical cord of cats (*in vivo*) to obtain the electrical conductivity along (0.47 S/m) and across fibers (0.08 S/m).

Bone, cortical and cancellous, has anisotropic structure and, in consequence, anisotropic dielectric properties. For cortical bone, the ratio of the conductivity in the axial and radial dimensions is 3.2 (Reddy and Saha 1984). Cancellous bone is less anisotropic; the conductivity is higher in the longitudinal direction compared to the lateral and anterior–posterior directions (Saha and Williams 1989).

Huo et al. (2013) carried a simulative study to determine the reliability of methods of measuring the dielectric properties of anisotropic tissue. Their analysis identified probe design features necessary to detect the isotropic behavior when present. This is an area of importance to electrophysiology; among other applications, it is also an area where data are scarce.

4.5.3.4 Variation of Dielectric Properties with Age

Significant changes in tissue water content or a drastic event, such as the destruction of the cellular membrane, result in predictable and observable changes in the dielectric properties. Age-related physiological and morphological changes to tissues are gradual and varied; the rate at which they occur depends on the species and the type of tissue. For example, fetal liver and kidney are much nearer to the biochemical composition of the adult organs than are skeletal muscles or skin (Widdowson et al. 1960). In recent years, the need for rigorous assessment of the exposure of children to electromagnetic fields from telecommunication devices necessitated a more quantitative assessment of the dielectric properties as function of age.

Peyman et al. (2001, 2002) and Peyman and Gabriel (2003) showed that for some head tissues (brain, skin, and skull of new-born to fully grown rat) the permittivity and conductivity at microwave frequencies decreased systematically with age. Similar findings were obtained (Peyman et al. 2005 and 2007b) for porcine tissue from animal weighing 10, 50, and 250 kg to cover the developmental stages from piglets to mature animals. In this case, no variations were observed in the dielectric data of gray matter, while statistically significant variations were observed for spinal cord and white matter (Figure 4.13). The observed

Properties of Biological Materials 131

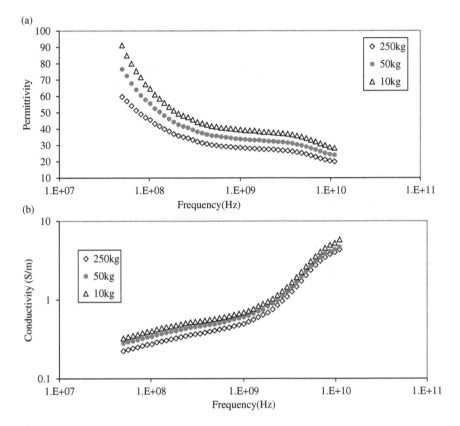

FIGURE 4.13
Dielectric properties of (a) Permittivity and (b) conductivity white matter and spinal cord, at 37°C. Data from recent studies compared to the prediction of the 1996 database.

variations are related to the process of myelination, which begins at birth and lasts till maturation. The skull bone of 10 and 50 kg pigs had the appearance of a soft tissue (wet to the touch, pitted and filled with red marrow) its dielectric properties were found to be closer to those of high water content tissues. This property appears peculiar to the skull bone of young pigs (Peyman et al. 2009). The skull bone of mature animals has a hard consistency and much lower conductivities (Figure 4.14).

Bone marrow was another tissue exhibiting systematic variation with age. The variation in dielectric properties correlated with the compositional variation of the tissue as it changes from red bone marrow, a relatively high water content tissue, to yellow bone marrow which is mostly a fatty tissue (Allen et al. 1995). Internal organs, (liver, kidney, heart, lung, and spleen) as well as cornea and tongue do not vary significantly throughout the lifespan.

The dielectric properties of fetal tissue have been measured at microwave frequencies by Peyman and Gabriel (2012). The study showed a trend of decrease in both permittivity and conductivity of rat embryo/fetus from 14 to 20 days (the total gestation period is 21–24 days). Although not very large, the change in dielectric properties reflects the decrease in total water content of the embryo/fetus as it develops. Furthermore, the dielectric properties of fetus are generally higher than those of adult muscle and brain tissues.

Dielectric properties of human pregnancy-related tissues have been studied by Peyman et al. (2011), indicating that the dielectric properties of placenta are higher than muscle

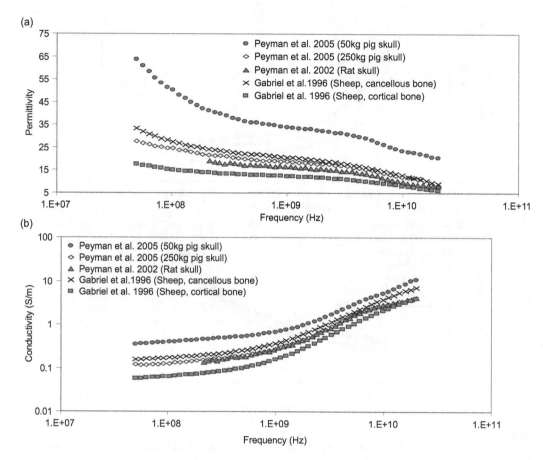

FIGURE 4.14
Permittivity and conductivity of white matter as a function of animal growth. The measurements were made *in vitro*, at 37°C. The lowest permittivity and conductivity spectra pertain to a fully grown 250 kg saw, the highest to a 10 kg piglet (data from Peyman et al. 2005).

and slightly lower than blood; generally closer to blood than muscle. The values recorded for permittivity and conductivity of umbilical cord, were higher than those of placenta. This could be due to the presence of many umbilical blood vessels and more importantly a thick and whitish substance called Wharton's jelly which cannot be found on any other part of human body.

Levy et al. (2017) found that the dielectric parameters of cytoplasmic water in stored red blood cells are sensitive to the age of the cells and coincides with age-related morphological change (transition from discocyte to echinocyte). From the analysis of the dielectric relaxation as a function of age, they postulated that the behavior is rooted in the interplay between bound and bulk water in the cellular interior.

4.5.3.5 Changes Following Death

Dielectric properties of tissues change postmortem as demonstrated by Haemmerich et al. (2002) and Pliquett et al. (2000) for porcine and canine liver in the range 10 Hz–1 MHz and 200 Hz–200 kHz, respectively. Their results showed that conductivity decreases after death and slowly increases again after 2 to 4 hours.

Properties of Biological Materials 133

Riedel et al. (2003) developed a contact-free inductive measurement procedure and demonstrated the system by carrying out conductivity measurements on liver tissue between 50 kHz and 400 kHz as a function of time after death. Although the absolute values of conductivity reported by this non-contact system had larger errors, the trend of change postmortem was similar to that observed by Haemmerich et al. (2002) and Pliquett et al. (2000).

4.5.3.6 Healthy versus Pathological Tissue

Changes to tissue structure and composition due to pathological conditions could, in principle, be monitored using dielectric measurements. Interest in this field of study is driven by the need to develop novel diagnostic and therapeutic tools using radio and microwave frequencies. Cancerous and ischemic tissues have been the subject of many investigations to establish differences between healthy and counterpart tissue that can serve as basis for clinical applications.

4.5.3.6.1 Cancerous Tissue

There is evidence that tumors have higher vascularity and water content and therefore higher permittivity and conductivity at microwave frequencies than the corresponding normal tissue as observed and reported by Schepps and Foster (1980), Foster and Schepps (1981), Rogers et al. (1983), Joines et al., (1994), Stauffer et al. (2003) and more recently O'Rourke et al. (2007), Lazebnik et al. (2007), and Peyman et al. (2015).

Morphological changes affect the dielectric properties in the frequency range of the β-dispersion and can be quite significant (Smith et al. 1986). Walker et al. (2000) used a finite element analysis to model the differences in impedivity between normal and precancerous cervical cells in the frequency range 100 Hz to 10 MHz. There results showed significant differences at frequencies lower than 10 kHz, basically in line with measurements carried out *in situ* with a four-electrode pencil probe. Polevaya et al. (1999) used time-domain dielectric spectroscopy to study the differences between normal and malignant white blood cells. They used a Maxwell–Wagner mixture formulation and a double-shell cell model to determine differences in cellular and nuclear membrane characteristics between normal and malignant cells. Their detailed analysis relates to some functional differences between membranes and provides some insight into the etiology of cancer.

Therapeutic and diagnostic applications emerged on the basis of the observed differences in dielectric properties. Radio and microwave hyperthermia are procedures whereby electromagnetic energy is preferentially absorbed by the cancerous tissue, usually as an adjunct to radiotherapy. Electromagnetic hyperthermia was an active field of study in the 1980s; it remains the domain of specialist medical centers. The advantages and limitations of the procedures are described by Stauffer and van Rhoon (2016) in the light of its use for the treatment of cancer of the bladder.

More recently, there has been a growing interest in applications geared toward the detection of cancerous legions using three-dimensional microwave tomography (MWT) procedures (Hagness et al. 1998 and 1999; Bulyshev et al. 2001; Wersebe et al. 2002). In brief, MWT is achieved using arrays of transmit and receive antennas around the subject and a demanding numerical analysis of the diffraction pattern to extract the dielectric properties and construct sectional maps of permittivity and conductivity. Semenov (2009) describes the technique, its successes, limitations, and potential for non-invasive assessment of functional and pathological conditions of soft tissues *in vivo*. Recently, improvement to both software and hardware by Grzegorczyk et al. (2012) enabled the development and deployment of the first clinical 3-D MWT system adequate for breast cancer screening and therapy monitoring. MWT remains an active field of research; its main strength is the wide range of dielectric properties, which allows for differentiation between tissue types and abnormalities (Meaney et al. 2013; Park et al. 2016). The ultimate goal remains to detect changes at the precancerous stage prior to their visibility by X-rays and to the emergence of serious clinical symptoms.

4.5.3.6.2 Ischemic Tissue

Ischemic changes develop in a tissue that is starved of its natural blood supply and nutrients. Ischemia can lead to irreversible damage to the cellular structure of the tissue that may be visible as changes to the dielectric spectrum in the region of the β-dispersion.

Ischemia in myocardial muscle is a matter of clinical importance in the assessment of myocardial infarction and has been the subject of many dielectric investigations. One of the drivers for this work is to test the possibility for using *in situ* impedance measurements to map the histological changes in tissue *in vivo*. There is also potential for non-invasive imaging provided that the electrical characteristics of both normal and ischemic tissue are well defined. Schaefer et al. (1999) and Miyauchi et al. (1999) observed changes in the α and β dispersions of normal and ischemic skeletal muscle. Schwartzman et al. (1999) investigated the properties of the border zone, which were found to be intermediate between healthy and infracted tissue in the case of chronically infarcted ventricular myocardium. Semenov et al. (2002) observed the dielectric properties of canine myocardium during acute ischemia and hypoxia to explore the potential for the clinical assessment of myocardial tissue using electrical impedance and MWT. One of the problems identified is the need to know and take into consideration the tissue electrical anisotropy.

Haemmerich et al. (2002) reported changes in the electrical resistivity of liver tissue during induced ischemia and postmortem. They observed increases in resistivity *in vivo* during occlusion. They analyzed the data in terms of intra- and extracellular resistance and cell membrane capacitance.

Strand-Amundsen et al. (2016) used impedance spectroscopy to measure changes in electrical parameters during ischemia in various tissues. They observed that the physical changes in the tissue at the cellular and structural levels after the onset of ischemia lead to time-variant changes in the electrical properties, which could provide means to assess the condition and the ischemic time duration. In the case of intestinal occlusion, they observed that changes in $\tan \delta$ $(=\varepsilon''/\varepsilon')$ measured at 31.6 kHz, within a 6-h period of the onset of ischemia correlates with physical changes in the tissue.

4.5.3.7 Species Specific Tissue: Skin

Published data on tissue dielectric properties pertain to human and animal tissue from many species. For example, data reported in Figures 4.7–4.9 correspond to human tissue as well as tissue from mouse, rat, cat, dog, pig, sheep, and others. In general, no systematic, species-specific variations are evident in the compiled data tissues. For most tissues, the variation in tissue properties within a species due to tissue inhomogeneity, age, viability, directionality exceed variations, if any, between species.

4.5.3.7.1 Skin

A notable exception to this general statement is skin, which is a species-specific organ. Within a species, skin varies depending on the part of the body and external conditions. Human skin has been the subject of many investigations as it is possible to carry out non-invasive, *in vivo* measurement using topical coaxial probes (Gabriel et al. 1996a, 1996b, 1996c;

Gabriel 1997; Raicu et al. 2000). However, the interpretation of the measured quantity as effective properties of the skin is not straightforward due to its layered structure (Lahtinen et al. 1997; Alanen et al. 1998). The outermost layer, the stratum corneum consists of several layers of dry cells; its purpose is to prevent dehydration from the inner layers of the epidermis and dermis. The stratum corneum can also absorb moisture from external application, which affects its dielectric properties and the measured effective dielectric properties of the skin (Gabriel 1997). Skin is the only tissue for which the dielectric data are available for both dry and moist conditions. Moistening provides good coupling to a topical measuring probe and reduces the effect of skin layers and affects the dielectric spectrum.

Raicu et al. (2000) carried out measurements on dry skin and on skin moistened with physiological saline, in the frequency range 100 Hz–100 MHz, the site of a very broad dispersion. They analyzed the data using a general dispersion model (equation 4.42) specially formulated to model this wide, multi-dispersion region. Their results are also consistent with the presence of a polarization originating at the stratum corneum/epidermis interface that occurs in dry skin, as suggested by Alanen et al. (1999), but not when saline moistened. It, therefore, appears that topical measurement on dry skin *in vivo* may not be proportionately representative of the inner layers.

In practice, the use of a coupling agent gives more reproducible results and leads to better agreement between data from the recent literature as evident from Figures 4.15–4.17 where recent data from the literature (Gabriel 1997; Raicu et al. 2000; Hwang et al. 2003; Petaja et al. 2003; Sunaga et al. 2002; Ghodgaonkar et al. 2000) collectively cover the frequency range 100 Hz to 100 GHz.

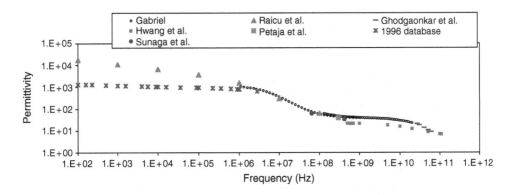

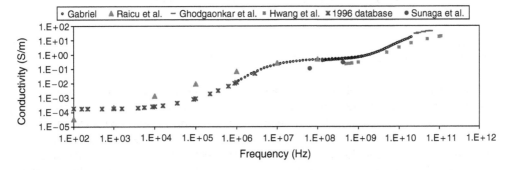

FIGURE 4.15
Permittivity and conductivity of skin (different parts of the body, excluding palms and soles). No moistening or contact gel was used. Different measurement techniques were used including open-ended coaxial probes of vastly different sizes.

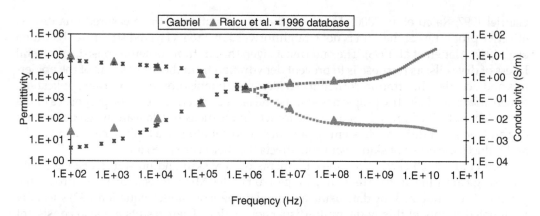

FIGURE 4.16
Permittivity and conductivity of skin (Raicu et al.: back of neck, moistened with physiological saline; Gabriel and database: ventral forearm, moistened with water). Open-ended coaxial probes of vastly different sizes were used.

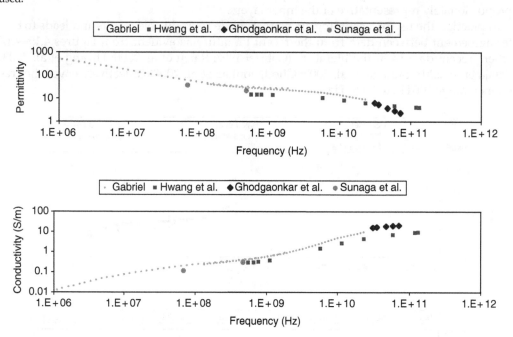

FIGURE 4.17
Permittivity and conductivity of palm, from independent studies.

The dielectric properties of skin have been widely investigated as monitors of various pathological conditions. Marzec and Wachal (1999) measured the conductance and susceptance of soles and calves of leg skin in healthy controls and patients with ischemia in the frequency range of 100 Hz to 100 kHz. Ischemia was found to have no effect on the admittance at frequencies lower than 10 kHz where the effect of the stratum corneum is dominant. Observed differences at frequencies in excess of 10 kHz are ascribed to ischemia in the underlying skin tissue.

Hayashi et al. (2005) in investigated the dielectric properties of human skin *in vivo* at frequencies up to 10 GHz to monitor the progress of the healing process of skin burns

Properties of Biological Materials 137

using water content as the determinant factor. Their measurement technique, time domain spectroscopy, and open-ended probe, is similar to that used by Gabriel et al. (1987), who reported the dielectric spectra of normal and wounded tissue and ascribed the differences to water content. Petaja et al. (2003) attempted to correlate the dielectric properties of skin at 300 MHz to body fluid changes after cardiac surgery and report limited success. Sunaga et al. (2002), investigated the variability in the dielectric properties of human skin of healthy volunteers, collagen disease patients, and dialysis patients over the frequency range of 1–450 MHz. No significant difference was detected in the dielectric properties among the three groups, some regional (abdomen, thigh, and forearm) dependence was observed.

Lindholm-Sethson et al. (1998) investigated the potential of using non-invasive skin impedance spectroscopy for the early detection of diabetic changes. They implemented a multivariate data analysis procedure to demonstrate how a regression model between the skin impedance and other diagnostic data for diabetic and control groups can be developed into a novel diagnostic tool for the early discovery of possible complications for diabetic patients. Statistical procedures are increasingly being applied to correlate dielectric parameters to structural or compositional elements of biological material, particularly in cases where there is a physical mechanism underpinning the effect that is obscured by noisy data (for example, Kent et al. 2002).

Dielectric spectroscopy is used to monitor damage to the skin caused by ionizing radiation to assess the side effects of clinical radiotherapy objectively and quantitatively. It appears that the changes to the skin during the acute stage cause both the permittivity and conductivity to decrease (Tamura et al. 1994; Nuutinen et al. 1998) while the reverse happens when radiation-induced fibrosis finally sets in Lahtinen et al. (1999). The initial decrease in permittivity, which also means a decrease in skin hydration, may be due to damage to skin capillaries resulting in a reduction in the effective microcirculation of the skin. In the long term, an increase in collagen and collagen-bound water is a likely explanation for the observed increase in the permittivity in line with a clinical indicator of subcutaneous fibrosis (Lahtinen et al. 1999).

4.5.4 Conductivity of Tissue at Low Frequency

There are limited, reliable dielectric data for body tissue at frequencies below 100 kHz. Some of the reasons relate to the dependence of the dielectric properties on the physiological state, degree of perfusion, time after death, and other biological parameters. There are also experimental difficulties, in particular, electrode polarization, which is a major source of systematic error at frequencies below 100 Hz even when precautions are taken to minimize its effects (Gabriel et al. 2009). Based on typical tissue dielectric data and a simple model for the electrode polarization, it is possible to estimate that it affects the permittivity more than the conductivity and that, for body tissue, the conductive rather than the capacitive component dominate their electrical admittance (Schwan 1992; Gabriel et al. 2009).

The conductivity of body tissue can be estimated by modeling on a cellular scale and applying appropriate mixture equations. Using this approach, Peters et al. (2001) evaluated the effective conductivity of several tissues such as cerebral cortex, liver, and blood. Such studies help place upper and lower bounds on the conductivity values based on cellular parameters and knowledge of the conductivity of the phases.

Faes et al. (1999) carried out a meta-analysis of review studies (Geddes and Baker 1967; Stuchly and Stuchly 1980; Duck 1990; Gabriel et al. 1996a and b) of tissue conductivity in the frequency range 100 Hz to 10 MHz. To make relative comparisons between different

TABLE 4.4

Conductivity (S/m) of Various Tissues in the Range of
40–70 Hz (from Gabriel et al. 2009)

Tissue	40–70 Hz
Muscle (0°)	0.15 ± 0.014
Muscle (90°)	0.19 ± 0.018
Muscle (transverse)	0.16 ± 0.037
Heart (atrium)	0.48 ± 0.13
Skull	0.32 ± 0.38
Fat	0.078 ± 0.019
Lung (inflated)	0.042 ± 0.014
Lung (deflated)	0.11 ± 0.069
Liver	0.091 ± 0.024
Urine	1.87 ± 0.69
CSF	1.59 ± 0.18
Bile	1.27 ± 0.15
Blood	0.60 ± 0.21

Note: *In vivo* measurements on 50 kg pigs. Body fluids measured *in vitro* immediately upon retrieval.

tissues, they calculated the mean and 95% confidence interval. They found large confidence intervals such that the conductivities of most high water content tissues (skeletal and cardiac muscle, kidney, liver, lung, spleen) were not statistically different from one another at that level of significance. By contrast, blood has higher conductivity while bone and fat have lower conductivities. The insignificance of differences in high water content tissues could, of course, imply an equality of their conductivities, but could also point at a large source of experimental variation which obscures real differences.

Data from Gabriel et al. (2009) are given in Table 4.4. In the case of skeletal muscle, the dimension of the sampling probe did not allow for the anisotropy of the conductivity of muscle tissue to be observed. The conductivity of bone (mid-sectional part of the skull of 50 kg pigs) is peculiar to young pigs (see Figure 4.14 and accompanying text).

4.5.5 Nonlinear Dielectric Properties

The polarization mechanisms discussed so far occur from interactions with weak fields eliciting linear responses. At high-field strength, nonlinear molecular and cellular polarization phenomena are predicted on theoretical grounds, on the basis of induced dipolar properties and classical electrodynamics. The threshold for initiating such effects is system and frequency dependent. As a general rule, as the frequency increases, so does the field level required to cause an effect. In general, at frequencies below the manifestation of the β dispersion, field strengths of the order of $10^{6\,V/m}$ may be capable initiating polarization mechanisms that affect the cellular function, higher fields may cause dielectric breakdown within the membrane, ultimately leading to cell destruction.

Under controlled conditions, high-field strength, nonlinear effects are the focus numerous applications in biotechnology. For example, dielectrophoresis or the motion of particles caused by electrical polarization effects in non-uniform fields, is used to separate and manipulate cells. For a review of this subject, see Pethig (1996). Another nonlinear phenomenon, electroporation, is a consequence of the electric breakdown of biological

Properties of Biological Materials   139

membranes resulting in the formation of pores and a significant increase in the membrane permeability to external ions and molecules. Under controlled conditions, electroporation could be reversible and used to advantage in therapeutic, drug-delivery applications. The basic principles can be found in mechanistic studies by Prausnitz et al. (1999), Pliquett and Weaver (1996), and many others.

The hypothesis that weak fields may trigger nonlinear effects in cells has been investigated in theory and practice (Woodward and Kell 1990; Weaver and Astumian 1990). The generation of harmonics is one aspect that can be used to monitor their occurrence (Woodward and Kell 1990); it also means that the dielectric properties are nonlinear, responding to harmonics as well to the fundamental frequency.

Balzano (2002) and Davis and Balzano (2010) proposed to use a similar approach to test whether biological cells exhibit nonlinear responses to weak fields, at microwave frequencies. They designed a resonant cavity capable of detecting a microwave signal at 1.8 GHz (2nd harmonic of 900 MHz) as weak as one microwave photon per cell per second. However, no second harmonic was detected from any of the cells or tissue tested at levels down to the noise floor of their system at about—160 dBm with a fundamental drive power into the cavity of 0 dBm (1 mW).

4.5.6 Electric Properties Tomography

"Electric Properties Tomography" (EPT) is a novel technique that derives the electric conductivity and permittivity of tissues, non-invasively, quantitatively, *in vivo* using a standard magnetic resonance (MR) system and standard MR measurements. Unlike MWT, EPT does not require externally mounted electrodes. Instead, the conductivity and permittivity are derived by post-processing the measured spatial magnetic field distribution B_1 of the RF transmit coil applied. The idea of EPT was first mentioned in an article from the early 1990s (Haacke et al. 1991), but systematic research started in earnest in 2009 spearheaded by the work of Katscher et al (2009). Katscher and van den Berg (2017) is comprehensive review of the subject to date.

The tissue dielectric properties and the measured B_1 are related by the so-called Helmholtz equation, which results from a combination of two of Maxwell's equations, Faraday's law and Ampere's law. The solution of this Helmholtz equation, however, requires the measurement of all three spatial components of B_1, however, MR imaging allows the measurement of only one of these three components. Assuming locally constant electric properties, which is sufficiently fulfilled within organs and tissue compartments, a "truncated" Helmholtz equation can be derived, which can be based on the single spatial B_1 component measurable with MR. Thus, the truncated Helmholtz equation is typically used for MR-based EPT investigations. Disregarding higher-order terms, the conductivity relates to the phase of B_1, and permittivity relates to the magnitude of B_1. So far, clinical EPT studies were focusing on B_1-phase-based conductivity determination, since the phase of B_1 can be measured much easier, faster, and more accurate than the magnitude of B_1. The dielectric properties obtained with EPT correspond to the Larmor frequency of the MR system used, which in turn depend on B_0, the static magnetic field strength. Typically, 64 MHz (for $B_0 = 1.5$ T), 128 MHz ($B_0 = 3$ T), sometimes also 21 MHz ($B_0 = 0.5$ T) or 300 MHz ($B_0 = 7$ T).

EPT has been evaluated by investigating phantoms with different, *a priori* known electric properties, typically yielding a high correlation between expected and measured values. EPT studies of healthy volunteers yielded electric properties in line with the expected values (1996 database). The observed inter-subject variability of measured electric properties is typically somewhat above 10%, the intra-subject variability somewhat below 10%.

Clinical EPT studies currently focus on tumors in breast (Kim et al. 2016) and brain (Tha et al. 2017). These pilot studies indicate a correlation between malignancy and conductivity. On one hand, the observed tumor conductivity is typically clearly larger than conductivity of surrounding healthy tissue. On the other hand, conductivity seems to be able to distinguish also between different tumor types, or between different malignancy grades. An additional evaluation of EPT is given in Tha et al. (2017) where *in vivo* tumor conductivity (measured with EPT) correlates with *ex vivo* conductivity (of the excised tumor specimen measured with an independent probe).

Furthermore, electric properties obtained with EPT are expected to be useful not only as biomarker, but also as input for patient-individual estimation of the Specific Absorption Rate (SAR) important in the framework of MR safety management (Liu et al. 2017) as well as input for hyperthermia treatment planning (Balidemaj et al. 2016).

4.6 Magnetic Properties of Matter

The magnetic properties of matter are a measure of their interaction with an externally applied magnetic field. The interaction occurs at the level of moving subatomic particles and their associated atomic currents and magnetic dipole moments. In as much as all matter contains moving subatomic particles all matter has some inherent magnetization. The relative permeability μ is a measure of the magnetization in the material compared to free space.

Another parameter used to characterize magnetic materials is the magnetic susceptibility χ_m with $\chi_m = \mu - 1$, where the subscript m is to differentiate it from the dielectric susceptibility [5].

For linear, isotropic materials, the relation $B = \mu\mu_0 H$ can also be written as:

$$B = \mu_0 (H + M) \text{ and } M = \chi_m H \tag{4.54}$$

where M is the magnetization per unit volume in the material, that is, the sum total of magnetic moments per unit volume. These expressions mirror the relationship between polarization and electric field parameters (Equations 4 and 5). By definition, in free space, $\mu = 1$ and $\chi_m = 0$.

In time dependent, harmonic fields of angular frequency ω, $\chi_m(\omega) = M(\omega)/H(\omega)$ if the magnetization and magnetizing field experience a phase difference, the susceptibility is expressed as a complex number with an in-phase, real component χ'_m and an out-of-phase, imaginary component χ''_m (van Berkum et al. 2013). However, for biological materials, the frequency dependence of χ_m is not, at present, a matter of practical interest, the assumption is that $\chi_m(\omega) \approx \chi_m(0)$ for human tissues. The basis of this assumption is that for static and low frequencies, the induced magnetic field is determined by the magnetizing field and the magnetic susceptibility, at high frequencies, magnetic susceptibility loses its relevance because the electric component is dominant in determining both the induced electric and magnetic fields. Consequently, in situations of human exposure to electromagnetic fields it is acceptable to assume $\mu = 1$ and $\chi_m = 0$ for all tissues. However, the magnetic susceptibility is determined by the material structure and composition, so different tissues have different magnetic susceptibilities. In recent years, it has become possible to determine these properties and use the differences to great advantage in numerous biological applications. The new techniques have extended to the determination of magnetic anisotropy in certain tissues.

Properties of Biological Materials

4.6.1 Molecular origin

Magnetization has its origin in the atomic and molecular configuration and the tendency of their atomic constituents to behave as magnetic dipoles. For instance, electrons orbiting a nucleus are equivalent to a circulating current and have a magnetic moment similar to that for a current loop. There are larger magnetic moments associated with the electronic spin.

In quantum mechanical terms, electrons may assume two possible spin states: spin +1/2 or spin –1/2. These may also be referred to as "spin up" and "spin down." The Pauli exclusion principle states that no two electrons may occupy the same energy state in an atom. This means that no two electrons may have the same set of values for the quantum numbers as they would then be indistinguishable. As electrons are added, they fill up each possible state in a given shell before filling the shell associated with the next higher energy state. The filling of the shells is governed by Schrödinger's wave equation and the quantum numbers.

Electrons are added to subshells in parallel spin configurations first according to Hund's rule. If all electrons are paired, there is no spin magnetic moment. These materials are still magnetic though, because of the orbital motion of the electron. In most materials of biological origin, electron spin motion is cancelled, allowing electron orbital motion to dominate.

The spin structure of the transition series elements (iron in particular) is most important for the magnetic properties of biological materials. This is due to the presence of uncompensated spins in the 3D orbital, which gives rise to a spin magnetic moment. The spin moment is much stronger than the orbital moment and is aligned parallel to an applied field.

Atomic nuclei have much smaller magnetic moments than electrons; their contribution to the susceptibility is negligible. However, the study of their interaction with very high magnetic fields, magnetic field gradients, and RF fields, illicit resonant effects (Nuclear Magnetic Resonance) and has many important academic and practical applications. Recently, MRI technology has been used to map the magnetic susceptibility of tissues *in vivo*. This emerging technology, quantitative susceptibility mapping (QSM) is fast becoming an important source of information about the magnetic properties of biological tissues.

Anisotropy in magnetic properties originates from certain molecular configurations as, for example, when biomolecules have non-spherical distribution of electrons. When such molecules are spatially ordered within a tissue to form elongated substructures, the tissue exhibits a bulk anisotropic susceptibility.

The origin of the magnetic moment—spin and orbital motion of electrons—and their interactions determines the magnetic behavior and the classification of matter into one of three categories: diamagnetic, paramagnetic, or ferromagnetic.

The different types of magnetic materials will be briefly described followed by the implications for biological materials.

4.6.2 Diamagnetic Materials

Diamagnetism originates from the non-cooperative behavior of orbiting electrons. Diamagnets are materials in which all electron spins are paired, the paired spin magnetic moments cancel out and do not contribute to the susceptibility. The magnetic properties of diamagnets are determined solely by the electron orbital motion. There is no net magnetic moment when there is no applied field.

When subjected to an external magnetic field those electrons in orbit planes at a right angle to the field will experience a force in accordance with Faraday's Law of electromagnetic induction. This leads to a change in their angular momentum and magnetic moment. The individual magnetic moments no longer cancel completely and the material acquires an induced magnetic moment that is opposite in direction to the applied field in accordance with Lenz's Law; this behavior defines diamagnetism. The magnetic susceptibility is negative and small.

Diamagnetic materials are repelled by a magnet, but the effect is imperceptibly small for all practical purposes in weak and moderate fields. The magnetic susceptibility is of the order of 10^{-6} to -10^{-5} and is independent of temperature.

Water and most organic materials are diamagnetic. So are sodium and chlorine ions and their salts. Inert gases and some metal such as gold, copper, and mercury fall in that category too. In fact, all materials experience a diamagnetic response, however, the effect being weak, cannot be observed in the presence of other types of magnetic responses such as paramagnetism.

4.6.3 Paramagnetic Materials

Paramagnetic materials are those in which individual atoms, ions, or molecules have a number of uncompensated spins and thus a permanent net-spin magnetic moment, which are randomly oriented because of thermal agitation. As previously stated, the spin moment is much larger than the orbital moment, so we would therefore expect that the behavior of paramagnetic materials when placed in a magnetic field will be governed by the behavior of the spin magnetic moments. This is indeed the case.

When paramagnetic substances are placed in an external magnetic field, the uncompensated spin moments tend to align, to some degree, parallel to the applied field direction (Figure 4.18). The magnetic energies involved in this alignment are relatively small, and the energy associated with thermal agitation tends to work against the alignment, having a randomizing effect. The degree of alignment of the uncompensated spins with the applied magnetic field depends, therefore, on the strength of the field (the stronger the field, the greater the degree of alignment up to very high fields) and the temperature (the hotter the material, the lower the degree of alignment in the same applied field).

Since the spin moments in paramagnetic materials align with the applied field in this classical model, they add to it, so that the net effect is that these materials are attracted to a magnetic field (and they have a positive magnetic susceptibility). The inverse temperature dependence of the magnetic susceptibility in paramagnetic materials is known as Curie's law:

$$\chi_m = \frac{C}{T} \tag{4.55}$$

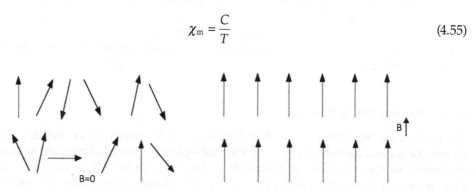

FIGURE 4.18
Orientation of spins in a paramagnet in the absence of a magnetic field (left) and in the presence of a strong magnetic field (right).

where T is the absolute temperature, and C is the Curie constant and is related to the magnetic properties of the material.

In paramagnetic materials, the individual dipole spin moments of the ions may be thought of as non-interacting (in other words, the magnetic moment of one atom has no effect on its neighboring atoms in the material). Because of the non-interaction of the magnetic moments, this fairly weak effect (paramagnetism) is lost upon removal of the external field. Therefore, when a paramagnetic material is not in an external magnetic field, the net-magnetic moment in the material is zero because of the randomizing effects of thermal agitation.

The susceptibility is small and positive, typically of the order of $+10^{-5}$ to $+10^{-3}$. Examples of paramagnetic materials include some metals like aluminum and platinum; some diatomic gases like oxygen; some biologic molecules like hemoglobin. Paramagnetic materials are attracted to a magnet but the effect is almost as weak as diamagnetism.

Diamagnetism and paramagnetism are the most common types of magnetism, between them they account for most elements in the periodic table. In a way, they are magnetic equivalent to non-polar and polar materials.

4.6.4 Ferromagnetic Materials

As in paramagnets, in ferromagnetic materials, there are also uncompensated spins; however, these spins are coupled, giving rise to strong magnetic effects. Ferromagnetism may be thought of as a group phenomenon, where groups of spin moments act in concert, whereas paramagnetism may be thought of as an individual phenomenon, where the moment of one atom has little or no effect on the moment of neighboring atoms.

In ferromagnetic materials, as in paramagnets, the magnetic susceptibility is positive, and these materials acquire a positive magnetization when placed in an applied field because of alignment of the spin moments in the material with the field. Unlike paramagnets, however, the net magnetization is not lost upon removal of the field (as long as the material is below a certain temperature, which will be discussed in a moment), and the induced moment in the material may be very strong (Figure 4.19). This is to say that ferromagnetic materials exhibit hysteresis.

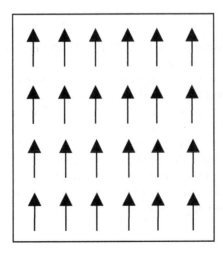

FIGURE 4.19
In ferromagnets, all spins are coupled and aligned, even in the absence of an applied field. This is the origin of remanent magnetization (i.e., hysteresis) in materials.

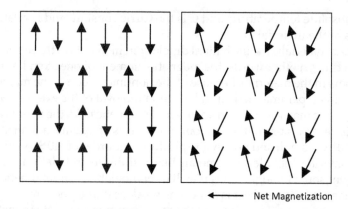

FIGURE 4.20
Pure anti-ferromagnetic behavior in which spins are coupled antiparallel to each other (left) and an antiferromagnet with a canted spin structure that gives rise to a net magnetization even in the absence of an applied field (right).

The mechanism responsible for coupling of the spin magnetic moments in neighboring atoms in a material is due to quantum mechanical phenomena and is governed by the Pauli exclusion principle. The uncompensated spins in individual atoms of a ferromagnetic material may couple either directly (direct exchange) or through an intermediate anion—usually oxygen (super-exchange). In ferromagnetic materials, this gives rise to a net-magnetic moment because of the coupling of spins in a preferred orientation. Keep in mind that this coupling is quantum mechanical in nature and not purely due to magnetic forces acting between uncompensated spins in neighboring atoms.

The susceptibility is positive and large at temperatures below the Curie point.

There are also special cases of ferromagnetism in which neighboring spins are coupled, but not necessarily in the same direction. We will examine two of these cases, anti-ferromagnetism and ferrimagnetism, as they are important to biological materials, though there are others.

4.6.4.1 Anti-ferromagnetism

For some ferromagnetic materials, the exchange coupling between neighboring lattice elements is such that the spins are aligned opposite to each other. This is called anti-ferromagnetism, and the exchange coupling arises from super exchange according to the Pauli exclusion principle and Hund's rule (Figure 4.20).

In this case, the spin moments will still align themselves to an external applied field, only some will be parallel to the applied field and those exchange coupled to them will be antiparallel. This would normally give rise to a material with no net-magnetic moment if for every spin up it was coupled to a spin down. This is not, however, always the case. In some materials, there is a canted anti-ferromagnetic spin structure (Figure 4.21) or lattice defects and frustrated surface spins (in very fine particles), which can give rise to a net moment in the absence of an applied field.

4.6.4.2 Ferrimagnetism

In addition to anti-ferromagnetic materials, it is also possible for the neighboring lattice subunits to have unequal numbers of uncompensated electrons coupled antiparallel to

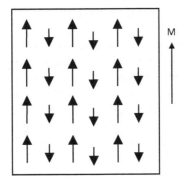

FIGURE 4.21
Electron spin configuration for a ferrimagnet. M = magnetization.

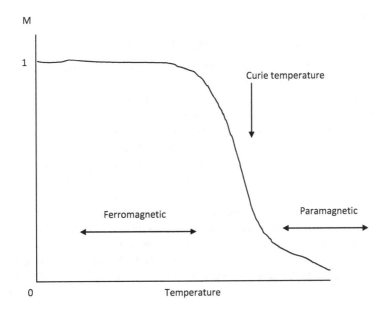

FIGURE 4.22
Magnetization as a function of temperature for a ferromagnet. Above the Curie temperature, spin coupling breaks down, and the material behaves as a paramagnet.

each other. This is the case for magnetite (Fe_3O_4), which contains both Fe^{2+} and Fe^{3+} in its lattice structure. The unequal distribution of the two neighboring iron ions gives rise to a net moment (again, even in the absence of an applied field) since one sublattice will have a magnetic moment of greater magnitude than the other, as shown in Figure 4.22. This type of material is called ferrimagnetic.

4.6.5 Temperature Dependence of Ferromagnetism

Since ferromagnetism results from the interaction of atomic moments in materials, there is an exchange energy associated with coupling of the spin moments. At room temperature, this exchange energy is much greater than the energy due to randomizing thermal effects (kT). If thermal energy exceeds the spin coupling (exchange) energy, the coupling breaks down, and the material behaves as a paramagnet. This temperature is dependent on the material and is called the Curie temperature (or, in the case of anti-ferromagnetic materials, the Néel temperature) (Figure 4.22).

Finally, materials that are superparamagnetic are generally very small (on the order of nanometers), and the electron spins may be coupled either parallel (ferromagnet) or anti-parallel (ferri- or anti-ferromagnet). In the case of these materials, however, thermal considerations are dominant. Superparamagnetic materials are named as such because thermal energy causes them to behave—even though this is a special class of ferromagnetism—like a paramagnet. The difference is that, because of coupling of the spin moments, thermal energy causes the spins to flip rapidly as a group rather than individually, as is the case for paramagnetism. On a macroscopic level, the behavior of the two is very similar, except at low temperatures when the thermal energy is sufficiently reduced.

4.7 Magnetic Susceptibility of Biological Materials

There are very few reports of direct measurements of the susceptibility of tissues because: the susceptibility is very small, tissues are heterogeneous and difficult to work with in a susceptometer (Schenck 1996). There have, however been studies of some tissue components for example water, hemoglobin, and lipids. Water is a main constituent and has a susceptibility of -9.05×10^{-6}; and most tissues have susceptibilities within $\pm 20\%$ of that of water. However, the body contains iron and trace amounts of several paramagnetic metal ions such as copper, manganese, and cobalt. Adult humans have about 40–50 mg iron/ kg body weight. Most of it is in the blood as hemoglobin, the rest in organs such as liver, spleen, and brain as ferritin deposits, there are also trace amounts in the myoglobin of skeletal muscle. If uniformly distributed throughout the body, this amount of iron, even in its most magnetic configuration, would have a negligible effect on the susceptibility; as it is concentrated in certain tissues, these can have positive susceptibilities. The susceptibilities of some biological materials were reported by Schenck (1996) as summarized and adapted in Table 4.5. Susceptibility values can also be found in Sood et al. (2016) who reported

TABLE 4.5

Susceptibilities of Some Biological Materials (Adapted from Schenck 1996 and Deistung et al. 2017)

Material	$\chi_m \times 10^6$
Ca^{2+}	−14.83
Human tissues (except for specific tissues known to contain large amount of iron)	~(−11.0 to −7.0)
Lipids (stearic acid), phospholipids, sphingolipids	−10, −9.68, −10.03
Apohemoglobin (iron-free protein) and other apoproteins	−9.91
Water	−9.05
Cortical bone	−8.86
Liver	−8.7
Whole blood (deoxygenated)	−7.9
Red blood cell (deoxygenated)	−6.52
Liver (severe iron overload)	~0.0
Hemoglobin	+0.15
Ferritin (whole molecule)	+520

Properties of Biological Materials

data for different parts of the brain; so did Lin et al. (2014) who have also shown a trend of increasing susceptibility with age for some brain tissue.

4.7.1 Factors that Affect the Magnetic Susceptibility of Tissue

The composition and structure of tissue are the determinant of its intrinsic dielectric and magnetic properties. In terms of composition, water, the main constituent of tissue is responsible for the overall diamagnetic property of tissue. Iron, the element with highest magnetic impact, and tissue structure, are the main determinants of their magnetic property.

4.7.1.1 Iron

Iron is essential to the proper functioning of living organisms; it plays an important role in energetic biochemical reactions. In the body, it is either stored in organs in the form of ferritin, attached to protein as in hemoglobin, or, as recently discovered in the form of biogenic magnetite.

4.7.1.1.1 Ferritin

The accepted model of ferritin molecule consists of a 12-nm hollow spherical protein shell made up of 24 subunits. The core of ferritin protein is 8 nm in diameter, and it can hold up to 4500 iron atoms in the form of ferrihydrite ($5Fe_2O_3 \cdot 9H_2O$). Iron is transported into and out of the core through three- and fourfold channels in the shell. During transport, highly toxic Fe(II) is oxidized to Fe(III) for storage as ferrihydrite (Harrison and Arosio 1996). The specific iron biochemistry of ferritin is complex and is not completely understood (e.g., Yang et al. 1998 and Zhao et al. 2001). Ferrihydrite is a superparamagnetic anti-ferromagnet at body temperature, and as such, its magnetic properties are important determinant of the magnetic properties of ferritin-rich tissues.

4.7.1.1.2 Hemoglobin

A molecule of hemoglobin has four protein chains each containing one paramagnetic iron ion Fe^{++}. When combined with four paramagnetic oxygen molecules, the resultant oxyhemoglobin molecule has no net spin and is slightly more diamagnetic than water (Schenck 1996). The paramagnetic susceptibility of deoxyhemoglobin (Table 4.5) arises from the paramagnetic properties of the four iron atoms moderated by the diamagnetic susceptibility of the apoprotein matrix. Hemoglobin in blood cells is diluted by intracellular water, which accounts for the diamagnetic properties of deoxygenated red blood cells.

4.7.1.1.3 Magnetite (and Other Ferromagnetic Compounds)

Kirschvink et al. (1992) discovered the presence of biogenic magnetite in the human brain tissue. Later work demonstrated that this magnetic iron biomineral is present in several organs in the human body, including the heart, liver, and spleen (Grassi-Schultheiss et al. 1997). Dobson and Grassi (1996) found magnetite in tissue removed from the hippocampi of epileptic patients. Magnetite (Fe_3O_4)—a ferromagnetic iron oxide—is also known as lodestone and is a mineral more commonly associated with sedimentary rocks and volcanoes.

Magnetite crystals produced by living systems have unique features that distinguish them from geologically produced crystals; their characteristics include single domain size, chemical purity, crystallographic perfection (Strbak et al. 2011) and have been found in many organisms. A well-known example is the magnetotactic bacterium. These bacteria use chains of single-domain, biogenic magnetite arranged in chains in order to sense the

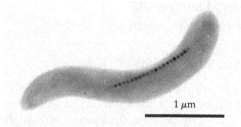

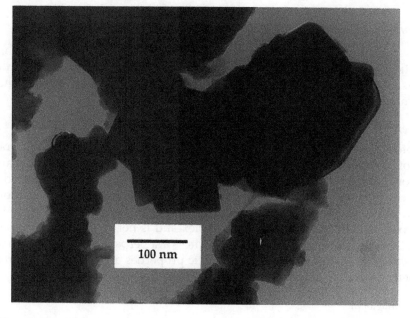

FIGURE 4.23
Transmission electron micrograph of the magnetotactic bacterium MS-1 (top). (From www.calpoly.edu/~rfrankel/mtbphoto.html) Biogenic magnetite extracted from the human hippocampus (bottom). (From Schultheiss-Grassi, PP, R Wessiken, and J Dobson (1999) *Biochim. Biophys. Acta* 1426: 212–216. With permission.)

geomagnetic field and use it for navigation—much like a compass needle (Blakemore, 1975) (Figure 4.23). Although the mechanism by which these organisms produce perfect magnetite crystals is not well understood, it has recently been shown that the process appears to be mediated by specific proteins (Arakaki et al. 2003). Magnetite has been found in a wide variety of animals from bacteria to humans, and in some cases, as with magnetotactic bacteria, it appears to be used for navigation (e.g., Walker and Bitterman 1989; Walker et al. 1997; Wiltschko and Wiltschko 2002 and for a review, see Kirschvink and Hagadorn 2000).

Although magnetite and ferrihydrite are two of the most ubiquitous magnetic materials in organisms, they are not the only ones. Greigite (Fe_7S_8) is a ferrimagnetic iron sulfide found in some iron-reducing bacteria (Posfai et al. 1998). It has a strong magnetic moment similar to magnetite and is thought to be produced as a by-product of iron reduction. Hematite (Fe_2O_3) and wüstite-like (FeO) iron phases also have recently been found within human ferritin (Quintana et al. 2004). And hemosiderin (FeOOH) is a goethite-like iron oxyhydroxide that is anti-ferromagnetic and is found primarily in pathogenic liver tissue (St. Pierre et al. 1998).

Properties of Biological Materials 149

4.7.1.2 Structure of Tissue (Magnetic Anisotropy)

Aligned tissue structures and microstructures give some tissues anisotropic magnetic susceptibilities. For example, the lipid organization of myelin in white matter contributes to its bulk susceptibility and its anisotropy. The anisotropy of white matter has been demonstrated by Lee et al. (2010) who reported a difference of 0.012 ppm between the parallel and transverse susceptibility of the corpus callosum, an inner part of the brain white matter characterized by high myelin content. More recently, van Gelderen et al. (2015) confirmed and quantified the magnetic anisotropy of white matter with direct measurements and analysis of the torque acting on human spinal cord samples exposed to magnetic fields. Differences in susceptibilities along and across the samples varied between 0.014 and 0.019 ppm. Magnetic anisotropy has also been observed in tissues outside the central nervous system as reported by Dibb and Liu (2017) for renal, cardiac, and collagen tissue.

4.7.2 MRI Techniques for Magnetic Susceptibility Mapping

In MRI, small variations in the susceptibility of different tissues have long been considered an unavoidable source of image distortion due to their effect on the local field. Recently, these subtle field distortions have been utilized to double advantage; to obtain information about tissue magnetic susceptibility and as a novel contrast procedure in MRI. Based on the realization that variations in phase shifts at a point are sensitive to the susceptibility of the substance, a relatively new MRI technique, QSM has developed; it extracts spatial susceptibility distribution of the objects or tissue from local field data.

4.7.2.1 Quantitative Susceptibility Mapping (QSM)

In the broadest possible terms, the bulk magnetic susceptibility distribution in the volume of interest is determined by deconvoluting the internal magnetic field at a point with the corresponding point dipole response. Deistung et al. (2017) is a comprehensive and well-referenced overview of the subject (other reviews include: Haake et al. 2014 and Reichenbach et al. 2015). Because phase is sensitive to susceptibility, combining magnitude and phase of the internal field is referred to as susceptibility-weighted imaging (SWI) whereby the image contrast is enhanced by the differences in tissue bulk (assumed isotropic) magnetic properties. A more recent development STI (susceptibility tensor imaging) treats susceptibility as anisotropic determined from multiple orientation measurements. As such, it has limited *in vivo* applicability but is useful for the characterization of animal and post-mortem tissue samples. QSM and STI are active areas of research including attempts to overcome the need for multiple orientation scans for the assessment of anisotropy. A recent review of magnetic anisotropy by Dibb and Liu (2017) suggests that despite the challenges and limitations of these techniques, including object reorientation and prolonged scan time, quantitatively assessing susceptibility anisotropy is a promising method for studying healthy and diseased organ tissues.

4.7.2.2 QSM versus SQUID Susceptometry

SQUID (superconducting quantum interference device) susceptometry is a well-established technique for susceptibility measurement. It is a planar method that uses electronic magnetometers sensitive to nearby magnetized tissues. By contrast, QMS provides 3D spatial maps of the susceptibility distribution. Sharma et al. (2017) carried out a comparative study of the techniques with measurements, *in vivo*, on patients with liver iron overload. SQUID is particularly well suited to such measurement; it provides the magnetic susceptibility throughout the entire liver. Both techniques are sensitive to the iron content in the liver but differ significant in the methodology used to derive the susceptibility values. Nevertheless, QSM data demonstrated a very strong linear correlation to SQUID measurements.

QSM is a developing technique where much remains to be standardized (Deistung et al. 2017); there are still unanswered questions about its possible dependence on the imaging parameters (Sood et al. 2016), there are challenges in field-to-susceptibility conversion and questions about absolute accuracy. As with any measurement on heterogeneous biological systems, reproducibility is an important issue in current research (see, for example, Santin et al. 2016).

4.7.2.3 Magnetic Susceptibility in Diagnostic Applications

Although iron is essential for the proper function of organisms, excessive accumulation of iron in the body is toxic and can lead to multiple health complications, including liver and heart damage, pancreatic dysfunction, and growth failure through pituitary dysfunction. Abnormalities in iron and ferritin expression have been observed in many types of cancer (Brem et al. 2006). Direct susceptibility measurement or QMS are capable of quantifying the iron content as demonstrated by Sharma et al. (2017) for liver.

SWI is especially sensitive to deoxygenated blood and intracranial mineral deposition and, for that reason, has been applied to image various pathologies including intracranial hemorrhage, traumatic brain injury, stroke, neoplasm, and multiple sclerosis Liu et al. (2015).

Excess iron accumulation in the brain has been associated with neurodegenerative diseases including Parkinson's, Alzheimer, multiple sclerosis, and other progressive neurological diseases (Deistung et al. 2017). Associated changes in magnetic susceptibility in specific parts of the brain were observed. The expectation is that the developing techniques, QSM and STI will have the potential to provide diagnostic information and clinical follow-up on these neurodegenerative diseases.

Acknowledgments

One of us (CG) is most grateful to Dr. Ulrich Katscher, Senior Scientist, Philips GmbH, Hamburg, Germany, for personal communication regarding EPT and input on the subject.

References

Alanen E, Lahtinen T, Nuutinen J. 1998. Variational formulation of open-ended coaxial line in contact with layered biological medium. *IEEE Trans Biomed Eng* 45(10): 1241–1248.

Alanen E, Lahtinen T, Nuutinen J. 1999. Penetration of electromagnetic fields of an open-ended coaxial probe between 1 MHz and 1 GHz in dielectric skin measurements. *Phys Med Biol* 44: N169–N176.

Properties of Biological Materials

Allen JE, Henshaw DL, Keitch PA, Fews AP, Eatough JP. 1995. Fat cells in red bone marrow of human rib: their size and spatial distribution with respect to the radon-derived dose to the haemopoietic tissue. *Int J Radiat Biol* 68: 669–678.

Arakaki A, Webb J, Matsunaga T. 2003. A novel protein tightly bound to bacterial magnetic particles in Magnetospirillum magneticum strain AMB-1. *J Biol Chem* 278(10):8745–8750.

Balidemaj E, Kok HP, Schooneveldt G, van Lier AL, Remis RF, Stalpers LJ, Westerveld H, Nederveen AJ, van den Berg CA, Crezee J. 2016. Hyperthermia treatment planning for cervical cancer patients based on electrical conductivity tissue properties acquired in vivo with EPT at 3 T MRI. *Int Journal Hyperthermia* 32: 558–568.

Balzano Q. 2002. Proposed test for detecting nonlinear responses in biological preparations exposed to RF energy. *Bioelectromagnetics* 23(4): 278–287.

Bao JZ, Lu ST, Hurt WD. 1997. Complex dielectric measurements and analysis of brain tissues in the radio and microwave frequencies. *IEEE Trans Microwave Theory Tech MTT* 45(10): 1730–1741.

Barthel J, Buchner R, Munsterer M. 1995. The dielectric properties of water in aqueous electrolyte solutions. In: *Chemistry Data Series 12*, Kreysa G, Ed., DECHEMA, Frankfurt.

Bateman JB, Gabriel C. 1987. Dielectric properties of aqueous glycerol and a model relating these to the properties of water. *J Chem Soc Faraday Trans* 2(83): 355–369.

Bateman JB, Gabriel C, Grant EH. 1990. Permittivity at 70 GHz of water in aqueous solutions of some amino acids and related compounds. *J Chem Soc Faraday Trans* 2(86): 3577–3583.

Bergman DJ. 1978. The dielectric constant of a composite material. *Phys Rep C* 43: 377.

Bianco B, Chiabrera A, Giordano S. 2000. DC-ELF characterization of random mixtures of piecewise nonlinear media. *Bioelectromagnetics* 21: 145–149.

Blakemore R. 1975. Magnetotactic bacteria. *Science* 190(4212): 377–379. Bibcode:1975Sci...190..377B. PMID 170679. doi:10.1126/science.170679.

Böttcher CJF, Bordewijk P. 1978. *Theory of Electric Polarization*. Elsevier, Amsterdam.

Brem F, Hirt AM, Winklhofer M, Frei K, Yonekawa Y, Wieser HG, Dobson J. 2006, Magnetic iron compounds in the human brain: A comparison of tumour and hippocampal tissue. *J R Soc Interface* 3(11): 833–841.

Buchner R, Hefter GT, May PM. 1998. Dielectric relaxation of aqueous NaCl solutions. *J Phys Chem A* 103: 1–9.

Buckmaster HA. 1990. Precision microwave complex permittivity measurements of high loss liquids. *J Electromagn Waves Appl* 4: 645–656.

Bulyshev AE, Semenov SY, Souvorov AE, Svenson RH, Nazarov AG, Sizov YE, Tatsis GP. 2001. Computational modeling of three dimensional microwave tomography of breast cancer. *IEEE Trans Biomed Eng* 48(9): 1053–1056.

Burdette EC, Cain FL and Seals J. 1980. In vivo probe measurement technique for determining dielectric properties at VHF through microwave IEEE Trans. *Microw Theory Tech* 28: 414–427

Chassagne C, Dubois E, Jiménez ML, van der Ploeg JPM and van Turnhout J. 2016. Compensating for electrode polarization in dielectric spectroscopy studies of colloidal suspensions: Theoretical assessment of existing methods. *Front Chem* 4: 30.

Cole KS, Cole RH. 1941. Dispersion and absorption in dielectrics. I. Alternating current characteristics. *J Chem Phys* 9: 341–351.

Davidson DW, Cole RH. 1951. Dielectric relaxation in glycerol, propylene glycol and n-propanol. *J Chem Phys* 19: 1484–1490.

Davis, CC, Balzano, Q. (2010). The brain is not a radio receiver for wireless phone signals: Human tissue does not demodulate a modulated radiofrequency carrier. *Comptes Rendus Physique* 11(9–10): 585–591.

Debye, P. 1929. *Polar Molecules*, Dover, Mincola, N.Y.

Deistung, A, Schweser, F, Reichenbach, JR. (2017) Overview of quantitative susceptibility mapping. *NMR Biomed* 30(4): e3569. doi: 10.1002/nbm.3569. Epub 2016 Jul 19.

Dibb, R, Liu, C. (2017). Joint eigenvector estimation from mutually anisotropic tensors improves susceptibility tensor imaging of the brain, kidney, and heart. *Magn Reson Med* 77: 2331–2346. doi:10.1002/mrm.26321.

Dissado LA. 1990. A fractal interpretation of the dielectric response of animal tissues. *Phys Med Biol* 35(11): 1487–1503.

Dobson J, Grassi P. 1996. Magnetic properties of human hippocampl tissue: evaluation of artefact and contamination sources. *Brain Res Bull* 39: 255–259.

Dobson J. 2004. Magnetic iron compounds in neurological disorders. *Ann N Y Acad Sci* 1012: 183–192.

Duck FA. 1990. *Physical Properties of Tissue: A Comprehensive Reference Book*, Academic Press, London.

Dukhin SS. 1971. Dielectric properties of disperse systems. *Surface Colloid Sci* 3: 83.

Dukhin SS, Shilov VN. 1974. *Dielectric Phenomena and the Double Layer in Disperse Systems*, John Wiley & Sons, New York.

Ellison WJ, Lamkaouchi K, Moreau J. 1996. Water: A dielectric reference. *J Mol Liq* 68: 171–279.

Epstein BR, Foster KR. 1983. Anisotropy in the dielectric properties of skeletal muscle. *Med Biol Eng Comput* 21: 51–55.

Faes TJC, Meij HA, Munk JC, Heethaar RM. 1999. The electric resistivity of human tissues (100 Hz–10 MHz) a meta-analysis of review studies. *Physiol Meas* 20: R1–R10.

Fallert MA, Mirotznik MS, Bogen DK, Savage EB, Foster KR, Josephson ME. 1993. Myocardial electrical impedance mapping of ischemic sheep hearts and healing aneurisms. *Circulation* 87: 188.

Farrugia L, Wismayerb P, Zammit Mangiona L, Sammuta CV, 2016, Accurate in vivo dielectric properties of liver from 500 MHz to 40 GHz and their correlation to ex vivo measurements, *Electromagn Biol Med* 35(4): 365–373.

Fixman M. 1980. Charged macromolecules in external fields. 1. The sphere. *J Chem Phys* 72: 5177.

Fixman M. 1983. Thin double layer approximation for electrophoresis and dielectric response. *J Chem Phys* 78: 1483.

Foster KR, Schepps JL. 1981. Dielectric properties of tumor and normal tissues at RF through microwave frequencies. *J Microwave Power* 16(2): 107–119.

Foster KR, Schwan HP. 1989. Dielectric properties of tissues and biological materials: A critical review. *Crit Rev Biomed Eng* 17(1): 25–104.

Fröhlich H. 1955. *Theory of Dielectrics*, Oxford University Press, Oxford.

Gabriel C, Sheppard RJ, Grant EH. 1983. Dielectric properties of ocular tissues at 37°C. *Phys Med Biol* 28: 43–49.

Gabriel C, Grant EH and Young IR. 1986. Use of time domain spectroscopy for measuring dielectric properties with a coaxial probe. *J Phys E Sci Instrum* 19: 843.

Gabriel C, Bentall RH, Grant EH. 1987. Comparison of the dielectric properties of normal and wounded human skin material. *Bioelectromagnetics* 8: 23–28.

Gabriel C, Chan TYA, Grant EH. 1994. Admittance models for open ended coaxial probes and their place in dielectric spectroscopy. *Phys Med Biol* 39: 2183–2200.

Gabriel C, Gabriel S, Corthout E. 1996a. The dielectric properties of biological tissues: I. Literature survey. *Phys Med Biol* 41: 2231–2249.

Gabriel S, Lau RW, Gabriel C. 1996b. The dielectric properties of biological tissues: II. Measurements in the frequency range of 10 Hz to 20 GHz. *Phys Med Biol* 41: 2251–2269.

Gabriel S, Lau RW, Gabriel C. 1996c. The dielectric properties of biological tissues: III. Parametric models for the dielectric spectrum of tissues. *Phys Med Biol* 41: 2271–2293.

Gabriel C. 1997. Comments on 'dielectric properties of the skin'. *Phys Med Biol* 42(8): 1671–1673.

Gabriel C, Peyman A. 2006. Dielectric measurement error analysis and assessment of uncertainty. *Phys Med Biol* 51: 6033–6046.

Gabriel C, Peyman A, Grant EH. 2009. Electrical conductivity of tissue at frequencies below 1 MHz. *Phys Med Biol* 54: 4863–4878.

Geddes LA, Baker LE. 1967. The specific resistance of biological material - A compendium of data for the biomedical engineer and physiologist. *Medical and Biological Engineering* 5: 271–293.

Galejs J. 1969. *Antennas in Inhomogeneous Media*, Pergamon Press.

Ghodgaonkar DK, Gandhi OP, Iskander MF. 2000. Complex permittivity of human skin in-vivo in the frequency band 26.5–60 GHz. *IEEE Antennas and Propagation Society Symposium Proceedings*, Salt Lake City, UT, USA, July 16–20, 2000, Vol. 2, pp. 1100–1103.

Gimsa J, Wachner D. 1998. A unified resistor–capacitor model for impedance, dielectrophoresis, electrorotation, and induced transmembrane potential. *Biophys J* 75: 1107–1116.

Gimsa J, Wachner D. 1999. A polarization model overcoming the geometric restrictions of the Laplace solution for spheroidal cells: Obtaining new equations for field-induced forces and transmembrane potential. *Biophys J* 77: 1316–1326.

Gimsa J, Wachner D. 2001a. Analytical description of the transmembrane voltage induced on arbitrarily oriented ellipsoidal and cylindrical cells. *Biophys J* 81: 1888–1896.

Gimsa J, Wachner D. 2001b. On the analytical description of transmembrane voltage induced on spheroidal cells with zero membrane conductance. *Eur Biophys J* 30: 463–466.

Grant E, Shack R. 1967. Complex permittivity measurements at 8.6 mm wavelength over the temperature range 1–60 degrees centigrade. *Br J Appl Phys* 18: 1807–1814.

Grant EH, Sheppard RJ. 1974. Dielectric relaxation in water in the neighbourhood of 4°C. *J Chem Phys* 60: 1792–1796.

Grant E, Buchanan T, Cook H. 1957. Dielectric behaviour of water at microwave frequencies. *J Chem Phys* 26: 156–161.

Grant EH, Sheppard RJ, South GP. 1978. *Dielectric Behaviour of Bilogical Molecules in Solution*, Clarendon Press, Oxford.

Grant EH, Szwarnowski S, Sheppard RJ. 1981. Dielectric properties of water in the microwave and infrared regions. In: *Biological Effects of Nonionising Radiation*, Illinger KH, Ed., American Chemical Society Symposium Series, Washington, DC, vol. 157, pp. 47–56.

Grassi-Schultheiss PP, Heller F and Dobson J, 1997, Analysis of magnetic material in the human heart, spleen and liver. *BioMetals* 10: 351–355.

Greffe JL, Grosse C. 1992. Static permittivity of emulsions. *Prog Electromagn Res* 41.

Grosse C. 1988. Permittivity of a suspension of charged spherical particles in electrolyte solution. II. Influence of the surface conductivity and asymmetry of the electrolyte on the low and high frequency relaxations. *J Phys Chem* 92: 3905–3910.

Grosse C, Foster KR. 1987. Permittivity of a suspension of charged spherical particle in electrolyte solution. *J Phys Chem* 91: 3073.

Grzegorczyk TM, Meaney PM, Kaufman PA, diFlorio-Alexander RM, Paulsen KD. 2012. Fast 3-D tomographic microwave imaging for breast cancer detection. *IEEE Trans Med Imaging* 31(8): 1584–1592.

Haggis GH, Hasted JB, Buchanan TJ. 1952. The dielectric properties of water in solutions. *J Chem Phys* 20: 1452–1465.

Hagness SC, Taflove A, Bridges JE. 1998. Two-dimensional FDTD analysis of a pulsed microwave confocal system for breast cancer detection: fixed-focus and antenna-array sensors. *IEEE Trans Biomed Eng* 45(12): 1470–1479.

Hagness SC, Taflove A, Bridges JE. 1999. Three-dimensional FDTD analysis of a pulsed microwave confocal system for breast cancer detection: Design of an antenna-array element. *IEEE Trans Antennas Propagat* 47(5): 783–791.

Haacke EM, Pepropoulos LS, Nilges EW, Wu DH. 1991. Extraction of conductivity and permittivity using MRI. *Phys Med Biol* 36: 723–734.

Haake EM et al. 2014. QSM; current status and future directions. *Magn Reson imsging* 33(1): 1–25.

Hammerich D, Ozkan OR, Tsai JZ, Staelin ST, Tungjitkusolmun S, Mahvi DM, Webster JG. 2002. Changes in electrical resistivity of swine liver after occlusion and postmortem. *Med Biol Eng Comput* 40: 29–33.

Hanai T. 1968. *Emulsion Science*, Sherman P, Ed., New York Academic Press.

Hanai T, Zhang HZ, Sekine K, Asami K. 1988. The number of interfaves and the associated dielectric relaxations in heterogeneous systems. *Ferroelectrics* 86: 191.

Harrison PM, Arosio P. 1996. The ferritins: Molecular properties, iron storage function and cellular regulation. *Biochimica et Biophysica Acta* 1275: 161–203.

Hasted JB, El Sabeh. 1953. The dielectric properties of water in solutions. *Trans Faraday Soc* 49: 1003–1011.

Hasted JB, Husain SK, Frescura FAM, Birch JR. 1985. Far-infrared absorption in liquid water. *Chem Phys Lett* 118(6): 622–625.

Havriliak SJ, Negami S. 1966. A complete plane analysis of dispersion in some polymer systems. *J Polym Sci Polym Symp* 6: 99–117.

Hayashi Y, Miura N, Shinyashiki N, Yagihara S. 2005. Free water content and monitoring of healing processes of skin burns studied by microwave dielectric spectroscopy in vivo. *Phys Med Biol* 50: 599–612.

Hill NE, Vaughan WE, Price AH, Davies M. 1969. *Dielectric Properties and Molecular Behaviour.* Van Nostrand, London.

Hill RM, Jonscher AK. 1983. The dielectric behaviour of condensed matter and its many-body interpretation. *Contemp Phys* 24(1): 75–110.

Hodgetts TE. 1989. The open-ended coaxial line: A rigorous variational treatment, royal signals and radar establishment, *Memorandum* 4331.

Huo X, Shi X, You F, Fu F, Liu R, Tang C, Lu Q, Dong X. 2013, Reliability of in vivo measurements of the dielectric properties of anisotropic tissue: A simulative study. *Phys Med Biol* 58(10): 3163–3176.

Hwang H, Yim J, Cho J, Cheon C, Kwon Y. 2003. 110 GHz broadband measurement of permittivity on human epidermis using 1 mm coaxial probe. *IEEE MTT S Digest*: 399–402.

Irimajiri A, Suzaki T, Asami K, Hanai T. 1991. Dielectric modeling of biological cells. Models and algorithm. *Bull Inst Chem Res Kyoto Univ* 69(4): 421–438.

Jenkins S, Hodgetts TE, Symm GT, Warhamm AGP, Clarke RN. 1992. Comparison of three numerical treatment for open ended coaxial line sensor. *Electron Lett* 24: 234.

Joines WT, Zhang Y, Li C, Jirtle RL. 1994. The measured electrical properties of normal and malignant human tissues from 50 to 900 MHz. *Med Phys* 21: 547–550.

Jonscher AK 1983. *Dielectric Relaxation in Solids*, Chelsea Dielectrics Press, London.

Kaatze U. 1986. The dielectric spectrum of water in the microwave and near-millimetre wavelength region. *Chem Phys Lett* 132(3): 291–293.

Kaatze U. 1988. Complex permittivity of water as a function of frequency and temperature. *J Chem Eng* 34: 371–374.

Kaatze U. 1989. Complex permittivity of water as function of frequency and temperature. *J Chem Eng Data* 34: 371–374.

Kaatze U, Giese K. 1980. Dielectric relaxation spectroscopy of liquids: Frequency domain and time domain experimental methods. *J Phys E: Sci Instrum* 13: 133–141.

Katscher U, Voigt T, Findeklee C, Vernickel P, Nehrke K, Dössel O. 2009. Determination of electrical conductivity and local SAR via B1 mapping. *IEEE Trans Med Imag* 28: 1365–1374.

Katscher U, van den Berg CAT. 2017. Electric properties tomography: Biochemical, physical and technical background, evaluation and clinical applications. *NMR Biomed* 30: 3729.

Kent M, Peyman A, Gabriel C, Knight A. 2002. Determination of added water in pork products using microwave dielectric spectroscopy. *Food Control* 13: 43–149.

Kim SY, Shin J, Kim DH, Kim MJ, Kim EK, Moon HJ, Yoon JH. 2016. Correlation between conductivity and prognostic factors in invasive breast cancer using MREPT. *Eur Radiol* 26: 2317–2326.

Kirkwood JG. 1936. On the theory of dielectric polarization. *J Chem Phys* 4(9): 592–601.

Kirschvink JL, Kobayashi-Kirschvink A, Woodford BJ. 1992. Magnetite biomineralization in the human brain 89(16). doi:10.1073/pnas.89.16.7683.

Kirschvink JL, Hagadorn JW. 2000. *A Grand Unified Theory of Biomineralization, The Biomineralisation of Nano- and Micro-Structures*, Wiley-VCH Verlag GmbH, Weinheim, Germany, pp. 139–150.

Lahtinen T, Nuutinen J, Alanen E. 1997. Dielectric properties of the skin. *Phys Med Biol* 42:1471–1472.

Lahtinen T, Nuutinen J, Alanen E, Turunen M, Nuortio L, Usenius T, Hopewell JW. 1999. Quantitative assessment of protein content in irradiated human skin. *Int J Radiat Oncol Biol Phys* 43(3): 635–638.

Lane JA, Saxton, JA. 1952. Dielectric dispersion in pure polar liquids at very high radio frequencies. *Proc R Soc Lond* 213: 400–408.

Latikka J, Kuurne T, Skola H. 2001. Conductivity of living intracranial tissues. *Phys Med Biol* 46: 1611–1616.

Properties of Biological Materials

Lazebnik M, Popovic D, McCartney L, Watkins CB, Lindstrom, MJ, Harter J, Sewall S, Ogilvie T, Magliocco A, Breslin TM, Temple W, Mew D, Booske JH, Okoniewski M, Hagness SC. 2007. A large-scale study of the ultrawideband microwave dielectric properties of normal, benign and malignant breast tissues obtained from cancer surgeries. *Phys Med Biol* 52:6093–6115.

Lee J, Shmueli K, Fukunaga M, van Gelderen P, Merkle H, Silva AC, Duyn JH. 2010 Sensitivity of MRI resonance frequency to the orientation of brain tissue microstructure. *Proc Natl Acad Sci U S A* 107(11): 5130–5135.

Levy E, Puzenko A, Kaatze U, Ishai PB, Feldman Y. 2012. Dielectric spectra broadening as the signature of dipole-matrix interaction. I. Water in nonionic solutions. *J Chem Phys* 136: 114502–114505.

Levy E, David M, Barshtein G, Yedgar S, Livshits L, Ishai PB, and Feldman Y. 2017. Dielectric response of cytoplasmic water and its connection to the vitality of human red blood cells. II. The influence of storage. *J Phys Chem* 121: 5273–5278.

Liebe HJ, Hufford GA, Manabe T. 1991. A model for the complex permittivity of water at frequencies below 1 THz. *Int J Infrared Millimeter Waves* 12: 659–660.

Lin PY, Chao TC, Wu ML. 2014. QSM of human brain at 3T: A multisite reproducibility study. doi:10.3174/ajnr.org.

Lindholm-Sethson B, Han S, Ollmar S, Nicander I, Jonsson G, Lithner F, Bertheim U, Geladi P. 1998. Multivariate analysis of skin impedance data in long term type 1 diabetic patients. *Chemom Intell Lab Syst* 44: 381–394.

Liu C, Li W, Tong KA, Yeom KW, Kuzminski S. (2015) Susceptibility-weighted imaging and quantitative susceptibility mapping in the brain. *J Magn Reson Imaging* 242(1): 23–24. Published online 2014 Oct 1. doi: 10.1002/jmri.24768.

Liu J, Wang Y, Katscher U, He B. (2017). Electrical properties tomography based on B1 maps in MRI: Principles, applications and challenges review, *IEEE Trans Biomed Engin*, in press.

Mandel M, Odjik T. 1984. Dielectric properties of polyelectrolyte solutions. *Annu Rev Phys Chem* 35: 75–108.

Marzec E, Wachal K. 1999. The electrical properties of leg skin in normal individuals and in-patients with ischemia. *Bioelectrochem Bioenerg* 49: 73–75.

Marcuvitz N. 1951, *Waveguide Handbook*, IET, Technology & Engineering, London, UK.

Marzec E, Wachal K. 1999. The electrical properties of leg skin in normal individuals and in-patients with ischemia. *Bioelectrochem Bioenerg* 49: 73–75.

Meaney PM, Kaufman PA, Muffly LS, Click M, Poplack SP, Wells WA, Schwartz GN, di Florio-Alexander RM, Tosteson TD, Li Z, Geimer SD, Fanning MW, Zhou T, Epstein NR, Paulsen KD, 2013. Microwave imaging for neoadjuvant chemotherapy monitoring: initial clinical experience. *Breast Cancer Res* 15: R35.

Milton GW. 2002. *Theory of Composites*, Cambridge University Press, Cambridge.

Miyauchi T, Hirose H, Sasaki E, Hayashi M, Mori Y, Murakawa S, Takagi H, Yasuda H, Kumada Y, Iwata H. 1999. Predictability of dielectric properties for ischemic injury of the skeletal muscle before reperfusion. *J Surg Res* 86: 79–88.

Munoz San Martin S, Sebastian JL, Sancho M, Miranda JM. 2003. A study of the electric field distribution in erythrocyte and rod shape cells from direct RF exposure. *Phys Med Biol* 48: 1649–1659.

Nevels RD, Butler CM, Yablon W. 1985. The annular slot antenna in a lossy biological medium IEEE Trans. *Microw Theory Tech* 33: 314–319.

Nicholson PW. 1965. Specific impedance of cerebral white matter. *Exp Neurol* 13: 386–401.

Nicholson C, Freeman JA. 1975. Theory of current source-density: Analysis and determination of conductivity tensor for anuran cerebellum. *Neurophysiol* 38: 356–368.

Nightingale NR, Goodridge VD, Sheppard RJ, Christie JL 1983. The dielectric properties of the cerebellum, cerebrum and brain stem of mouse brain at radiowave and microwave frequencies. *Phys Med Biol* 28(8): 897–903.

Nuutinen J, Lahtinen T, Turunen M, Alanen E, Tenhunen M, Usenius T, Kolle R. 1998. A dielectric method for measuring early and late reactions in irradiated human skin. *Radiother Oncol* 47: 249–254.

Onsager L 1936 Electric moments of molecules in liquids. *J Am Chem Soc* 58: 1486–1493.

O'Rourke AP, Lazebnik M, Bertram JM, Converse MC, Hagness, SC, Webster JG, Mahvi DM. 2007. Dielectric properties of dielectric properties of human normal, malignant and cirrhotic liver tissue: In vivo and ex vivo measurements from 0.5 to 20 GHz using a precision open-ended coaxial probe. *Phys Med Biol* 52: 4707–4719.

Park Y, Woo Kim H, Yun J, Seo S, Park CJ, Lee JZ, Lee JH. 2016. Microelectrical impedance spectroscopy for the differentiation between normal and cancerous human urothelial cell lines: Real-time electrical impedance measurement at an optimal frequency. *BioMed Res Int* 2016, Article ID 8748023.

Peters MJ, Stinstra JG, Hendriks M. 2001. Estimation of the electrical conductivity of human tissue. *Electromagnetics* 21: 545–557.

Pethig R. 1996. Dielectrophoresis: Using inhomogeneous AC electrical fields to separate and manipulate cells. *Crit Rev Biotechnol* 16(4): 331–348.

Peyman A, Rezazadeh AA, Gabriel C. 2001. Changes in the dielectric properties of rat tissue as a function of age at microwave frequencies. *Phys Med Biol* 46: 1617–1629.

Peyman A, Rezazadeh AA, Gabriel C. 2002. Changes in the dielectric properties of rat tissue as a function of age at microwave frequencies- Corrigendum. *Phys Med Biol* 47: 2187–2188.

Peyman A, Gabriel C. 2003. Age Related Variation of the Dielectric Properties of Biological Tissues. Final technical report, RRX88. UK Department of Health.

Peyman A, Holden S, Gabriel C. 2005. Dielectric properties of biological tisues at microwave frequencies. Final technical report MTHR Department of Health UK, www.mthr.org.uk/research_projects/documents/Rum3FinalReport.pdf.

Peyman A, Gabriel C, Grant EH. 2007a. Complex permittivity of sodium chloride solutions at microwave frequencies. *Bioelectromagnetics* 28(4): 264–274.

Peyman A, Holden SJ, Watts S, Perrott R, Gabriel C. 2007b. Dielectric properties of porcine cerebrospinal tissues at microwave frequencies: In vivo, in vitro and systematic variation with age. *Phys Med Biol* 52: 2229–2245.

Peyman, A, Gabriel, C, Grant, EH, Vermeeren, G, Martens, L. 2009. Variation of the dielectric properties of tissues with age: The effect on the values of SAR in children when exposed to walk-ieetalkie devices. *Phys Med Biol* 54: 227–241.

Peyman A, Gabriel C, Benedickter HR, Fröhlich J. 2011, Dielectric properties of human placenta, umbilical cord and amniotic fluid. *Phys Med Biol* 56(7): N93–N98.

Peyman A, Gabriel C. 2012. Dielectric properties of rat embryo and foetus as a function of gestation. *Phys Med Biol* 57: 2103–2116.

Peyman A, Kos B, Djokić M, Trotovšek B, Limbaeck-Stokin C, Serša G, Miklavčič D, 2015. Variation in dielectric properties due to pathological changes in human liver. *Bioelectromagnetics* 36(8): 603–612.

Petaja L, Nuutinen J, Uusaro A, Lahtinen T, Ruokonen E. 2003. Dielectric constant of skin and subcutaneous fat to assess fluid changes after cardiac surgery. *Physiol Meas* 24: 383–390.

Pliquett U, Weaver JC. 1996. Transport of a charged molecule across the human epidermis due to electroporation. *J Controlled Release* 38: 1–10.

Pliquett U, Gersing E, Pliquett F. 2000. Evaluation of fast time-domain based impedance measurements on biological tissue. *Biomed Tech (Berl).* 45(1–2): 6–13.

Polevaya Y, Erunolina I, Schlesinger M, Ginzburg BZ, Feldman Y. 1999. Time domain dielectric spectroscopy study of human cells II. Normal and maligant white blood cells. *Biochemic Biophysica Acta* 1419: 257–271.

Pósfai, M, Buseck, PR, Bazylinski, DA, Frankel, RB. (1998) Reaction sequence of iron sulfide minerals in bacteria and their use as biomarkers. *Science* 280: 880–883.

Prausnitz MR, Pliquett U, Vanbever R. (1999). *Mechanistic studies of skin electroporation using biophysical methods in Electrically Mediated Delivery of Molecules to cells – Electrochemotherapy, Electrogenetherapy, and Transdermal Delivery by Electroporation*, Jaroszeski MJ, Gilbert R, Heller R, Eds., Humana Press, Totowa, NJ, pp. 214–235.

Puzenko A, Levy E, Shendrik A, Talary MS, Caduff A. et al. 2012. Dielectric spectra broadening as a signature for dipole-matrix interaction. III. Water in adenosine monophosphate/adenosine-5'-triphosphate solutions. *J Chem Phys* 137: 194502–194508.

Quintana C, Cowley JM, Marhic C. 2004. Electron nanodiffraction and high-resolution electron microscopy studies of the structure and composition of physiological and pathological ferritin. *J Struct Biol* 147(2): 166–178.

Raicu. 1999. Dielectric dispersion of biological matter: Model combining Debye-type and "universal" response. *Phys Rev E* 60(4): 4677–4680.

Raicu V, Kitagawa N, Irimajiri A. 2000. A quantitative approach to the dielectric properties of the skin. *Phys Med Biol* 45: L1–L4.

Ranck JB, BeMent SL. 1965. The specific impedance of the dorsal columns of cat: An anisotropic medium. *Exp Neurol* 11: 451–463.

Reddy GN, Saha S. 1984. Electrical and dielectric properties of wet bone as a function of frequency. *IEEE Trans Biomed Eng* 31: 296–303.

Reichenbach JR, Schweser F, Serres B, Deistung A. 2015, Quantitative susceptibility mapping: Concepts and applications. *Clin Neuroradiol* 25(Suppl. 2): 225–230.

Riedel CH, Keppelen M, Nani S, Dössel O. 2003. Postmortem conductivity measurement of liver tissue using a contact free magnetic induction sensor. *EMBC IEEE*: 3126–3129.

Rogers JA, Sheppard RJ, Grant EH. 1983. The dielectric properties of normal and tumour mouse tissue between 50 MHz and 10 GHz. *Br J Radiol* 56: 335–338.

Saha S, Williams PA. 1989. Electric and dielectric properties of wet human cancellous bone as a function of frequency. *Ann Biomed Eng* 17: 143–158

Santin M, Didier M, Valabregue R, Lehericy S. 2016. Reproducibility of R2* and QSM reconstruction methods in the basal ganglia of healthy subjects. *NMR Biomed*. doi: 10.1002/nbm.3491.

Semenov SY, Svenson RH, Posukh VG, Nazarov AG, Sizov YE, Bulyshev AE, Souvorov AE, Chen W, Kasell J, Tatsis GP. 2002. Dielectrical spectroscopy of canine myocardium during acute ischemia and hypoxia at frequency spectrum from 100 kHz to 6 GHz. *IEEE Trans Medical Imaging* 21(6): 703–707.

Schaefer M, Gross W, Ackemann J, Gebhard MM. 2002. The complex dielectric spectrum of heart tissue during ischemia. *Bioelectrochemistry* 58: 171–180.

Schafer M, Kirlum HJ, Schlegel C, Gebhard MM. 1999. Dielectric properties of skeletal muscle during ischemia in the frequency range from 50 Hz to 200 MHz. *Ann NY Acad Sci* 873: 59–64.

Sharma SD, Fischer R, Schoennagel BP, Nielsen P, Kooijman H, Yamamura J, Adam G, Bannas P, Hernando D, Reeder SB. 2017. MRI-based QMS and R2* mapping of liver iron overload: comparison with SQUID-based biomagnetic liver susceptometry. *Magn Reson Med* 78(1): 264–270. doi: 10.1002/mrm.26358. Epub 2016 Aug 11.

Schenck JF. 1996. The role of magnetic susceptibility in magnetic resonance imaging: MRI magnetic compatibility of the first and second kinds. *Med Phys* 23(6): 815–850.

Schepps JL, Foster KR. 1980. UHF and microwave dielectric properties of normal and tumor tissues: variation in dielectric properties with tissue water content. *Phys Med Biol* 25: 1149–1159.

Schmid G, Neubauer G, Illievich UM, Alesch F. 2003a. Dielectric properties of porcine brain tissue in the transition from life to death at frequencies from 800 to 1900 MHz. *Bioelectromagnetics* 24: 413–421.

Schmid G, Neubauer G, Mazal PR. 2003b. Dielectric properties of human brain tissue measured less than 10 h post-mortem at frequencies from 800 to 2450 MHz. *Bioelectromagnetics* 24: 423–430.

Schwan HP, Kay CF. 1957. Capacitive properties of body tissues. *Circ Res* 5: 439–443.

Schwan HP. 1992. Linear and nonlinear electrode polarization and biological materials. *Ann Biomed Eng* 20: 269–288.

Schwan HP, Sheppard RJ, Grant EH. 1976. Complex permittivity of water at 25°C. *J Chem Phys* 64: 2257–2258.

Schwan HP. 1992. Linear and nonlinear electrode polarization and biological materials. *Ann Biomed Eng* 20: 269–288.

Schwartzman D, Chang I, Michele JJ, Mirotznik MS, Foster KR. 1999. Electrical impedance properties of normal and chronically infarcted left ventricular myocardium. *J Interv Card Electrophysiol* 3: 213–224.

Sebastian JL, Munoz S, Sancho M, Miranda JM. 2001. Analysis of the influence of the cell geometry, orientation and cell proximity effects on the electric field distribution from direct RF exposure. *Phys Med Biol* 46: 213–225.

Semenov SY, Svenson RH, Posukh VG, Nazarov AG, Sizov YE, Bulyshev AE, Souvorov AE, Chen W, Kasell J, Tatsis GP. 2002. Dielectrical spectroscopy of canine myocardium during acute ischemia and hypoxia at frequency spectrum from 100 kHz to 6 GHz. *IEEE Trans Med Imaging* 21(6): 703–707.

Semenov S. 2009. Microwave tomography: Review of the progress towards clinical applications. *Philos Trans A Math Phys Eng Sci* 367(1900): 3021–3042.

Sihvola AH. 1989. Self-consistency aspects of dielectric mixing theories. *IEEE Trans Geosci Remote Sensing* 27(4): 403.

Sihvola AH, Lindell IV. 1992. Polarizability modeling of heterogeneous media. *Prog Electromagn Res PIER* 06: 101–151.

Smith SR, Foster R, Wolf GL. 1986. Dielectric properties of VX-2 carcinoma versus normal liver tissue. *IEEE Trans Biomed Eng* 33(5): 522–524.

Sood S, Urriola J, Reutens D, O'Brien K, Bollmann S, Barth M, Vegh V. 2016. Echo time-dependent QSM containing information on tissue properties. *Magn Reson Med* 77(5): 1946–1958.

St. Pierre, TG, Chuaanus, W, Webb, J, Macey, D, Pootrakul, P. 1998. The form of iron oxide deposits in thalassemic tissues varies between different groups of patients—A comparison between Thai beta-thalassemia/hemoglobin-E patients and Australian beta-thalassemia patients. *Biophys Biochim Acta* 1407: 51–60.

Stauffer PR, Rossetto F, Prakash M, Neuman DG, Lee T. 2003. Phantom and animal tissues for modelling the electrical properties of human liver. *Int J Hyperthermia* 19(1): 89–101.

Stauffer PR, van Rhoon GC. 2016. Overview of bladder heating technology: matching capabilities with clinical requirements. *Int J Hyperthermia* 32(4): 407–416.

Steel MC, Sheppard RJ. 1988. The dielectric properties of rabbit tissue, pure water and various liquids.

Strand-Amundsen RJ, Tronstad C, Kalvøy H, Gundersen Y, Krohn CD, Aasen AO, Holhjem L, Reims HM, Martinsen Ø, Høgetveit JO, Ruud TE, Tønnessen TI. 2016. In vivo characterization of ischemic small intestine using bioimpedance measurements. *Physiol Meas* 37: 257–275.

Strbak O, Kopcansky P, Frollo I. 2011. Biogenic magnetite in humans and new magnetic resonance hazard questions. *Measurement Science Review* 11(3): 85–91.

Stuchly MA, Stuchly SS. 1980. Dielectric properties of biological substances—tabulated. *J Microwave Power* 15(1): 19–26.

Sunaga T, Ikehira H, Furukawa S, Shinkai H, Kobayashi H, Matsumoto Y, Yoshitome E, Obata T, Tanada S, Murata H, Sasaki Y. 2002. Measurement of the electrical properties of human skin and the variation among subjects with certain skin conditions. *Phys Med Biol* 47: N11–N15.

Takashima S. 1989. Electrical properties of proteins. I. Dielectric relaxation. In: *Physical Principles and Techniques of Protein Chemistry*, Leach JS, Ed., Academic Press, New York.

Tamura T, Tenhunen M, Lahtinen T, Repo T, Schwan HP. 1994. Modelling of the dielectric properties of normal and irradiated skin. *Phys Med Biol* 39: 927–936.

Tha KK, Katscher U, Yamaguchi S, Stehning C, Terasaka S, Fujima N, Kudo K, Kazumata K, Yamamoto T, Van Cauteren M, Shirato H, 2017, Noninvasive electrical conductivity measurement by MRI: A test of its validity and the electrical conductivity characteristics of glioma, EurRad, e-publication ahead of print

Tinga WR. 1992. Mixture laws and microwave material interactions. *Prog Electromagn Res* 6: 1–40.

Tsai JZ, Cao H, Tungjitkusolmun S, Woo EJ, Vorperian VR, Webster JG. 2000. Dependance of apparent resistance of four-electrode probes on insertion depth. *IEEE Trans Biomed Eng* 47(1): 41–48.

Tsai JZ, Will JA, Stelle SHV, Cao H, Tungjitkusolmun S, Choy YB, Haemmerich D, Vorperian VR, Webster JG. 2002. In-vivo measurements of swine myocardial resistivity. *IEEE Trans Biomed Eng* 49(5): 472–483.

Van Beek LKH. 1967. Dielectric behaviour of heterogeneous systems, *Prog Dielectr* 7: 69–114.

Van Berkum S, Dee JT, Philipse AP, Erné BH 2013. frequency-dependent magnetic susceptibility of magnetite and cobalt ferrite nanoparticles embedded in PAA hydrogel. *Int J Mol Sci* 14: 10162–10177.

Van Gelderen P, Mandelkow H, de Zwart JA, Duyn JH. 2015. A torque balance measurement of anisotropy of the magnetic susceptibility in white matter. *Magn Reson Med* 74: 1388–1396.

Walker MM, Bitterman ME. 1989. Conditioning analysis of magnetoreception in honeybees. *Bioelectromagnetics* 10(3): 261–275.

Walker MM, Diebel CE, Haugh CV, Pankhurst PM, Montgomery JC, Green CR. 1997. Structure and function of the vertebrate magnetic sense. *Nature* 390(6658): 371–376.

Walker DC, Brown BH, Hose DR, Smallwood RH. 2000. Modelling the electrical impedivity of normal and prealignant cervical tissue. *Electron Lett* 36(19): 1603–1604.

Wei Y Z, Sridhar S. 1991. Radiation-corrected open-ended coax line technique for dielectric measurements of liquids up to 20 GHz IEEE Trans. *Microw Theory Tech* 39: 526–531

Wei YZ, Sridhar S. 1993. A new graphical representation for dielectric data. *J Chem Phys* 99(4): 3119–3124.

Wersebe A, Siegmann K, Krainick U, Fersis N, Vogel U, Claussen CD, Muller-Schimpfle M. 2002. Diagnostic potential of targeted electrical impedance scanning in classifying suspicious breast lesions. *Invest Radiol* 37(2): 65–72.

Widdowson EM, Dickerson JWT. 1960. The effect of growth and function on the chemical composition of soft tissues. *Biochem J* 77: 30–43.

Wiltschko W, Wiltschko R. 2002. Magnetic compass orientation in birds and its physiological basis. *Naturwissenschaften* 89(10): 445–452.

Woodward AM, Kell DB. 1990. On the nonlinear dielectric properties of biological systems Saccharomyces cerevisiae. *Bioelectrochem Bioenerg* 24: 83–100.

Yang, X, Chen-Barrett, Y, Arosio, P, Chasteen, ND. 1998. Reaction paths of iron oxidation and hydrolysis in horse spleen ferritin and recombinant human ferritins. *Biochemistry* 37: 9763–9750.

Zhang ZH, Sekine K, Hanai T, Koizuni N. 1983. Dielectric observations on polystrene microcapsules and the theoretical analysis with reference to interfractal polarization. *Colloid Polym Sci* 261: 381.

Zhao G, Bou-Abdallah F, Yang X, Arosio P, Chasteen ND. 2001, Is hydrogen peroxide produced during iron(II) oxidation in mammalian apoferritins? *Biochemistry* 40(36): 10832–10838.

5

Interaction of Static and Extremely Low-Frequency Electric Fields with Biological Materials and Systems

Frank Barnes

University of Colorado Boulder

CONTENTS

5.1 Introduction 161
5.2 Physics of the Interactions of Electric Fields with Biological Materials 162
5.3 Changes in Chemical Reaction Rates 171
    5.3.1 Changes in Collision Rates 172
    5.3.2 Changes in Polarization with Electric Fields 173
    5.3.3 Changes in Energy 173
5.4 Water and Proteins 175
5.5 Protein–Protein Reactions 176
5.6 Conduction of Electrons in Large Molecules 178
5.7 Competing Chemical Reactions 179
5.8 Biological Amplification 179
5.9 Feedback Amplifiers and Processes 180
5.10 Parametric Amplifiers 183
5.11 Stochastic Resonance 184
5.12 Effects of Electric Fields on Cell Membranes 185
5.13 Nonlinear Effects of AC Fields on Cells 191
    5.13.1 Introduction 191
    5.13.2 Rectification by Cell Membranes 191
5.14 Thermal Effects 203
5.15 Natural Fields, Man-Made Fields, Noise, and Random Fluctuations 207
5.16 Discussion and Summary 212
Acknowledgments 212
References 212

5.1 Introduction

The fact that electrical currents can affect the behavior of biological systems has been known for more than 2000 years. Electric shocks have been used to treat a wide variety of ailments since the 18th century. However, our knowledge of how these fields and the resulting currents influence biological systems is surprisingly incomplete. Electrical signals are clearly important in the control of biological processes and in carrying information from one part of the body to another. Nerve cells propagate electrical signals from sensors of pressure, temperature, light, sound, etc., to the brain and return control signals

162   *Electromagnetic Fields*

to muscles and other tissue. Yet, if we choose to stimulate these processes with external electrical inputs, we have a relatively limited understanding of how a given electrical signal will affect various biological organs; what the safe limits of exposure are (particularly overextended periods of time); and how electrical signals are carried across cell membranes, are propagated along nerves, or affect growth processes and cell division.

The purpose of this review is to bring together some of the physical concepts that underlie the interaction between electric fields and biological materials with the objective of providing background for determining safe levels of exposure and new applications for the use of electricity in therapy. This is the first step in a long chain of events that lead from externally applied electric field forces to significant biological changes. An objective of this chapter is to provide a background for some of the other chapters that cover both possible health effects and some therapeutic applications of electric and magnetic fields. While this chapter emphasizes processes effective for static and low frequency fields, most are also applicable to higher frequencies as well, though the coupling of the electric and magnetic fields at high frequencies introduces other phenomena as well. Some of these are identified in Chapter 7 of this volume and in Chapter 2 of BMA.

We will start by assuming that the values for the electric and magnetic field at the desired location in the biological system can either be calculated from Maxwell's equations or measured. Some approximate solutions for Maxwell's equations are given in the introduction and much more detailed approaches to solving these equations are given in Chapter 9 of this volume. The issues in making measurements of electric and magnetic fields are discussed in Chapter 10 of this volume.

In this chapter, the force equations are used to develop equations for the conductivity and the dielectric constant. It is organized to begin at the lowest level of complexity by examining some of the forces that are exerted on charged particles in fluids, and it then proceeds to some of the effects of electric fields on chemical reaction rates. At the next level of complexity, some effects of externally applied electric fields on currents through membranes and membrane nonlinearities are described. Some effects of high-level fields and electroporation are described in Chapter 7 in *BMA*. This is followed by a discussion of some long-term adaptive processes and secondary effects of current flow due to heating and by a description of a few effects on whole animals. This information is presented with the objective of specifying the general level or intensity of fields, currents, and temperatures where one can expect to observe a given class of biological responses. Much more data are presented in *BMA*. The next section contains data on the levels of typical naturally occurring and man-made fields. This section also includes a comparison of some externally applied fields, fundamental noise levels, and signals generated in the body. J. Weaver and M. Bier present a more complete treatment of some of the noise sources in biological cells in Chapter 8 in this volume.

5.2 Physics of the Interactions of Electric Fields with Biological Materials

Biological systems consist of complex physical subsystems. In an attempt to understand them, we will start at the most elementary level. Perhaps the simplest level, that is already surprisingly complicated, is the effect of electric fields on biological fluids. These fluids contain a large number of components, including ions, polar molecules such as water,

Static & Low-Frequency Electric Fields
163

proteins, lipids, hormones, and colloidal particles. Current flow in these fluids is given by the sum of the drift and diffusion currents for each of the charged components of the fluid. At low current densities the system is linear; however, at moderate to high current densities nonlinearities are observed [1]. In addition, the fields can change the orientation of molecules with dipole moments, induce dipoles by distorting electron orbits, and change the relative positions of some of the atoms within the molecule producing polarization, that is, a separation of the positive and negative charges within something that is overall electrically neutral. This is discussed in the introduction and also in Chapter 4. This, in turn, leads to changes in the dielectric constant. The next level of complexity involves the interaction of the fields with membranes that behave like porous solids for fields applied perpendicularly to their surface and like viscous liquids for fields in the plane of the membrane [2,3]. Membranes are inhomogeneous so that different portions of them may be affected differently by the perturbing fields. Additionally, membranes are involved in active chemical reactions that change their porosity to various ions selectively. Both electrical potentials and chemical signals may change the membranes' conductivity by orders of magnitude and transmit signals across membranes. The next level of complexity occurs in the interactions between the biological fluids and the membranes in the presence of electric fields. Electric fields affect the selective transport of ions or molecules through the membrane. They change the buildup of charged ion layers at the surface and change the way new molecules are incorporated into the membrane or are bound to its surface. The result of changes in the transport of molecules or ions across cell membranes is changes in the performance of the cells and, in turn, of the organs of which they are a part. They can also lead to changes in the rate of exchange of electrons between molecules in the membrane and ions or molecules in the fluid [4]. For example, a biasing electric voltage across a pacemaker cell in the heart will change its firing rate and thus the pumping rate of the heart.

The fundamental law describing the forces on charged particles is given by

$$\vec{F} = q(\vec{E} + \vec{v} \times \vec{B}) \tag{5.1}$$

where $\vec{F}$ is the force, q is the charge on the particle, and $\vec{v}$ is the velocity of the particle. $\vec{E}$ and $\vec{B}$ are coupled by Maxwell's equations so that a time-varying magnetic field generates an $\vec{E}$ field and vice versa. This force may lead to ion currents and changes in the orientation of dipoles in molecules, and it may also lead to transitions between energy levels, to shifts in their spacing and induced dipole moments, $\vec{P}$. Additionally, if nonlinearities or time-varying impedances are present, alternating currents (AC) can be rectified to produce direct current (DC), frequencies at the second and higher harmonics, and sum and difference frequencies with biological or molecular oscillations. Direct magnetic field effects may occur through the term $\vec{v} \times \vec{B}$. For example, for a Na^+ moving at a thermal velocity of 4×10^2 m/s in the earth's magnetic field of about 5×10^{-5} T, this term has a magnitude of 2×10^{-2} V/m, and the force is at right angles to both the field and the velocity.

In addition to the forces on charged particles, electric fields can induce forces on polarizable atoms, molecules, ions, and molecules with dipole moments. The first order of these forces is described by

$$\vec{F}_d = (\vec{P}_0 \cdot \vec{\nabla})\vec{E} \tag{5.2}$$

$$\vec{F}_L = \alpha V(\vec{E} \cdot \vec{\nabla})\vec{E} \tag{5.3}$$

where $\vec{F}_d$ is the force on a molecule with a permanent dipole moment $\vec{P}_0$, and $\vec{\nabla}\vec{E}$ is the gradient of the electric field. $\vec{F}_L$ is the force on a molecule with an induced dipole moment $\vec{P}_i = \alpha\vec{\nabla}\vec{E}$, where α is the tensor polarizability and V is the volume [5]. Note that biological materials are highly inhomogeneous and that there are large electric field gradients at the boundaries between the fluids and membranes. Additionally, for induced dipole moments, when the sign of the dipole reverses with an alternating field, the force along the gradient of the field can be in a constant direction.

The current flow $\vec{J}_i$ of a given molecule or ion, in molecules or ions per second per meter square, has both drift and diffusion components that may be given by

$$\vec{J}_i = N_i\mu\vec{E} + qD\vec{\nabla}N_i \tag{5.4}$$

where N_i is the ion concentration, μ is the electrical mobility in meters squared per second per volt (m^2/s V), D is the diffusion constant in meter square per second, and $\vec{\nabla}N_i$ is the gradient of the concentration. For charged particles, the force has two components [6]:

$$\vec{F} = q\vec{E} + (\vec{M} \cdot \vec{\nabla}\vec{E}) \tag{5.5}$$

where $\vec{M}$ is the sum of the permanent and induced dipole moments.

The drift portion of the ion currents takes the form:

$$\vec{J} = \sum q_i N_i \mu_i \vec{E} + \sum N_i \mu_i (\vec{M} \cdot \vec{\nabla})\vec{E} \tag{5.6}$$

The conductivity $\sigma = \sum q_i N_i \mu_i$, and N_i is the concentration of each ion, μ_i is the mobility, and $\vec{M}_i$ is the dipole moment. Table 5.1 shows some typical values of mobility.

TABLE 5.1

Typical Values of Biological Ionic Mobilities Atkins [7]

Cations	Mobilities	Anions	Mobilities
Ag+	6.42	Br^-	8.09
Ca^{2+}	6.17	$CH_3CO_2^-$	4.24
Cu^{2+}	5.56	Cl^-	7.91
H^+	36.23	CO32–	7.46
K^+	7.62	F^-	5.70
Li^+	4.01	$\left[Fe(CN)_6\right]^{3-}$	10.5
Na^+	5.19	$\left[Fe(CN)_6\right]^{4-}$	11.4
NH_4^+	7.63	I^-	7.96
$\left[N(CH_3)_4\right]^+$	4.65	NO_3^-	7.40
Rb^+	7.92	OH^-	20.64
Zn^{2+}	5.47	SO_4^{2-}	8.29
Particles	**Mobilities**		
Proteins	10^{-10} to 10^{-8}		

Ionic mobilities in water at 298 K, $u/\left(10^{-8}\,\mathrm{m}^2/\mathrm{s/V}\right)$ $u = \lambda/zF$

Static & Low-Frequency Electric Fields 165

The conductivity of biological fluids such as blood, which contains cells, is in the vicinity of $\sigma = 0.6$ S/m, while for physiological saline it is approximately 1.4 S/m. For more detailed material on the conductivities and dielectric constants of biological materials, see Chapter 4 in this volume by C. Gabriel. If the fluid channels between cells are relatively thick and the fluids are relatively good conductors, the channels tend to short circuit the voltages that might otherwise appear across the perpendicular component of the cell membranes that typically have conductivities at least a thousand times smaller.

The total dielectric constant for a material includes the sum of the induced polarizabilities of the components and interaction terms between them. It is sometimes useful to think of the dielectric constant as a way of describing the fraction of the electric field that is shorted out by the bound charges. This can be shown by considering an ideal parallel plate capacitor where the outside plates are separated by a distance l. The capacity for these plates is given by

$$C_0 = \frac{\varepsilon_0 A}{l} \tag{5.7}$$

where ε_0 is the permittivity of free space.

If an ideal thin metal plate of thickness w is inserted halfway between these plates, then the resulting capacity is given by

$$C = \frac{C_0}{(1 - w/l)} = \frac{\varepsilon A}{l} \tag{5.8}$$

The corresponding dielectric constant is given by

$$\varepsilon = \frac{\varepsilon_0}{(1 - w/l)} \tag{5.9}$$

In this example, it is apparent that as the fraction of the field that is shorted out by the metal plate of thickness w increases, so does the effective dielectric constant. The electrons or ions forming an induced dipole moment can be thought of as doing the same thing. If there is a significant time lag for the movement of the charge, the effective value of w is reduced. The very large values of the dielectric constants of some tissues at low-frequencies can be thought of as the resulting motion of ions that are trapped inside highly resistive membranes. At higher frequencies, the ions can no longer move fast enough to fully charge the surfaces of the membranes, and the effective dielectric constant for the tissue decreases. If energy is absorbed in inducing the dipole moments, then the dielectric constant becomes a complex number.

The forces applied by an electric field superimpose on the much larger random thermal velocity, a drift velocity in the opposite directions for positively and negatively charged particles. These forces can lead to a redistribution of ions or molecules as a result of the differences in mobility and to an increase in the concentration of ions at interfaces. The average drift velocity $\vec{v}$ for a charged particle is given by

$$\vec{v} = \mu_i \vec{E} \tag{5.10}$$

The separation of molecules as a result of the different velocities in a DC electric field is known as electrophoresis and is frequently used to identify large molecules or charged colloidal particles [8,9]. The separation of particles in an AC field gradient is known as dielectrophoresis [5]. For a spherical particle in a homogenous insulating fluid the mobility μ_i in an E field is given by

$$\mu_i = q / 6\pi\eta a \qquad (5.11)$$

provided that the particle is significantly larger than the background particles of the fluid, where η is the viscosity of the fluid and a is the radius of the particle. In a conducting medium, counterions, ions with a charge opposite to that of the particle, and molecules with dipole moments are attracted to it. They change the effective radius of the particle and then partially shield its charge. Additionally, small counterions may flow in the direction opposite to the particle motion, exerting a viscous drag. The theory for motion of a rigid sphere through a conducting liquid is complicated if all these effects are taken into account. Often some of the parameters, including the charge on the sphere, are not measurable. However, a relatively simple expression for the electrophoretic mobility is often used:

$$\mu_i = \frac{\varepsilon_i \zeta}{4\pi\eta} \qquad (5.12)$$

where ε_i and η are the dielectric permittivity and the viscosity of the fluid (in kg/m s), respectively, and ζ is the electrical potential drop from the particle surface across the bound fluid to the interface where the liquid begins to flow under the shear stress. Stated another way the "zeta potential," ζ, is the potential at the surface boundary between the stationary fluid and the liquid that is moving with the particle. It should be noted that ζ is less than the total potential ψ across the charge double layer surrounding the charged particle. Also, note that water molecules bind to the ions, increase the effective diameter, and reduce the effective charge. This, in turn, makes the mobility less than that which might be expected at first from the atomic size and Stokes' law. Stokes' Law calculates the viscous drag force $\vec{F}_{dr}$ on a spherical particle in terms of the radius a, the viscosity η and the velocity of the particle $\vec{v}$.

$$\vec{F}_{dr} = 6\pi a \eta \vec{v} \qquad (5.13)$$

Computer simulations show a rather large number of configurations for bound water that surrounds some of the ions which are of most interest in the study of the effects of electric fields on biological systems. The results of a few of these simulations are shown in Figure 5.1.*

It may be more appropriate to think of the motion of individual ions as being scattered by the water molecules in a lattice with different scattering cross-sections rather than as spheres moving through a viscous fluid. However, there are enough adjustable parameters, including the choice of an effective radius a, so that the Stokes' Law approach gives useful results. Note that both H^+ and OH^- have very high mobility's that result from this hydrogen-bonded lattice. See Table 5.1 [7].

The separation of molecules as a result of the different velocities in a DC electric field is known as electrophoresis and is frequently used to identify large molecules or charged colloidal particles. Proteins are usually denatured in the presence of a detergent such as sodium dodecyl sulfate/sodium dodecyl phosphate (SDS/SDP) that coats the proteins with a negative charge [11]. This is done so that the molecules are stretched out in the presence

---

* See Marechal [10] for an extensive review of the structure of water.

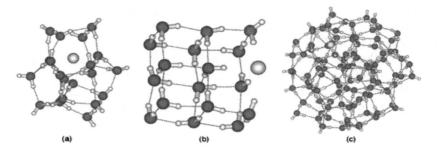

FIGURE 5.1
Structures for the putative global minimum: (a) $Na^+(H_2O)_{20}$, (b) $Cl^-(H_2O)_{17}$, and (c) $Na^+(H_2O)_{100}$ [9].

of the field and the effective charge on the different molecules is the same and the mobilities are proportional to the mass (also see Bier [8]). The separation of particles in an AC field gradient is known as dielectrophoresis [5]. In this case, the force on the molecules is proportional to the induced dipole moment and the gradient of the field.

In a uniform AC field, a charged particle oscillates about its mean position, and the electrical energy added to the solution is largely converted to heat via local collisions. If there is a gradient in the field, as is to be expected in biological materials, which are highly inhomogeneous, then the gradient of the field can lead to a net charge displacement if the fields are large enough to lead to nonlinearities in the mobility or induced dipole moments. For large E the velocity saturates and mobility varies as:

$$\mu_i = \frac{\mu_0'}{|\vec{E}|} \tag{5.14}$$

and Equation 5.10 yields

$$|\vec{v}| = \mu_0' \tag{5.15}$$

Most biological systems are highly inhomogeneous, and the induced currents will vary rapidly in space. For the case of an induced dipole moment and an ideal dielectric sphere with a permittivity ε_2 and a conductivity $\sigma_2 = 0$ in an ideal dielectric fluid with a dielectric permittivity ε_1 and a conductivity $\sigma_1 = 0$ and a nonuniform electric field prior to inserting the sphere, the force:

$$\vec{F}_L = \alpha V(\vec{E} \cdot \vec{\nabla})\vec{E} = 4\pi a^2 \varepsilon_1 \left\{ \frac{\varepsilon_2 - \varepsilon_1}{\varepsilon_2 + 2\varepsilon_1} \right\} \{((\vec{E}_1 \cdot \vec{\nabla})\vec{E}_1)\} \tag{5.16}$$

where $\vec{E}_1$ is the field in the fluid prior to insertion of the sphere. Written another way

$$\vec{F}_L = (3/2)V\varepsilon_1 \left\{ \frac{\varepsilon_2 - \varepsilon_1}{\varepsilon_2 + 2\varepsilon_1} \right\} \vec{\nabla} |\vec{E}_1|^2 \tag{5.17}$$

If we assume that the viscous drag on a spherical particle is given by Stokes' law, then the mobility μ_i is given by:

$$\mu_i = (2a^2/3\eta)\varepsilon_1 \left\{ \frac{\varepsilon_2 - \varepsilon_1}{\varepsilon_2 + 2\varepsilon_1} \right\} \vec{\nabla}\vec{E}_1 \tag{5.18}$$

Dielectrophoresis may also be used for identifying molecules, and a more general treatment of the forces needs to take into account the conductivity or a complex dielectric constant for both the fluid and the particle [12,13].

For particles with dipole moments to change their distribution under the influence of an electric field gradient the force $\vec{F}$ must be large enough to overcome other forces. One of these forces that frequently must be overcome is due to osmotic pressure or diffusion. The osmotic pressure can be thought of as the force per unit area arising from diffusion or the random motion of the particles and is given by:

$$\Pi = N_i kT \tag{5.19}$$

where k is Boltzmann's constant and T is the absolute temperature [14]. The average differential force on a particle is proportional to the gradient of the osmotic pressure and is given by

$$\vec{F}_{os} = -\frac{1}{N_i}\vec{\nabla}\Pi = \frac{kT\vec{\nabla}N_i}{N_i - k\vec{\nabla}T} \tag{5.20}$$

If we consider the case of a spherical volume with a radial concentration gradient at constant temperature, the force is given by:

$$\vec{F}_{os} = -kT\,\frac{\Delta N_i}{N_i}\cdot\frac{r_0}{\Delta r} \tag{5.21}$$

where r_0 is the unit vector, ΔN_i is the incremental change in concentration, and Δr is the incremental change in distance. The maximum change is given by:

$$\frac{\Delta N_i}{N_i} = 1 \tag{5.22}$$

when the presence or absence of a particle occurs at a distance $\Delta r = 2a$, where a is the particle radius. In this case, we get the maximum force:

$$\left|\vec{F}_{os(max)}\right| = -\frac{kT}{2a} \tag{5.23}$$

To get an idea of the size of these forces, consider a particle of fat with $a = 1$ μm in water. The maximum osmotic pressure at $T = 300$ K is $|F_{os(max)}| = 2 \times 10^{-13}$ N. The dielectric constant for water is approximately $\varepsilon_1 = 80\varepsilon_0$ and for a fat particle, $\varepsilon_2 = 2\varepsilon_0$, where $\varepsilon_0 = 8.854 \times 10^{-12}$ F/m. To get a dielectric force greater than the maximum osmotic force, we need a value of $\vec{\nabla}\,|\,\vec{E}_1\,|^2 > 10^{12}\,V^2\,/\,m^3$. This is approximately given by a voltage of 100 V across a 5 mm gap when the $\vec{E}$ field goes from zero to a peak value of 5×10^4 V/m over the same gap. For a particle with a single charge in a uniform field, we would need a field of $E = 1.3 \times 10^4$ V/m to get an equal force.

The electric current densities generated by a concentration gradient are given by

$$\vec{J}_d = -qD\vec{\nabla}N_i \tag{5.24}$$

Static & Low-Frequency Electric Fields

where D is the diffusion constant and is given by

$$D = vkT \tag{5.25}$$

where v is the hydrodynamic mobility with the dimensions of velocity/force and D has the dimensions of m²/s. The diffusion coefficient D is related to the mobility μ by $\dfrac{D}{\mu} = \dfrac{kT}{q}$.

For rigid spherical particles of radius a, where $a \gg a_{H_2O}$, the Einstein–Stokes equation gives

$$D = \frac{kT}{6\pi\eta a} \tag{5.26}$$

This is only a first-order approximation because D varies slightly with concentration, departure of the molecule from a spherical shape, and other factors. η is the viscosity in (kg/m s).

It is sometimes of interest to estimate the ratio of the drift to the diffusion current in order to estimate the level of the applied fields or the applied field gradients that lead to biological changes. This ratio is approximately given by [6]

$$\frac{\vec{J}_{i,\text{diffusion}}}{\vec{J}_{i,\text{drift}}} = \left(\frac{kT}{F_i}\right) \cdot \left(\frac{\nabla N_i}{N_i}\right) \tag{5.27}$$

where $\vec{F}_i$ is the force on the particle due to both the charge on the particle and the gradient of the field on the dipole moment. If we assume that, the maximum change in N_i goes from N_i in the solution to zero at the membrane surface over a distance of the diameter of the molecule of N_i and that this is the same distance over which the field goes from the field in the fluid to the field at the surface of the membrane, then

$$\frac{\vec{J}_{i,\text{diffusion}}}{\vec{J}_{i,\text{drift}}} = \frac{kT}{W_i} \tag{5.28}$$

where W_i is the energy acquired by the particle moving through the field and its gradient. At room temperature the thermal energy $kT \cong 0.026$ eV. A voltage drop from an externally applied source across the membrane liquid boundary on the order of 2×10^{-3} V would be required in order to make the drift current significant with respect to the total diffusion current under these assumptions. One way in which smaller drift currents and smaller voltages could be significant is if the ions with low velocities perpendicular to the membrane are the most important in binding to the membrane. Slow molecules stay close to the membrane for longer times, and these molecules are most affected by the applied forces [6].

For different boundary conditions the results will be quite different. If, for example, the boundary was nearly perfectly reflective, then the concentration gradient in the region adjacent to it would be nearly zero, and so would the net diffusion current. Additionally, the gradient in the concentration may occur over a larger distance than the gradient of the electric field. At steady state the concentration at the membrane can be expected to increase until the diffusion current and the drift current balance each other so that the net current is equal to the rate at which the molecules are bound to the membrane or pass through it [6]. Voltages as small as 5×10^{-5} V/m applied at the minimum concentration of the oscillating NAD(P)H concentrations have been shown to lead to amplification and, applied at the peak, leads to attenuation [15].

There are four forces that may become important when considering the interaction between two particles in a fluid. These are the osmotic diffusion force, the electrostatic force, the van der Waals force, and the hydration force [16,17]. These forces may all become important in considering the interaction between particles or bilipid membranes in an aqueous fluid. Electrostatic or coulomb forces between particles of like charge are repulsive. Because the charged particles attract free ions of the opposite sign, which produces a double layer, they are effectively shielded or are screened by the charged ions of the opposite sign when immersed in a conducting fluid. This force decays exponentially or

$$\vec{F}_c = \vec{F}_0 \exp\left[\frac{-r}{\lambda_d}\right]$$

(5.29)

where λ_d is known as the Debye screening length [16,17]

$$\lambda_d = \left[\frac{2q^2 n}{\varepsilon kT}\right]^{1/2}$$

(5.30)

where n is the density of the ion species doing the shielding, q is the charge and ε is the dielectric constant of the solution, k is Boltzmann's constant, and T is the absolute temperature. For physiological saline solution of approximately 0.14 M, the Debye length is approximately 0.83 nm [19]. Thus, the electrostatic forces are important only at very short ranges.

For like particles, the Van der Waals forces are repulsive at short distances (0.1–0.2 nm) and attractive at longer ranges. These forces may be thought of as being generated by transient electromagnetic fields because of fluctuations that occur as a result of thermal agitation or natural uncertainties in the position and momentum of the electrons and atomic nuclei. If one thinks of the local transient fluctuations in terms of the underlying contributions from oscillations at all possible frequencies, it can be shown that the strength of the contributions due to the local fluctuations at a given frequency is proportional to the absorption of light at that frequency by the material. For an individual atom these forces fall off very rapidly as $1/r^7$ [17]. However, when they are integrated over the surface of a membrane, which is thick compared to an atomic layer, they are correlated over many atoms, as the wavelengths are large compared to an atomic diameter.

A calculation of these fields has been performed starting with quantum field theory [18]. The size of the forces and the rate at which they decay depend on the distance between the membranes and the difference of the bulk polarizability of the membrane and the aqueous gap in a complex way. All frequencies of the charge fluctuations contribute to the attraction, and each gives rise to a different relationship between energy and the distance of separation. For many simple cases and for a classical explanation of these forces and potential distributions, see Ref. [17].

One case of interest is for two membranes with a distance d_w across the aqueous gap between them. The thickness of the membranes is assumed to be large compared to the spacing. The force between these two membranes is approximately given by

$$\vec{F}_w = \frac{H}{6d_w^3}$$

(5.31)

Static & Low-Frequency Electric Fields

where H is the Hamaker coefficient [17]. In a typical situation, the distances over which the van der Waals forces are estimated to be important extend out to separations of 10–20 nm, which is substantially longer than a Debye length or the rate of falloff for the electrostatic or coulomb forces. The hydration forces are repulsive forces that rise extremely rapidly as the membrane bilayers approach a separation distance of approximately an atomic spacing. Experimentally, these forces can be expressed in the form [20]

$$\vec{F}_H = \vec{F}_{H_0} \exp - d_w / \Lambda \tag{5.32}$$

where Λ is a scaling constant. In the case of egg phosphomonoesterase bilayers, $\vec{F}_{H0} \approx 7 \times 10^{-13} N / m^2$ and $\Lambda = 0.256$ nm. This force may be important up to about 2 nm and is assumed to come about as a consequence of the work required to remove water from the hydrophilic surface of the membrane.

Long-range attractive forces have been observed between hydrophobic surfaces [19,20]. These forces are proportional to the contact area and may be orders of magnitude larger than the van der Waals forces. They may also have decay lengths up to 25 nm. The magnitude and range of these forces depends on the temperature and the length of the surfactant's chain, and they appear only when the chains are in a fixed ordered state. These forces appear to be generated when the fields emanating from one surface induce a larger polarization in the other surface layer than in the intervening medium. Some relatively complex expressions for these attractive forces have been worked out [20].

These forces are important in self-organizing processes such as protein folding, ligand binding to hydrophobic receptor sites, and transformation of membrane structures. All these forces act over relatively short ranges in typical biological fluids. The ion densities are so large that charge neutrality is maintained everywhere except very close to charged surfaces.

The effect of an electric field, or an electric field gradient in a fluid, is to superimpose a small drift velocity on a relatively large random thermal velocity. For example, if we apply an electric field of 10^3 V/m to a Na^+ ion, we would expect a drift velocity of about 5×10^{-5} m/s as compared to a thermal velocity of about 4×10^2 m/s. For a protein, we would expect a drift velocity approximately one-tenth of the speed of the Na^+ ion, although at higher fields. This means that if we are to transport proteins or other small charged particles over appreciable distances of a few millimeters, we can expect it to take minutes or longer. In the case of bacteria, we have measured drift velocities of 10^{-6} m/s at 100 Hz in fields of about 10^4 V/m and gradients of 5×10^6 V/m² or about 0.2% of the velocity of the Na ions in the same field [4,21].

5.3 Changes in Chemical Reaction Rates

This drift velocity may also change chemical reaction rates if the rate is limited by the availability of one of the charged components. Consider the case of a chemical reaction that takes place in a homogenous fluid if the chemical reaction has the form

$$(A) + (B) \underset{k_2}{\overset{k_1}{\longleftrightarrow}} (C) \tag{5.33}$$

where (A) and (B) are the concentrations of the two input chemical reactants and k_1 is the reaction rate for A + B to C and k_2 is the rate for the back reaction of C to A and B. If we simplify the system and let k_2 be small, then the initial reaction rate may take the form [7,22]

$$k_1 = k(A)^n (B)^m \tag{5.34}$$

where n and m refer to the order of the reaction. In order to find the values of n and m, one can make the concentration of one of the reactants small so that it takes the form

$$k_1 = k(A_0)^n (B)^m \tag{5.35}$$

where we have made the concentration (A_0) large enough so that it is approximately constant, and the changes in the reaction rate can be measured by varying (B). The value of k is given by

$$k = zpe^{\frac{-\Psi}{RT}} = zpe^{-\frac{qV}{k_BT}} \tag{5.36}$$

where z is the collision frequency and p is the steric factor, which is <1 and reflects the fact that not all collisions occur with the right orientation of the molecules to react. Additionally, there may only be specific sites on a molecule such as a protein or DNA where the two molecules react or bind. ψ is the activation energy, R is the gas constant, and T is the absolute temperature.

In other units, the activation energy can be given by the charge q times the potential energy V and the average thermal energy is given by k_B Boltzmann's constant times the absolute temperature.

5.3.1 Changes in Collision Rates

For many cases the collision frequency is proportional to the current density, and thus there are terms that are proportional to both the drift and the diffusion currents. For example, consider the case of an enzyme reaction on a charged substrate such as a biological membrane. The total current density for a given ion in the fluid incident on the membrane is given by Equation 5.4. If the chemical reaction rate is limited by the number of ions arriving at the membrane surface with enough energy to overcome the barrier required to initiate the reaction, then a DC drift current may either add to or subtract from the diffusion current. If the field direction is such that it prevents the ion from reaching the surface, then the chemical reaction is blocked. If the direction is reversed, the rate can grow exponentially. These changes in chemical reaction rates with the direction of the electric field are likely to be responsible for changes in the growth and reabsorption of neurites [23]. They are also likely to be involved in the mobility of cells such as leukocytes and fibroblasts [24,25].

AC drift currents will add to the diffusion currents. For the AC fields, the drift current can be thought of as increasing the volume covered by a particle executing a random walk as a result of Brownian motion. Thus, in an asymmetrical environment an electric field oscillating in the x direction may increase the number of particles that will strike the y–z plane in a fixed period of time and can increase the chemical reaction rate for a catalytic reaction at the y–z plane. Seto and Hsieh show that AC fields as low as 5 V/m can increase enzyme reaction rates by a factor of 5 [26]. For a 60 Hz field, the peak to-peak displacement for Ca^{2+} resulting from this field is estimated to be about 1.6 nm or about twice

Static & Low-Frequency Electric Fields 173

the thickness of the Debye layer. AC magnetic fields have also been shown to change the growth rate of corn roots at field levels of 5×10^{-3} T. It is likely that these fields are inducing significant currents [27]. The enhancement of the sorption reaction rate for charged reactants onto a reactive colloidal particle is shown to be proportional to $E^2 \omega^{1/2}$ for values of $\omega < 10^{10}$ rad/s and small applied fields. At high frequencies, $\omega > 10^{10}$ rad/s, the sorption reaction rate goes as $E^2 \omega^{-2}$ [28].

5.3.2 Changes in Polarization with Electric Fields

The angle at which two molecules collide can determine whether or not a chemical reaction occurs. For proteins, this factor, p, is usually a very small number—meaning there is only a very small, solid angle for contact that will result in the chemical reaction occurring. An electric field exerts a force on a molecule with a dipole moment to align the molecule along the field. This effect is in a constant direction for an induced dipole moment and to first order varies with the square of the electric field. The average orientation is governed by the Langevin equation [29]

$$< \cos (\theta) >= \coth\left[\frac{W_{DEP}}{k_B T}\right] - \frac{k_B T}{W_{DEP}} \tag{5.37}$$

where θ is the angle between the electric field and the dipole moment. The size of the induced dipole moment, and thus W_{DEP}, the energy acquired from the field, will also be dependent on θ. For the weak fields W_{DEP} is small compared to $k_B T$ and

$$< \cos (\theta) >\approx \frac{W_{DEP}}{3 k_B T} \tag{5.38}$$

In order to get an average change in orientation of $5°$ at room temperature, $W_{DEP} \approx 7$ meV.

5.3.3 Changes in Energy

Because of the large collision rate for ions and molecules in a fluid ($\approx 10^{12}$/s), the mean free paths are very short ($\approx 10^{-9}$/m), and these particles redistribute the energy acquired from an electric field rapidly to the particles around them. The energy distribution at thermal equilibrium for these particles is approximately described by a Boltzmann distribution function which in turn leads to the ratio of the number of particles N_2 with energy W_2, to the number of particles N_1 with energy W_1 so that

$$N_2 = N_1 e^{-\frac{\Delta W}{k_B T}} \tag{5.39}$$

where k_B is Boltzmann's constant. $\Delta W = W_2 - W_1$ is the difference in energy between the two particles. T is the absolute temperature. For small electric fields, the redistribution of energies reaches steady state so rapidly that the distribution can be described by a slightly increased value for T. The quantum of energy for a single photon at radio and microwave frequencies has an energy of hf where h is Planck's constant and f is the frequency. This energy, for the frequencies of interest, is much smaller than the thermal energy $k_B T$ at room temperature so that $N_2 \cong N_1$ at thermal equilibrium. Note that living biological systems

174   *Electromagnetic Fields*

are not in thermal equilibrium and these populations may not be equal. The distribution functions for electrons, ions, and molecules may be described by different values of T, and this is typically the case in plasma where the electrons may be described by a much larger value of T than the ions or molecules. The temperature T can be thought of as a convenient way of describing a distribution function.

In a solid, the distribution of energy for electrons is described by a Fermi function where the reference level for ΔW is the Fermi level, W_c, and where all the electrons lie below W_c for $T = 0$.

$$N_2 = N_1 \frac{1}{\exp(\frac{\Delta W}{k_B T}) + 1} \tag{5.40}$$

To get a significant change in energy we often need to add enough energy to overcome the activation energy for the chemical reaction. The activation energy is typically more than 0.1 eV so that it is enough larger than the thermal energy of about 0.026 eV to minimize the probability of thermal activation. Because of the very short mean free path between collisions, providing this much energy takes a large electric field. The activation energy can be reduced by a catalyst that reduces the barrier for the chemical reaction and has a binding energy that is small enough so that the resulting molecule is released by the thermal energy. This then frees the binding site on the catalyst to react with the next molecule of the reactants and the process is repeated.

An additional mechanism by which AC or DC electric or magnetic fields can effect chemical reactions is by shifting the energy level and the distribution of particles in them. DC electric fields can shift the energy level by an amount that is given by the change in the dipole moment, ΔM, and in the polarizability, $\Delta\alpha$, associated with the transition. A DC field can either stretch or compress a dipole depending on its orientation with respect to the field, thus increasing or decreasing the energy levels for atoms or molecules with different orientations. It also can modify its rate of rotation, speeding it up when the dipole is pointed in the direction of the field and slowing it down when it is pointed away from the field [30]. In a vacuum, the modifications of the rotational states have been worked out from the quantum mechanics for relatively simple molecules and can lead to a relatively complex set of allowed energy states that are a function of the applied field [30]. In a solid or a membrane the energy differences between the states corresponding to the different orientations shift by different amounts for each state as a function of the applied field. This is known as the Stark effect [31]. The frequency corresponding to this energy shift with a fixed orientation is given by

$$h\Delta f = -\Delta \vec{M} \cdot \vec{E} - \frac{1}{2}\vec{E} \cdot \Delta\alpha \cdot \vec{E} \tag{5.41}$$

where Δf is the frequency splitting between levels, $\Delta \vec{M}$ is the change in the dipole moment, $\Delta\alpha$ is the change in polarizability, and h is Plank's constant. These terms give the linear and quadratic Stark effects for a transition in a uniaxially oriented system. These energy levels will be in homogenously broadened by the random orientation of the dipoles with respect to the applied field and by the thermal energy. Since the quantum of energy, hf, at microwave and lower frequencies is very much smaller than almost all thermal quanta, low-lying energy levels are approximately equally populated. However, higher-energy

Static & Low-Frequency Electric Fields 175

states may be preferentially excited by chemical reactions or optical photons so that different excited states may contain different populations.

These states may be further defined by the magnetic field and separated by the background magnetic field or a Zeeman splitting. Thus, radio- and low-frequency fields corresponding to energy separation between these states may excite transitions between levels that are separated by the Stark, Zeeman, or other splitting and change the population distribution in these excited states. Thermal or other relaxation processes may re-equalize the distributions. However, induced transitions by electromagnetic field at frequencies such that $hf = \Delta W$ corresponding to energy gap between levels can lead to absorption or emission depending on the difference in the population of the two energy levels. The transition rate between an excited molecule and its terminal energy state depends on the overlap between the energy levels of the two states. Thus, the application of an electric field can shift the energy levels so as to either increase or decrease this overlap and the transition rate. If an AC field is applied so that $hf \cong \Delta W$, then transitions between energy levels may be excited. The first-order shifts in energy for electronic dipole moments are given by $\Delta W = \vec{P} \bullet \vec{E} = hf$, where $\vec{P}$ is the electric dipole moment for a molecule. For typical molecules, $\vec{P} = 3.3 \times 10^{-30}$ to 6.6×10^{-30} cm. Thus, the fields across a membrane that are on the order of 2×10^7 V/m would lead to energy level splitting of a few kilohertz. It is to be noted that many molecules have rotational and vibration levels that are separated by energies corresponding to frequencies in the radio and microwave spectrum and that transitions between these levels can change reaction rates [30]. Some examples are introduced with respect to how electric field might interact with water, proteins, and protein-protein reactions in the following two sections.

5.4 Water and Proteins

Water performs important functions in determining the shape and function of proteins. Proteins typically have both hydrophobic and hydrophilic regions. In the hydrophobic regions, the water molecules form structures that form a shield so that this region is not soluble in water. In the hydrophilic regions, the charged regions of the proteins of the proteins strongly attract water molecules. The regions in water that are affected by hydrophobic forces can form stable water structures that exclude solutes and micro spheres out to distances of 200 µm [32]. In proteins, the hydrophilic regions repel water and the protein folds to exclude water from these regions. Water is also hydrogen bonded to other regions and forms a diffuse shell around the protein that increases its size and decreases its mobility in a way that is similar to that previously described for simple ions. Water may also be folded into the interior of a protein so that it is not in contact with the bulk water in which it is dissolved. Some of this enclosed water is bound to fixed positions in the protein structure and some appears to be free to tumble. The bound water is important in determining the shape of the proteins and therefore their biological function. Additionally, the bound water H bonds may be dynamically connected to each other forming water structures that connect water molecules that are bonded to specific sites on the protein. The dynamic nature of the water structures provides flexibility to the proteins. Water is also important in catalyzing the chemical reactions with oxygen that provide the energy for living systems [33].

5.5 Protein–Protein Reactions

Protein–protein reactions are important biochemical reactions. Protein binding between two proteins may take place in at least two ways. The first is a force fit where one protein modifies the configuration of the other. The second is configuration recognition where one protein reacts with the other only when it is in a particular configuration. An illustration for these processes is shown in Figure 5.2.

The energy diagram depicted is the simplest case. The binding partners may have an affinity for a number of protein sub-states that would further modify the structural energy landscape. For the case of ubiquitin, conformation selection seems to be sufficient to explain most of the complexes it forms with other proteins [34].

Typical proteins have a very large number of possible configurations. Even small proteins with 100 base pairs may have 10^{89} possible configurations [36]. Many of these configurations have nearly the same energy and there is a dynamic equilibrium with the molecules taking on many of these configurations over time. A case which has been examined in

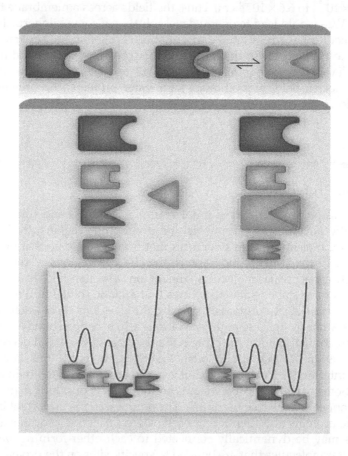

FIGURE 5.2
Molecular recognition mechanisms in proteins. Induced fit assumes an initial interaction between a protein and its binding partner (top left), followed by conformational changes that act to optimize the interaction (top right). In conformational selection, a weakly populated, higher-energy conformation interacts with the binding partner, stabilizing the complex. Relative populations of conformations are indicated by size. In the structural ensemble presented by Ref. [35], different conformations may interact with distinct protein-binding partners [36].

considerable detail is the binding of small ligands to myoglobin (Mb) [37]. Myoglobin is a protein that reversibly stores O_2 and also binds to CO. The conformational sub-states can be divided into three sub-groups or tiers with significant energy barriers ($\approx$0.2 eV between them. Each of the sub-groups has the same amino acid sequence but differs in the geometry for the bound CO and binds to CO at different rates, as indicated in Figure 5.3.

Within each of the sub-groups or tiers are a large number of conformations with nearly equal energies and occupation of these states is best described by a distribution function.

An external electric field would provide a bias that would shift the midpoint of these distributions. Small AC fields can change the distribution of particles in the configurations' tiers by stochastic resonances. In this process, a small AC signal increases the probability that the noise energy leads to the movement of a particle from one energy state to another over an intervening energy barrier [38]. This process can lead to both amplification of the AC signal and increase in the signal-to-noise ratio by as much as 25 dB. This process has

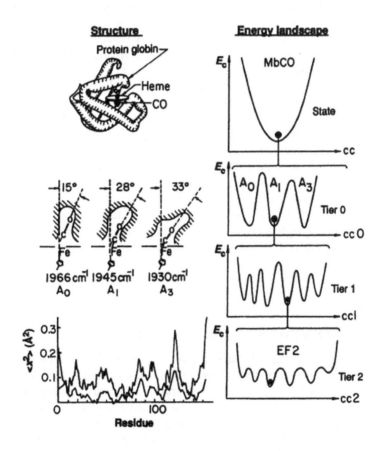

FIGURE 5.3
Structure and conformational energy landscape of MbCO (myoglobin containing carbon monoxide). The top row shows (left) the coarse structure of MbCO and (right) an overall picture of the conformational energy E, as a function of a conformational coordinate, cc. The second row (right) depicts three sub-states of tier 0. The three conformational states, CSOs, have different orientations of the bound CO with respect to the heme; possess different enthalpies, entropies, and volumes; and are separated by high barriers. The third row (left) shows the mean-square deviations for MbCO at 300 K (upper curve) and 80 K (lower curve) (15). The plot of E versus ccl for tier 1 is vastly oversimplified. In reality, E is a hypersurface in a conformational space of very high dimensions and the number of valleys is extremely large. Valleys and barriers can no longer be characterized individually but must be described by distributions. The same remark applies to lower tiers, such as CS_2 [36].

been shown to be used by crayfish in their sensing system in murky water [39] and applies to a number of other biological systems, as well [38].

One of the best-known biological effects of changes in protein configurations with voltages or electric fields is the opening and closing of channel proteins in membranes for controlling the Na^+, K^+, and Ca^{++} currents. The Na^+ channel proteins change configurations as the voltage across the membrane shifts from -90 to $-70\,mV$ and the current increases from approximately 10%–90% [40]. For the Na^+ channels the opening of the channels corresponds to the movement of at least four charges across the membrane and the creation of an opening that allows for the selective passage of the Na^+ ions [41].

Proteins fold into complex configurations and the configurations can determine their biological functions. Some configurations, for example, can expose parts of the molecule that act as a catalyst and others are inactive. There are multiple paths by which this folding may take place in order to reach an energetically stable state and there may be more than one stable state or configuration. The process of folding has been compared to water flowing down a mountainside where small obstacles can change the direction of the stream [43]. Thus it can be hypothesized that relatively small electric- or magnetic-induced energies might change the configurations of some proteins during their formation process or for refolding after a denaturing event.

Another aspect to consider is the catalytic process. It works by lowering the energy barrier for the formation of the resulting compound or molecule. In a typical case, component molecules are absorbed on a metal surface, but not so strongly that they cannot move around over the surface with the help of thermal energy. The metal surface may contribute an electron to one of the components and lower the energy barrier for the two components to combine. The resulting molecule has a lower binding energy to the metal surface and evaporates to leave sites for the process to repeat [42].

Enzymes may also serve as catalysts by stabilizing the transition states and lowering the energy barrier for the formation of the product or splitting the peptide bonds [42]. This process often involves multiple steps and both electron and ion transfers from one position to another on the enzyme and the molecule M modified.

5.6 Conduction of Electrons in Large Molecules

Long conjugated molecules can conduct electrons. This has been demonstrated in DNA and soluble donor-bridge-acceptor systems [45,46]. For short lengths less than 4 nm, tunneling is the main mechanism for conduction and the resistance is exponentially dependent on the length. For the short wires, the tunneling is voltage driven. For longer lengths, the mechanism is hopping. The activation energy for electron hopping is about 0.28 eV and the electron transport is field driven. The hopping activation energy corresponds to the barrier for rotation of the aromatic ring, which transiently couples the conjugated sub-units [44]. Molecules of phenylene ethynylene oligomers may switch from low- to high-conductance states through conformational changes [45]. These electron conduction processes are most likely to be important in membranes where high electric fields exist and where the applied electric fields can be amplified by approximately half the ratio of the length of the biological cells to the membrane thickness. The conduction of electrons through a protein that penetrates the cell membrane is a potential mechanism for transmitting signals from the outside to the inside of a cell. The possibility that external electric

Static & Low-Frequency Electric Fields 179

fields can affect biological processes by modifying the charge transport through a molecule is discussed by Martin Blank [46].

5.7 Competing Chemical Reactions

Two competing biological processes going on at the same time with different time constants can result in a resonance. This can occur when the chemical reaction generating a compound has a slower rate constant than the one destroying it. If the nonlinear rate equation is expanded to second order, the Fourier transformation of the expansion associated with the energy perturbation of the electric field results in a Lorentzian decrease in response to the perturbation with increasing frequency. The difference between these two response curves for the generation and destruction of the compound results in resonance with maximum perturbation at a frequency below that for the 3 dB roll of frequency of the slower generation rate constant. Thus, we can expect processes that have more than one rate constant to have resonant responses that have a maximum response at a given frequency for the externally applied signal [47].

5.8 Biological Amplification

There are a wide variety of amplification and signaling processes in biological systems. The basic characteristic of amplifiers is that a small signal is used to extract energy from another system to perform a function that requires more energy than is in the original signal. Electronic amplifiers typically work by allowing a small signal to extract energy from a DC power source and convert it into a larger signal that replicates the input. However, other sources of energy such as AC signals and noise may be used as the sources of power for the amplification of small signals, as for example in parametric and stochastic resonance amplifiers. In many biological systems, chemical energy from metabolic processes are used to maintain the concentration balance of Na^+, K^+, and other ions so that the interior of a quiescent cell lies in the range of -50 to $-90\,mV$. The energy is supplied by hydrolysis of an ATP molecule, which leads to the flow of three sodium ions out of a cell and two potassium ions into the cell. In nerve cells, the energy stored in this potential difference can then be released, triggered by an input stimulus, as an action potential that propagates along the nerve and signals additional biological responses such as activating muscles. Similar signal/responses can be seen in many other systems, often when one molecule causes release of other, different ones.

As another example of such a nerve signal, consider that the input from many dendrites can be summed in a pyramidal cell to trigger an action potential that is larger than any of the input signals [41]. The input from a single synaptic junction might change the cell resting potential by 0.5–1 mV, and 10–20 inputs might be required to fire an action potential of 50–100 mV [41]. Additionally, sub-threshold inputs can lead to the release of neural transmitters that, in turn, can release from 2 to 10,000 Ca^{2+} ions from internal stores. These neural transmitters may remain bound to the postsynaptic membrane for up to 4 s and reduce the threshold for the firing of successive pulses [41]. Feedback from the postsynaptic membrane to the presynaptic membrane can further reduce the firing potential for the synaptic junction.

Biological sensing systems are followed by amplifiers and signaling systems that transmit a signal to a system that responds further. For example, light, heat, and acoustic inputs get translated to nerve impulses. These nerve impulses may activate muscles or other systems. The inputs from dendrites get summed to fire an action potential which in turn propagates along an axon to a synapse. There are two kinds of synapse and both can be affected by electric fields. Electrical synapses may connect cells by means of gap junctions. At a gap junction, voltage activated channels open the connection between cells and voltage gain results if the depolarizing current pulse flows from a larger cell into a smaller cell with a larger resistance. If the voltage changes resulting from summing the currents from multiple gap junctions is large enough to trigger an action potential, a large number of nerves can be fired rapidly. Gap junctions can conduct currents in both directions and can be closed by lowering the cytoplasmic pH or increasing the cytoplasmic Ca^{2+}. Their response can also be modulated by the release of neural transmitters from nearby cells [48,49].

Most of the biological sensing systems have negative feedback, that is, the system's output modifies the input so as to reduce the subsequent output. The gain of the amplification system can be calculated from the size of the correction that is made to a perturbation. For example, the gain in the control system for maintaining body temperature is approximately –33 and the gain for controlling arterial blood pressure is –2 [48].

Chemically gated synapses release neural transmitters. There are more than 40 different neural transmitters such as acetylcholine (Ach). These neural transmitters can be released from vesicles in the presynaptic cell by changing the potential in the presynaptic cell. The neural transmitters diffuse across the synaptic cleft and bind to receptors of the postsynaptic cell. A single vesicle in a presynaptic cell can release thousands of stored neural transmitter molecules. Typically, only two molecules are required to open a single postsynaptic ion channel. Therefore, the opening of one synaptic vesicle can release enough neural transmitters to open thousands of ion channels which in turn can lead to an action potential. Different neural transmitters can either amplify or inhibit the firing of an action potential [50,51]. Other biological amplification processes occur in the replication of DNA and cell growth.

5.9 Feedback Amplifiers and Processes

An extensive review of how feedback loops shape cellular signals in space in time is presented by Brandman and Meyer [52]. It is to be noted that there are over 3000 signaling proteins and over 15 second messengers that lead to hundreds of cell specific signaling systems. The multiple feedback loops lead to a wide variety of responses including oscillations, bistability, and system stabilization. The multiple feedback loops often make it hard to separate cause and effect. One of the second messengers is Ca^{2+}, which is involved in bone regrowth and has been shown to be modified by electric fields. (See Chapter 8 in *BMA*.) The details of the physics and chemistry of these effects are yet to be understood.

It is to be noted that many biological feedback processes occur with a time delay in the feedback loop. This includes such things as the activation of the immune system, the activation of the repair processes for wound healing and generation of antioxidants to reduce oxidative stress. Depending on the process these time delays can range from fractions of

Static & Low-Frequency Electric Fields

a microsecond for atomic or molecular transitions to days or years. See Table 5.2 for the properties of some typical cells [53].

For example, heart rates are typically in the range from 40 to 150 beats per minute and cell growth rates for some cancer cells lead to cell division rates that occur with periods of hours. For processes with time delays in the feedback loop, if we apply periodic electric or magnetic fields to stimulate the process, the timing or the frequency and phase of the stimulus are important. This can be seen if we look at a simple circuit model for a feedback amplifier with time delay in the feedback as shown in Figure 5.4 [51]. We can set the input of the amplifier $V_1(t)$ equal to the sum of the input voltage $V_s(t)$ and the feedback β from the output voltage at $(t - \tau)$ so that

$$V_1(t) = V_s(t) + \beta V_o(t - \tau) \tag{5.42}$$

TABLE 5.2

Typical Parameter Values for the Bacterial E. coli Cell, the Single-Celled Eukaryote *Saccharomyces cerevisae* (Yeast), and a Mammalian Cell (Human Fibroblast) [53]

Property	E. coli	Yeast (S. cerevisae)	Mammalian (Human Fibroblast)
Cell volume	~1 μm³	~1000 μm³	~10,000 μm³
Proteins/cell	~4 × 10⁶	~4 × 10⁹	~4 × 10¹⁰
Mean size of protein	5 nm		
Size of genome	4.6 × 10⁶ bp	1.3 × 10⁷ bp	3 × 10⁹ bp
	4500 genes	6600 genes	~30,000 genes
Size of: Regulator binding site	~10 bp	~10 bp	~10 bp
Promoter	~100 bp	~1000 bp	~10⁴ to 10⁵ bp
Gene	~1000 bp	~1000 bp	~10⁴ to 10⁶ bp (with introns)
Concentration of one protein/cell	~1 nM	~1 pM	~0.1 pM
Diffusion time of protein across cell	~0.1 s $D = 10\ \mu m^2/s$	~10 s	~100 s
Diffusion time of small molecule across cell	~1 ms, $D = 1000\ \mu m^2/s$	~10 ms	~0.1 s
Time to transcribe a gene	~1 min 80 bp/s	~1 min	~30 min (including mRNA processing)
Time to translate a protein	~2 min 40 aa/s	~2 min	~30 min (including mRNA nuclear export)
Typical mRNA lifetime	2–5 min	~10 min to over 1 h	~10 min to over 10 h
Cell generation time	~30 min (rich medium) to several hours	~2 h (rich medium) to several hours	20 h—nondividing
Ribosomes/cell	~10⁴	~10⁷	~10⁸
Transitions between protein states (active/inactive)	1–100 μs	1–100 μs	1–100 μs
Timescale for equilibrium binding of small molecule to protein (diffusion limited)	~1 ms (1 μM affinity)	~1 s (1 nM affinity)	~1 s (1 nM affinity)
Timescale of transcription factor binding to DNA site	~1 s		
Mutation rate	~10⁻⁹/bp/generation	~10⁻¹⁰/bp/generation	~10⁻⁸/bp/year

bp: base-pair (DNA letter).

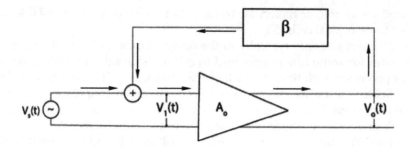

FIGURE 5.4
A simple operational amplifier with a time delay τ in the feedback circuit β.

and

$$V_o(t) = A_o V_1(t) \tag{5.43}$$

Substituting Equation 5.43 into 5.42 and eliminating $V_1(t)$ yields

$$\text{So that} \quad \frac{V_o(t)}{V_s(t)} = A_o + \frac{\beta A_o V_o(t-\tau)}{V_s(t)} \tag{5.44}$$

where $V_o(t)$ is the output voltage at time t. $V_s(t)$ is the input signal at time t. β is the feedback coefficient, A_o is the gain of the amplifier and $V_o(t-\tau)$ is the output voltage at a time τ seconds earlier than t.

If we apply a step function input to an amplifier with negative gain A_o and content feedback with a time delay τ we get an output voltage that decays exponentially in steps with intervals of τ. If we assume that the input signal is given by $V_s = V_{in} \cos(\omega t)$ and $V_o \cos(\omega t - \theta)$ where $\theta = \omega \tau$, the steady state equation can be rewritten as:

$$A_f = \frac{V_o(t)}{V_s(t)} = \frac{A_o}{1 - \beta A_o \dfrac{\cos(\omega t - \theta)}{\cos \omega t}} = \frac{A_o}{1 - \beta A_o (\cos \theta + \tan \omega t \sin \theta)} \tag{5.45}$$

From this equation, it is easy to see that that the sign of the feedback changes as the phase angle θ changes. The term $\tan \omega t \sin \theta$ varies from zero to infinity with ωt so that our overall gain A_f oscillates between zero and $A_f = \dfrac{A_o}{1 - \beta A_o \cos \theta}$ in time with ωt. When $\beta A_o \cos \theta = 1$ the system breaks into oscillation with no externally applied signal. As θ is frequency dependent, the response of our amplifier system is also frequency dependent. If we examine the system at times when $t = 2n\pi$, the term $\beta A_o \cos(\omega \tau)$ changes sign with frequency and A_f will increase or decrease from the value for a system with zero time delay with changes in frequency. A more realistic model that describes the effects of time delays in the control of the frequency in biochemical oscillators is presented by Novak and Tyson [54].

An example of the effects of a system where delayed feedback leads to either amplification or attenuation of NAD(P)H, reactive oxygen, and nitric oxide oscillations depending on the timing of the applied electric field stimulus is given by Rosenpire et al. [15] for human neutrophils. In this chapter, they show that electric fields as weak as 5×10^{-5} V applied at

Static & Low-Frequency Electric Fields

the minimum concentration of the oscillating NAD(P)H concentrations lead to amplification and applied at the peak lead to attenuation. In this case the period of oscillation was approximately 25 s and the electric fields were generated by time varying magnetic fields or by applying a voltage between a pair of platinum electrodes [15].

The behavior of these systems is determined by the nonlinearity of the rate equations, the delay time between the rate of synthesis and the rate of degradation. For the system to oscillate the time delay τ must be sufficiently long and the negative feedback signal must overshoot the stable operating point. Oscillating systems of this type are important for many biological processes.

5.10 Parametric Amplifiers

Parametric amplifiers utilize the nonlinear characteristics of devices such as membranes to convert energy from a higher frequency to energy at a lower frequency. The fundamentals are discussed in the classic paper by Manley and Rowe [55]. In its simplest form the two basic equations are the conservation of energy and momentum. On a per photon basis for the simple case of three frequencies f_1, f_2, f_3 coupled by a nonlinear reactance the conservation of energy is given by

$$hf_3 = hf_1 + hf_2 \text{ or } f_3 = f_1 + f_2 \tag{5.46}$$

where h is Planck's constant. See Figure 5.5. The conservation of momentum is given by

$$k_3 = k_1 + k_2 \tag{5.47}$$

where the k's are the propagation constants and are given by

$$n_3 f_3 = n_1 f_1 + n_2 f_2 \tag{5.48}$$

where the n's are the indexes of refraction at the specified frequencies.

These devices have been extensively studied at radio and optical frequencies for use as low noise amplifiers and second harmonic generation. Early discussions of these

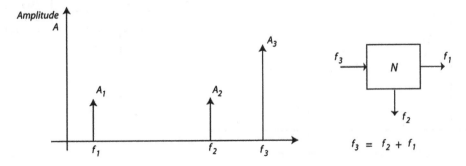

FIGURE 5.5
Amplitude versus frequency for a parametric amplifier with the driving power at f_3, the signal at f_1, and the idler frequency at f_2.

amplifiers are contained in the references by Heffner and Wade [56] An extensive discussion of the electronic circuits used in these amplifiers has been carried out by Louisell [57] and Penfield [58]. Nonlinear dielectric constants are used to build both low noise optical parametric amplifiers and tunable optical oscillators [59].

Parametric processes have been proposed to describe observations for the effects of combinations of AC and DC magnetic fields on PC 12 cells [60]. Tributsch has proposed parametric energy conversion as a possible way to describe a wide variety of biological processes [61]. Parametric amplification of neural signals by noise has been described theoretically by Balkarey et al. [62] and observed in flies in reference [63].

5.11 Stochastic Resonance

An additional mechanism for amplifications is stochastic resonance. Stochastic resonance differs from the foregoing mechanisms of amplification in that the energy is extracted from the noise. Consider, for example, a small, externally applied sinusoidal electric field incident on an ion in a potential well. If the energy acquired from the external signal is not large enough to exceed the potential barrier, the ion stays trapped in the potential well. However, if noise is added to the system, then when the sum of the applied electric field and the noise are large enough to provide enough energy to exceed the height of the potential barrier, the ion may escape the potential well (see Figure 5.6). This happens most frequently at the peaks of the applied electric field so that the signal is amplified at the applied frequency. Gains on the order of 20–30 dB (factors of 100–1000 in power) and increases in the signal-to-noise ratio of 18 dB have been observed for stochastic resonance amplifiers [64]. For an extensive review of this subject and some applications to neuronal systems, see Gammaitoni [38]. For a bistable system, such as a pacemaker cell that is driven by both noise and a periodic signal, it has been shown that the signal-to-noise ratio can be enhanced by the addition of noise to a weak periodic signal and that power can be extracted from the noise.

A strong periodic signal can be generated for input signal-to-noise ratios <1 [64,65]. This phenomenon occurs when two energy states are separated by a barrier, and the probability

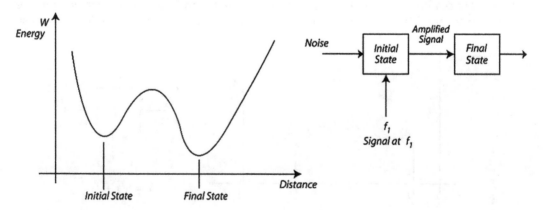

FIGURE 5.6
A potential energy level diagram for the movement of a particle from an initial state to the final state with the aid of noise.

Static & Low-Frequency Electric Fields 185

of a transition increases exponentially with increasing noise power. For periodic signals that are insufficient to cause a transition over the barrier but periodically increase the energy of the particle, the transition rate at the signal frequency first increases with increased noise power up to some maximum. The amount of amplification and the signal to noise ratio depends exponentially on the ratio of the barrier height to the noise energy. The maximum signal to noise ratio occurs when the noise energy is half the barrier energy [65,66]. When the noise power is increased above this level, the output signal becomes more random.

Energy from thermal noise and other noise sources can be used to amplify small electrical signals by providing the energy needed to overcome energy barriers that are needed to initiate a chemical reaction. A simple example is the case of a small electrical pulse which increases the energy with which two particles collide. If the energy acquired from the electrical pulse is not enough to overcome the barrier, nothing happens. However, if we add the fluctuating thermal energy, the probability that there will be enough energy to overcome the barrier increases with the temperature. If we assume that there is a Gaussian distribution of velocities, this probability increases exponentially with temperature. For a periodic sequence of pulses, an exponential increase in the average chemical reaction rate occurs during the pulse with respect to the period between pulses.

The noise enhancement of the power spectral density by crayfish mechanoreceptors has been measured to be 4.5 dB at the optimal noise intensity [38]. It has also been shown that stochastic amplification and signaling enzymatic futile cycles can lead to bistability and oscillations [67].

The subject of noise is discussed further in Chapter 8 of this volume.

5.12 Effects of Electric Fields on Cell Membranes

Electric fields play a very important role in the normal biological functioning of membranes. Membranes are complex structures containing lipids, voltage-activated ion channels, and proteins. It would be surprising if externally applied fields did not affect the membrane behavior. First, an electric field exerts a mechanical force on a membrane by means of the force exerted on charges in the Debye layer on either side of it and on charged proteins that may protrude from the lipid bilayer. Note that although as a first approximation the membrane is often modeled as a smooth planar or spherical surface, it is highly inhomogeneous, and the charges are sparsely disturbed. Thus, the field on a protein may be widely different from the average field. See Figure 5.7a and b for a partial indication of a membrane and cell complexity.

The effects of fields in the plane of the membrane, where large molecules such as proteins are free to move as in a viscous fluid, are significantly different from the effects of fields in the transverse direction, where the membrane components are bound in a layer typically 5–15 nm thick.

The field distribution incident on a particular part of a cell membrane is a function of its geometry, frequency, and the cells around it. As can be seen from the models in Figure 5.8a,b, a wide variety of environments may exist.

The currents that flow through and along the membranes are dependent on the geometry and frequency. A variety of equivalent circuits have been used to model both the impedance of the membrane and the extracellular fluids. The simplest of these are a resistor and

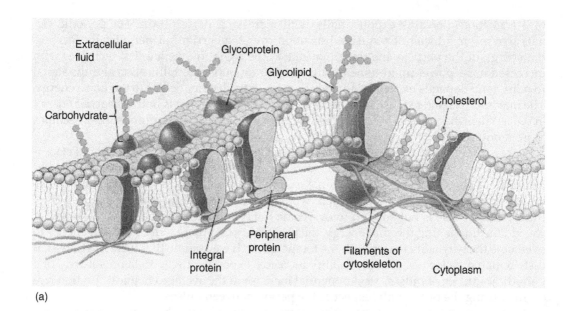

(a)

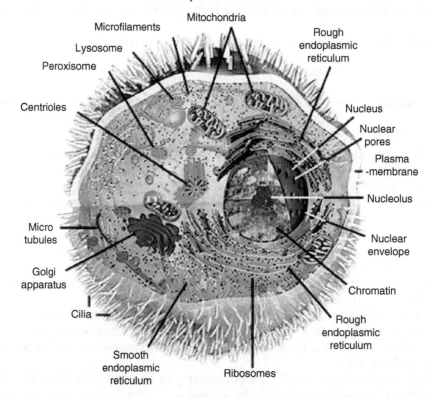

(b)

FIGURE 5.7
(a) Model of a cell membrane. (From Chiras, D., Human Biology, © 5th edition, 2006, Jones and Baretlett Publishers, Boston. With permission.) (b) Anatomy of the animal cell. (From Molecular Expression, http://microscopy.fsu.edu, accessed September 30, 2005; drawing © M.W. Davidson and Florida State University. With permission.)

Static & Low-Frequency Electric Fields

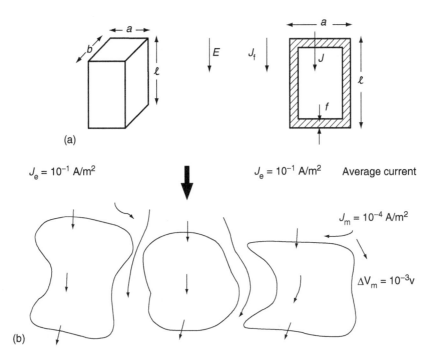

FIGURE 5.8
(a) Current distribution in a hypothetical rectangular cell. (b) Partition of 60-Hz currents through and around cells for an average current density $J = 102$ A/m². J_c is the current density between cells, and J_f is the current density through the membrane. (From Wachtel, H., private communication. With permission.)

capacitor in parallel. At very low-frequencies a collection of cells can be modeled with resistors.

The interiors of cells are normally negatively biased in relation to the surrounding fluid by 30–150 mV, which leads to average transverse electric fields up to tens of millions of volts per meter [68]. Some typical values for the potential inside a number of cells are given in Figure 5.9 [69].

It is to be noted that cancer and growing cells are less negatively biased than quiescent cells. The effective membrane resistance (R_m) per unit area takes on values of 0.14–15 Ω/m² in the transverse direction. This corresponds to resistivities in the range of $p_m = 10^7$–10^9 Ω m. The relative dielectric constant for the membrane is typically in the range of 2–4. Both the surrounding fluid and the interior of a cell have resistivities ρ_f of about 2 Ω m and a relative dielectric constant of 50–80. This means that the cell membrane tends to shield the interior of a cell very effectively from externally applied fields at frequencies below a few kilohertz and becomes almost a short circuit in the multi-megahertz region of the spectrum. In most cells, the interior of the cell contains complex structures that are functions of time as the cell grows and divides. See Figure 5.7b.

Consider the case of an oversimplified hypothetical rectangular cell as shown in Figure 5.8a. At low-frequencies, an external field $\vec{E}$ causes a current density $\vec{j}_f = \vec{E}/\rho_f$ to flow in the external medium, where ρ_f is the resistivity of the fluid. The corresponding voltage drop is $V = \vec{E} = j_f \rho_f L$, which we can consider to be applied to the cell. This voltage is distributed across the cell length as

$$+V = \left[\rho_m 2t + \rho_f (L - 2t)\right] |J_m| \tag{5.49}$$

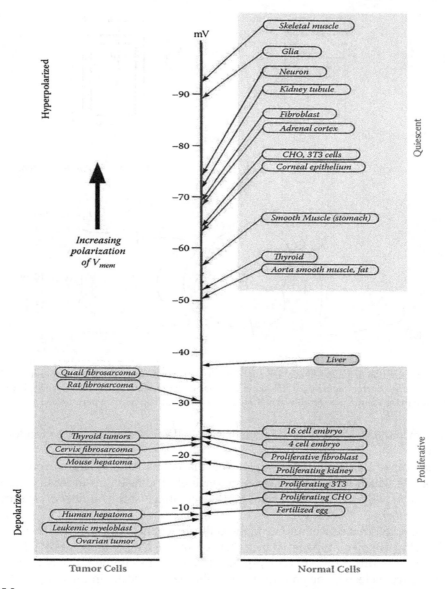

FIGURE 5.9
Typical values for cell potentials. (From Levin, M., *Trends Cell. Biol.*, 17, 262–71, 2007b. In Levin, M. Chapter 3: Endogenous bioelectric signals as morphogenetic controls of development, regeneration, and neoplasm. In *The Physiology of Bioelectricity in Development, Tissue Regeneration and Cancer*, Pullar, C., Ed. CRC Press, Boca Raton, FL, 2010 [69].)

where $\vec{j}_m$ is the current density through the cell and ρ_m is the resistivity of the membranes. Typical cell membrane thicknesses are 6–10 nm, and typical dimensions are 10–150 μm. Setting $L = 100$ μm and

$$\rho_m 2t = 10 \ \Omega m^2 \tag{5.50}$$

$$V = \left(10 \ \Omega m^2 + 2 \times 10^{-6} \Omega m^2\right) |J_m| \tag{5.51}$$

Static & Low-Frequency Electric Fields

This shows that essentially all of the transverse voltage drop occurs across the membrane at low-frequencies and the interior of the cell is almost completely shielded from external fields. A more complete theory for long cells that accounts for the internal resistance of the cell is given by Cooper et al. [70]. Note that in accord with Maxwell's equations, fields parallel to the cell membrane will cross into and through the membrane without attenuation. Muscles, nerves, and a number of other cells may be much longer than 100 µm and may have dimensions in centimeters. Additionally, blood vessels form long, low-resistance paths that may concentrate currents due to externally applied fields.

The anisotropic characteristics of cells are reflected in the anisotropy of the dielectric and conductive properties of tissue, which may give variations of as much as 10 to 1 in conductivity, depending on the direction of measurement relative to cell orientation [71]. A number of fish, including sharks, have been shown to use very long cells and to sum signals in both series and parallel to increase the voltage drop across a sensitive membrane in order to sense fields as low as 10^{-6} V/m [72–74]. The long cell may be thought of as an antenna that concentrates the field across a very thin, voltage-sensitive detector membrane. This membrane appears to have a built-in amplifier that allows detection of signals that are only a little above the natural electrical noise.

Membranes are not just simple linear resistors; they usually are nonlinear and, in the case of nerve cells, they are time varying as well. For a passive membrane in which the membrane potential is primarily determined by the concentration gradient of a single ion such as K^+, the Nernst equation predicts a diode-rectifying characteristic of the form [68]

$$I = I_0 \left[\exp\left(\frac{V_m}{\eta V_T} \right) - 1 \right] \tag{5.52}$$

where V_T is given by

$$V_T = \frac{kT}{q} = 0.026 \text{ V} \tag{5.53}$$

at $T = 300$ K. Here, q is the charge on the electron, V_m is the voltage across the membrane, I_o is the value for ideal back-biased current in amperes, and η is a dimensionless constant. Thus, for currents flowing through a membrane in one direction, the current is nearly constant, whereas for flow in the other direction the current increases exponentially with voltage. In addition to passive currents, cells also use the energy from metabolic processes for the active transport of ions against the fields established by the concentration gradients. These processes are usually modeled as current sources and described as pumps [68]. A thermodynamic approach to pumping shows that ions can be pumped if they form a compound with a material that can flow through the membrane and that is created on one side of the membrane and destroyed on the other [75]. A large variety of models have been generated to characterize the effects of externally applied fields on the transport of ions through membranes [76–78]. However, the details of the pumping process are not well understood. Recently, an approach to treating the behavior of these cells as phase changes in the interior of the cells as a gel has been developed by Pollack [79]. This book challenges the concept of ion channels and pumps for maintaining ionic balances in cells. It provides arguments against the existence of pumps in terms of the channel size for excluding small ions while passing large ones and the large amount of energy required to operate a large number of different pumps for different ions.

In this approach, the solubility of the gel for Na+, K+, and other ions changes with the phase of the gel which in turn can lead to the inflow and out flow of these and other ions based on their hydrated size. Although this approach needs development and is not generally accepted in the biological literature, it has significant experimental backing. Additionally, a thermodynamic treatment of the propagation of nerve pulses that includes changes in nerve cell diameter has been developed by Heimburg and colleagues [80]. In addition to ion transport, electrical fields can change the binding of ions or molecules to the membrane surface.

In the case of pacemaker cells, there are also feedback processes that lead to an oscillating membrane potential and a membrane resistance that is a function of time. The current flow for these cells is described empirically by the Hodgkin–Huxley equation [68]. An alternate approach that treats the nerve pulse like a plasma instability has been proposed by Triffet and Green and by Vaccaro and Green [81,82]. Na+ and K+ currents are the dominant carriers for the propagation of nerve impulses along a cell. It is generally believed that the Na+ and K+ currents that flow through the membrane in opposite directions are carried through separate channels. Ca^{2+} ion currents are involved in the activation of at least a portion of the K+ currents and are voltage gated. By activating the K+ currents, the Ca^{2+} ions shorten the length of time the cell is depolarized and thus speed up the firing cycle [83]. A statistical approach to the formation of protein channels in the membrane by Baumann and colleagues predicts many of the observed characteristics [84–86].

During the firing of a nerve cell, the Na+ current pulse precedes the K+ current pulse, which returns the cell to its resting potential [68]. In this model, the overall concentration balances are maintained by active ion pumps. Cl-, Mg^{2+}, and possibly OH- and H+ ions may also be involved in the current flow across a cell membrane.

The firing of a nerve cell typically involves voltage spikes of 0.1 V and peak current densities of 1.5 A/m². Changes in the firing rate can be induced by the injection of charge through a microelectrode of $<10^{-9}$ A for a few milliseconds. However, in cases where electrodes are used to stimulate muscles or to control epilepsy, the current is injected through a series of cell membrane fluid boundaries at a distance from the controlling nerve fiber. Thus, typical injected currents to produce behavioral changes in cells are in milliamperes and current densities are 10 A/m² or higher.

For fields parallel to the plane of the membrane, it is possible to obtain electrophoresis or a rearrangement of charged particles. This has been shown by Poo in a striking fashion in cultured embryonic *Xenopus* myotomal muscle cells [87,88]. Receptors on the surface of the cell were labeled with a fluorescent dye and allowed to uniformly distribute themselves. Exposures to electric fields of 10^2–10^3 V/m were sufficient to concentrate the fluorescent-labeled receptors on the side of the anode in about 10 min. After shutting off the field, diffusion returned the dye to its uniform distribution in about 2 h. This corresponds to an in-plane diffusion constant of about 3×10^{-12} m²/s. The force on the receptor molecules or particles in the membrane includes not only $q\bar{E}$ but also any viscous drag that may be generated by the flow of ions of the opposite sign moving along the surface in the opposite direction. The direction of motion for a given charged particle seems to depend on whether it has a larger or smaller zeta (ζ) potential than the potential across the charged double layer at the interface between the cell surface and the fluid (see Equation 5.10).

Additional work has shown that the distribution of acetylcholine (ACh) receptors is changed by external fields [88]. These receptors are concentrated on the cathode-facing surface of the cell in fields of 10^3 V/m over a period of 30 min by literally rearranging channels already existing in the cell membrane. The concentration or clustering persists for at least 5 h after the field has been turned off, indicating that the clustering is relatively

Static & Low-Frequency Electric Fields

stable. Single-channel patch measurements show both a higher density of ACh channels in the clusters near the cathode and a longer mean duration of the pulses through the transmembrane channels. The length of the current pulse near the anode does not differ from the controls, indicating that the field itself does not have a direct effect on the channel kinetics. The lateral diffusion coefficient, D, of ACh receptors in the plasma membrane of cultured *Xenopus* embryonic muscle cells is estimated to be 2.6×10^{-6} m^2/s at 22°C [87,88]. Lateral concentration gradients in lipid monolayers have been shown to be induced by externally applied electric field gradients. For binary mixtures of dihydrocholesterol and dimyristoylphosphatidylcholine, the application of an electric field gradient at pressures below the critical pressure produces a liquid–liquid phase separation in a monolayer that is otherwise homogenous [89]. This separation occurs at field levels on the order of 10^7 V/m and gradients of 10^9–10^{11} V/m^2.

5.13 Nonlinear Effects of AC Fields on Cells

5.13.1 Introduction

The application of an AC electric field to nonlinear systems, which can be described by either a nonlinear resistance or capacitance, leads to at least partial rectification of the input signal and the generation of harmonics. If two or more signal frequencies are applied, it also leads to frequency mixing of the form

$$f_o = \pm m f_1 \pm n f_2 \tag{5.54}$$

where f_o is the output frequency, f_1 and f_2 are input frequencies, and m and n are integers. The rectified component of the AC current can, in turn, lead to ion accumulation at interfaces, which results in changes in ion concentration [90,91]. These changes in ion concentration, in turn, can affect biological function. Another important additional effect is the dependence of the dielectric constant on frequency. This leads to changes in the electric field distributions in tissue with frequency. Thus, both the electrophoretic and the dielectrophoretic forces become both size and frequency dependent. A third—possibly important—additional effect is the excitation of frequency-sensitive biological systems in a resonant manner. By driving systems near their resonant frequency, we may change the effective amplitude of the stimulating signal and change the frequency of the nerve cells firing.

In this section, we will review the rectification process at the cell membrane in some detail. Additionally, we will show that cell nonlinearities lead to frequency-dependent effects such as injection phase locking of pacemaker cells. We will also briefly examine some problems associated with the exposure of cells to very low, extremely low-frequency (ELF) fields and the application of large ELF fields to biological systems.

5.13.2 Rectification by Cell Membranes

The rectification of currents flowing across membranes has been studied by many authors, beginning with Katz in 1949. Much of this work is referenced by Hayashi and Fishman in their paper on the inward rectifier K$^+$ channel kinetics [90].

For many passive cell membranes, an approximate relation for the transmembrane current can be derived from the Nernst equation as given in Equation 5.41 [91]. If we apply an AC signal across the membrane of the form $+V_M = V_0 + V_1 \cos \omega t$, the resulting current can be approximated for small values of V_M (i.e., $qV_m < \eta kT$) by a Taylor series yielding

$$I = \frac{I_0}{\eta V_T}\left(V_0 + \frac{V_1^2}{4\eta V_T} + V_1 \cos \omega t + \frac{1}{4\eta V_T}V_0 V_1 \cos \omega t + \frac{V_1^2}{4\eta V_T}\cos 2\omega t + \ldots\right) \qquad (5.55)$$

It is to be noted that the second term in the expression is the first approximation to the fraction of the applied AC voltage V_1 that yields a DC current component ΔI

$$\Delta I = \frac{I_0}{4}\left(\frac{V_1}{\eta V_T}\right)^2 \qquad (5.56)$$

or an offset voltage V_{DC} given by

$$V_{DC} \approx \frac{I_0}{4}\left(\frac{V_1}{\eta V_T}\right)^2 R_m \qquad (5.57)$$

where R_m is the membrane impedance. This predicted voltage offset for an applied AC current has been measured by Montaigne and Pickard [92]. In their experiments, an AC signal was applied to a large plant cell by a strip line, and the measured voltage shift was obtained through microelectrodes located outside the applied AC fields. For an applied AC field of about 0.2 V, they measured a DC offset of 1 to $\times 2 \times 10^{-4}$ V. For frequencies above 2.5 kHz, the effects of the membrane capacitance must be taken into account, and the effective driving voltage is reduced to

$$(V_1)_{\mathit{eff}} = \left[\sqrt{2}a\sigma_e \bar{E}_{1rms}\right]\left[(\sigma_e + aG)^2 + (a\omega C)^2\right]^{-1/2} \qquad (5.58)$$

where a is the cell radius, σ_e, is the conductivity of the medium, $\bar{E}_{1rms}$ is the electric field strength in the medium surrounding the cell, G is the membrane conductance per unit area, ω is the frequency, and C is the membrane capacitance per unit area [93]. This leads to the usual roll-off in the measured DC offset with increasing frequency. Note that the DC effect gets still smaller at higher frequencies (above 1 MHz) because of transit time limitations for ion flow across the membrane [94].

The relaxation times for a typical K^+ channel in an *Aplysia* membrane has been measured to be from 2 to 8 ms [95]. Rectification has also been demonstrated in thin lipid membranes [96]. In these systems, both the conductivity of the membrane and the ion concentration differences across it can be controlled. The Nernst equation was shown to apply to the I vs. V curve over a range of voltages from −60 to +40 mV. Depending on the ion concentration and membrane doping, the values of η ranged from 1 to 0.25.

AC field has been carried out by Franceschetti and Pinto and by Casaleggio et al. [96,97]. Both these groups have expanded the Nernst equation in a Volterra series that takes into account memory of the preceding state of the cell. They have also treated the cell in spherical rather than planar geometry. The inclusion of a spherical cell requires that the total current into and out of the cell be equal to zero, and thus loops are formed circulating through the cell membrane (see Figure 5.10). All the theoretical treatments predict a DC component

Static & Low-Frequency Electric Fields

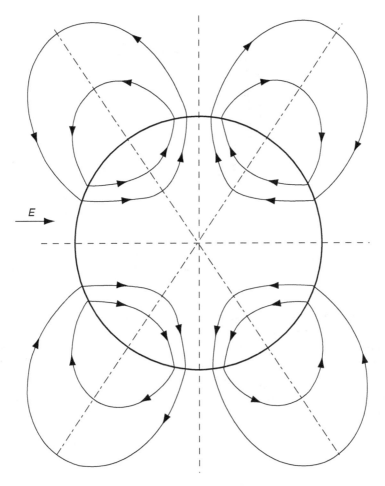

FIGURE 5.10
Induced DC current distribution in a spherical cell. (From Bisceglia and Pinto, I., personal communication, 1984 [99].)

that varies as the square of the input signal V and tends to hyperpolarize the cell or make the interior of the cell more negative.

Cain has considered the effects of an AC field on nonlinearities of the nerve cell by numerical analysis of the Hodgkin–Huxley equation [98].* He applied a voltage

$$V_m = V_0 + V_1 \cos \omega t \left[u(t) - u(t - \tau) \right] \quad (5.59)$$

across the membrane, where $u(t)$ and $u(t-\tau)$ are unit step functions that define an AC pulse of length τ. For the case where the AC frequency is large compared to the reciprocal of the pulse length, if a 7 mV depolarizing pulse is also applied to the membrane, the action potential is obtained as shown in Figure 5.11. Cain has assumed coefficients appropriate to the giant squid axon. Increasing V_1 first delays, and then suppresses, the action

---

* Bisceglia and Pinto have applied a Volterra series expansion to the Hodgkin–Huxley equations. This approach gives an alternate method to Cain's of computing the current shifts resulting from applied AC signals [99].

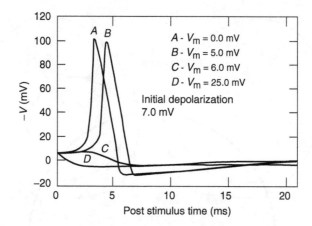

FIGURE 5.11
Computed membrane action potentials in response to an initial membrane depolarization of 7 mV for different values of V_m. Curves are solutions to the Hodgkin–Huxley equations. (From Cain, C.A., *Bioelectromagnetics*, 2, 23, 1981. With permission [98].)

potential. If no depolarizing pulse is applied, the predicted changes in g_{Na} and g_K and the deviation V from the resting potential are as shown in Figure 5.12 for a 10 m s AC pulse with $V_1 = 25$ mV. Note that the applied AC frequency is assumed high enough not to be resolved in these figures. From these results, it is clear that AC signals can induce substantial changes in the operating characteristics of nerve cells at moderate to high levels of applied voltage. Although the appropriate coefficients were not measured in order to make a direct comparison between theory and experiments, Wachtel's results on *Aplysia*

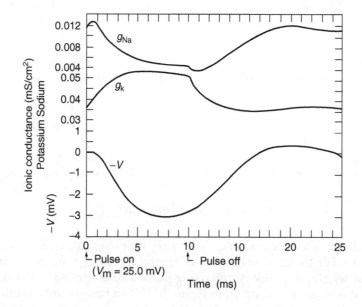

FIGURE 5.12
Response of model axon to a pulsed oscillating component of membrane electric field (10-ms pulse, $V_m - 25$ mV). The membrane potential and the sodium and potassium conductances are shown. These curves are solutions of the Hodgkin–Huxley equations. (Note: 1 mS/cm² = 10 S/m².) (From Cain, C.A., *Bioelectromagnetics*, 2, 23, 1981. With permission [98].)

at frequencies above the lock-in range would appear to support Cain's theoretical predictions [100].

Wachtel has made a series of measurements that demonstrate the nonlinear characteristics of pacemaker cells from *Aplysia* [100]. First, he measured the current input through a microelectrode that changed the firing rate of the cell. The current threshold for a minimum detectable change was approximately 6×10^{-10} A at frequencies between 0.8 and 1 Hz (see Figure 5.13). The natural firing rate for this cell is about 0.8 Hz, and an increasing current is required to synchronize the cell to the injected signal as the frequency deviates from the natural firing rate. A theory for injection locking of electronic oscillators predicts that the signal required for locking an oscillator to an external signal increases linearly as the difference between the two $\Delta \omega$ frequencies [101]. The signal required for lock-in according to this theory is given by

$$I_t \approx |A\Delta\omega| I \qquad (5.60)$$

where I_t is the injected signal current and I is the peak unperturbed oscillator current. $A = \partial\phi/\partial\omega$ is the rate of change of phase with respect to frequency in the unperturbed oscillator. $\Delta\omega_0$ is equal to the difference between the frequency of the free-running oscillator and the injected signal. This expression is applicable as long as

$$\Delta\omega_0 \leq \frac{2\pi}{\tau} \qquad (5.61)$$

where τ is the time constant for adjusting the gain of the circuit. The time constant τ for the *Aplysia* cells varied between 0.1 and 0.5 s, and this corresponds to a maximum measured lock-in frequency of about 10 Hz. The results in Figure 5.13 show the threshold for one-to-one locking up to about 2 Hz. In the range from 2 to 10 Hz, Wachtel observed a lower threshold for subharmonic locking than one-to-one locking. At frequencies above 80 Hz, he observed a constant shift in the firing rate of the neuron in response to the injected transmembrane AC signal. The natural firing rate would be restored by also

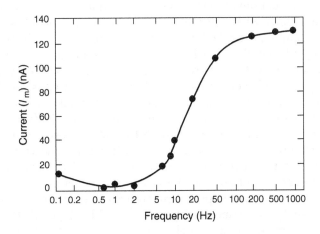

FIGURE 5.13
Intracellular (transmembrane) currents I_m (in nA) needed at different frequencies to produce firing-pattern changes (in a pacemaker neuron). Note that the detectable changes take on different forms at different frequencies. (From Wachtel, H., *Proceedings of the 18th Annual Hansford Life Science Symposium*, Technical Information Center, U.S. Department of Energy, Richland, WA, 132, 1978. With permission [100].)

injecting a transmembrane DC signal equal in amplitude to about 1% of the peak-to-peak value of the AC current. This DC current was in the depolarizing direction, making the exterior of the cell more negative with respect to the cell cytoplasm to increase the firing rate, i.e., to restore it to its natural value. Apparently, the applied transmembrane AC current was partially rectified so as to hyperpolarize the membrane, making the interior of the cell more negative with respect to the external fluid. The details of how the applied field modifies the ion flow are only partially understood, but one characteristic is an increase in the conductivity for K^+, which increases its flow out of the cell. Wachtel also injected low-frequency currents into the seawater surrounding the cell preparation through external electrodes [100]. In this case, the minimum current densities flowing in the vicinity of the cell preparation for injection locking were estimated to be about 10^{-2} A/m^2, and there was about a 30–1 variation between the maximum and minimum sensitivities for changes in angle between the applied field and the cells. At frequencies above 100 Hz, a minimum of about 0.35 A/m^2 was necessary to obtain a detectable change in firing rate.

These studies have been extended by Barnes et al. (102), and injection locking at harmonic and subharmonics has been shown to occur. It is suggested that phase locking may provide a mechanism for narrow banding or time averaging so that a weak coherent signal may be distinguished from noise by a cell. In an electronic circuit model, we showed we could phase lock an oscillator at signal-to-noise ratios <1 [102]. Extensive modeling of phase locking for a squid axon using two versions of the Hodgkin–Huxley equations has been carried out by Fohlmeister et al. [103]. They show that phase locking can occur for a wide variety of frequencies with AM-modulated signals at injected current densities greater than 0.1 A/m^2 [103]. For natural oscillation frequencies less than the externally applied signal, the system may be treated as a parametric process. For parametric amplification, a phase stability such that

$$\frac{d\phi}{dt} < \Delta\omega - KV_s \tag{5.62}$$

is required for injection locking of the frequency of oscillation to an external signal, where $d\phi/dt$ is the rate of change of the phase, $\Delta\omega$ is the frequency offset, K is the linear control characteristic in units of $(2\pi\,\mathrm{Hz/V})$ and is closely related to the loop gain, and V_s is the injected signal [101]. Stated in words, this equation requires that the amplified signal, KV_s be large enough to correct for the random frequency fluctuations $d\phi/dt$ generated by the noise for the system to become phase locked to a signal that is displaced by $\Delta\omega$ (see Figure 5.12 for some examples of injection locking of pacemaker cells to an external signal) [104,105]. An increase in the sensitivity to electromagnetic fields has also been shown in isolated frog hearts for signals that approach the natural resonant frequency or firing rate [106]. In these experiments, the firing rate of the heart was shown to increase as much as 30% when a signal in the vicinity of 10–20 V/m was applied through Ringer's solution to the isolated frog hearts at a frequency between 0.5 and 1 Hz. The natural firing rate of these excised hearts started out at approximately 1 Hz and dropped to about 0.5 Hz over a period of 2 h, where they remained stable for at least 5 h. To get a 30% increase in firing rate at 60 Hz, it was necessary to apply field strengths of 60–80 V/m. Thus, we have additional evidence that electric fields with repetition rates near the natural biological signaling frequencies are more likely to induce changes than those of higher frequencies and that signal strengths required for a given shift increase approximately linearly up to some cutoff, as shown in Figure 5.14.

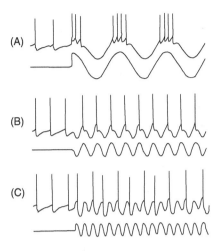

FIGURE 5.14
Examples of several modes of synchrony between an imposed ELF field and neuronal patterns. In each case, the ELF current is shown below the transmembrane potential recording. (A) For ELF frequencies well below FR_0, several nerve impulses (spikes) are locked to each ELF half cycle. (B) ELF frequencies slightly above FR_0 are effective in phase locking the rise of neuronal spikes on a one-to-one basis. (C) For ELF frequencies several times greater than FR_0, phase locking can take the form of spikes occurring on alternate cycles (two-for-one synchrony). (From Barnes, F.S., *Bioelectromagn. Suppl.*, 1, 67–85, 1992. With permission [104].)

For weak fields, it has been shown that cells can respond differently to signals that are both space and time coherent than they do for signals that look like the background noise. Litovitz et al. have shown that the application of 10 µT magnetic fields at either 55 or 65 Hz doubles the specific activity of ornithine decarboxylase (ODC) in L929 cells if the signals are coherent for periods of 10 s or longer during the course of a 4 h exposure [107]. The applied signal and the corresponding ODC response as a function of the coherence time are shown in Figure 5.15. The ODC response of the cell can be fitted to an exponential curve of the form

$$(ODC) = 1 + 1.26\left[1 - \exp\left(\frac{\tau_{coh}}{\tau_{cell}}\right)\right] \tag{5.63}$$

where τ_{coh} is the length of the time between shifts in frequency and the introduction of a random phase shift and τ_{cell} is the effective time constant of the cell [107]. τ_{cell} has a value of about 8 s for these cells. If a spatially coherent noise signal with a power spectral density ranging from 30 to 90 Hz is superimposed on the coherent signal, the increased ODC response decreases with a decreasing signal-to-noise ratio and is less than 10% at a signal-to-noise ratio of 1 [108]. This work has been extended to show that temporally incoherent magnetic fields inhibit 60 Hz-induced changes in the ODC activity of developing chick embryos [109].

For the exposure geometry used in these experiments, the magnetic field induced a corresponding electric field of 4 µV/m. This signal is well below the calculated thermal noise field of 0.02 V/m for a 20 µm cell diameter. The combined results of the experiments cited above indicate that both space and time coherence may be used by cells to separate useful signals from larger natural background noise signals. For example, to get a significant biological response, some threshold number of channels or receptor molecules may need to be activated within a given period of time; this, in turn, requires nearly simultaneous activation over a significant fraction of the cell surface. Similar results have been obtained

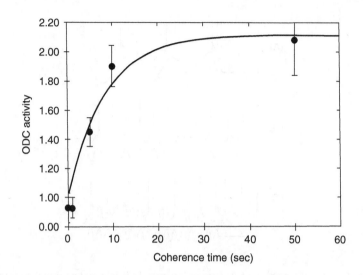

FIGURE 5.15
Plot of the enhancement of ODC activity (exposed/control) as a function of the coherence time, τ_{coh}, of the applied field. The solid line is the best fit to the mathematical function given by Equation 5.50, where τ_{cell} is found to be 8.2 s. The experimental points shown represent a minimum of six different exposures. (© Academic Press; From Litovitz, T.A., Krause, D., and Mullins, J.M., *Biochem. Biophys. Res. Commun.*, 178, 3, 862, 1991. With permission [107].)

for developing chick embryos, where weak coherent signals lead to an increased incidence of abnormalities [110]. In this work, Litovitz and his colleagues show an increase in the incidence of abnormalities of approximately a factor of 3 for White Leghorn chicken embryos incubated in periodic magnetic fields with peak field strength of 1 μT (100 Hz repetition rate, 500 μs pulse duration, 2 μs rise, and decay times) when compared with the controls. This increased rate of the incidence of abnormalities was nearly eliminated with the addition of band-filtered noise with a spectrum running from 30 to 100 Hz and a root mean square value of 1 μT. Thus, Litovitz makes a strong case for a requirement of both space and time coherence for biological systems to detect signals below the natural noise environment.

A number of experiments indicate that at least two mechanisms are involved in the effects of low-level time-varying magnetic fields on membrane transport. The first of these is through Faraday's law or the induced electric field, which, in turn, induces electric currents. In these experiments, one would expect to get the same effects by introducing electric fields with electrodes at levels that induce the same current densities. The second group of experiments indicates that the background DC magnetic field is also important and that the combined effects of AC and DC magnetic fields are observed.

The initial experiments by Walleczek and Liburdy showed an enhanced uptake of Ca^{2+} in Con. A-activated rat thymocytes with exposures of 1 h to 60 Hz magnetic fields of 22 mT and induced current densities of 0.16 A/m² [111]. In this paper, the exposure system consisted of concentric rings on cell culture plates, which, in turn, were placed in a water-cooled solenoid that produced a uniform magnetic field. This was followed by a group of experiments by Liburdy on Ca^{2+} transport across mitogen-activated lymphocyte membranes [112]. In these experiments, both the DC and the AC magnetic fields were controlled so that the DC geomagnetic field and the ambient 60 Hz fields were perpendicular to the exposed and control plates. The results show an increase in the Ca^{2+} influx during the plateau phase of the calcium signaling for Con. A-activated lymphocytes, which was a function of the induced electric field and which could be reproduced by applying the electric fields across the cells with a salt bridge at levels between 0.1 and 0.17 V/m. This corresponds to induced current levels of 0.168–0.28 A/m² in the fluid surrounding the cells, which had a conductivity, σ = 1.68 S/m, that is approximately a hundred times larger than the current densities observed around growing cells. Thus, the approximately 20%–25% increase in the initial Ca^{2+} uptake is the result of a relatively large external current. In other experiments it was also shown that the response is dependent on the age of the animals from which cells are taken [113].

Most other reported experiments have not been done in a way to sort out the differences between possible direct effects of the magnetic fields and the induced electric fields. Yost and Liburdy [114] have also conducted experiments in the same system that shows a direct dependence of the calcium uptake on the DC magnetic field.

The experiments by McLeod et al. [115] show both a frequency dependence and a dependence on the electric field strength across the cell membrane. They exposed neonatal bovine fibroblast cells to electric fields in culture through a media bridge. The fibroblasts populated a collagen matrix that enabled the cells to be grown with a dominant orientation and exposed to a well-defined current. An estimate of newly synthesized protein was made by measuring the incorporation of (³H) proline into macromolecules after a 12-h exposure to current densities ranging from 10^{-3} to 10 A/m² and frequencies from 0.1 Hz to 1 kHz. The results in Figure 5.15 show an approximately 30% reduction in the ³H counts with current densities as low as 10^{-2} A/m². This reduction is interpreted as a reduction in the incorporation of newly synthesized protein into the extracellular matrix rather than as a change in the cell number. The frequency specificity for this threshold is shown in Figure 5.16; the peak sensitivity was recorded at 5×10^{-3} A/m² and 10 Hz.

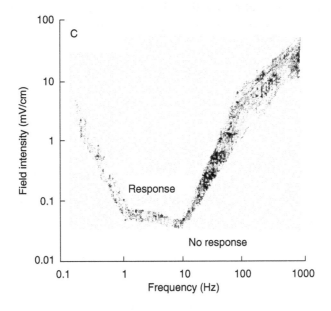

FIGURE 5.16
Minimum field intensity for a detectable response. Summary of results for all tested frequencies and current densities. Current densities were converted to peak field intensities by using the measured media resistivity of 65 Ωcm. The lower boundary of the gray region represents the highest field intensity at which no significant change in extracellular protein accumulation was detected; the upper boundary represents the lowest intensity evoking a statistically significant change (n = 6). (From McLeod, K.J., Lee, R.C., and Ehrlich, H.P., *Science*, 136, 1465–1469, 1987 [115].)

The corresponding peak electric field intensity was 4.5 mV/m. The fractional change in the (^{3}H) proline was nearly independent of the current density for increases in current density up to two orders of magnitude above 10^{-2} A/m^2. The cell membranes have a resistance many times higher than the resistance of the matrix as a whole. The cells are also asymmetric, with a ratio of major to minor axes of about 7–10. Thus, the current through the cell membranes would be expected to be at a maximum when the long axes of the cells are parallel to the applied field. For randomly oriented cells, current densities of 3 mA/m^2 produced no significant effect on the rate of proline incorporation. However, when the cells were oriented parallel to the electric field that was estimated at 2 mV/m and 10 Hz, a little more than a 30% reduction was observed. The estimated transmembrane potential was 0.5 µV. With the cell oriented perpendicular to the field, no significant change in proline incorporation was measured at 5 mA/m^2.

In addition to the nonlinear conductances associated with Na$^+$ and K$^+$ currents, membranes also exhibit nonlinear (i.e., potential dependent) and frequency-dependent capacitances and inductances. It is sometimes useful to think of these effects in terms of a phasor diagram as shown in Figure 5.17, where the electric field vector $\vec{E}$ is rotating at a velocity ω, and ϕ is the phase angle between $\vec{E}$ and the current density $\vec{J}$. If there is, for example, a fixed time delay between the field activation of a current gate and the current flow, then, depending on the frequency, $\vec{J}$ may be in any of the four quadrants and appear capacitive or inductive or even present a negative resistance to an external driving source.

Nonlinear inductive effects seem to be associated with the time delay for the onset of the K$^+$ currents under excitation in a typical excitable membrane, and they have been studied in the giant squid axon [50]. The nonlinear capacitive effects are difficult to measure at frequencies below a few kilohertz. Extra care needs to be exercised to minimize the series resistance and the end effects of the wire being used to measure the capacitance or inductance. Additionally, corrections must be made in the calculations of the membrane

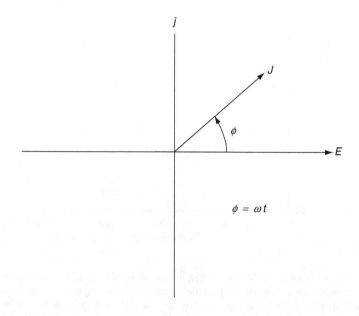

FIGURE 5.17
Steady-state vector characterization of electric fields $\vec{E}$ versus current density $\vec{J}$ in polar form. ϕ is the phase angle between the sinusoidal electric field $\vec{E}$ and the resulting current density $\vec{J}$.

capacitance to take into account the appropriate variations in the frequency response that these terms introduce. However, when this is done, it can be shown that the membrane capacitance has both frequency- and voltage-dependent terms. The capacitance of giant squid axons is shown in Figures 5.18 and 5.19 as a function of frequency and membrane voltage.

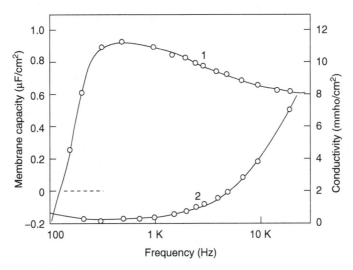

FIGURE 5.18
Membrane capacitance (Curve 1) and conductivity (Curve 2) of squid giant axon at various frequencies. Note the anomalous behavior at low-frequencies. (Note: 1µF/cm².) (From Takashima, S., in Illinger, K.H., Ed., *Biological Effects of Nonionizing Radiation*, ACS Symposium Series, No. 157, 133–145, 1981. [116])

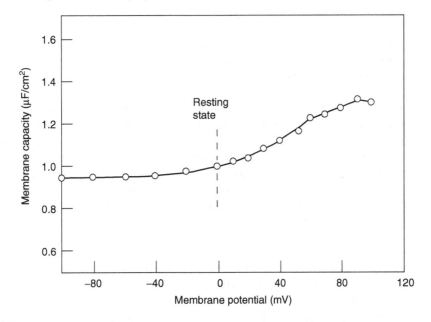

FIGURE 5.19
Membrane capacitance of squid giant axon at various membrane potentials. Membrane potential was shifted by injecting currents. The abscissa shows the actual potential across the membrane in millivolts. (From Takashima, S., in *Biological Effects of Nonionizing Radiation*, ACS Symposium Series, No. 157, Illinger, K.H., Ed., 133–145, 1981. [116])

Variation of the capacitance of these membranes with frequency and amplitude differs from that of a simple bilipid membrane that has nearly constant capacitance. The variation appears to be associated with changes in the conformation of the proteins associated with the Na^+ conductance channels. Nonlinearity in conductance and capacitance can be induced into a bilipid membrane by the addition of Alamethicin. The nonlinear inductance or capacitance may also generate both sum and difference frequencies if two signals are applied. For the case of the single signal, a DC term is added to the current density that is proportional to membrane potential and the square of the applied AC signal [116,117]. The effects due to nonlinear membrane capacitance thus far observed are small. They appear likely to be more important in providing an understanding of the possible gating mechanism in membranes than as a mechanism for introducing rectification.

Another form of nonlinearity in the electrical response of cells comes about in what is often described as adaptive processes. For example, we found that repetitive exposures of pacemaker cells (taken from the ganglion of an *Aplysia*) to microwave pulses resulted in a decreasing reduction in the firing rate by successive pulses. This kind of change has also been shown to occur in neurons that have been conditioned with repetitive stimulation. Studies of conditioning have shown decreases in potassium ion conductance through membranes, thus raising the internal potential and enhancing the excitability [118,119]. The decrease in resistance between adjacent cells can occur in two ways. First, the resistance of gap junctions may be reduced by repetitive electrical stimulation, which increases the electrical coupling between the cells by up to 62%. Second, repetitive electrical stimulation can modify the chemical excitatory postsynaptic potential by amounts ranging from 31% to 140% [119]. This change is associated with the movement of protein kinase C from the interior of the cell into the membrane. An accompanying change in Ca^{2+} concentrations and the movement of a second messenger, diacylglycerol, into the membrane reduce the potassium ion flow. This enhanced excitability reduces the voltage or the charge required to initiate an action potential. If charge is transferred efficiently between cells, either actively or passively, cell length is effectively multiplied in the linear model by the number of cells in the chain; this, in turn, reduces the external electric field required to generate a given voltage across a terminating membrane.

An interesting speculation that is raised by these adaptive processes is whether or not a neural network can be trained to identify a repetitive signal such as 60 Hz in the presence of larger electric fields generated by the surrounding biological material. To test this hypothesis, we programmed a computer to simulate a neural network as shown in Figure 5.20 [102]. Using a backpropagation algorithm to adjust the connecting weights between neurons, a sigmoidal summing junction to model the neurons, and a pseudorandom noise generator, we measured the number of runs required to train the network to recognize a 60 Hz signal with 97% accuracy as a function of the input signal-to-noise ratio. The results in Figure 5.19 show that the training time increased from about 200 runs to about 1400 runs as the signal-to-noise ratio decreased from 1 to 0.001. The way the noise is presented to this network during the training makes a difference. For example, if you want the network to separate 59 Hz from 60 Hz, it helps to tell the network that 59 Hz is noise. This computer network model is clearly too simple to describe a biological nervous system, but it may provide a clue to one way in which a collection of cells may be able to respond to weak, externally applied electric fields, but a single cell would not.

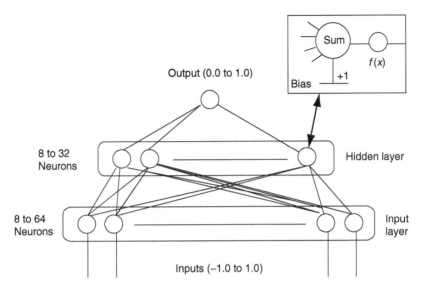

FIGURE 5.20
Backpropagation neural network. (From Barnes, F.S., *Bioelectromagn. Suppl.*, 1, 67–85, 1992. With permission [104].)

5.14 Thermal Effects

One important effect of current flow due to electric fields is heating. The power input to a given volume of material can be expressed by $P' = I^2R$, where I is the total current and R is the resistance of the sample. For many calculations, a more useful expression is given by the power per unit volume or $P = \sigma E^2$, where σ is the conductivity, E is the electric field intensity. (For a more complete treatment of heating, see Chapter 9 of *BMA*.) The temperature rise resulting from this heat input is determined by the thermal capacity of the volume and the mechanisms for carrying the heat energy away. Typically, these thermal loss mechanisms include a combination of conduction and convection processes. For short current pulses, the heat dissipation is usually dominated by thermal conduction, and the basic equation for the rate of change of temperature is given by

$$\frac{\partial T}{\partial t} = \frac{P}{\rho' C_p} - \frac{T - T_0}{\tau_c} \qquad (5.64)$$

where T is the temperature, T_0 is the initial temperature, t is time, and P is the power supplied per unit volume. ρ' is the density of the material (in kg/m³), C_p is the specific heat under constant pressure, and τ_c is the thermal relaxation time.

If we consider a homogenous sphere of radius a immersed in an infinite fluid, the thermal conductive relaxation time is approximately given by

$$\tau_c = \frac{a^2}{4\bar{K}} \qquad (5.65)$$

where $\bar{K}$ is the thermal diffusivity and is measured in meter square per second [120]. The thermal diffusivity is given by

$$\bar{K} = \frac{K'}{\rho' C_p} \tag{5.66}$$

where K' is the thermal conductivity (in cal/m s °C), ρ' is the material density (in kg/m³), and C_p is the thermal capacity (in cal/°C kg). If an applied current pulse is short compared to τ_c, the maximum temperature change is given by

$$\Delta T_{max} = \left(\frac{3}{2\pi e}\right)^{3/2} \frac{\bar{H}}{\rho' C_p a^3} \tag{5.67}$$

where $\bar{H}$ is the total input energy in calories and e is the base of natural logarithms [120]. For current inputs that are long compared to the thermal relaxation time τ_c, the peak temperature is determined by a balance between the input power and the dissipation process controlled by conduction and convection including blood flow. It is interesting to note that if we assume the thermal properties of water as a first approximation to various kinds of tissue, then τ_c for a sphere with a equal to 1 μm is a little less than 2 μs. Since a sphere has the smallest surface to volume ratio, Equation 5.65 gives an upper bound on τ_c, and Equation 5.67 gives an upper bound on the peak temperature excursion for small structures and pulses that are short compared to τ_c. Simply stated, it takes high power densities and large differential absorption coefficients to get significant differential temperature rises in small biological structures.

For situations where the volume involved is a cubic millimeter or larger, the thermal time constant is controlled by the amount of blood flowing through the volume. In these cases, temperatures may be more easily measured than calculated since a complicated thermal and electrical boundary value problem would have to be solved to calculate the temperature rise. This is particularly true since the viscosity η and other thermal and electrical parameters such as ρ, C_p, $\bar{K}$, etc. are functions of temperature. For example, C_p for an artificial bilipid membrane is shown in Figure 5.22 [121]. Another example of the importance of change in temperature is the electrical conductivity of saline,

$$\sigma \approx C_1 \left[10^{[(1/T)+\alpha](1/b)} \right] \times 10^{-4} S / m \tag{5.68}$$

where C_1 is the concentration of NaCl in milligram equivalents per liter, T is the absolute temperature, $\alpha \approx 6.23 \times 10^{-3}$ degrees⁻¹, and $b \approx 1.4 \times 10^{-3}$ degrees⁻¹ [122]. In the range around 37.5°C, this means that a 5°C change in temperature corresponds to a little less than 9% change in conductivity [122].

Changes in temperature are important, not only because they change transport properties such as viscosity, mobility, and the diffusion coefficient D, but also because they change chemical reaction rates. Typical biochemical reactions can be described by an equation of the form

$$\frac{dS}{dt} = -K'S \tag{5.69}$$

where S is the fraction of the material that has undergone the chemical reaction, t is the time, and K' is the reaction rate [123]. K' is often given by

$$K' = \frac{kT}{h} \exp\left(\frac{+\Delta H' - T\Delta S'}{R'T}\right) \tag{5.70}$$

Static & Low-Frequency Electric Fields

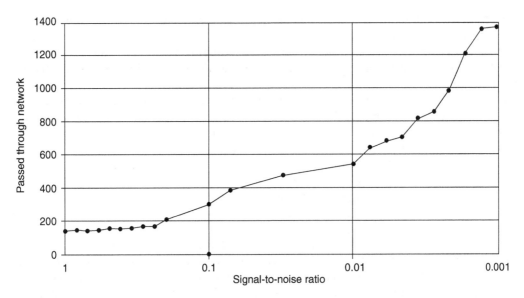

FIGURE 5.21
The learning response of a neural network with 64 input neurons, 8 neurons in the hidden layer, and 1 output neuron to a 60 Hz input signal and a pseudorandom noise signal with a decreasing signal-to-noise ratio. (From Barnes, F.S., *Bioelectromagn. Suppl.*, 1, 67–85, 1992. With permission [104].)

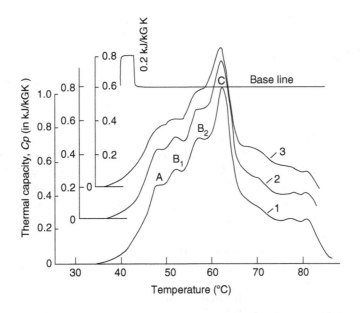

FIGURE 5.22
Differential changes in the heat capacity, C_p, of erythrocyte membranes as a function of temperature in 5 mmol/L sodium phosphate with pH 7.4 and a concentration of 5 mg protein per milliliter. The changes at A, B, B_2, and C correspond to changes in the structure of the membrane with temperature and are irreversible. Curve 1: intact membranes. Curve 2: irradiated at 330 MHz for 5 min (SAR 9 W/kg). Curve 3: irradiated at 300 MHz for 30 min (SAR W/kg). (From Shuyrou, V.L., Zhodan, G.G., and Akorv, I.G., Academy of Science, Institute of Biophysics, Pushchino, Moscow Region, Russia, personal communication, 1984. With permission [121].)

where k is the Boltzmann constant, T is the absolute temperature, H' is the free energy, S' is the entropy, h is Plank's constant, and R' is the gas constant. The significant feature is that the reaction rate K' varies exponentially with temperature, and $\Delta H'$ and $T\Delta S'$ are large numbers. Thus, very small changes in temperature can lead to big changes in chemical reaction rates.

In addition to chemical reaction rate changes, there may be changes in the binding of the proteins to cell membranes that lead to a shedding of proteins with a small increase in temperature. An exponential temperature dependence of the binding to membrane receptors is to be expected just as it is for chemical reactions [124].

A rule of thumb that the author uses to estimate whether or not significant biological changes are likely is to see if ΔT is >10°C for 10^{-6} s, 5°C for 1 s, or 2°C for hours. If the ΔTs are larger, then they can be expected to lead to important changes in the biological system. Typical mammalian temperature regulatory systems will hold the internal body temperature constant to within ±0.5°C.

In addition to the magnitude of the temperature change, it can be shown that the rate of temperature rise, dT/dt, is important and can induce current to flow across membranes. Changes in the firing rate of pacemaker cells from the ganglion of *Aplysia* have been induced by total temperature changes of as little as 1/10°C when the rates of change are about 1°C/s [125]. This change of the firing rate corresponds to the injection of approximately 1 nA into the cell. By taking the time derivative of the Nernst equation, which describes the passive equilibrium potential across a membrane for a single ion, it can be shown that a current proportional to the temperature derivative is to be expected, or

$$ I = -qV'_1C_1\left(\frac{\phi}{\phi_T}\right)\left(\frac{\dot{\phi}}{\phi} - \frac{\dot{T}}{T}\right) \tag{5.71} $$

where q is the charge of the ion, V'_1 is the volume of the cell, C_1 is the concentration of ions inside the cell, ϕ is the resting potential, ϕ_T is given by $f_T = \dfrac{kT}{q}$, $\dot{\phi}$ is the derivative of the membrane potential with respect to time, T is the temperature, and $\dot{T}$ is the temperature derivative with respect to time [126].

Bol'shakov and Alekseyev [127] have observed similar changes in the firing rate of pacemaker cells taken from the large parietal ganglion of the central nervous system of *Limnea stagnalis*. In their experiments they observed a slow increase in temperature (1°C/min or slower) to increase the firing rate of the pacemaker cell and a rapid increase in temperature (0.1°C/s or faster) to decrease or stop the firing. They ascribe these changes to changes in the Na^+ pump as the rapid temperature effect was completely blocked by adding ouabain to the solution. In addition to the changes in the Na^+ currents, Ca^+ currents have been shown to be sensitive to rapid changes in temperature [128]. The rate of rise has also been shown to be significant in exciting a brain slice from a mouse with pulses of 10^{-3} s and peak temperature rises of less than 0.5°C [129].

Temperature rises also lead to thermal expansion, and rapid temperature rises lead to the generation of acoustic waves [130]. These acoustic waves, in turn, can affect stretch receptors in nerve cells and other tissue and thus generate a biological response that may be at a considerable distance from the electrical heating [131].

To get an idea of the magnitudes of both heating (as described in Equation 5.64) and the effect of the rate of rise (as given by Equation 5.71), consider the case of liver tissue with $\sigma = 0.14$ S/m and a field strength in the tissue of 2×10^3 V/m. The rate of temperature rise is

Static & Low-Frequency Electric Fields 207

approximately 13°C/s assuming no conduction or convection heat losses and the thermal capacity of water. For this high field, a significant temperature rise occurs in about 1/2 s. However, the rate of rise has been shown to be significant in exciting a brain slice from a mouse with pulses of 10^{-3} s [132].

5.15 Natural Fields, Man-Made Fields, Noise, and Random Fluctuations

It is of interest to compare man-made with naturally occurring fields. First, we would like to know the approximate magnitudes of the fields that occur in nature outside man or the biological system of interest. Second, we would like to have values for the internal or physiological fields.

The natural electric fields at the surface of the earth have both DC and AC components [133]. One may think of the earth as a spherical capacitor where the surface is negatively charged with respect to an electrical conducting ionosphere that is about 50 km above the surface. This capacitor is being continuously charged by about 100 lightning strokes per second from thunderstorms worldwide. Since the atmosphere is a finite conductor, it also discharges with an RC time constant of about 18 s. The result is an average electric field of about 130 V/m. This field is not uniform with height and typically falls off to 30 V/m at 1 km above the surface. The local values vary widely with temperature and humidity. In the Sahara during dust storms caused by winds in the dry season, a field of 1500 V/m has been measured with the polarity reversed from the normal. In thunderstorms, fields of up to 3000 V/m have been measured without lightning, and the polarity has been known to reverse in minutes. Storms as far as 50 km away have been shown to affect local fields. See also Chapter 1 in this volume.

The atmosphere is a relatively poor conductor and as such will suspend a significant number of charged ions, dust particles, etc. This helps to contribute to local field variations of 20% to 50% over the course of the day and is a normal characteristic of our environment. The level of natural AC fields in the atmosphere falls very rapidly from a DC value of about 130 V/m [133]. The average value of the vertical component of the electric field above 1 Hz has a typical value of 10^{-4} V/m Hz$^{1/2}$. However, this value fluctuates widely with the time of day, the season of the year, and location. Additionally, the Schumann resonances impose multiple-cavity resonances on this spectrum with a periodicity of about 10 Hz. These resonances may be explained in terms of standing waves in a cavity formed by the earth and the atmosphere. These very low levels of the natural fields are one of the reasons why electronic communications in the ELF band are useful for ships at sea and submarines. However, because of the very low level of the natural atmospheric fields at frequencies above a few hertz, there is very little reason for biological organisms to develop natural protection against perturbations at these frequencies. It also means that biological systems could communicate internally at these frequencies using very low signal power levels and still maintain a good signal-to-noise ratio.

Many of signals generated within the body are the result of nerve firing and other cell activity. A typical nerve cell fires with an action potential of 50–100 mV and transmits a current pulse about 0.4 ms long [134]. The rise time for this current spike is approximately 0.1 ms, and the fall time is about 0.5 ms. Each pulse is followed by a refractory period that is typically on the order of 1–3 m s. The longitudinal fields along the exterior of a nerve cell membrane are estimated to have a maximum value of about 5×10^{-2} V/m during an action potential when the cell is surrounded by a relatively high conductivity fluid of 5 S/m [50]. If we look at these signals closely, it will be noted that the interspike interval along any given nerve cell fluctuates in time. Additionally, variations in the beat-to-beat intervals for the ECG are random or chaotic, and the period can vary up to 30%. This is frequently seen, particularly at slow heart rates.

In looking at the natural fields in the body, we have two concerns. The first is how large an external signal is needed to perturb the ongoing natural signal that is being used to communicate or control some biological process [135]. The second is how much of the signal field typically leaks away from active nerve fibers or bundles to form a background noise environment for surrounding tissue and processes. Regarding the first of these questions, it is interesting to look on the microscopic level at the electrical noise, i.e., the fluctuations that occur fundamentally as a result of the electrical process itself. See Chapter 8 in this volume for more information the detection of signals in the presence of noise.

The first of several sources of noise that are always present is blackbody radiation, or Johnson noise, which is given by

$$P_n = kTB \qquad (5.72)$$

where P_n is the noise power, k is the Boltzmann constant, T is the absolute temperature, and B is the bandwidth [136,138]. The voltage equivalent of this noise power, which can be delivered to a matched load (one where the resistance of the source is equal to the resistance of the load; in the case of complex impedances the source and the load are complex conjugates), or the mean squared voltage fluctuation $\bar{V}_n^2$ across a resistance R, is given by [136–138]

$$\bar{V}_n^2 = 4kTBR \qquad (5.73)$$

or by the mean squared current fluctuations

$$\bar{i}_n^2 = \frac{4kTB}{R} \qquad (5.74)$$

Johnson noise applies to systems at thermodynamic equilibrium. Living systems are not at thermodynamic equilibrium. Thus, the foregoing expressions must be applied with caution to only those portions of biological systems where thermodynamic equilibrium is a good approximation. In the case of lasers, the spontaneous emission noise associated with the nonequilibrium population inversion of the energy levels can be obtained from Planck's radiation law by defining a negative temperature that assumes a Boltzmann distribution of atoms with N_2 atoms in the excited energy level E_2, which is greater than the N_1 atoms in the energy level E_1, such that

$$\frac{N_1}{N_2} = \exp\left[\frac{E_2 - E_1}{kT}\right] \qquad (5.75)$$

In this case, the spontaneous emission noise $P_n = hvB$, where h is Planck's constant and v is the frequency of the radiation corresponding to a transition from E_2 to E_1 [136]. In those situations, where the nonequilibrium characteristic may be described by an amplifier that can be modeled by a negative resistor or by energy storage in an inverted population distribution, the concept of a negative temperature may be a useful approach. Note that an equivalent temperature, T, is a convenient way to describe the energy distribution of a

Static & Low-Frequency Electric Fields

large number of particles. A much more complete description of nonequilibrium noise is given in Chapter 8 in this volume.

The second source of noise that is also present is the shot noise, which is given by

$$\overline{i_n^2} = 2q\overline{I}_{DC}B \tag{5.76}$$

where $\overline{i_n^2}$ is the mean-squared current fluctuation. This noise comes about because of the discreteness of the electronic charge q and the assumption that the motion of each charge is independent. With negative feedback, this noise may be reduced, as has been shown for space charge-limited diodes. Shot noise results in an AC fluctuation, $\overline{i_n^2}$, which is proportional to the average value of the current, $\overline{I}_{DC}$.

A third source of noise is $1/f$ noise. This noise may be generated by many processes, some of which are described in Chapter 8 in this volume. $1/f$ noise can be synthesized from Gaussian noise by filtering it with a circuit that requires about one low pass state variable per decade for the period of time over which the model is used to generate noise with a power density spectrum $S(f) = (C/f^\alpha)$, where C is a constant and α is a constant between 1 and 2 [139]. We can expect to find this kind of noise for processes that evolve with time and/or have memory. $1/f$ noise describes the power spectral density of the fluctuations at low-frequencies in such diverse phenomena as transistors, quartz crystal oscillators, the closing Dow Jones Averages for the stock market, and the weather. It is also generated by the flow of ion currents through an orifice and thus is a fundamental part of the transport of current through channels in membranes [140,141]. Measurements of the noise voltage across a 10 μm hole in a 6 μm Mylar film showed that for a wide range of ionic concentrations the voltage noise spectral density $S(f)$ is given by

$$\frac{S_\phi(f)}{\phi^2} = \frac{a}{bnr^3 f} \tag{5.77}$$

where b is a numerical geometric factor, n is the density of ions in the solution, r is the radius of the hole, a is a constant, and ϕ is the applied voltage. The data showed that $2.5 < a < 40$ with a mean value of 10 for a wide range of solutions including HCl, KCl, and AgNO, with concentrations from 0.05 to 5 mol.

For natural membranes, this noise has been shown to take the form of

$$S_E(f) = \frac{C_E}{f^\alpha} \tag{5.78}$$

where $0.7 < \alpha < 1.2$ with a mean close to $\alpha = 1$. For the frog node of Ranvier, the noise is a function of the membrane voltage as shown in Figure 5.23 [142]. The dominant source of this noise appears to be the K^+ current, and it has a minimum when the membrane is biased, so that this K^+ current is biased to zero.

To get an estimate of the size of these noise sources, let us consider a pacemaker cell from the abdominal ganglion of *Aplysia*. This cell fires 20-ms pulses at about 1 Hz/s. It has a resting voltage of about 50 mV and a resistance R, measured with a microelectrode between the inside of the cell and the surrounding solution, of approximately 10^6 Ω. If we assume a system bandwidth of 100 Hz and $T = 300$ K, the Johnson noise voltage would be $\overline{V}_n \approx 3 \times 10^{-6}$ V. This gives a resting potential-to-noise ($\overline{V}$) ratio of about 4×10^4. The peak current flow in these cells is estimated to be about 10^{-7} A, and thus the estimated shot noise current is $\overline{i_n} \approx 2 \times 10^{-12}$ A, and the ratio of the peak current to the noise current is

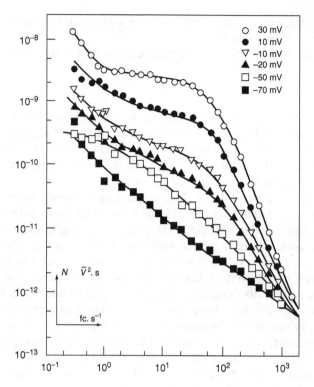

FIGURE 5.23
Voltage noise spectra of a frog node of Ranvier at different levels of membrane potential. (From Sichenga, E. and Verveen, A.A., in *Proceedings of the 1st European Biophysics Congress*, Vol. 5, Verlag Wiener Medizinischen Akademic, Vienna, Austria, 219, 1971. With permission [140].)

about 2×10^4. We do not have the available value $S(f)$ for the *Aplysia*, $\bar{v}_\phi = \sqrt{S(f)B}$, where B is the bandwidth. If it is assumed that the maximum value of the noise is the same as that of the frog node of Ranvier, then for a bandwidth of 1 Hz we get $\bar{v}_\phi = 1.4 \times 10^{-5}$ V at a center frequency of 1 Hz from the curve for −50 mV in Figure 5.21. This is about a factor of 10^3 greater than the Johnson noise. It is likely that $1/f$ noise is the largest source of noise at the cell membranes for frequencies below 160 Hz [143,144].

These fundamental sources of noise, which are generated by random fluctuations in the position of ions and their transport through channels, are spatially incoherent [142]. For many processes the important quantity in deciding whether or not an electrical signal is biologically important is the signal-to-noise ratio S/N where S is the power in the signal and N is the noise power. Typically, it is assumed that a signal-to-noise ratio of one is required for an externally applied signal to be detectable. In the foregoing discussion for both thermal and shot noise the movement of each charge was assumed to be statistically independent of each other. If, for an externally applied signal, the openings of the channels in a cell are excited in parallel and coherently and the noise is generated by incoherent random firing, then the signal-to-noise ratio increases with the square root of the number of channels. Similarly, the signal-to-noise ratio for a bundle of nerves would be expected to increase with the square root of the number of nerves for a signal applied externally to the whole bundle. Thus, a collection of cells can be expected to detect smaller signals than a single cell.

In addition to the electrical noise generated by currents and voltages that are part of the single-cell operation, electrical signals propagate through the body as a result of the

Static & Low-Frequency Electric Fields

incomplete confinement of electrical signals propagating in nerve cells. In a sense, these signals may be thought of as noise if they are not pertinent to the activity in that portion of the body through which they are propagating. If, on the other hand, they are used by tissue within the organism at some distance from the source, they must be thought of as signals. In the brain, the fraction of these signals that reach the scalp is called the electro-encephalogram (EEG). The EEG is obtained by placing two or more conducting electrodes on the scalp and measuring the voltage between them. For electrodes placed 5 cm apart, the peak-to-peak voltages range up to 30 μV [143]. The author views this voltage as the integral of the vector sum of the leakage fields from the firing of the nerve cells in the brain between the two electrodes. Since there are a very large number of cells firing, most of the 50 mV signals from an isolated nerve are canceled by summing over many like cells firing at different times and by the attenuation caused by propagation through the tissue. Estimates of surface potential gradients along a nerve fiber range from 3×10^{-4} to 5×10^{-2} V/m, and the corresponding current densities external to the nerve cells range from 5×10^{-2} to $4 A/m^2$ [145,146]. The EEG voltage has a strong periodic component (particularly during sleep) near 10 Hz, which is known as the alpha (α) wave. Peak amplitude of this component may be as large as 50 μV when measured at the surface of the scalp. It is interesting to note that the EEG signal contains significant information on the brain's activity, and a few individuals have been trained to control these signals so as to control a computer in way that allows them write messages.

At the surface of the chest, a signal may be recorded between two electrodes known as the ECG or EKG (electrocardiogram). This signal results from the highly coordinated firing of the cells in the heart and has a definite wave shape that is closely related to the operation of the heart. The peaks of the so-called R wave in this signal may range up to 2.5 mV and are typically 0.5–1.5 mV, depending on the placement of the electrodes, the amount of body fat, etc. The pulse repetition rate is usually in the range of 1–2 Hz, and the "QRS spike" of the typical cardiogram is 40 ms long. Again, the signal measured at the urface of the skin is the result of leakage from electrically active cells located at a distance. The estimated current density near the firing heart cell ranges up to 1 A/m^2 [145,146]. In this case, the shape of the signal reaching the skin is so closely related to the activity of the heart that it provides detailed information on heart function.

One result of electric discharges in the atmosphere, as well as natural ionizing radiation, is the creation of small positive and negative ions in the atmosphere. In clean country or mountain air, the typical ion density is about $10^{10}/m^3$ with an average ion lifetime of a few minutes [147]. When a hot dry wind is blowing, positive ions created by the shearing forces can increase in concentration significantly. It has been shown that increases in the negative ion concentration reduce the amount of serotonin (5-HT) in mice and rabbits, possibly by accelerating the enzymatic oxidation process [147]. A similar result has been demonstrated in the oxidation of cytochrome c. Positive ions appear to block monoamine oxidase action, thus raising the concentration of free 5-HT. Changes in 5-HT levels produce significant changes in the central nervous system, with high levels of positive ions raising the anxiety levels under stress. Other effects of increased positive ion concentration include a decrease in the survival rate of mice exposed to a measured dose of influenza virus, while an increase of negative ions reduced the mortality rate [147].

The significance of these results is that it is relatively easy to change the ion concentration in air using high-voltage DC systems where a leakage current of 1 mA from a burr or other sharp point would correspond to the generation of about 10^{12} ions per second.

Relatively few high-voltage DC transmission lines compared to AC lines are in use today for distribution of power although this number is increasing as a result of the advances that have been made in power electronic inverters. Because the shocks resulting from a short contact across a high DC or AC voltages are so painful and obviously dangerous, these systems are nearly always shielded when direct contacts with the wires is likely such as for buried underground distribution lines. One is rarely exposed to AC or DC electric fields >10^3 V/m as the height of transmission lines is increased as the voltages on the lines are increased. An additional feature of this exposure is that air is such a good insulator that the currents flowing through the body in a noncontacting situation are very small, as explained in the Introduction. For example, 1000 V across a 1-cm gap would yield a current density of approximately 10^{-7} A/m^2 flowing across the air gap. Thus, the principal hazards from DC or AC fields at low frequencies are most likely to occur when parts of the body make contact with a conductor.

5.16 Discussion and Summary

In this review, some of the physical mechanisms by which DC and time-varying electric fields affect biological systems are presented. A few typical values of electric field strengths and current densities that are known to affect the biological system are compared with those of natural fields and other forces. Some values of electric fields and their gradients that are shown to modify the currents and shift energy levels are given. These in turn are shown to modify chemical reaction rates, which can lead to changes in the growth cells and other characteristics of biological systems. It is hoped that this information will help the readers to make their own estimates of when a given exposure to electric fields will be significant in modifying biological systems and provide a basis for understanding some of the biological results presented in other chapters of this handbook.

Acknowledgments

The author wishes to express appreciation to Mikhail Zhadin, Howard Wachtel, Maria Stuchly, Ross Adey, Mike Marron, Elliot Postow, Charles Polk, and many students for their many helpful comments and suggestions and to Adam Sadoff for help in the preparation of the text. He also wishes to express his appreciation to the Office of Naval Research under Contract N00014-81-K-0387, the Mobile Manufactures Form, the University of Colorado, the National Science Foundation under NSF# 000416452 and the Milheim Foundation for financial support of his work in this area.

References

1. Barnes, F.S. and Hu, C.L. Nonlinear interactions of electromagnetic waves with the biological materials. In *Nonlinear Electromagnetics*, Uslenghi, P.L.L., Ed. Academic Press, New York, 391–426, 1980.

Static & Low-Frequency Electric Fields

2. Singer, S.J. and Nicolson, G.L. The fluid mosaic model of the structure of cell membranes. *Science*, 175, 720–731, 1972.

3. Poo, M. In situ electrophoresis or membrane components. In *Annual Review of Biophysics and Bioengineering*, Vol. 10, Mullins, L.J., Ed. Academic Press, New York, 245–276, 1981.

4. Kyriacous, D. *Modern Electroorganic Chemistry*. Springer-Verlag, Berlin, 1994.

5. Pohl, H.A. Dielectrophoresis, the Behavior of Neutral Matter. In *Nonuniform Electric Fields*. Cambridge University Press, Cambridge and New York, xii, 579 pp. 1978.

6. Kwon, Y. and Barnes, F. A theoretical study of the effects of RF fields in the vicinity of membranes. *Bioelectromagnetics*, 26(2), 118–124, 2005.

7. Atkins, P.W. *Physical Chemistry*, 4th ed. W.H. Freeman Co., New York, Chapter 26, 1990.

8. Bier, M. *Electrophoresis: Theory, Methods, and Applications*, Vol. 2, Bier, M., Ed. Academic Press, New York, 1967.

9. Burnham, C.J. et al. The properties of ion-water clusters. II. Solvation structures of Na+, Cl–, and H+clusters as a function of temperature. *Journal of Chemical Physics*, 124(2), 024327, 2006.

10. Marechal, Y. *The Hydrogen Bond and the Water Molecule*. Elsevier, Oxford, 2007.

11. Berg, J.M., Tymoczko, J.L., and Stryer, L. *Biochemistry*, 5th ed. WH Freeman, 2002. www.ncbi.nlm.nih.gov/books/bv.fcgi?&rid=stryer.section.438#455.

12. Gascoyne, P.R. and Vykoukal, J.V. Dielectrophoresis-based sample handling in general-purpose programmable diagnostic instruments. *Proc. IEEE*, 92(1), 22–41, 2004.

13. Pethig, R. *Dielectrophoresis, Theory,Methodology and Biological Applications*. Wiley, Hoboken, NJ, 2017.

14. Rand, E.P. Interacting phospholipids bilayers: measured forces and induced structural changes. In *Annual Review of Biophysics and Bioengineering*, Vol. 10, Mullins, L.J., Ed. Academic Press, New York, 227–314, 1981.

15. Rosenspire, A., Kindzelskii, A., Simon, B., and Petty, H. Real-time control of neutrophil metabolism by very weak ultra-low frequency pulsed magnetic fields. *Biophysical Journal*, 88, 3334–3347, 2005.

16. Pethig, R. *Dielectric and Electronic Properties of Biological Materials*. John Wiley & Sons, New York, 184, 182–185, 1979.

17. Iralelachvili, J. *Intermolecular and Surface Forces*, 2nd ed. Academic Press, San Diego, CA, 1992.

18. Lifshitz, F.M. Zh. Eksp. Teor. Fiz., 29, 95, 1955: Sov. Phys. *JETP* 2, 73, 1956.

19. Parsegian, J. Long range physical forces in the biological milieu. In *Annual Review of Biophysics and Bioengineering*, Mullins, L.J., Ed. Academic Press, New York, 221, 1973.

20. Tasao, Y.T., Evan, D.F., and Wennerstrom, H. Long-range attractive force between hydrophobic surfaces observed by atomic force microscopy. *Science*, 262, 547–550, 1993.

21. Barnes, F.S., Ginley, H., and Shulls, W. AC electric field effects on bacteria. Presented at the Third Annual Conference, Bioelectromagnetics Society (BEMS), Washington, DC, 1981.

22. Zumdahl, S.S. *Chemistry*, 2nd ed. D.C. Health Co., Lexington, MA, 546, 1989.

23. McCaig, C.D. Spinal neurite reabsorption and regrowth *in vitro* depend on the polarity of an applied electric field. *Development*, 100, 31–41, 1987.

24. Nuccitelli, R. Physiological electric fields can influence cell motility, growth, and polarity. *Advances in Molecular and Cell Biology*, 2, 213–233, 1988.

25. Erickson, C.A. and Nuccitelli, R. Embryonic fibroblast motility and orientation can be influenced by physiological electric fields. *Journal of Cell Biology*, 98, 296–307, 1984.

26. Seto, Y.J. and Hsieh, S.T. Electromagnetic induced kinetic effects on charged substrates in localized enzyme systems. *BiotechnologyM and Bioengineering*, XVIII, 813–837, 1976.

27. Muraji, M., Nishimura, M., Tatebe, W., and Fujii, T. Effect of alternating magnetic field on the growth of the primary root of corn. *IEEE Transactions on Magnetics*, 28(4), 1996–2000, 1992.

28. Raudino, A. and Larter, R. Enhancement of sorption kinetics by an oscillatory electric field. *Journal of Chemical Physics*, 98, 4, 1993.

29. Kuznetsov, A. *Stochastic and Dynamic Views of Chemical Reaction Kinetics in Solutions*, Lausanne: Presses Polytechniques et Universitaires Romandes, 265 pp.

30. Townes, C. and Schawlow, A. *Microwave Spectroscopy*. McGraw-Hill, New York, 255–283, 1955.

31. Bublitz, G.U. and Boxer, S.G. Stark spectroscopy: applications in chemistry, biology, and materials science. *Annual Review of Physical Chemistry*, 48, 213–242, 1997.
32. Zheng, J., Chin, W., Khijniak, E., Khijniak, E., Jr., Gerald, H., and Pollack, G. Surfaces and interfacial water: Evidence that hydrophilic surfaces have long-range impact. *Advances in Colloid and Interface Science*, 127, 19–27, 2006.
33. Voeikov, V. and Del Giudice, E. Water respiration—The basis of the living state*Water*, 1, 52–75, 2009.
34. Lange, O., Lakomek, N., Fares, C., Schroder, G., Walter, K., Becker, S., Meiler, J., Grubmuller, H., Griesinger, C., and de Groot, B. Recognition dynamics up to microseconds revealed from an RDC-derived Ubiquitin ensemble in solution. *Science*, 320, 1471–1475, 2008.
35. Boehr, D.D. and Wright, P.E. How do proteins interact? *Science*, 320, 1329–1430, 2008.
36. Creighton, T. Chapter 1: The protein folding problem. In *Mechanisms of Protein*, Pain, R.H. Ed. New York: Oxford University Press, 1–22, 1994.
37. Frauenfelder, H., Sligar, S., and Wolynes, P. The energy landscapes and motions of proteins. *Science*, 254, 1598–1602, 1991.
38. Gammaitoni, L., Hanggl, P., Jung, P., and Marchesoni, F. Stochastic resonance. *Reviews of Modern Physics* 70(1), 223–287, 1998.
39. Douglass, J., Wilkens, L., Pantazeloul, E., and Moss, F. Noise enhancement of information transfer in crayfish mechanoreceooptors by stochastic resonance. *Nature*, 365, 337–340, 1993.
40. Catterall, W. Structure and function of voltage-sensitive ion channels. *Science*, 242, 50–60, 1988.
41. Kandel, E., Schwartz, J., and Jessell, T. *Principles of Neural Science*, 4th ed. McGraw Hill, 2000.
42. Branden, C. and Tooze, J. *Introduction to Protein Structure*, 2nd ed. New York: Garland Publishing. 205–221, 1999.
43. Murphy, C., Arkin, M., Jenkins, Y., Ghatlia, N., Bossmann, S., Turro, N., and Barton, J. Long-range photoinduced electron transfer through a DNA helix. *Science*, 262, 1025–1029, 1993.
44. Choi, S., Kim, B., and Frisbie, C. Electrical resistance of long conjugated molecular wires. *Science*, 320, 1482–1486, 2008.
45. Donhauser, Z., Mantooth, B., Kelly, K., Bumm, L., Monnell, J., Stapleton, J., Price Jr, D., Rawlett, A., Allara, D., Tour, J., and Weiss, P. Conductance switching in single molecules through conformational changes. *Science*, 292, 2303–2407, 2001.
46. Blank, M. and Soo, L. Electromagnetic acceleration of electron transfer reactions. *Journal of Cellular Biochemistry*, 81, 278–283, 2001.
47. Robertson, B. and Astumian, R. Frequency dependence of catalyzed reactions in a weak oscillating field. *Journal of Chemical Physics*, 94(11), 1, 1991.
48. Guyton, A.C. *Textbook of Medical Physiology*, 8th ed. W.B. Saunders, Philadelphia, PA, 47, 1991.
49. Barnes, F.S. A model for the detection of weak ELF electric and magnetic fields. *Bioelectrochemistry and Bioenergetics*, 47, 207–212, 1999.
50. Alkon, D. and Rasmussen, H. A spatial-temporal model of cell activation. *Science*, 26, 998–1004, 1988.
51. Barnes, F. and Kandala, S. Effects of time delays on biological feedback systems and electromagnetic field exposures. *Bioelectromagnetics*, 39, 249–252, 2018.
52. Brandman, O., and MeTyer, T. Feedback loops shape cellular signals in space and time. *Science*, 322, 390–395, 2008.
53. Alon, U. *Introduction to Systems Biology, Design Principles of Biological Circuits*. Chapman and Hall/CRC Press, London, 2006
54. Novak, B. and Tyson, J. Design principles of biochemical oscillators. *Nature Reviews Molecular Cell Biology*, 9(12), 981–991, 2008. doi:10.1038/nrm2530.
55. Manley, J. and Rowe, H. Some general properties of nonlinear elements i general energy relations. *Proc. IRE* 44, 904–913, 1956.
56. Heffner, H. and Wade, G. Gain, bandwidth and noise characteristics of the variable parameter amplifier. *Journal of Applied Physics*, 29, 1321–1331, 1958.
57. Louisell, W. *Coupled Mode and Parametric Electronics*. Hoboken: John Wiley and Sons, 1960.

Static & Low-Frequency Electric Fields

58. Penfield, P. Jr. and Rafuse, R. *Varactor Applications*. MIT Press, 1962.

59. Yariv, A. and Yeh, P. *Photonics. Optical Electronics in Modern Communications*, 6th ed. New York: Oxford University Press, 2007.

60. Trillo, M., Ubeda, A., Blanchard, J., House, D., and Blackman, C. Magnetic fields at resonant conditions for the hydrogen ion affect neurite outgrowth in PC-12 cells: A test of the ion parametric resonance model. *Bioelectromagnetics*, 17(1), 10–20, 1996.

61. Tributsch, H. Parametric energy conversion—A possible universal approach to energetics in biological structures. *Journal of Theoretical Biology*, 52, 17–56, 1975.

62. Balkarey, Y., Nagoutchev, O., Evtikhov, M., and Elinson, M. Parametric amplification of signals by noise in neurons and neural networks. *Neural Processing Letters*, 12, 215–223, 2000.

63. Brenner, N., Agam, O., Bialek, W., and De Rauter van Steveninck, R.R. Universal statistical behavior of neural spike trains. *Physical Review Letters*, 81, 4000–4003, 1998.

64. Moss, F. Stochastic resonance. *Berichte der Bunsengesellschaft für physikalische Chemie*, 95(3), 302–311, 1991.

65. McNamara, B. and Wiesenfeld, K. Theory of stochastic resonance. *Physical Review A*, 39(9), 4854–4869, 1989.

66. Bulsara, A. and Gammaitoni, L. Tuning in to noise. *Physics Today*, 39–45, March 1996.

67. Samoilov, M., Plyasunov, S., and Arkin, A. Stochastic amplification and signaling in enzymatic futile cycles through noise—Induced bistability with oscillations. *PNAS*, 102(7), 2310–2315, 2005.

68. MacGregor, R.J. and Lewis, E.R. *Neural Modelling*. Plenum Press, New York, 1977.

69. Levin, M. Chapter 3: Endogenous bioelectric signals as morphogenetic controls of development, regeneration, and neoplasm. In *The Physiology of Bioelectricity in Development, Tissue Regeneration and Cancer*, Pullar, C., Ed. CRC Press, Boca Raton, FL, 2010.

70. Cooper, M.S., Miller, J.P., and Fraser, S.E. Electropheretic repatterning of charged cytoplasmic molecules within tissues coupled by gap junctions by externally applied electric fields. *Developmental Biology*, 132, 170–188, 1989.

71. Epstein, B.R. and Foster, K.R. Anisotropy in the dielectric properties of skeletal muscle. *Medical & Biological Engineering & Computing*, 21, 51, 1983.

72. Kalmijn, A.J. Electric and magnetic field detection in elasmobranch fishes. *Science*, 281, 916–918, 1982.

73. Kalmijn, A.J. Chapter 6: Detection of weak electric fields. In *Sensory Biology of Aquatic Animals*, Atema, E.J. et al., Eds. Springer-Verlag, Berlin, 1987.

74. McCleave, J.D, Rommel, S., and Cathcart, A.S. Weak electric and magnetic fields in fish orientation. In *Orientation: Sensory Basis*, Vol. 188, Adler, H.E., Ed. New York Academy of Sciences, New York, 270–281, 1971.

75. Ransom, B.P. and Eyring, H. Membrane permeability and electrical potential. In *Ion Transport across Membranes*, Clarke, H.J. and Nachmansohn, D., Eds., Academic Press, New York, 103, 1954.

76. Tsong, T.Y., Liu, D.S., and Chauvin, R. Electroconformational coupling (ECC): An electric field induced enzyme oscillation for cellular energy and signal transductions. *Bioelectrochemistry and Bioenergetics*, 21, 319–331, 1989 (a section of J. Electroanal. Chem. and constituting Vol. 275, Elsevier Sequoia, S.A., Lausanne, Switzerland, 1985).

77. Liu, D.S., Astumian, R.D., and Tsong, T.Y. Activation of Na+ and K+ .pumping modes of (Na, K)-ATPase by an oscillating electric field. *Journal of Biological Chemistry*, 265(13), 7260–7267, 1990.

78. Horn, L.W. A novel method of the observation of membrane transporter dynamics. *Biophysical Journal*, 64, 281–289, 1993.

79. Pollack, G. *Cells, Gels and the Engines of Life*. Ebner and Sons publisher, Seattle, WA 2001.

80. Andersen, S., Jackson, A., and Heimburg, T. Towards a thermodynamic theory of nerve pulse propagation. *Progress in Neurobiology*, 88, 104–113, 2009.

81. Triffet, T. and Green, H.S. Information and energy flow in a simple nervous system. *Journal of Theoretical Biology*, 86, 3, 1980.

82. Vaccaro, S.R. and Green, H.S. Ionic processes in excitable membranes. *Journal of Theoretical Biology*, 81, 771, 1979.
83. Eckert, R. and Ewald, D. Residual calcium ions depress activation of calcium-dependent current. *Science*, 216, 730, 1982.
84. Baumann, G. and Easton, G., Modeling state-dependent sodium conductance data by memory-less random process. *Mathematical Biosciences*, 60, 265, 1982.
85. Schauf, C.L. and Baumann, G. Experimental evidence consistent with aggregation kinetics in sodium current of myxicola giant axons. *Biophysical Journal*, 35, 707, 1981.
86. Baumann, G. and Easton, G. Charge immobilization linked to inactivation in the aggregation model of channel gating. *Journal of Theoretical Biology*, 99, 249, 1982.
87. Poo, M. Rapid lateral diffusion of functional Ach receptors in embryonic muscle cell membrane. *Nature*, 295, 332, 1982.
88. Poo, M. and Lam, J.W. Lateral electrophoresis and diffusion of concanavalin, a receptor in the membrane of embryonic muscle cells. *Journal of Cell Biology*, 76, 483, 1978.
89. Lee, K.Y.C., Lingler, J.B., and McConnell, H.M. Electric field-induced concentration gradients in lipid monolayers. *Science*, 263, 655, 1994.
90. Hayashi, H. and Fishman, H., Inward rectifier K^+ channel from analysis of the complex conductance of aplysia neuronal membrane. *Biophysical Journal*, 53, 747–757, 1988.
91. Barnes, F.S. and Hu, C.L. Model for some non thermal effects of radio and microwave fields on biological membranes. *IEEE Transactions on Microwave Theory Techniques*, 25, 742, 1977.
92. Montaigne, K. and Pickard, W.F. Offset of the vascular potential of characean cells in response to electromagnetic radiation over the range of 250 Hz to 250 kHz. *Bioelectromagnetics*, 5, 31, 1984.
93. Pickard, W.F. and Rosenbaum, F.J. Biological effects of microwaves at membrane level: two possible athermal electrophysiological mechanisms and a proposed experimental test. *Mathematical Biosciences*, 39, 235, 1978.
94. Pickard, W.F. and Barsoum, Y.H. Radio-frequency bioeffects at the membrane level: separation of thermal and athermal contributions in the Characeae. *The Journal of Membrane Biology*, 61, 39, 1981.
95. Kalkwarf, D.R., Frasco, D.L., and Brattain, W.H. Current rectification and action potentials across thin lipid membranes. In *Physical Principles of Biological Membranes*, Snell, F., Wolken, J., Iverson, G., and Lam, J., Eds. Gordon & Breach, New York, 1970.
96. Franceschetti, G. and Pinto, I., Cell membrane nonlinear response to applied electromagnetic field. *IEEE Transactions on Microwave Theory and Techniques*, 32, 7, 1984.
97. Casaleggio, A., Marconi, L., Morgavi, G., Ridella, S., and Rolando, C. Current flow in a cell, with a nonlinear membrane, stimulated by an electric field, personal communication, 1985.
98. Cain, C.A. Biological effects of oscillating electric fields: Role of voltage sensitive ion channels. *Bioelectromagnetics*, 2, 23, 1981.
99. Bisceglia and Pinto, I. Volterra series solution of Hodgkin-Huxley equation, personal communication, 1984.
100. Wachtel, H. Firing-pattern changes and transmembrane currents produced by low frequency fields in pacemaker neurons. In *Proceedings of the 18th Annual Hansford Life Science Symposium*, Technical Information Center, U.S. Department of Energy, Richland, WA, 132–147, 1978.
101. Adler, R. A study of locking phenomena in oscillators. *Proceedings of the IEEE*, 34, 351, 1946.
102. Barnes, F.S., Smoller, A., and Sheppard, A. Injection locking of pacemaker cells. In *Proceedings of the 9th Annual Conference*, IEEE Engineering in Medicine and Biology Society, 1986.
103. Fohlmeister, J.F., Adelman, W.J., Jr., and Poppele, R.E. Excitation properties of the squid axon membrane and model systems with current stimulation. *Biophysical Journal*, 30, 79–98, 1980.
104. Barnes, F.S. Some engineering models for interactions of electric and magnetic fields with biological systems. *Bioelectromagnetics*, 1, 67–85, 1992.
105. Kroupa., V.F. *Frequency Synthesis*. John Wiley & Sons, New York, 1973.
106. Koss, D.A. and Carstensen, E.L. Effects of ELF electric fields on the isolated frog heart. *IEEE Transactions on Biomedical Engineering*, 30, 347, 1983.

107. Litovitz, T.A., Krause, D., and Mullins, J.M. Effect of coherence time of the applied magnetic field on ornithine decarboxylase activity. *Biochemical and Biophysical Research Communications*, 178(3), 862–865, 1991.
108. Mullins, J.M., Krause, D., and Litovitz, T.A. Simultaneous application of a spatially coherent noise field blocks use response of cell cultures to a 60 Hz electromagnetic field. *Proceedings of the 1992 World Congress on Bioelectromagnetism, Bioelectromagnetics Society*, Orlando, FL, 1992.
109. Farrell, J.M., Barber, M., Krause, D., and Litovitz, T.A. The superposition of a temporally incoherent magnetic field inhibits 60 Hz-induced changes in the ODC activity of developing chick embryos. *Bioelectromagnetics*, 19, 53–56, 1998.
110. Litovitz, T.A., Montrose, C.J., Doinov, P., Brown, K.M., and Barber, M. Superimposing spatially coherent electromagnetic noise inhibits field induced abnormalities in developing chick embryos. *Bioelectromagnetics*, 15(2), 105–113, 1994.
111. Walleczek, J. and Liburdy, R.P. Nonthermal 60 Hz sinusoidal magnetic-field exposure enhances $^{45}Ca^{2+}$ uptake in rat hymocytes: Dependence on mitogen activation. *Federation of European Biochemical Societies*, 271(1/2), 157–160, 1990.
112. Liburdy, R.P. Calcium signaling in lymphocytes and ELF fields. *Federation of European Biochemical Societies Letters*, 301(1), 53–59, 1992.
113. Liburdy, R.P. Biological interactions of cellular systems with time-varying magnetic fields. *Annals of the New York Academy of Sciences*, 649, 74–94, 1992.
114. Yost, M.G. and Liburdy, R.P. Time-varying and static magnetic fields act in combination to alter calcium signal transduction in the lymphocyte. *Federation of European Biochemical Societies*, 296(2), 17–122, 1992.
115. McLeod, K.J., Lee, R.C., and Ehrlich, H.P. Frequency dependence of electric field modulation of fibroblast protein synthesis. *Science*, 136, 1465–1469, 1987.
116. Takashima, S., Non-linear properties of nerve membranes. *Biophysical Chemistry*, 11, 447, 1980.
117. Berkowitz, G.C. and Barnes, F.S. The effects of nonlinear membrane capacity on the interaction of microwave and radio frequencies with biological materials. *IEEE Transactions on Microwave Theory and Techniques*, 27, 204, 1979.
118. Alkon, D.L. Memory storage and neural systems. *Scientific American*, 261, 42–50, 1989.
119. Yang, X., Korn, H., and Faver, A.S. Long-term potentiation of electronic coupling at mixed synapses. *Nature*, 348, 542–545, 1990.
120. Hu, C.L. and Barnes, F.S. The thermal chemical damage in biological materials under laser irradiation. *IEEE Transactions on Biomedical Engineering*, 17, 220, 1970.
121. Shuyrou, V.L., Zhodan, G.G., and Akrov, I.G. Effects of 330 MHz radio frequency, Academy of Science, Institute of Biophysics, Pushchino, Moscow Region, Russia, personal communication, 1984.
122. Trautman, E.D. and Newbower, R.S. A practical analysis of the electrical conductivity of blood. *IEEE Transactions on Biomedical Engineering*, 30, 141, 1983.
123. Johnson, F.D, Eyring, H., and Stover, B.J. *The Theory of Rate Processes in Biology and Medicine*. John Wiley & Sons, New York, 1974.
124. Liburdy, R.P. and Penn, A. Microwave bioeffect in erythrocyte are temperature and pO dependent action permeability and protein shedding occur at the membrane phase transition. *Bioelectromagnetics*, 5, 283–291, 1984.
125. Chalker, R. The effect of microwave absorption and associated temperature dynamics on nerve cell activity in Aplysia. M.S. thesis, University of Colorado, Boulder, CO, 1982.
126. Barnes, F.S. Cell membrane temperature rate sensitivity predicted from the Nernst equation. *Bioelectromagnetics*, 5, 113, 1984.
127. Bol'shakov, M.A. and Alekseyev, S.I. Change in the electrical activity of the pacemaker neurons of *L. stagnalis* with the rate of their heating. *Biophysics*, 31, 569–571, 1986.
128. Alekseyev, S.I., IL'in, V.I., and Tyazhelov, V.V. Effect of electromagnetic radiation in decimeter wavelength range on calcium current of mollusk neurons. *Biophysics*, 31(2), 290–295, 1986.
129. Philippova, T.M., Novoselov, V.I., Bystrova, M.F., and Alekseyev, S.I. Microwave effect on camphor binding to rat olfactory epithelium. *Bioelectromagnetics*, 9, 347–354, 1988.

130. Bushanam, S. and Barnes, F.S. Laser generated thermoelastic shock waves in liquids. *Journal of Applied Physics*, 46(5), 2074–2082, 1975.

131. Mihran, R.T., Barnes, F.S., and Wachtel, H. Temporally-specific modification of myelinated axon excitability *in vitro* following a single ultrasound pulse. *Ultrasound in Medicine and Biology*, 16(3), 297–309, 1990.

132. Ady, G., McNaughton, B.L., and Wachtel, H. A system for recording microwave effects on isolated mammalian brain slices. *Presented at the 5th Annual Conference, Bioelectromagnetics Society*, Boulder, CO, 1983.

133. Polk, C. Sources, propagation amplitude and temporal variations of extremely low frequency (0–100 Hz) electromagnetic fields. In *Biological and Clinical Effects of Low-Frequency Magnetic and Electric Fields*, Llaurado, J.G., Sances, A., Jr., and Battocletti, J.H., Eds. Charles C Thomas, Springfield, IL, 21, 1974.

134. Plonsey, R. *Bioelectric Phenomena*, McGraw-Hill, New York, 1969.

135. Barnes, F.S. and Seyed-Madani, M. Some possible limits on the minimum electrical signals of biological significance. In *Mechanistic Approaches to Interactions of Electric and Electromagnetic Fields with Living Systems*, Blank, M. and Findl, E., Eds. Plenum Press, New York, 339–349, 1987.

136. Yariv, A. *Introduction to Optical Electronics*. Holt, Reinhart & Winston, New York, 1976.

137. MacDonald, D.K.C. *Noise and Fluctuations: An Introduction*. John Wiley & Sons, New York, 1962.

138. Beck, A.H.W. *Statistical Mechanics, Fluctuations, and Noise*. Edward Arnold, London, 1967.

139. Keshner, M.F. 1/f noise. *Proceedings of the IEEE*, 70(3), 212–218, 1982.

140. Sichenga, E. and Verveen, A.A. The dependence of the 1/f noise intensity of the diode of Ranvier on membrane potential. In *Proceedings of the 1st European Biophysics Congress*, Vol. 5, Verlag Wiener Medizinischen Akademic, Vienna, 219, 1971.

141. Dorset, D.L. and Fishman, H.M. Excess electrical noise during current flow through porous membranes separating ionic solutions. *The Journal of Membrane Biology*, 21, 291–301, 1975.

142. Verveen, A.A. and DeFelice, L.J. Membrane noise. *Progress in Biophysics & Molecular Biology*, 28, 189, 1974.

143. Nuney, P.L. and Katznelson, R.D. *Electric Fields of the Brain—The Neurophysics of EEG*. Oxford University Press, New York, 1981.

144. Verveen, A.A. and Derksen, H.E. Fluctuation phenomena in nerve membrane. *Proceedings of the IEEE*, 56, 906, 1968.

145. Bernhardt, J. The direct influence of electromagnetic fields on nerve and muscle cells of man within the frequency range of 1 Hz to 30 MHz. *Radiation and Environmental Biophysics*, 16, 309, 1979.

146. Beckwith, J.R. and McGuire, L.B. *Basic Electrocardiography and Vector Cardiography*, Raven Press, New York, 1982.

147. Krueger, A. and Reed, E. Biological impact of small air ions. *Science*, 193, 1209, 1976.

6

Magnetic Field Interactions with Biological Materials

Frank Barnes

University of Colorado Boulder

CONTENTS

6.1 Introduction 219
6.2 Some Basic Physics 219
6.3 Induced Electric Fields from Time-Varying Magnetic Fields 221
6.4 Energy Effects of Magnetic Fields 221
6.5 Generation of Free Radicals in Solution 222
6.6 Generation of Radicals by Fragmentation of a Large Molecule 225
6.7 Radicals and Paramagnetic Molecules 228
6.8 Summary 229
References 230

6.1 Introduction

Magnetic fields have been used as mechanism for coupling electromagnetic energy into biological systems for a large number of applications. Among the most common uses for time-varying magnetic fields are inducing electric fields that may be used to heat the biological material, stimulate nerves, and activating bone growth. Magnetic pulses are used to induce electric fields that in turn stimulate bone growth and for transcranial stimulations of brain cells. These applications are discussed in other chapters. In this chapter, and in Chapter 7, BBA, an outline of some of the mathematics that describes the physics of the interaction of magnetic fields on biological systems and some effects of weak magnetic fields on the generation of radical are presented. Radicals are molecules or ions with unpaired spins such as reactive oxygen and nitrogen. Both are important signaling molecules in biological systems and can also do damage that is associated with aging, cancer, and Alzheimer's (Droge 2002). The effects of weak magnetic fields on radicals in cell cultures are also discussed in Chapters 7 in this volume and Chapter 1 in BMA, which include many additional references.

6.2 Some Basic Physics

Magnetic fields interact with biological materials both by applying torques to the dipole moments, by changing the energy levels and their occupation by electrons. The torques

219

220   *Electromagnetic Fields*

can change the orientation of the dipole moments that can in turn change chemical reaction rates.

The fundamental law describing forces on charged particles is given by

$$\vec{F} = q\left(\vec{E} + \vec{v} \times \vec{B}\right)$$ (6.1)

These fields may also lead to transitions between energy levels and shift the separation between energy levels. $\vec{F}$ is the force, q is the charge on the particle, $\vec{v}$ is the velocity of the particle, $\vec{E}$ is the electric field, and $\vec{B}$ is the magnetic flux density. $\vec{E}$ and $\vec{B}$ are coupled by Maxwell's equations so that a time-varying magnetic field generates an $\vec{E}$ field and vice versa. This force may lead to ion currents and changes in the orientation of dipoles in molecules and changes in molecular configuration. As indicated in the Introduction to this volume, time-varying magnetic fields lead to induced electric fields and these induced electric fields lead to time-varying current flows. It is often difficult to separate the direct effects of magnetic fields from those resulting from the induced electric fields. As indicated in Chapter 5 electric fields as small as 10^{-7} V/m (Kalmijn 1988) can be detected by sharks and exposures of human neutrophils to fields as small as 10^{-4} V/m (Rosenspire et al. 2005) have been shown to result in significant biological effects.

The magnetic field $\vec{H}$ is related to the magnetic flux density $\vec{B}$ by $\vec{B} = \mu\vec{H}$ where μ is the magnetic permeability. Magnetic dipole moments in magnetic fields experience a torque $\vec{\tau} = \vec{\mu}_{mff} \times \vec{B}$ where μ_{meff} is the effective magnetic dipole moment. The translational force on a magnetic material is given by

$$\vec{F}_x = \vec{M}\frac{\partial \vec{B}}{\partial x}$$ (6.2)

$\vec{M}$ is the magnetization of the material. The magnitude of the magnetization vector is equal to the magnetic moment per unit volume. $\vec{B} = \mu_o(\vec{H} + \vec{M})$. μ_o is the permeability of free space. For materials without permanent dipole moments the magnetization to first order is given by $\vec{M} = \chi\vec{H}$ where χ is the susceptibility tensor per unit volume. In an inhomogeneous field, the material will experience a translational force in the direction of the increasing or decreasing field strength depending on the sign of χ

$$\vec{F} = \chi V \vec{H} \nabla \vec{H}$$ (6.3)

V is the volume occupied by the material. The sign of χ is positive for paramagnetic and negative for diamagnetic materials (Frankel 1996). It is some times more convenient to write this expression in terms of the magnetic flux density and its gradient

$$\vec{F} = \frac{\chi}{\mu_o}\vec{B}\nabla\vec{B}$$ (6.4)

It is to be noted that force on paramagnetic materials and diamagnetic materials are much smaller than those of ferromagnetic materials. Time-varying magnetic fields induce electric fields as shown in the introduction and these induced electric fields and corresponding currents may be used to stimulate nerve cells and other biological processes.

Magnetic Fields & Biomaterials 221

6.3 Induced Electric Fields from Time-Varying Magnetic Fields

The induced voltage V around a closed path is given by

$$V = \oint E \cdot dl = - \iint \frac{\partial B}{\partial t} \cdot ds \qquad (6.5)$$

where E is the field induced by the time-changing magnetic field in accord with Maxwell's equations. The integration $\oint E \cdot dl$ is over the appropriate conducting path, $\partial B/\partial t$ is the time derivative of the magnetic flux density, and the "dot" product with the surface element, ds, indicates that only the component of $\partial B/\partial t$ perpendicular to the surface, i.e., parallel to the direction of the vector ds, enclosed by the conducting path, induces an E field. Note that the change in magnetic flux across the area enclosed by the path may be caused either by the change in time of B or by a change due to motion of a part of the path.

As the value for the magnetic permeability, μ in most biological materials is equal to μ_o, it is relatively easy to calculate the magnetic field distribution in a biological system for an incident magnetic field, especially since and in many cases to a first approximation, the field is uniform over the area of interest. For example, in exposing cell in a petri dish to a uniform vertical magnetic field at an angular frequency ω for a circular path about the center of the dish the induced electric field increases with radius. The induced current density had clearly been shown to affect the growth rates of P815 mastocytoma cells by Bingham (1996)

$$E = \frac{\omega B r}{2} \qquad (6.6)$$

$$J = \sigma E = \frac{\sigma \omega B r}{2} \qquad (6.7)$$

where σ is the conductivity of the fluid.

Rosenspire et al. (2005) have shown that induced electric fields as small as 10^{-4}V/m can be important in the control of neutrophil metabolism. In bone repair, the induced electric fields from magnetic pulses with fast rise times have the advantage of being noninvasive compared to applying the electric fields by inserting electrodes across the breaks, which includes the possibility of causing infections. See Chapter 8 BMA. Note, however, that the local geometry and tissue properties can strongly affect the magnitude and direction of induced currents in actual situations. For example, Greenebaum (2012) simulated the E fields and current densities of a pulsed magnetic field on simplified models of a bone fracture and found that their direction was always through the fracture gap, independent of the direction of the applied field, though the E field and current densities were much stronger for magnetic fields parallel to the bone. Large rapidly varying magnetic field pulses are also used to induce electric fields for transcranial stimulation of the brain as discussed in Chapter 10 in BMA.

6.4 Energy Effects of Magnetic Fields

In a magnetic field, the energy of a molecule is modified by the interaction of the magnetic field with the magnetic dipole moments of the electrons, protons, and neutrons. This leads to shifts in the energy levels with the magnetic field, called the Zeeman Effect. Generally, for molecules with no net electronic angular momentum, these effects are generally small by comparison to the energy level shifts with electric fields or the Stark effect. Exceptions are molecules that have electronic angular momentum and are paramagnetic. The magnetic moments for paramagnetic molecules are generated by the sum of angular momentum of the electrons, their spin and nuclear magnetic moments (Townes and Schawlow 1955). The magnetic field coupling between the nuclear magnetic moments and the electrons leads the hyperfine shifts in the energy levels for the electrons. For weak magnetic fields when the hyperfine energy levels are separated by more than the thermal energy the changes in magnetic field energy $g\mu_B B$ are given by

$$\Delta W = g\mu_B B \tag{6.8}$$

g is a constant that can be calculated quantum mechanically from the rotational, vibrational energy levels, etc. and their projections on the axis of rotations and the static magnetic field (SMF). It often has a value of about 2. μ_B is the Bohr Magneton and $\mu_B = 9.27 \times 10^{-24}$ J/T. For magnetic fields on the order of the Earth's magnetic field ($\approx 45\,\mu$T) the changes in energy with the weak magnetic fields will remove the zero field degeneracy between the triplet states for the hyperfine levels. Because of the small energy differences between these energy levels at thermal equilibrium the population densities in each of these energy levels will be approximately equal.

In a typical molecule, the spins of the electrons in the outer orbits are paired in a singlet state. In the singlet state, S, the spins are aligned in opposite directions ↑↓ or spin up and spin down so that the energy level does not change with weak externally applied magnetic fields. In the triplet state both spins are aligned parallel to each other so that they have a net magnetic moment. This means that the energy levels as a function of magnetic field vary depending on if the spins are aligned parallel, antiparallel, or perpendicular to the external magnetic field. The triplet levels T_+, T_-, and T_0 have an unpaired spin so that the energy of the external magnetic field may add, subtract, or not interact with the internal energy. The size of the separation between energy levels corresponds in the classical description to the Larmor precession frequency, f, For the electron spins, $f = \dfrac{g\mu_B B}{h}$, where g is a factor that is a function of the angular momentum and other quantum numbers related to the orientation of the net magnetic moment and the direction of the externally applied magnetic field, and B is the magnetic flux density. Note we have assumed in this section that $B = \mu_0 H$ where μ_0 is the permeability of free space. Transitions between levels are coupled by the nuclear spins and can be driven by AC fields such that hf corresponds to the difference in the energy between adjacent levels (Timmel and Henbest 2004).

6.5 Generation of Free Radicals in Solution

Radical molecules are defined to be chemically bonded ions or molecules with uncompensated spin. They have been found with both one and two uncompensated spins (Wadas 1991). These molecules are paramagnetic and they are typically characterized by measuring the electron spin resonance spectra. Free radicals are chemically very active and often have short lifetimes as they react with lipids and many other biological molecules.

Radical may be generated in a variety of ways including ionizing radiation, chemical reaction, and thermal decompositions. In this section, we consider the case where a molecule is split to form a free radical pair so that each of molecular fragments contains an outer electron with an unpaired spin. Free radicals can be carbon centered and formed in a number of common compounds including a variety of methyl and alkyl radicals. They can also be formed in a wide variety of other compounds including radicals centered on nitroxide, phosphorus, oxygen, and sulfur.* Free radicals that are important in metabolic processes include O_2^-, HO•, H_3O^+, NO and others (Halliwell and Gutteridge 2015). Free radicals are chemically important parts of many biological processes.

The S and T levels are defined by the orientation of the spins in the two different fragments. The energy level gap between the S and T level as shown in Figure 6.1 (Steiner and Ulrich 1989, Figure 5) is larger at zero magnetic field than it is at larger values of the B field for T levels that are less than four times the value of the exchange energy J.

The lifetime for transitions between the S and T states typical range from (10^{-6} to 10^{-10} s). The coupling between the electrons and the magnetic moment of the nucleus leads to the hyperfine levels. It is difference in the coupling between the nuclear spins and the electronic spins that leads to the conversion of electrons in a free radical pair from an S to a T state or from a T to an S state. The conversion from S to T states is a function of both the coupling between the nuclei and the outer electrons in each of the fragments and the diffusion lifetime. Both the conservation of angular momentum and the conservation of energy must be satisfied for recombination and this leads to the selection rules for the allowed transitions. The allowed transitions are for the S to all T states and between T_+ and T_- and T_0 but not between T_+ and T_-. Radical pairs in the T states with the spins aligned parallel to

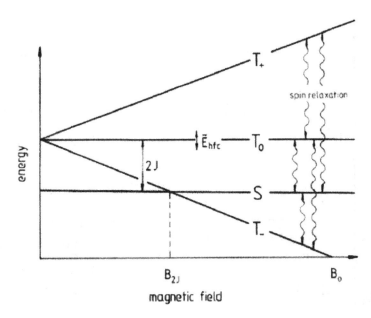

FIGURE 6.1
Energy diagram of electronic spin states of a radical pair in a magnetic field. E_{hfc} is an average level width due to hyperfine coupling, and J is the exchange integral (Steiner and Ulrich 1989 figure 5.).

---

* See Fossey [1995] for the chemical description of a large number of free radicals and their reaction rates.

each other are not allowed to recombine by the Pauli Exclusion Principle. Thus, they have more time to diffuse away from their initial partner and combine with other molecules.

Changes in free radical concentrations as a function of magnetic field are predicted to take on one of the several shapes as shown in Figure 6.2.

Calculations for changes in free radical lifetimes and concentrations in small magnetic fields have been carried out by (Brocklehurst and McLauchlan 1996; Timmel et al. 1998 Timmel and Henbest 2004), and includes a much more detailed description of the coupling between the nuclear magnetic spin energy levels and the orbital electrons. The coupling constant can vary from 0.01 to 3 mT for carbon centered free radicals. The corresponding separation between hyperfine energy levels for carbon-centered free radicals can vary from about 1.2×10^{-9} eV to about 3×10^{-7} eV. Detailed calculations of these effects show a curve for free radical concentrations similar to that shown in Figure 6.2 and Figure 6.3 (Brocklehurst and McLauchlan 1996, Figure 4). This inverted J-shaped curve leads to an increase in the lifetime for conversion of singlet born pairs of free radicals as the magnetic

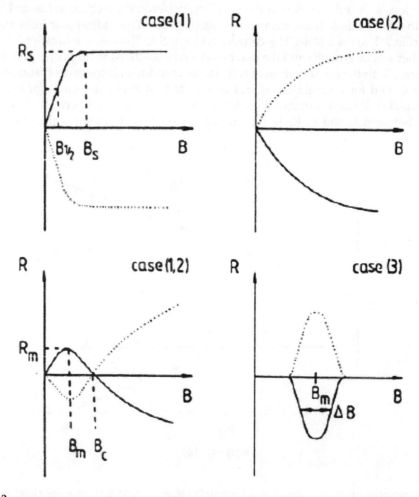

FIGURE 6.2
Phenomenological cases of MFD of reaction yields. Dotted lines indicate sign inversion of effects when changing the precursor multiplicity in the radical pair mechanism (Adapted from Sakaguchi et al. 1980; Steiner and Ulrich 1989, Figure 6.).

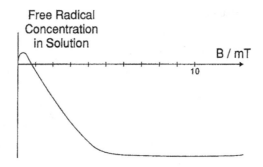

FIGURE 6.3
A schematic representation of the experimentally observed field effect in the pyrene/1,3-DCB system. At the lowest low field values, including that of the geomagnetic field, the effect of the field is to increase the proportion of radicals which survive the geminate period and diffuse into the surroundings, but at high field the reverse happens. The schematic presentation is used since the actual published results measured the derivative of this curve, and to display them would introduce an unnecessary complication (Batchelor et al. 1993; Brocklehurst and McLauchlan 1996.)

fields increases form zero and thus an increase in the number of free radicals in the triplet state that can diffuse from the site of origin to react with other molecules. As the magnetic field increases in this example a maximum concentration of free radicals occurs at a value below 300 µT. Changes in free radical concentrations in the forgoing example saturate for changes in magnetic fields at higher values (1–100 mT).

It is to be noted that energy shifts, $\mu_B B$, that are small compared to $k_B T$ can lead to large changes in chemical reaction rates if the initial states are in excited energy level (Steiner and Ulrich 1989). Excitations by electric fields keep particles that start in a singlet state stay in a singlet state or an excited singlet state.

6.6 Generation of Radicals by Fragmentation of a Large Molecule

Free radicals may be created by splitting a molecule so that the surviving fragments each have an odd number of electrons in an orbit. This can be done by hemolytic cleavage of bonds, or thermolysis in solution leading to a pair of radicals in singlet states, and by photolysis in either singlet or triplet states. In a typical molecule, there is an even number of electrons in outer orbits and, when they are split one fragment has an electron with spin up and the other with spin down. These two fragments often recombine in periods of 10^{-7} to 10^{-10} s. However, if one of the spins flips, then recombination is forbidden by the Pauli Exclusion Principle and fragments typically survive for about 10^{-5} s. This in turn increases the probability that the fragments may drift apart and diffuse through the solution as free radicals. The relative energies of the singlet and triplet states of a radical pair in a magnetic field as a function of distance between the pair particles are shown by Fossey et al. (1995).

The energy level diagrams for typical biological molecules are much more complicated than that for deuterium, shown in Figure 6.4. Figure 6.4 provides an illustration of the way in which the energy levels may shift with magnetic fields and possible transitions between them.

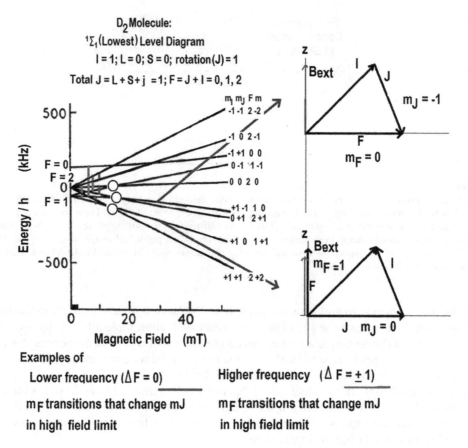

FIGURE 6.4

Left: Energies of D2 molecule states as a function of magnetic field with low-field (F, m) and high-field (m_j, m_I) quantum number labels. m_J amd m_I are the projections of the electron angular moment and nuclear spin on the external magnetic field I. Note linearity of curves in low-field region, where $F = J + I$ is a good quantum number, and curvature as well as crossovers as field increases [after Ramsey (1956)]. Vertical lines indicate allowed transitions. Relative orientations of one transition's upper and lower state angular momenta are shown (Right upper and lower). In left diagram, circles indicate possible level-crossing transition points and double arrow indicates region of possible zero-field transitions.

If time-varying magnetic fields at a frequency f are applied such that $hf = \Delta W$ where h is Planck's constant and ΔW is the energy between the levels, transitions between levels may be induced. This in turn can change the population distribution in these levels. A hypothetical energy diagram for a radical pair is shown in Figure 6.5 for two values of the static magnetic fields SMF. The recombination rates increase when the energy levels for the two fragments approach each other. The maximum rates occur when the energy levels are equal and the angular momentum quantum numbers for the active electrons are such that recombination does not violate the Pauli Exclusion Principle. This can happen for more than one value of the magnetic field and both increase and decrease in radical concentrations have been observed with varying the values of SMFs from the background of 45 μT (Bruzon et al. 2017). Energy level splitting associated with the magnetic dipoles is given to first order by $\Delta W = g\mu_B B$. $\mu_B = 9.27 \times 10^{-24}$ J/T. g is a number near unity and is approximately 2 for many chemically active electrons. Thus, earth's magnetic field of about 50 μT leads to transitions with a resonant frequency at about 1.4 MHz. The separation between energy

Magnetic Fields & Biomaterials

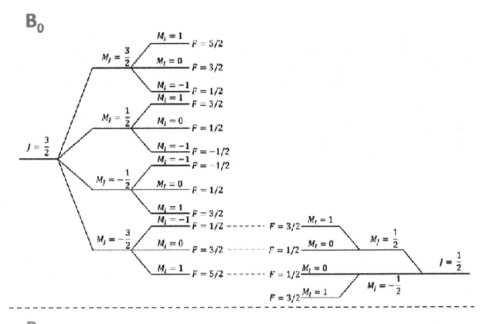

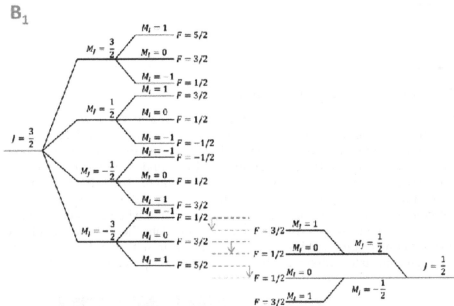

FIGURE 6.5
A hypothetical energy level diagram for two radicals showing the effects of external magnetic fields.

levels and the resonant frequency change with the SMF, and this changes the recombination rate for the radial pair which in turn changes the resulting radical concentration.

In Figure 6.5 for B_0 the energy levels line up for several different states of the two radicals and they can recombine rapidly. For B_1 the states do not line up and there is an energy barrier for recombination. Additionally for recombination the angular momentum transitions must be allowed. $F = I+J$ and is the quantum number for the sum of the nuclear and the total electronic magnetic moment. I is the nuclear spin quantum number, S is the electronic spin quantum number, and L is the quantum number for the electronic orbital angular momentum. $J = L+I$ and is the total electronic angular momentum quantum number. The projection of each angular momentum along the direction of the applied magnetic field is given by M_I, M_S, and M_L. As shown in Figure 6.5, increasing the DC magnetic flux can either increase or decrease the energy required for the energy levels in the two fragments to match.

The population distribution can also be modified by the application of magnetic fields at the resonant frequencies. The required power is usually quite small, and when the populations become equal and the net absorption goes to zero. For example, when the change in the population for nuclear spin states is given by

$$n'_{eq} = \frac{n_{eq}}{1 + \gamma^2 B_1 T_2 T_1} \tag{6.9}$$

where n_{eq} is the number of radicals in the initial state, n'_{eq} is the population difference between the upper and lower energy levels, γ is the gyromagnetic ratio, B_1 is the magnitude of the AC magnetic flux density, T_1 is the relaxation time between states, and T_2 is the nuclear spin relaxation time (Bovey et al. 1988). Depending on assumptions with respect to relaxation times and γ we have calculated values for B of from 10^{-5} to 10^{-9} T will reduce n'_{eq} by a factor of two (Barnes and Greenebaum 2015).

6.7 Radicals and Paramagnetic Molecules

Radicals are paramagnetic and they are typically characterized by measuring the electron spin resonance spectra. Organic molecules that contain Fe^{+2}, Fe^{+3}, Ni^{+2}, Mn^{+3}, Mn^{+2}, Cu^{+3}, and related cations are also paramagnetic and are important in biological processes. Iron, Fe^{+2}, is present in the largest quantities and is found in almost every human cell. These paramagnetic ions are often contained in diamagnetic structures. For example, iron is important in hemoglobin's ability to transport oxygen and is located in the interior of the molecule (see Figure 6.6). Hemoglobin is diamagnetic when it contains oxygen and paramagnetic without oxygen. In the paramagnetic state the effective dipole moment $\mu_{eff} = 5.35\ \mu_B$ per heme group. With O_2, it is in the low spin state with $S = 0$ and without O_2, it is in a high spin state with $S = 2$. This reduces the energy required to take on oxygen.

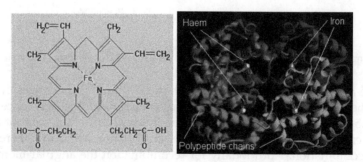

FIGURE 6.6
The structure of hemoglobin, www.elp.manchester.ac.uk

Magnetic Fields & Biomaterials

Additionally, with the uptake of O_2, the complex shrinks the average distance between Fe^{2+} ions from 3.41 to 3.235 nm. The minimum potential energy for hemoglobin with O_2 and paired spins is less than the minimum potential energy without O_2 and uncompensated spins and occupies a smaller volume. It releases 6×10^4 calories/mole on attaching O_2 and requires the same amount of energy to release it (Wadas 1991). It is to be noted that both O_2 and hemoglobin without O_2 are paramagnetic. The chemical reaction involves both an electrical interaction and magnetic dipole-dipole interaction. Paramagnetic ions may be contained in both enzymes and coenzymes.

The paramagnetic enzymes and coenzymes act as accelerators for biochemical reactions. For example, weak 50 Hz magnetic fields have been shown to reduce the number of free-oxygen radicals in rat lymphocytes *in vitro* when the applied field reduces the earth's magnetic field to near zero for at least part of the cycle (Zmyslony et al. 2004). One hour exposures to 50 Hz fields at levels between 25 and 100 µT have been shown to increase the levels of super oxide radical anions in the human leukemia cell line K562 along with transiently increased HSP70 levels (>twofold), compared to sham controls (Mannerling et al. 2010). Additionally, it has been shown that low levels of magnetic fields can be a stimulus for immune relevant cells (e.g., macrophages) to release free radicals. Simkó et al. (2004) and Martino et al. (2008, 2010) have shown that growth rate of human umbilical vein cells (HUVECs) and two kinds of cancer cells increases as the DC magnetic field is increased from less than a few microtesla to the earth's magnetic field of about 45 µT. They have also shown that they could decrease the growth rates of the HUVECs cells by adding the antioxidant, superoxide dismutase (SOD) indicating that increasing the magnetic field may be changing the number of free radicals in the cell culture. Usselman et al. (2014) have shown that they can modulate the O_2^- and H_2O_2 concentrations by exciting the hyperfine transition for mixing the S and T states with 50 µT SMFs combined with 1.4 MHz, 20 μT_{rms} radiofrequency (RF) magnetic fields at Zeeman resonance in experimental samples. These changes were dependent on the angle between the static and RF fields. An extensive review of free radical chemistry and the effects of both low- and high-frequency electric and magnetic fields is given by Georgiou (2010). This reference also contains over 200 references.

A related effect is an increase in the release by ferritin molecules of Fe^{+2} from stored nanoparticles of Fe^{+3} with the aid of 6-hydroxidopamine upon the application of RF fields in the 10–100 µT range at 3–10 MHz. In this case, the energy absorbed from the RF fields by the nanoparticle is likely to contribute to both the conversion for Fe^{+3} to Fe^{+2} and a change in the configuration of the ferritin (Ueno et al. 2008).

Enzymes may also serve as catalysts by stabilizing the transition states and lowering the energy barrier for the formation of the product or splitting the peptide bonds (Branden, and Tooze 1999). This process often involves multiple steps and both electron and ion transfers from one position to another on the enzyme and in the molecules being modified.

6.8 Summary

A brief review of some of the physical mechanisms by which magnetic fields can lead to changes in biological systems has been presented. These changes may be amplified by the biological system so that small changes in magnetic fields can lead to changes in a variety of biological processes including growth rates of cells, wound healing, bone growth rates, etc. Additional material on magnetic field effects is presented in Chapters 7 BBA, 1 BMA, 8 BMA, 10 BMA, and 11 BMA.

References

Barnes, F., and Greenebaum, B. 2015. The effects of weak magnetic fields on radical pairs. *Bioelectromagnetics* 36:45–54.

Batchelor, S., Kay, C., McLauchlan, K., and Shkrob, I. 1993. Time-resolved and modulation methods in the study of the effects of magnetic fields on the yields of free radical reactions. *J. Phys. Chem.* 97:13250–13258.

Bingham, C. 1996. The effects of DC and ELF AC magnetic fields on the division rate of mastocytoma cells. PhD Thesis, University of Colorado, Boulder.

Bovey, F. 1988. *Nuclear Magnetic Resonance Spectroscopy*, 2nd ed. Cambridge, MA: Academic Press, p. 29.

Branden, C., and Tooze, J. 1999. *Introduction to Protein Structure*, 2nd ed. New York: Garland Publishing, pp. 205–221.

Brocklehurst, B., and McLauchlan, K. 1996. Free radical mechanism for the effects of environmental electromagnetic fields on biological systems. *Int. J. Radiat. Biol.* 69:3–24.

Bruzon, R., Gurhan, H., Xiong, Y., and Barnes, F. 2017 Oxidative stress as an initial step in the biological effects induced by magnetic fields. *Bioelectromagmetics Meeting*, Hangzhou, China, June 5–9.

Droge, W. 2002. Free radicals in the physiological control of cell function. *Physiol. Rev.* 82:47–95.

Fossey, J., Lefort, D., and Sorba, J. 1995. *Free Radicals in Organic Chemistry*. New York: Wiley.

Frankel, R., and Liburdy, R. 1996. Chapter 3: Biological effects of static magnetic fields. In *Handbook of Biological Effects of Electromagnetic Fields*, 2nd ed., C. Polk and E. Postow, eds. Boca Raton: CRC Press.

Georgiou, C. 2010. Oxidative stress-induced biological damage by low-level EMFs: Mechanism of free radical pair electron spin polarization and biochemical amplification. In *Non-thermal Effects and Mechanisms of Interaction between Electromagnetic Fields and Living Matter*, L. Giuliani and M. Soffritti, eds. *Eur. J. Oncol.—Library* 5:63–113

Greenebaum, B. 2012. Induced electric field and current density patterns in bone fractures. *Bioelectromagnetics* 33:585–593.

Halliwell, B., and Gutteridge, J. 2015. *Free Radicals in Biology and Medicine*, 5th ed. Oxford University Press, Chapter 1, pp. 1–30.

Kalmijn, A. 1988. Detection of weak electric fields. In *Sensory Biology of Aquatic Animals* Editors: Atema, J., Fay, R., Popper, A., Tavolga, W. New York: Springer, pp. 151–186.

Mannerling, A.C., Simkó, M., Mild, K.H., and Mattsson, M.O. 2010. Effects of 50-Hz magnetic field exposure on superoxide radical anion formation and HSP70 induction in human K562 cells. *Radiat. Environ. Biophys.* 49:731–741.

Martino C., Belchenko, D., Ferguson, V., Preiss, S., and Oi, J. 2008. The effects of pulsed electromagnetic fields on cellular activity of SaOS-2 cells. *Bioelectromagnetics* 29(2):125–132.

Martino, C., McCabe, K., Portelli, L., Hernandez, M., and Barnes, F. 2010. Reduction of the earth's magnetic field inhibits growth rates of model cancer cell lines. *Bioelectromagnetics* 8:649–655.

Ramsey, N.F. 1956. *Molecular Beams*. Oxford: Clarendon Press, p. 237.

Rosenspire, A., Kindzelskii, A., Simon, B., and Petty, H. 2005. Real-time control of neutrophil metabolism by very weak ultra-low frequency pulsed magnetic fields. *Biophys. J.* 88:3334–3347.

Sakaguchi, Y., Hayashi, H., and Nagakura, S. 1980. Classification of the External Magnetic Field Effects on the Photodecomposition Reaction of Dibenzoyl Peroxide. *Bull. Chem. Soc. Jpn.* 53:39–42.

Simkó, M. Mattsson, M.-O. 2004. Extremely low frequency electromagnetic fields as effectors of cellular responses in vitro: Possible immune cell activation. *J. Cell Biochem.* 93(1):83–92. Available at: www.ncbi.nlm.nih.gov/pubmed/15352165.

Sipka, S., Szollosi, I., Batta, G., Szegedi, G., Illes, A., Bakeo, G., and Novak, D. 2004. Decreased chemotaxis in human peripheral phagocytes exposed to strong static magnetic field. *Acta Physiol. Hung.* 91(1):59–65.

Steiner, U., and Ulrich, T. 1989. Magnetic field effects in chemical kinetics and related phenomena. *Chem. Rev.* 89:147–151.

Timmel, C., and Henbest, K. 2004. A study of spin chemistry in weak magnetic fields. *Phil. Trans. R Soc. London Ser. A* 362:2573–2589.

Timmel, C., Till, U., Brocklehurst, B., McLauchlan, K., and Hore, P. 1998. Effects of weak magnetic fields on free radical recombination reactions. *Mol. Phys.* 95:71–89.

Townes, C., and Schawlow, A. 1955. *Microwave Spectroscopy.* New York: McGraw Hill, p. 290.

Ueno, S., and Cespedes, O. 2008. Effects of radio frequency magnetic fields on the iron release in: Cage Proteins via 6-Hydroxydoopamine. BEMS Annual meeting Abstract.

Usselman, R.J., Hill, I., Singel, D.J., and Martino, C.F. 2014. Spin biochemistry modulates reactive oxygen species production by radio frequency magnetic fields. *PLoS One* 9:e101328.

Wadas, R. 1991. *Biomagnetism.* Hemel, Hemstead, UK: Ellis Horwood Limited and Polish Scientific Publishers.

Zmyslony, M., Rajkowska, E., Mamrot, P., Politanski, J., and Jajte, J. 2004. The effect of weak 50 Hz magnetic fields on the number of free oxygen radicals in rat lymphocytes in vitro. *Bioelectromagnetics* 25:607–661.

7

Mechanisms of Action in Bioelectromagnetics

Ben Greenebaum
University of Wisconsin-Parkside

CONTENTS

7.1 Introduction 234
7.2 Generally Accepted Interactions 235
    7.2.1 Heating 235
    7.2.2 Specialized Sensory Organs 236
    7.2.3 Magnetite 236
    7.2.4 Nerves and the Nervous System 236
    7.2.5 Vibration Detection 237
7.3 Radical Recombination Rates and Related Quantum Mechanical Phenomena 237
    7.3.1 Introduction 237
    7.3.2 Theoretical Background 238
        7.3.2.1 Hyperfine Interaction-Induced Singlet-to-Triplet Conversion 240
        7.3.2.2 High-Field Regime: Spin Rephrasing through the Δg Mechanism 242
        7.3.2.3 Low-Field Effect: $B < 1$ mT 242
        7.3.2.4 Time-Varying Fields; Resonant Transitions 243
    7.3.3 General Characteristics of the Free Radical Mechanism 244
        7.3.3.1 Experimental Discrimination of Free Radical Models 244
    7.3.4 Free Radicals in Biology 245
        7.3.4.1 Biological Transduction Mechanisms 245
        7.3.4.2 Role of Freely Diffusing Radicals 246
        7.3.4.3 Animal Navigation Models Based on Free Radicals 246
        7.3.4.4 Coenzyme B12-Dependent Reactions 247
        7.3.4.5 Other Experimental Observations 247
    7.3.5 Summary 248
7.4 Other Proposals Involving Quantum Mechanics 249
    7.4.1 Precession Changes 249
7.5 Proposals Involving Direct Electromagnetic Forces 249
    7.5.1 Effects at the Cell Surface 250
        7.5.1.1 Ligand Binding 250
        7.5.1.2 Electromechanical Models 250
    7.5.2 Direct Effects of Electromagnetic Forces on Charges and Currents 251
        7.5.2.1 Isolated Ions and Molecules 252
        7.5.2.2 Electroporation 252
        7.5.2.3 Ion Cyclotron Resonance and Related Ideas 252
7.6 Electromagnetic Forces Interacting with Other Properties 253
    7.6.1 Water-Related Effects 253
    7.6.2 Phase Transitions 254

7.1 Introduction

Because the interaction of applied magnetic fields with atomic and molecular moments is relatively weak and most often involves energies that are equal or less than thermal noise or other interferences, theoretical models of the interactions must find a way to isolate the moment or the molecule. But for the field interaction to have an influence on subsequent biological processes, the isolation cannot be complete.

The basic physics involving electromagnetic fields is rather well understood. It is outlined in the Introduction and Chapters 5 and 6, as well as elsewhere in these volumes. Furthermore, much about the biological systems themselves is well understood and further understanding is evolving rapidly. Therefore, it is reasonable to seek to explain the effects of electromagnetic fields on biological systems by inferring that if a physical interaction produces a change in something that is important for a sequence of biological reactions, a biological change in the end result of the sequence will occur. However, biological systems incorporate many feedback and other control processes, so that a change at one stage of a process may or may not result in a change in the final outcome. In addition, the outcome may differ, depending on the state of the organism and its current surroundings. Although essentially all "explanations" in science have stronger and weaker links in their chains of evidence, the weak links are so far more prevalent in bioelectromagnetics. The inconsistencies that plague the bioelectromagnetics literature are due in part to these complications. Therefore, these inferred explanations of bioelectromagnetic influences can be speculative, incomplete, or at least open to question.

It is clear from the various chapters in these volumes that there are few instances where there is a full understanding of the complete series of processes by which a physical interaction with a field leads to a predictable biological outcome. Simko and Mattsson also discuss this issue in their introduction to Chapter 1 in BMA. One successful explanation is the way the earth's field exerts a force on chains of magnetite in certain bacteria that orients them to swim toward the muck at the bottom of the water in which they live, where conditions are best (Frankel and Blakemore, 1989). But in general, the chain of reasoning and experiment is less strong. This is true even for what is presently considered the strongest candidates to explain many bioelectromagnetic phenomena: that a magnetic field can alter the recombination rate of radical pairs to affect various biological end points. For example, magnetic fields are considered to affect radical recombination rates in birds, presumably in cryptochromes in the retina, producing information used in navigation during migration (Rodgers and Hore, 2009). The physics behind the initial interaction is solid; and it has been shown that fields affect cryptochromes *in vitro* and in various organisms, that cryptochromes are important in the functioning of the birds' retinas, and that fields alter birds' sense of direction. So the mechanism has become accepted even though the chain of evidence is partly experimental, partly theoretical, and partly based on inference that has yet to be backed by experiment.

Many scientists have proposed various interaction mechanisms, both for specific bioelectromagnetic effects and more general scenarios. In general, the chains of evidence supporting them are less complete than those for magnetotactic bacteria or bird migration. The ultimate goal in bioelectromagnetics, of course, is to find one or more (probably more

Bioelectromagnetic Mechanisms of Action 235

than one) mechanisms that explain all bioelectromagnetic effects. Where a satisfactory explanation can be agreed upon, not only would presently used applications of fields in the applicable parts of biology and medicine be fully understood and become capable of being refined, but new applications would become known, and electromagnetic fields might become powerful tools for medical diagnostics and treatment and also for probing how various biological processes actually work.

The purpose of this chapter is to describe briefly a number of the proposed mechanisms, beginning with the two mentioned above. In some cases, it will point out both successes in explaining experimental observations, at least in part, and some inherent problems. Most attention will be paid to ideas involving weak and moderate magnetic fields, since much of the concern over environmental effects lie in this region and very strong fields are rarely encountered. Similarly, less attention will be paid to electric fields, since in the absence of direct contact with an electrode or other current source, electric fields are strongly shielded at the surface of the body. Some of these cases are treated in other chapters.

Binhi's book (2002) analyzes a great many proposed interaction mechanisms using the tools of physical theory, pointing out strengths and weaknesses. A number of authors have analyzed the proposals and pointed out their weaknesses. Adair (1991, 1992, 1999) in particular used basic physics and relatively simple models to show that a number of proposed influences may be too weak to explain observed biological effects, although his models may oversimplify some biological situations.

Since many proposals have similar characteristics, they are presented in somewhat arbitrary groups: Proposals, mostly for strong fields, that are generally accepted; proposals based on specialized biological organs or structures; proposals based on quantum mechanical features of atoms and molecules; proposals based directly on electromagnetic forces, such as those based on the Lorentz magnetic force or the effects of strong electric fields on charged structures; and proposals based on electromagnetic forces in combination with other factors.

7.2 Generally Accepted Interactions

7.2.1 Heating

An electric field will exert a force on a charged object and, unless the object is firmly fixed in place, cause it to move. Furthermore, electric and magnetic fields will cause electric or magnetic dipoles to rotate unless they are firmly fixed. In general, the energy associated with these motions will be dissipated as heat, and it is well established that heating can result from application of strong electromagnetic fields. A microwave oven is an everyday example. Heating and its biomedical applications are discussed further in Chapter 9 in BMA.

While there is no question that strong enough fields can cause biological effects through heating, a more controversial question is the threshold below which the amount of heat deposited by a field is of no biological consequence or whether there might be situations where very local heating may occur, perhaps briefly, even though the extra heat energy may be rapidly dispersed through normal biological processes. This is discussed in Chapter 5 and will not be covered here.

7.2.2 Specialized Sensory Organs

It has long been known that certain organisms are sensitive to electric or magnetic fields, and in some of these organisms the specialized sensory organs have been identified. Examples include the sensors distributed on the surfaces of fish, skates, and sharks, which enable them to sense disturbances in self-generated electric fields or those generated by nearby prey or predators. Often, the animal senses and interprets the very small voltage difference between specialized cells at different positions on the skin (Kalmijn, 1988; Nelson and MacIver, 1999). In skates and sharks, the cells are the ampullae of Lorenzini, physiologically related to hair cells in the inner ear. Some fish generate high-frequency signals and sense changes in these fields with tuberous electroreceptor organs (Nelson and McIver, 1999). Similar organs are used in other aquatic species to sense mechanical disturbances in the water through their lateral lines.

7.2.3 Magnetite

Magnetite, Fe_3O_4, is a naturally occurring, highly ferromagnetic substance and small-enough grains such as are found in these animals are single-domain, that is, entirely magnetized in a single direction. Most biological materials are weakly diamagnetic or paramagnetic and do not interact with external magnetic fields in strengths that are anywhere comparable to the general thermal background noise. However, a number of animals have grains of magnetite distributed in various ways in their bodies. Such a magnetite grain will experience a force in an external magnetic field that tends to orient it and its internal magnetic field parallel to the external one. In some bacteria and other microorganisms, these grains form chains; and the forces are sufficient to allow the organisms to, for instance, orient and migrate along the earth's field to bury themselves in the bottom of a pond, where growth conditions are best (Frankel et al., 1979, Frankel and Blakemore, 1989). Another example is the honeybee, where magnetite is present in the abdomen (Walker and Bitterman, 1989), though in bees, detection of electric fields is also important, as discussed below. Experiments in fish have also indicated structures of some length that are magnetic field-sensitive (Kirschvinck et al., 2001). Isolated magnetite grains occur in many other species including mammals, birds, and possibly humans. Their role, if any, is not clear; they may in some way be associated with orienting the organism for foraging or even migration. However, in higher animals, the grains occur in isolation; and a chain of grains appears to be needed to provide a force that is strong and stable enough to act as a signal in the presence of thermal noise (Adair, 1991; Kirschvinck et al., 2001; see also Chapter 8 in BBA). In the case of birds, a mechanism involving radicals appears to be a better interpretation for bird migration behavior as discussed below, though other mechanisms involving light and perhaps other factors also seem involved.

7.2.4 Nerves and the Nervous System

Since the days of Galvani, it has been known that electrical stimulation of nerve and muscle cells is possible. In addition to simply making a quiescent cell function, properly timed pulses can entrain a nerve, changing its normal timing somewhat so that it follows the external stimulus. External electric stimulation has been used for purposes ranging such as regulation of heartbeats, amelioration of pain, or making muscles function after nerve injuries (Coster and Celler, 2003; Peckham and Knutson, 2005; Zaghi et al., 2010). The principle behind these applications is the depolarization of the nerve membranes (Saunders and Jefferys, 2002).

Nerve cells depolarize their membranes to produce an electrical impulse and send signals to other parts of the nervous system throughout the body, mediating cell-to-cell communication with chemical neurotransmitters. External fields can change the transmembrane potential to stimulate these impulses, usually though introducing internal electric fields or currents. A large body of experimental work links physiological and behavioral outcomes to field exposure, which are both frequency and intensity dependent. Examples include the stimulation of magneto- or electrophosphenes (perceived light flashes) in the eye and other neural stimulation (Wood, 2008). Direct contact with strong voltage or current sources can produce electric shock, muscle contractions, and various RF effects. Both of these mechanisms have had roles in published rationales for setting standards for human exposure to electromagnetic fields (ICNIRP, 1998, 2010; IEEE, 2002, 2005). Nerve cell interactions with fields and the effects of these interactions are discussed at length in Chapters 5 in BBA and 15 in BMA, as well as elsewhere, and will not be discussed further here.

7.2.5 Vibration Detection

Many animals have thin flexible appendages that are used to sense aspects of their surroundings, such as the vibrissae ("whiskers") around the nose area of rats and other species. One function of these is to sense the dimensions of small passages in the dark. Stell et al. (1993) discuss their and others' findings that rat vibrissae have been observed to move in 60 Hz electric fields above about 7.5 kV/m. However, Stell et al. also find that moving air does not affect rats' ability to detect the fields, possibly indicating another detection mechanism. Bees are known to become electrically charged as they fly, and this is known to help them find flowers, which also can be electrically charged, and attract pollen to their bodies upon arrival (Clarke et al., 2013). Greggers et al. (2013) have shown that the time-changing fields due to beating of their electrically charged wings are used to communicate information between bees in the waggle dance inside the dark hive. Field detection is apparently through sensing motion of the flagellum, the outer part of the antennae, which also picks up a charge. In strong DC fields, body hair is also known to be attracted and may in some cases act as a sensor.

7.3 Radical Recombination Rates and Related Quantum Mechanical Phenomena[*]

7.3.1 Introduction

The physical chemistry of spin-correlated free radical pairs and related phenomena offers several mechanisms explaining how magnetic fields may influence biochemical processes. The mechanisms are classified on the basis of the dominating contribution to how the pair's spins evolve, and they cover a wide range of field strengths. Radicals and related phenomena such as electron transfer reactions are important in biochemistry, including in reactions involving reactive oxygen species (ROS) and enzymes. Of particular interest is what is called the low-field mechanism, which has been extensively developed over the

---

[*] Section 3 is edited and updated by B. Greenebaum from the previous edition of this Handbook (Engstrom, 2007).

last decade and is now considered capable of explaining many biological effects induced by magnetic fields well below 1 mT.

The principal mechanism behind the free radical mechanism was discovered in the physical problem of magnetic field dependence on positronium decay (Deutsch and Brown, 1952; Halpern, 1954). However, the development of the radical pair mechanism in chemistry has its roots in the work of Kaptein and Oosterhoff (1969), Closs (1969), and Brocklehurst (1969).

An ambitious survey of the literature up to its date of publication concerning field effects on radicals and oxidative species and their reactions is the review of Steiner and Ulrich (1989), which lists some 775 references, 58 of which are themselves reviews on magnetokinetic phenomena. Another, now classic, reference on the subject is the book by Salikhov et al. (1984). More recent books include the extensive text by Halliwell and Gutteridge (2015) and Hayashi (2004); McLauchlan and Steiner (1991) published a review including the possible mechanisms at lower fields. The review by Grissom (1995) explored the higher-field mechanisms with particular attention to the context of biological systems. A didactic paper geared toward the issues in biological systems is that of Brocklehurst and McLauchlan (1996). There are also some recent reviews on the free radical mechanism in general (Woodward, 2002) and with particular attention to biological systems (Brocklehurst, 2002) and cell function (Droge, 2002). Buchachenko (2016) summarizes many experimental results that provide both support or sometimes add confusion to understanding the mechanisms. Hore and Mouritsen (2016) review the radical pair mechanism basics with particular reference to cryptochromes and bird migration.

7.3.2 Theoretical Background

A radical is an atom or a molecule with an unpaired electron. It tends to be highly reactive, a property that defines radicals' best known roles in biology. Especially notable radicals for biology are many (not all) of the ROS, a group that includes radicals like superoxide ($O_2^{\bullet-}$— the $\bullet$ symbol indicates the unpaired electron), hydroxyl ($OH^\bullet$), and carbonate ($CO_3^{\bullet-}$) as well as reactive but non-radicals like hydrogen peroxide (H_2O_2) and many others. Other elements also form reactive species, some of which are radicals, such as the reactive nitrogen species (RNS), radical nitric oxide ($NO^\bullet$) and the non-radical RNS nitroxyl anion (NO^-) (Halliwell and Gutteridge, 2015).

A spin-correlated (or geminate) radical pair is typically created by cleavage of a covalent bond, where each molecule retains one of the electrons that formed the broken chemical bond. The electron spins may remain correlated as they were before the bond was broken for a significant time (microseconds) after the pair's creation and are most frequently antiparallel (S or singlet state). As the radicals separate, the electron interaction term becomes small, and the electron states of the pair will fluctuate between where the electron spin angular momenta are antiparallel, with total spin angular momentum S = 0 (singlet or S state),[*] and parallel (S = 1, triplet or T state) (Figure 7.1). The relative spins evolve coherently through the hyperfine interactions between the electron spin and the nuclei. There is a chance of reencounter between the spin-correlated radicals. Reforming the bond is only permitted by quantum spin selection rules if the electron spins are oriented in the singlet

---

[*] Note that S is used here in two ways, stemming from conventions for values of two separate but related concepts: the spin quantum number and a type of atomic or molecular quantum mechanical state that contributes to a single spectral line (as opposed to double, triple, etc.) due to its particular combination of spin and other quantum numbers.

Bioelectromagnetic Mechanisms of Action

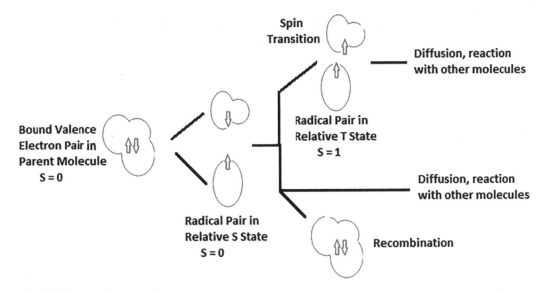

FIGURE 7.1
A molecule is split into two radicals. After diffusion and possible spin interconversion into a relative T state, the radicals may reencounter while still spin correlated. If the encounter occurs in the S state (bottom), the radicals may recombine. Otherwise, recombination cannot occur, and the radicals will diffuse apart again and eventually lose their spin correlation, reacting with other molecules. A magnetic field can influence this reaction by changing the rate of spin interconversion as long as the singlet and triplet products have different chemical fates.

state and can be as fast as a few nanoseconds. Otherwise, the radicals will react with other molecules, possibly after diffusing a short way from each other; their lifetime is typically short but can range from a few tens of nanoseconds to as much as a few microseconds (Grissom, 1995).

Magnetic fields can affect the electron state in the time before the reencounter; and if singlet and triplet pairs have different chemical fates, we have a basis for magnetic field effects on free radical chemistry. In exemplifying the process, we will assume that the radical pair is formed in the singlet state, the normal case for biologically relevant reactions (Eveson et al., 2000).

In weak external magnetic fields, atomic magnetic moments are characterized in the quantum mechanical Hamiltonian by the vector sum of its various angular momenta $F = J + I$, where J is the total electronic angular momentum, itself the vector sum of orbital and spin angular momenta, and I is the total nuclear angular momentum. In molecules, other terms, such as rotational angular momentum, need to be included. When external field strengths approach the relevant internal fields due to various spins and motions, this coupling breaks down and the Hamiltonian begins to have separate terms in I, J, and other quantities (Herzberg, 1950; Townes and Schalow, 1955). In low and high fields, the energies of the various levels are linear functions of the external field and internal moments. The transition between the low field coupling and separate consideration of the moments in the strong field coupling scheme, contributes to the curved part of the graph of the Zeeman energy levels as a function of applied field (Figure 7.2). Although the transition between low field and high field coupling of the moments is discussed in a great many theoretical articles, many detailed examples only consider the moments separately, although the low field coupling is more clearly used in the papers by Kaptein (1972), McLauchlan and

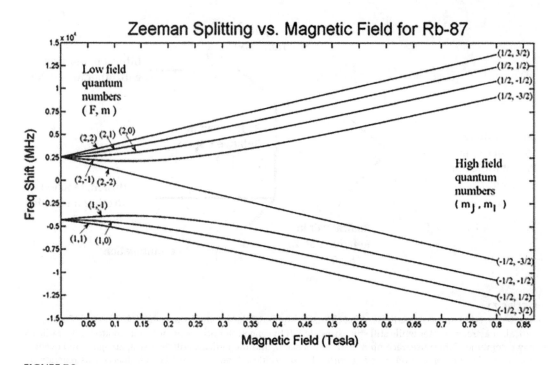

FIGURE 7.2
The Zeeman energy levels of rubidium-87, showing the transition from low-field coupling, where spins and orbital angular momentum couple and $F = I + J$ is a good quantum number, to high field where nuclear spin I and atomic electron spin J interact with the external field individually. $I = 3/2$ for this isotope. [Danskii 14. Creative Commons copyright (CC BY-SA 3.0)].

Steiner (1991), and in the experimental and theoretical analysis of resonance spectra of NO by Gallagher et al. (1954).

Many physical transduction mechanisms proposed to explain magnetic field effects in biology are very vulnerable to the randomizing effects of thermal noise at normal temperatures of living systems (Binhi and Savin, 2003). The free radical mechanism is uniquely resistant to this obstacle since it is a nuclear effect; the hyperfine interaction is between the electronic and nuclear spins and is not strongly coupled to the thermal bath (Adair, 1999).

A quantum mechanical formulation of the free radical mechanism contains many possible contributions to the Hamiltonian; Steiner and Ulrich (1989) provide a good categorization of the main components. The stochastic Liouville equation (SLE) is a tool for addressing the problem of simultaneous spin mixing and diffusion, but simplified models in which these two components are treated separately are often useful for the great reduction in problem complexity (Brocklehurst and McLauchlan, 1996). Recently, analytical results using a backward SLE have been presented (Pedersen and Christensen, 2004). Letuta et al. (2017) perform a spin-density calculation of theoretical magnitude of spin effects for the hyperfine and Δg mechanisms described below.

7.3.2.1 Hyperfine Interaction-Induced Singlet-to-Triplet Conversion

The direction of a magnetic moment vector in a magnetic field will precess about the field vector; precession can be visualized as the moment vector's tip rotating so it describes a circle the about the field vector while the two are at a constant angle. This is the Larmor precession; its frequency is the product of the magnetic field, the magnetic moment and the Landé g-factor, which depends the spins involved (Townes and Schalow, 1955). Hyperfine interactions between the spins of the electron and the nucleus stem from the electron spin moments within a radical precessing about field from its nuclear spin. Singlet-to-triplet conversion between the pair of radicals occurs as the precession rates in the two members of the radical pair are not the same.

The triplet state has a net magnetic moment, and in the presence of an external magnetic field the energy levels of the triplet states that have a moment aligned parallel or antiparallel to the magnetic field (T_+ and T_-, respectively) will be separated by Zeeman splitting. As the applied field strength is increased, the T_+ and T_- energy levels will be shifted away from the singlet state so much that they are decoupled from the spin interconversion process between singlet and triplet states, and only the remaining triplet state (T_0), which has a magnetic moment that is oriented perpendicular to the field, is capable of participating in the spin conversion process. In this way, the magnetic field can reduce the number of triplet states that can be converted into singlet states and subsequently reform the original chemical bond (Figure 7.3). This is the "normal" magnetic field effect on free radical chemistry. It becomes relevant for external fields larger than the effective field driving the hyperfine interaction mixing, typically 1–10 mT.

Another way in which singlet-to-triplet conversion can be facilitated is when an applied field causes the T_- energy level of one member of the radical pair to cross its nonmagnetic singlet level, which occurs when the Zeeman differential matches the electron exchange interaction energy (cf. Figure 7.3). This effect has been observed for fields as low as 3.6 mT (Werner et al., 1993), but it can in principle be observed for much lower fields if the radical pairs are fixed with an appropriate separation. In this case, the radical may change states (assuming angular momentum conservation can be observed), and may become in a position to more easily recombine with the other member of the pair.

In addition, it should be noted that as the applied field approaches zero, the energy differences between the triplet states also approach zero. When the nuclear spin of an atom is non-zero, it interacts with the electronic moment through the hyperfine effect, which

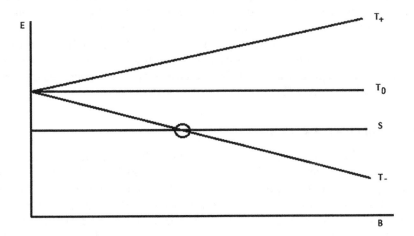

FIGURE 7.3
Energy level diagram for singlet and triplet states of a radical pair. At high fields T_+ and T_- states are completely disconnected from the singlet state and only the T_0 state is available for spin interconversion. Note that at a specific B field the Zeeman splitting causes the T_- state to closely match the singlet state (circled), increasing the probability of a transition between the two.

produces an energy difference between atomic S and the three T states, including at zero applied field. However, when this and the additional energies due to an external field are below the zero-field splittings, quantum rules governing the transitions between the levels are different and make the states more of a mixture of each other, rather than less as at higher external fields. As a result, recombination at low fields is less likely, the so-called low-field effect (McLauchlan and Steiner, 1991).

In addition, when the energy difference between quantum mechanical states is less than their natural width due to the uncertainty principle and other factors, they are said to be degenerate and become described mathematically as a mixture of the degenerate states (McLauchlan and Steiner, 1991). Therefore, an electron may appear to have spontaneously changed spin direction if a new field is applied. This may perhaps be more easily envisioned by thinking that, at zero applied field, there is no preferred direction along which to identify the spin orientation and so orientation is lost. Significant differences have been noted in many systems when the net external magnetic field approaches zero (Binhi and Prato, 2017). The momentary cancellation of the earth's field during each cycle of a parallel alternating field of similar or greater amplitude offers a repeated opportunity for mixing of levels, but it may well occupy too little a fraction of the total cycle time to have a noticeable effect.

Differences between in their internal couplings and electronic structures between different species of atoms and molecules mean that an applied magnetic field creates different shifts due to Zeeman or other interactions in the energy of quantum levels. Therefore, at the proper field strength, a pair of radicals may find that quantum states in each that are otherwise allowed to recombine, have their relative energies shifted to reduce or increase the energy barrier to recombination, shifting the radical concentrations.

7.3.2.2 High-Field Regime: Spin Rephrasing through the Δg Mechanism

Similar, but separate from the rephrasing of spin precession in the internal hyperfine fields of one of a radical pair, this process involves differences in spin precession frequency between the two members. As noted, the product of the magnetic field, the moment and the Landé g-factor determines the rate of Larmor precession of the unpaired electron spin, especially in the absence of a contribution independent of the hyperfine such as when no non-zero nuclear spins are present (Timmel and Henbest, 2004). If the two radicals have slightly different g-factors, this provides an additional source of spin conversion. Differences are usually quite small, so this mechanism typically becomes significant only for quite large fields, B > 0.1–1 T.

7.3.2.3 Low-Field Effect: B < 1 mT

At fields below the hyperfine interaction energy, it is still possible to see effects of external fields under certain circumstances. It was found by Brocklehurst (1976) that the selection rules of the hyperfine-induced spin mixing are more restrictive in zero field than when a field is applied (McLauchlan and Steiner, 1991; Brocklehurst and McLauchlan, 1996). This becomes relevant, even for a very small field, as long as the coherence of the pair's state is maintained for long periods (100 ns to 1 µs). A helpful vector model to visualize this effect, along with some illustrative numerical examples, is given by Till et al. (1998).

The low-field effect (LFE) occurs as correlations between electron and nuclear spins in radical pair are upset by a weak field, changing possible recombination possibilities (Timmel and Henbest, 2004). It can theoretically produce a large (40%) drop in the singlet

Bioelectromagnetic Mechanisms of Action

yield if the conditions are optimal (Timmel et al., 1998), but in practice only smaller effects attributed to this mechanism have been reported in the experimental literature.

Since long coherence times are required, it is necessary to understand spin relaxation effects and under what conditions they may be sufficiently long. Anisotropic hyperfine interactions provide noncoherent spin relaxation in solution, and it appears that the relaxation is slower in the low-field situation than has been generally thought (Fedin et al., 2001, 2003). It is becoming clear that understanding the local environment is crucial for evaluating LFEs (Eveson et al., 2000).

An important way to extend free radical magnetic field effects into the low-field region is to extend the lifetime of the spin-correlated pair. Integrating the magnetic field's influence over a longer time increases its ability to influence the spin evolution. Spin relaxation is not the primary problem here; rather, it is the reencounter probability that needs to be enhanced. There are several ways to achieve this:

1. Increased viscosity to restrict diffusion (Krissinel et al., 1999; Christensen and Pedersen, 2003; Kitahama et al., 2004)

2. Oppositely charged radicals that will oppose a tendency to diffuse apart (Adair, 1999)

3. Physically restricted mobility of the radicals through confining them to a surface or having the reaction taking place inside micelles, which are nanometerscale compartments that form and reform on microsecond timescales and are able to confine the radical pairs and increase the reencounter probability (Eveson et al., 2000).

7.3.2.4 Time-Varying Fields; Resonant Transitions

At low frequencies, the characteristic time for pair recombination or escape is short compared the rate at which the instantaneous field changes. Therefore, the low-frequency field is constant as far as the pair is concerned and the frequency itself is not important. Calculations generally average over the field's time average value (Brocklehurst and McLauchlan, 1996). However, hyperfine level splittings can be in the low frequency range, even in low fields; Barnes and Greenebaum (2015) give examples for NO in the earth's DC field ($45\,\mu T$) where resonant frequencies are in the 60–1000 Hz range in one instance and around 500 kHz in another.

For higher-frequency fields ($f > 1\,MHz$), the time modulation of the field starts to correspond to timescales present in the reaction dynamics, and a range of resonant interactions become available (Timmel and Hore, 1996). A detailed treatment of the coenzyme B12 system demonstrated resonant phenomena for relatively low-level radiofrequency (RF) fields using a variety of mathematical techniques (Canfield et al., 1994, 1995).

The frequency is important, however, in the case of resonant interactions, where the applied frequency f corresponds to the energy difference between two levels in a molecule ($\Delta E = hf$ where h is Planck's constant). Any such transition involves a change in the angular momentum of the molecule, which can affect the electronic spin state and therefore the recombination rate of a radical pair (Barnes and Greenebaum, 2015). Transitions can occur at almost any frequency. At weak magnetic fields, Zeeman splittings can be in the ELF or intermediate frequency ranges (Barnes and Greenebaum, 2015). Hyperfine transitions can be in the RF. A detailed treatment of the coenzyme B12 system demonstrated resonant phenomena for relatively low-level RF fields using a variety of mathematical techniques

(Canfield et al., 1994, 1995). Optical spectral lines, as is well-known, occur in transitions between electron orbital states.

7.3.3 General Characteristics of the Free Radical Mechanism

Free radical reactions are generally quite fast. There is evidence of picosecond reactions (Gilch et al., 1998; Musewald et al., 1999), but many known reactions occur over nanosecond timescales. If the free radical diffusion is constrained by micelles (Eveson et al., 2000; Christensen and Pedersen, 2003) or by Coulomb attraction (Horiuchi et al., 2003), it may be possible to extend the radical pair lifetimes to hundreds of nanoseconds or even microseconds.

Since the free radical mechanism is practically instantaneous when compared to the timescale of time-varying magnetic fields in the extremely low-frequency regime (<300 Hz), one would expect that the observable output from a biological detection of the field should depend only on the time-averaged absolute field amplitude (Scaiano et al., 1995). However, if there is a downstream system that is able to decode the low-frequency signal, this statement is not necessarily true (Engstrom, 1997; Engstrom and Fitzsimmons, 1999).

7.3.3.1 Experimental Discrimination of Free Radical Models

The relative orientation of a static and a much smaller oscillating field will provide a discriminating test for a free radical-based model as long as the timescale of the applied field is long compared to the lifetime of the radical pair. In an isotropic system, such as a liquid suspension, described by this field situation, only the amplitude of the magnetic field is relevant. While the smaller parallel field adds linearly to the larger static field, the perpendicular component is effectively reduced by the calculation of vector length and will cause a much smaller variation in field amplitude (Engstrom, 1997). For strictly parallel fields in which the alternating amplitude equals or exceeds that of the static field, there is a brief time where the net amplitude is zero and certain levels are degenerate, allowing mixing as discussed above.

For oriented systems in which the free radical chemistry steps have spatial preferences, it is possible to have angular dependence with respect to the angle of the applied field, $f(\theta)$. One can argue that some symmetry properties are very likely to be present in that kind of situation (Ritz et al., 2000). Polarity changes are not expected to be relevant, so $f(\theta + 180°) = f(\theta)$. Furthermore, due to the isotropic distribution of nuclear spins in the initial state of the radical pair, one also expects that $f(180° - \theta) = f(\theta)$.

If the free radical mechanism is active for low-frequency fields, one can also expect a response to RF fields in the same system, a property not expected by any other suggested physical transduction mechanisms for magnetic fields (Henbest et al., 2004). In a comparison between static fields in the range 0–2 mT, it was shown that a 300 μT, 5 MHz RF field applied perpendicularly or in parallel with the static field induced a response that was dependent on the magnitude of the static field (Henbest et al., 2004). There is also an angular dependence. Henbest et al. (2004) applied 5–50 MHz, 300 μT and parallel or perpendicular 0–4 mT static magnetic fields (SMFs) to a radical chemical reaction *in vitro* and found both enhancements and decreases as functions of both angle and field strength. There appeared to be an inflection point at all angles at the magnetic field corresponding a Zeeman resonance frequency. This is qualitatively, if not quantitatively, similar to the observation that the magnetic sense of migratory birds can be disrupted by a 470 nT, 7 MHz field when the field is applied at an angle with the geomagnetic field (Ritz et al., 2004).

Bioelectromagnetic Mechanisms of Action 245

Magnetic isotope effects involving non-zero nuclear spins are another possible discriminating character of free radical effects, and it is possible to differentiate this signature from pure mass effects (Brocklehurst, 1997).

7.3.4 Free Radicals in Biology

7.3.4.1 Biological Transduction Mechanisms

Direct detection methods for free radicals have been developed in chemistry only relatively recently (Woodward, 2002) but there is significant evidence for their role (Halliwell and Gutteridge, 2015). In biological systems, much experimental evidence for free radical involvement remains indirect. Generating hypotheses based on the signatures of free radical systems as outlined above are necessary to link free radical chemistry to magnetic field effects, but there is circumstantial evidence that free radical chemistry underlies some effects reported in the bioelectromagnetics literature. Jones (2016) reviews the basic physics described above but then goes on to discuss recent results regarding the radical-involved transitions in several types of biological reactions showing magnetic field effects *in vitro*, as well as reasons that some of these do not show downstream effects though others can. The examples include photosynthetic reactions, peroxidase enzymes, B12-dependent enzymes, photosynthetic reaction centers, enzymatic ATP synthesis, and cryptochromes.

It has been suggested that complex dynamical systems may have special sensitivity to magnetic field influences (Grundler et al., 1992; Walleczek, 1995). This idea has been elaborated in a series of theoretical models of oscillatory systems (Eichwald and Walleczek, 1996a,b; Kaiser, 1996). These models show that enzyme dynamics involving free radical chemistry may be frequency specific, although only for timescales comparable to or slower than the chemical kinetics of the system (Eichwald and Walleczek, 1997). Field amplitude can influence enzyme dynamics in some instances and this can be used to exert some control over enzyme systems (Eichwald and Walleczek, 1998).

The peroxidase–oxidase system has interesting, well-documented dynamical properties (Scheeline et al., 1997). Detailed modeling of this system has shown how a magnetic field-induced perturbation can affect its dynamical behavior (Eichwald and Walleczek, 1998; Moller and Olsen, 1999). The point of interaction in this system is suspected to be electron-transfer enzyme intermediates (Moller and Olsen, 2000; Moller et al., 2000).

Downstream effects from changes in chemistry must be taken into account to evaluate biological significance (Brocklehurst and McLauchlan, 1996). This can both facilitate detection (Walleczek, 1995) as well as introduce interventions that could block the biological significance of a physical detection event or produce an elevation of the final product in one situation and a depression in a slightly different one. Of particular interest may be the reactive oxygen and RNS, many of which are radicals, as well as other oxidation- or reduction- related radicals that may be affected by the processes outlined above. These important species have many roles, including as signaling and regulatory molecules, and are part of the way biological systems maintain proper balance and control. Changes in the concentration or lifetime of these and molecules with similar function are equivalent to changes in the amplification or time delay parameters in the feedback mechanism formalism discussed in Chapter 5.

It may be relevant that other enzyme systems have been studied in detail without the specific intention of addressing free radicals as a possible mechanism (Steiner and Ulrich, 1989). Magnetic field effects on bacterial photosynthesis (Werber et al., 1978) have long been observed and explained using a model of spin conversion in radicals (Haberkorn and Michel-Beyerle, 1979). Other examples include a electric and magnetic field effects in ATPase (Blank and Soo, 2001b). Myosin phosphorylation is another enzyme system that has shown sensitivity to time-varying (Markov et al., 1993) and SMFs (Markov and Pilla, 1994), as well as gradient-specific effects (Engstrom et al., 2002). Direct interactions with DNA have been suggested; and electron transfer reactions are proposed interaction targets (Blank and Goodman, 2000; Blank and Soo, 2001a).

In what follows, some examples of experimental findings involving radicals, including ROS, in various biological systems are given. Additional examples are given in Chapter 1 in BMA.

7.3.4.2 Role of Freely Diffusing Radicals

Free radicals observed in biology are most commonly oxygen or nitrogen based with an unpaired electron, leading to the terms ROS and RNS. A dominant role for these radicals is to act in immunological defense. They are secreted by macrophages and neutrophils and during attempts to kill bacteria, viruses, and tumors (Nathan, 1992). The highly reactive nature of the radicals also means that damage to normal cells is possible, and various defense mechanisms against this have evolved as well (Yu, 1994). This immunological weapon with checks and balances already suggests that there is a signaling system built around free radicals, but it seems that the ROS and RNS also have roles in intracellular cell signaling (Lander, 1997) as well as intercellular communication (Thannickal and Fanburg, 2000).

Consider a biochemical reaction producing a spin-correlated free radical pair in the singlet state. Depending on the specific mechanism at work, the ratio of singlet-to-triplet product at reencounter will be modified. This will increase or decrease the fraction of pairs that tend to recombine because of a reencounter finding the spins in singlet versus the triplet states. For the LFE, the triplet state is favored, and we would see an excess of escape product. The situation is the opposite for the "normal" field effect, in which the T_- and T_+ states are decoupled from the interconversion process, increasing the proportion of singlet reencounters leading to a larger amount of cage product and leaving fewer freely diffusing radicals. At higher fields the Δg mechanism creates enough difference in the Larmor frequencies of the pair to bring their moments alternately into S and T alignments, bringing T_- and T_+ states back into play and therefore again boosting the triplet-reencounter escape products.

Given the wide involvement of free radicals in signaling and biological function, it is clear that there is the potential of both subtle and not-so-subtle effects on biological systems if we are able to alter the production of free radicals and thereby change the dynamics of already ongoing processes. The conventional wisdom regarding the deleterious effects of magnetic field effects on free radical recombination has been that more escape product means more radical-induced damage. This may be an oversimplification since the direct effects on cage or escape products are typically fairly small, certainly not larger than tens of percent, implying that drastic biological effects must involve downstream responses that amplify this relatively slight modulation. The answer may lie in the signaling properties of free radicals.

7.3.4.3 Animal Navigation Models Based on Free Radicals

The free radical mechanism was the first mechanism suggested as an explanation of avian use of magnetic fields for navigation (Schulten et al., 1978; Schulten, 1982). This model has since undergone several iterations of refinement (Ritz et al., 2000; Cintolesi et al., 2003). Current understanding is reviewed by Hore and Mouritsen (2016). One interesting aspect of this work is a connection between photosensitivity and magneto-reception (Ritz et al., 2002). Dependence on light is a well-known feature of the avian magnetoreceptor (Deutschlander et al., 1999; Wiltschko et al., 2004a,b), but it has also appeared in other behavioral studies of animal magnetic field sensitivity (Prato et al., 1997, 1998).

The Ritz–Schulten model (Ritz et al., 2000) has an appealing geometrical application. Being integrated into the bird's retina, the suggested compass would appear as a modula-tion overlay on the bird's field of view. The mechanism operates through the so-called LFE, based on a single nuclear spin, and operates near the limit of the theoretical sensitivity, despite omitting degrading effects such as the presence of multiple nuclear spins, dipolar effects, and various spin relaxation process that will start to become relevant for the long radical pair lifetimes (>100 ns) considered in the model.

Cryptochromes in the birds' retinas provide one possible source of free radicals in a spatially ordered system (Ritz et al., 2002). A recent theoretical model for avian magne-toreception develops that idea by investigating a flavin–tryptophan radical pair with a high degree of homology to the cryptochromes (Cintolesi et al., 2003). This multinucleus model is realistic in that it still manages to provide sensitivity to fields in the geomagnetic field range. Interestingly, it does not operate through the LFE described above (the multi-nucleus approach appears to remove most signs of that mechanism), but rather it depends on immobilized radicals and assumes that the free radical pair may have a lifetime up to 5 μs.

The radical-based cryptochrome model has been criticized as a compass because it is sensitive to inclination but not polarity unless paired with a strong magnetic moment such as in magnetite. Qin et al. (2016) identify a protein-cryptochrome complex that seems to overcome this problem. Initially found in Drosophila, the magnetically sensitive iron-sulfur protein is linear and models show it can form a chain and a complex with crypto-chromes consistent with what is seen in birds' retinas.

7.3.4.4 Coenzyme B12-Dependent Reactions

Magnetic field effects in the coenzyme B12 are well explored experimentally with match-ing theoretical predictions (Harkins and Grissom, 1994; Grissom and Natarajan, 1997; Taoka et al., 1997). While most work on this model system has been concerned with inter-mediate and higher-field mechanisms, there are also detailed theoretical investigations suggesting that weak (<100 μT), relatively low-frequency (<100 kHz) fields, might be able to affect this system (Canfield et al., 1994, 1995, 1996).

7.3.4.5 Other Experimental Observations

The addition of iron ions or exposure to a 7-mT SMF did not affect the survival of rat lym-phocytes *in vitro* when performed in isolation, but combined exposure led to a significant increase in cell death (Jajte et al., 2002). One possible explanation of this behavior is that the addition of iron ions enhanced levels of ROS and that the field exposure further pro-moted the creation of free radicals, leading to cell death by both apoptosis and necrosis. An experiment with a similar rationale used added $FeCl_2$ to stimulate ROS production, and a 930 MHz, 5 W/m^2 cell phone-generated field affected a biological marker for ROS produc-tion. It should be noted that the vacuum magnetic field associated with this exposure is quite low (approximately 0.14 µT) and the frequency is a relatively unexplored region for this mechanism.

Proliferation of chick fibroblasts was observed to be enhanced by a 100-Hz, 0.7-mT sinusoidal magnetic field (Katsir et al., 1998). In a follow-up study it was found that free radical scavengers (Katsir and Parola, 1998) suppressed this effect, suggesting that the free radicals may have a role in mediating the magnetic field effect on proliferation.

Genotoxic effects from intermediate SMFs (250 mT) have been studied in Escherichia coli DNA, both *in vivo* and *in vitro* (Potenza et al., 2004). Free radical formation was stimulated, and the genetic damage was mapped as a function of exposure duration. *In vitro* experiments showed detectable genotoxic effects, but the *in vivo* assays did not, indicating that cellular protective responses may prevent damage in the intact system.

A reported effect on the oxidative burst in neutrophils by a 0.1-mT field was attributed to free radicals (Roy et al., 1995). In that study, the connection to free radicals lies in that the fluorescent probe used to study the neutrophil activity reacts specifically with free radical-derived oxidants that create the fluorescing compounds. Work in neutrophils in humans (Heine et al., 1999) using a much larger field (1.5 T) did not find any effects of magnetic fields on the respiratory burst of human neutrophils or on the production of radical species.

Phagocytosis was observed to be affected by 0.5–1.5-mT, 50-Hz sinusoidal magnetic fields (Simko et al., 2001). An attendant increase in superoxide production may be an indication that the field stimulated the system through a free radical process.

7.3.5 Summary

Free radical reactions are ubiquitous in biology, and recent developments of the low-field mechanisms (Timmel et al., 2001) and the consideration of detailed biochemical systems (Cintolesi et al., 2003) make this mechanism a strong contender for field effects down to geomagnetic field strengths. The physical transduction step is not vulnerable to thermal perturbations, a significant advantage over competing models. It has the distinct advantage of having a clear link between the physical interaction—changes in spin states that change the probability of a radical interaction with another molecule—and the subsequent step in the biochemical chain.

This model does not produce large (factors >2) changes at the initial field detection step. Theoretical models and direct experimental observations in the low-field region typically operate around or below the 10% level, so we should expect the physical detection mechanism to need cooperation from downstream processes for biologically relevant detection of magnetic fields with free radicals as the starting point. However, the role of ROS and RNS, as well as other radicals that act as signaling or control molecules in biological feedback processes, can mean that a small change in these populations or lifetimes can produce larger downstream changes and that the ultimate changes may either be increases or decreases. The literature mentioned above that summarizes observed field effects in biochemical reactions *in vitro* has generally been done with relatively strong magnetic fields, often with magnetic resonance techniques. It would be helpful for bioelectromagnetic researchers to survey this literature to identify similar experiments using weaker fields, such as that of Henbest et al. (2014); it would also be helpful if more such test-tube biochemical experiments were attempted. Additional theoretical work might consider how larger strengths could occur would be helpful, especially in cases that existing or future experimental results indicating field effects in radical-mediated reactions are found.

Bioelectromagnetic Mechanisms of Action

7.4 Other Proposals Involving Quantum Mechanics

7.4.1 Precession Changes

A magnetic moment will interact with a magnetic field, and the magnetic moments of particles or structures within atoms and molecules will interact with the internal magnetic fields due to the molecule's electronic structure as well as with external fields. The Larmor precession of a moment in a magnetic field is a simple example. In spectroscopy, the electronic moments produce the fine structure and the nuclear moments, the hyperfine structure energy differences that produce splittings of spectroscopic lines. There is a variety of suggestions that these interactions can produce changes, whether in polarization, structure, chemical reactivity, or some other property, which can themselves affect the molecule's interactions with its surroundings to produce downstream biological changes. Some proposals find a frequency dependence of the field effects that matches some experimental data. In the previous section, spin interactions with an external field alter radical concentrations which in turn may affect subsequent biochemistry enough to affect biological outcomes.

Some proposals, including many in the previous section, produce very approximate numerical estimates of how big a change will occur due to the field interaction. But many do not. Many proposals are not clear how the field-induced change interacts with the rest of the system to initiate possible downstream differences; and some authors have criticized various proposals as having too weak an influence to affect downstream processes, independent of the presence of various control, feedback, and other homeostatic downstream mechanisms.

The previous section's models of spin change affecting quantum state populations can be visualized semi-classically in terms of precessions of the magnetic moments about the net magnetic field at the moments' position in space (Brocklehurst and McLauchlan, 1996). Binhi (2016) has proposed that while the precession of moments in the earth's and internal molecular fields at a constant rate is a factor that evolution has accommodated and does not affect biochemistry, changes in the precession rate can affect reactions and have downstream effects. This will especially happen whenever the external field is drastically different from the earth's usual ~50 μT. Experimental effects in reactions have been noted when the earth's field is drastically reduced because of shielding, application of an opposing field, or a situation such as space travel (Binhi and Prato, 2017). Effects have also been observed when a strong field is applied (Steiner and Ulrich, 1989; Hayashi, 2004; Halliwell and Gutteridge, 2015). It is worth noting that Binhi (2016) calculates an effect size with zero external field of up to 10%–15%, depending on other parameters related to the precession. However, there is no indication of how these changes are transmitted to any subsequent part of the biochemistry or biological system. Similar effect sizes are estimated for spin-related mechanisms of the previous section under the "low field effect" (Brocklehurst and McLauchlan, 1996) and the mixing of quantum levels at zero field.

7.5 Proposals Involving Direct Electromagnetic Forces

The Introduction and Chapters 5 and 6 of this volume discuss most of the basic electromagnetic field interactions with single charges and currents; with a number of different configurations of multiple charges, such as dipoles and quadrupoles; or with structures carrying more than one charge in various configurations, such as a molecule. Chapter 5 also discusses how fields affect drift or diffusion of charged objects. This section discusses various proposals about how bioelectromagnetic effects might be produced as a result of direct consequences of these forces under weak fields. However, even though some of these proposals have been shown to act on cells or other biological entities *in vitro*, any implications of these actions for the cells or larger organisms are not clear.

7.5.1 Effects at the Cell Surface

Endogenous electric fields play important roles in cell and organismal physiology, as discussed in Chapter 1 in BMA. DC and low frequency electric fields external to an organism in air are generally drastically reduced at the outer surface of the skin due to polarization of the body's water-based fluids (Kaune et al., 1997), and fields within the body are similarly shielded by polarization by various cell membranes. Magnetic fields, in general, penetrate biological systems with little if any attenuation, at least at low and intermediate frequencies. In air the coupled electric and magnetic field strengths of higher frequency electromagnetic radiation decrease with distance below the body surface; and this decrease becomes more rapid as frequency increases. At the same time, shielding of the electric field by polarization at membranes also decreases at higher frequencies. As a result, some authors have investigated the consequences of interactions of fields at the cell surface.

7.5.1.1 Ligand Binding

Cells receive some information from their surroundings when a signaling molecule binds to a receptor on the cell surface, the receptor-ligand binding process. If the binding is affected by a the presence of the field, subsequent biochemistry is also affected, quite likely multiplied in effect because of the signaling nature of the ligand molecule. Chiabrera and Rodan (1984) assumed such an electromagnetic influence and analyzed the subsequent rate equations. The calculated curves compared favorably with measurements of parathyroid hormone-induced activation of adenylate cyclase. A subsequent analysis in context of the ion motion near the membrane in specific fields relevant to "cyclotron resonance" indicated that water viscosity changes, which can exist near the membrane, could produce effects (Biancno et al., 1988). As noted in Chapter 5, the probability equation for a chemical reaction occurring during a collision between two molecules includes a steric factor which represents whether molecules are in the correct range of relative orientation. This factor could change if applied fields affect the molecules so as to change this range.

7.5.1.2 Electromechanical Models

Hart et al. (2013) have developed an electromechanical model in which a rigid molecule anchored in the cytoskeleton extends through the cell membrane and is deflected by an external electric field directed parallel to the membrane surface, flexing the glycocalyx covering the cell surface and affecting motility. Under combined 1.6 or 160 Hz and DC fields with combined values varying between 40 and 160 V/m, directionality and to a lesser extent speed of migration of keratinocytes was observed. Hart and Palisano (2017) observe increased motility of amoebae under more or less similar conditions and interpret both experiments in terms of the model.

Bioelectromagnetic Mechanisms of Action

7.5.2 Direct Effects of Electromagnetic Forces on Charges and Currents

A magnetic field will exert a force on an electric current or moving charge or magnetic moment, as outlined in Chapter 5. Except in special circumstances, such as magnetic forces on ferromagnetic structures discussed above, any trend toward orientation of biological molecules, which usually are weakly paramagnetic or diamagnetic, due to external magnetic fields is overwhelmed by the random motion caused by the thermal noise background (Binhi, 2002).

An electric field will exert a force on a charge or ensemble of charges. In general, external electric fields also exert little perceptible influence on charges in biological molecules. First of all, polarization of the biological materials at the surface of the body or cell produces an attenuation of the external field; in the case of an animal exposed to an electric field in air, this attenuation is on the order of 10^{-7} (Kaune and Gillis, 1981). Furthermore, the charges are on atoms or ions bound in place by much stronger forces than the thermal background. Although external electric fields do not play a significant part, the endogenous electric fields inside the biological system, generated by the internal charge configurations are very important, but not part of this discussion (Levin, 2011).

Oscillating electromagnetic fields causing induced currents can heat tissues through dissipation of the energy transmitted by the fields, especially at intermediate and high frequencies. This is a time-honored medical application of fields and one of the few for which a mechanism of action is known.

Significant electric fields can be generated inside a biological system by direct application through electrodes or through induction by a rapidly changing magnetic field in accord with Faraday's Law, as outlined in Chapter 5 in BBA. These fields can have biological effects by creating electric currents or polarizing molecules or cells. Examples that use strong fields include electroconvulsive therapy, magnetic pulse stimulation of the brain, or use of pulsing magnetic fields to stimulate healing of recalcitrant fractures, as discussed in other chapters. However, the specific mechanisms by which these treatments are effective is not clear although the effects of local currents or membrane polarization are suspected.

Both external and intramolecular magnetic fields do have effects on the energy levels of molecules according to the Zeeman effect, and these form the basis of the model of bioelectromagnetic effects based on radicals and related phenomena, as discussed above. Electric fields can similarly alter energy levels according to the Stark effect, though this phenomenon has not been much studied to this author's knowledge. Endogenous electric fields are ever-present, can be rather strong, and play important roles in processes such as guiding embryo development, nerve growth, or cell migration. They also importantly influence molecular folding and biochemical function. However, since external low frequency electric fields are greatly attenuated at the surface of an organism or growth medium, as well as at cell and internal cell membranes, and penetration depth of high frequency fields depends on frequency. They do not seem to be intense enough to affect any Stark effect of the endogenous fields to a notable extent or to play another role, unless a strong voltage is applied directly through electrodes (which is likely to have disruptive direct effects). Theoretical analysis and computer modeling have shown that electric fields can affect biochemical reaction rates through changes in transport including diffusion, dielectrophoresis, etc. (Seto and Hsieh, 1976; Neumann, 1986; Barnes and Kwon, 2005) but at fairly strong applied external field strengths.

Since magnetic fields exert a force on moving charges, including ions, radicals, and other charged molecules, biological effects have been hypothesized from this magnetohydrodynamic effect. Binhi (2002) calculates this to be very small.

7.5.2.1 Isolated Ions and Molecules

As noted in Chapter 8 in BBA the effects of Brownian motion and other sources of noise are often much larger than those of putative electromagnetic field mechanisms, including many quantum mechanical effects. However, some authors have noted that ions, atoms, or molecules are in some instances isolated within a molecular structure or cluster of molecules, shielded from thermal noise. The microenvironment inside an ordered region of water, compared to the disordered outside may offer such an isolation (Zhadin, 1998; Del Giudice et al., 2002). The isolation cannot be total, however, because the interaction of the external field with the isolated structure must still somehow communicate with its surroundings to produce subsequent changes that eventually are manifested in a biological effect. Adair (1992) uses a model of transition probabilities to show that at low applied field intensities, four different factors limit how isolated structures can interact strongly enough with their surroundings to influence them. Interestingly, he finds that restrictions due to the non-overlap of quantum states vanishes at zero applied fields, consistent with mixing of states at zero field as discussed above and recent experiments with magnetic field shielding.

7.5.2.2 Electroporation

A locally strong electric field applied across a cell or intracellular membrane can produce a transient or even a permanent local disruption of the membrane, allowing ions and molecules to pass through the opening. This has become a means for inserting genetic material or drugs into cells and nuclei as well as for disrupting and producing cell death in tumors. It is covered in much more detail in Chapter 7 in BMA.

7.5.2.3 Ion Cyclotron Resonance and Related Ideas

Since the late 1970s, a large number of experiments have reported resonance-like effects in a combined weak DC magnetic field and a similar AC field at what is known as the ion cyclotron frequency, $f = qB_{DC}/2m$, where q and m are the charge and mass of an ion. Classically, this is the frequency with which a free ion makes one complete orbit in a plane perpendicular to B_{DC}; note that the cyclotron frequency is independent of the orbit radius, which does depend both on B_{DC} and the ion's energy. Effects were found for fairly narrow bands of AC field frequencies, but for broader bands of the strength of either magnetic field or the ratio between the two. Most work applied parallel AC and DC fields, but perpendicular fields have also been found to be effective. Calcium, potassium, and magnesium were the most common ion frequencies used, but effects have been reported for many others. Measured properties in these experiments ranged from changes in conductivity and transport in solutions through a wide variety of changes in cultured cells and tissues to whole changes in animals and plants (reviews include Liboff, 2005, 2007).

While the experimental resonant frequencies and the cyclotron resonance formula are in numerical agreement, that explanation is considered very unrealistic since it implies ion orbits much larger than a molecule and that a bare ion is being affected, isolated from its surroundings or molecular bonds or surrounding water of hydration. Most of the experiments were conducted in fields on the order of 0.01–1 mT, where the cyclotron orbit of an ion with biological-range energy has a radius of many centimeters.

No well-accepted explanation has been offered, though many alternatives have been proposed (Liboff, 2005, 2007). Probably for this reason, less attention has been paid to these

Bioelectromagnetic Mechanisms of Action

specific field combinations in recent years. Some have noted that the formula for the classical Larmor frequency for precession of the magnetic moment of a particle in a magnetic field is the same as the cyclotron frequency, but no well-accepted suggestions use this approach, either. In quantum mechanics, the Larmor frequency $f = g\ qB_{DC}/2m$, where the added Lande g factor depends on the spin and any orbital angular momenta of the particle and generally has a value in the range of 0.5–2; $|g| \sim 2$ for a free electron. Other suggestions include a parametric resonance process, splitting an ion oscillation frequency in a bond to a molecule like calmodulin, limiting orbit sizes through confinement in channels, fields changing interferences between quantum states, confined ions in small coherent water structures, and phase transitions (reviews include Blanchard and Blackman, 1994; Liboff, 2005, 2007; Zhadin and Giuliani, 2006; see also Lednev, 1991). As noted, to cause one of these apparent resonance effects, a very narrow band of frequencies but a broad band of B_{DC} is effective (Blackman et al., 1994, 1999). The narrow frequency band indicates a possible resonance for an isolated moment; the broad range of fields indicates that something else may also be involved.

7.6 Electromagnetic Forces Interacting with Other Properties

7.6.1 Water-Related Effects

Biological systems are strongly based on water, which constitutes a large fraction of their mass, whether inside a cell or one of its constituent parts or in intercellular spaces. Water molecules are highly polar, consisting of a line of two hydrogen atoms separated by an oxygen atom, bent at about $104°$ at the oxygen. The oxygen attracts the two hydrogen valence electrons, leaving it negatively and the hydrogens positively charged. As a result, water molecules have a strong tendency to form hydrogen bonds with each other or other charged or polarized species. In bulk water, there is a wide variety of small structured clusters, which fluctuate rapidly as well as a population of free, unorganized water molecules and small populations of reactive ions and radicals, including H^+, OH^-, $OH\bullet$, and H_3O^+ (Marechal, 2007; Tigrek and Barnes, 2010). A surrounding cloud of water molecules will be found around ions, radicals, and other charged or polarized molecules. These clouds have been hypothesized as one means for isolating their contents from the energy fluctuations caused by the surrounding medium's thermal noise, as well as possibly justifying use of the bare ion mass in ion resonance ideas, as discussed above.

Water also plays a role in several other proposed mechanisms. At magnetic field intensities on the order of Teslas, practical devices are used to purify water to prevent deposition of scale and for other purposes (Ambashta and Sillanpää, 2010). Apparently, effective ion resonance frequencies include those for hydrogen (Blackman et al., 1999) though it is not clear whether the protons involved are in water or other molecules. Binhi (2002) discusses proposals that water can be affected in magnetic fields by, among other methods, altering the way structural vacancies occur or move, transmitting energy along molecular chains via solitons, proposed by Davydov, or room temperature superconducting states, proposed using ideas of Frohlich and others.

Fields can also change the viscosity of water and other materials and affect the drift and diffusion of ions, radicals, and molecules. These mechanisms are discussed further in Chapter 5 and in Tigrek and Barnes (2010).

7.6.2 Phase Transitions

Materials change phases with changing external conditions, such as temperature and pressure but also electromagnetic fields. A common example is the transition of water into steam or ice. Other phase transitions are more subtle, such as the change between one crystalline form of ice to another as pressures increase. One such appeal to a phase difference is the hypothesized isolation of an ion in the microenvironment inside an ordered region of water, compared to the disordered outside (Zhadin, 1998; Del Giudice et al., 2002). Membranes are a double layer of fatty acid molecules with various proteins embedded in them. Changes in the ordering of the fatty acids in various regions of the membrane have been compared to different phases with different viscosities for diffusion of the proteins and changes in the proportions of the phases have been seen under applied fields (Phelan et al., 1992). Whether these are due to microheating in the case of RF fields and their implications for downstream processes is not clear.

7.7 Conclusions

This chapter has presented a number of theoretical proposals about how electric and magnetic fields may interact with biological systems. These proposals in general present ideas about the initial step that produces a change in the chain of biochemical and other reactions and finally results in a change in the biological system that is detectable and may be of consequence to the system. The system could be harmed, could benefit, or might just ignore the outcome. But for most of the proposals, a plausible initial interaction step is presented, but whether and if so, how that step affects the rest of the chain is unknown. This is true even if there is good evidence that there is a detectable consequence of having applied the fields. It is also true in cases where the experiment includes evidence that this consequence can be interfered with by something that blocks the action of a plausible intermediate step, since other steps and details of the interaction are usually not fully understood. In addition, it is often the case that similar experiments present different outcomes, one increasing and another either decreasing or showing no effect on the measured end point. So there remain many open questions that are both bioelectromagnetic and biological.

Acknowledgments

The author wishes to thank Prof. Frank Barnes for many helpful discussions and Dr. Stefan Engstrom for the use of material from his chapter in the 3rd Edition.

References

Adair R.K. 1991. Constraints on biological effects of weak extremely-low frequency electromagnetic fields. *Phys. Rev.* 43:1039–1048.

Adair R.K. 1992. Criticism of Lednev's mechanism for the influence of weak magnetic fields on biological systems. *Bioelectromagnetics* 13:231–235.

Adair R.K. 1999. Effects of very weak magnetic fields on radical pair reformation. *Bioelectromagnetics* 20:255–263.

Ambashta R.D. and Sillanpää M. 2010. Water purification using magnetic assistance: A review. *J. Hazard. Mater.* 180:38–49.

Barnes F. and Kwon Y. 2005. A theoretical study of the effects of RF fields in the vicinity of membranes. *Bioelectromagnetics.* 26(2):118–124.

Barnes F.S. and Greenebaum B. 2015. The effects of weak magnetic fields on radical pairs. *Bioelectromagnetics* 36:45–54.

Biancno B., Chiabrera A., Morron A., and Parodi M. 1988. Effects of magnetic exposure on ions in electric fields. *Ferroelectrics* 86:159–168.

Binhi V.N. 2002. *Magnetobiology: Underlying Physical Problems.* Academic Press: London and San Diego, 473 pp.

Binhi V.N. 2016. A primary physical mechanism of the biological effects of weak magnetic fields. *Biophysics* 61:170–176. (Original Russian in *Biofizika*, 2016, 61:201–208).

Binhi V.N. and Prato F.S. 2017. A physical mechanism of magnetoreception: Extension and analysis. *Bioelectromagnetics* 38:41–52.

Binhi V.N. and Savin A.V. 2003. Effects of weak magnetic fields on biological systems: Physical aspects. *Physics-Uspekhi* 46:259–291.

Blackman C.F., Blanchard J.P., Benane S.G., and House D.E. 1994. Empirical test of an ion parametric resonance model for magnetic field interactions with PC-12 cells. *Bioelectromagnetics* 15:239–260.

Blackman C.F., Blanchard J.P., Benane S.G., and House D.E. 1999. Experimental determination of hydrogen bandwidth for the ion parametric resonance model. *Bioelectromagnetics* 20:5–12.

Blanchard J.P. and Blackman C.F. 1994. Clarification and application of an ion parametric resonance model for magnetic field interactions with biological systems. *Bioelectromagnetics* 15:217–238.

Blank M. and Goodman R. 2000. Stimulation of the stress response by low-frequency electromagnetic fields: Possibility of direct interaction with DNA. *IEEE Trans. Plasma Sci.* 28:168–172.

Blank M. and Soo L. 2001a. Electromagnetic acceleration of electron transfer reactions. *J. Cell. Biochem.* 81:278–283.

Blank M. and Soo L. 2001b. Optimal frequencies for magnetic acceleration of cytochrome oxidase and Na, K-ATPase reactions. *Bioelectrochemistry* 53:171–174.

Brocklehurst B. 1969. Formation of excited states by recombining organic ions. *Nature* 221:921–923.

Brocklehurst B. 1976. Spin correlation in geminate recombination of radical ions in hydrocarbons. 1. Theory of magnetic-field effect. *J. Chem. Soc.—Faraday Trans. II* 72:1869–1884.

Brocklehurst B. 1997. Magnetic isotope effects in biology: A marker for radical pair reactions and electromagnetic field effects? *Int. J. Rad. Biol.* 72:587–596.

Brocklehurst B. 2002. Magnetic fields and radical reactions: Recent developments and their role in nature. *Chem. Soc. Rev.* 31:301–311.

Brocklehurst B. and McLauchlan K.A. 1996. Free radical mechanism for the effects of environmental electromagnetic fields on biological systems. *Int. J. Rad. Biol.* 69:3–24.

Buchachenko, A. 2016. Why magnetic and electromagnetic effects in biology are irreproducible and contradictory? *Bioelectromagnetics* 37:1–13. doi:10.1002/bem.21947.

Canfield J.M., Belford R.L., and Debrunner P.G. 1996. Calculations of Earth-strength steady and oscillating magnetic field effects in coenzyme B-12 radical pair systems. *Mol. Phys.* 89:889–930.

Canfield J.M., Belford R.L., Debrunner P.G., and Schulten K.J. 1994. A perturbation-theory treatment of oscillating magnetic-fields in the radical pair mechanism. *Chem. Phys.* 182:1–18 (see also Erratum *J. Chem. Phys.* 191:347, 1995).

Canfield J.M., Belford R.L., Debrunner P.G., and Schulten K.J. 1995. A perturbation treatment of oscillating magnetic-fields in the radical pair mechanism using the Liouville equation. *Chem. Phys.* 195:59–69.

Chiabrera A. and Rodan G.A. 1984. The effect of electromagnetic fields on receptor-ligand interaction: A theoretical analysis. *J. Bioelectricity* 3:509–521.

Christensen M. and Pedersen J.B. 2003. On the validity of the one-particle diffusion model of geminate recombination in micelles. *Chem. Phys.* 295:235–241.

Cintolesi F., Ritz T., Kay C.W.M., Timmel C.R., and Hore P.J. 2003. Anisotropic recombination of an immobilized photoinduced radical pair in a 50-mu T magnetic field: A model avian photomagnetoreceptor. *Chem. Phys.* 294:385–399.

Clarke D., Whitney H., Sutton G., and Robert D. 2013. Detection and learning of floral electric fields by bumblebees. *Science* 340:66–69.

Closs G.L. 1969. A mechanism explaining nuclear spin polarizations in radical combination reactions. *J. Am. Chem. Soc.* 91:4552–4554.

Coster A.C., and Celler B.G. 2003. Phase response of model sinoatrial node cells. *Ann. Biomed. Eng.* 31:271–283.

Del Giudice E., Fleischmann M., Preparata G., and Talpo G. 2002. On the "unreasonable" effects of elf magnetic fields upon a system of ions. *Bioelectromagnetics* 23:522–530.

Deutsch M. and Brown S.C. 1952. Zeeman effect and hyperfine splitting of positronium. *Phys. Rev.* 85:1047–1048.

Deutschlander M.E., Phillips J.B., and Borland S.C. 1999. The case for light-dependent magnetic orientation in animals. *J. Exper. Biol.* 202:891–908.

Droge W. 2002. Free Radicals in the Physiological Control of Cell Function. *Physiol Rev* 82: 47–95.

Eichwald C. and Walleczek J. 1996a. Activation-dependent and biphasic electromagnetic field effects: Model based on cooperative enzyme kinetics in cellular signaling. *Bioelectromagnetics* 17:427–435.

Eichwald C. and Walleczek J. 1996b. Model for magnetic field effects on radical pair recombination in enzyme kinetics. *Biophy. J.* 71:623–631.

Eichwald C. and Walleczek J. 1997. Low-frequency-dependent effects of oscillating magnetic fields on radical pair recombination in enzyme kinetics. *J. Chem. Phys.* 107:4943–4950.

Eichwald C. and Walleczek J. 1998. Magnetic field perturbations as a tool for controlling enzyme-regulated and oscillatory biochemical reactions. *Biophys. Chem.* 74:209–224.

Engstrom S. 1997. What is the time scale of magnetic field interaction in biological systems? *Bioelectromagnetics* 18:244–249.

Engstrom S. 2007. Magnetic field effects on free radical reactions in biology. In F. Barnes and B. Greenebaum, eds., *Bioengineering and Biophysical Aspects of Electromagnetic Fields*. Boca Raton, FL: CRC Press, pp. 157–168.

Engstrom S. and Fitzsimmons R. 1999. Five hypotheses to examine the nature of magnetic field transduction in biological systems. *Bioelectromagnetics* 20:423–430.

Engstrom S., Markov M.S., McLean M.J., Holcomb R.R., and Markov J.M. 2002. Effects of non-uniform static magnetic fields on the rate of myosin phosphorylation. *Bioelectromagnetics* 23:475–479.

Eveson R.W., Timmel C.R., Brocklehurst B., Hore P.J., and McLauchlan K.A. 2000. The effects of weak magnetic fields on radical recombination reactions in micelles. *Int. J. Rad. Biol.* 76:1509–1522.

Fedin M.V., Purtov P.A., and Bagryanskaya E.G. 2001. Anisotropic hyperfine interaction-induced spin relaxation in a low magnetic field. *Chem. Phys. Lett.* 339:395–404.

Fedin M.V., Purtov P.A., and Bagryanskaya E.G. 2003. Spin relaxation of radicals in low and zero magnetic field. *J. Chem. Phys.* 118:192–201.

Frankel R.B., and Blakemore R.P. 1989. Magnetite and magnetotaxis in microorganisms. *Bioelectromagnetics* 10(3):223–237.

Frankel R.B., Blakemore R.P., and Wolfe R.S. 1979. Magnetite in freshwater magnetotactic bacteria. *Science.* 203(4387):1355–1356.

Gallagher J.J., Bedard F.D., and Johnson C.M. 1954. Microwave spectrum of $N^{14}O^{16}$. *Phys. Rev.* 93:729–733.

Gilch P., Pollinger-Dammer F., Musewald C., Michel-Beyerle M.E., and Steiner U.E. 1998. Magnetic field effect on picosecond electron transfer. *Science* 281:982–984.

Greggers U., Koch G., Schmidt V., Durr A., Floriou-Servou A., Piepenbrock D., Gopfert M.C., and Menzel R. 2013. Reception and learning of electric fields in bees. *Proc. Royal Soc. B* 280:20130528.

Grissom C.B. 1995. Magnetic-field effects in biology—A survey of possible mechanisms with emphasis on radical-pair recombination. *Chem. Rev.* 95:3–24.

Grissom C.B. and Natarajan E. 1997. Use of magnetic field effects to study coenzyme B-12-dependent reactions. *Methods Enzymol.* 281:235–247.

Grundler W., Kaiser F., Keilmann F., and Walleczek J. 1992. Mechanisms of electromagnetic-interaction with cellular-systems. *Naturwissenschaften* 79:551–559.

Haberkorn R. and Michel-Beyerle M.E. 1979. On the mechanism of magnetic field effects in bacterial photosynthesis. *Biophys. J.* 26:489–498.

Halliwell B. and Gutteridge J.M.C. 2015. *Free Radicals in Biology and Medicine*, 5th Ed. Oxford: Oxford University Press, 905 pp.

Halpern O. 1954. Magnetic quenching of the positronium decay. *Phys. Rev.* 94:904–907.

Harkins T.T. and Grissom C.B. 1994. Magnetic-field effects on B-12 ethanolamine ammonia-lyase—Evidence for a radical mechanism. *Science* 263:958–960.

Hart F.X., Laird M., Riding A., and Pullar C.E. 2013. Keratinocyte galvanotaxis in combined DC and AC electric fields supports an electromechanical transduction sensing mechanism. *Bioelectromagnetics* 34:85–94.

Hart F.X. and Palisano J.R. 2017. Glycocalyx bending by an electric field increases cell motility. *Bioelectromagnetics* 38:482–493.

Herzberg G. 1950. *Molecular Spectra and Molecular Structure. I. Spectra of Diatomic Molecules*, 2nd Ed. Princeton, NJ: D. Van Nostrand, p. 308.

Heine J., Scheinichen D., Jaeger K., Herzog T., Sumpelmann R., and Leuwer M. 1999. Effect of magnetic resonance imaging on human respiratory burst of neutrophils. *FEBS Lett.* 446:15–17.

Henbest K.B., Kukura P., Rodgers C.T., Hore P.J., and Timmel C.R. 2004. Radio frequency magnetic field effects on a radical recombination reaction: A diagnostic test for the radical pair mechanism. *J. Am. Chem. Soc.* 126:8102–81.

Hayashi, H. 2004. *Introduction to Dynamic Spin Chemistry: Magnetic Field Effects upon Chemical and Biochemical Reactions*, Singapore: World Scientific Publisher, p. 268.

Henbest K.B., Kukura, P., Rodgers C.T., Hore P.J., and Timmel C.R. 2004. Radio Frequency Magnetic Field Effects on a Radical Recombination Reaction: A Diagnostic Test for the Radical Pair Mechanism. *J. Am. Chem. Soc.*, 2004, 126(26): 8102–8103.

Horiuchi M., Maeda K., and Arai T. 2003. Magnetic field effect on electron transfer reactions of flavin derivatives associated with micelles. *Appl. Magn. Reson.* 23:309–318.

Hore P.J., and Mouritsen H. 2016. The Radical-Pair Mechanism of Magnetoreception. *Annu Rev Biophys* 45:299–344.

ICNIRP. 1998. ICNIRP guidelines for limiting exposure to time-varying electric, magnetic and electromagnetic fields (up to 300 GHz). *Health Phys.* 74:494–522.

ICNIRP. 2010. ICNIRP guidelines for limiting exposure to time-varying electric and magnetic fields (1 Hz–100 kHz). *Health Phys.* 99:818–836.

IEEE. 2002. IEEE Std C95.6–2002: Standard for safety levels with respect to human exposure to electromagnetic fields, 0–3 kHz. New York: IEEE, 50 pp.

IEEE. 2005. IEEE Std C95.1–2005: Standard for safety levels with respect to human exposure to radio frequency electromagnetic fields, 3 kHz to 300 GHz. New York: IEEE, 250 pp.

Jajte J., Grzegorczyk J., Zmyslony M., and Rajkowska E. 2002. Effect of 7mT static magnetic field and iron ions on rat lymphocytes: Apoptosis, necrosis and free radical processes. *Bioelectrochemistry* 57:107–111.

Jones A.R. 2016. Magnetic field effects in proteins. *Mol. Phys.* 114:1691–1702. doi:10.1080/00268976.2016.

Kaiser F. 1996. External signals and internal oscillation dynamics: Biophysical aspects and modelling approaches for interactions of weak electromagnetic fields at the cellular level. *Bioelectrochem. Bioenerg.* 41:3–18.

Kalmijn A.J. 1988 Detection of Weak Electric Fields. In Atema J., Fay R.R., Popper A.N., Tavolga W.N., eds., *Sensory Biology of Aquatic Animals*. New York, NY: Springer, 151–186.

Kaptein R. 1972. Chemically induced dynamic nuclear polarization. X. On the magnetic field dependence. *J. Am. Chem. Soc.* 94:6269–6280.

Kaptein R. and Oosterhoff L.J. 1969. Chemically induced dynamic nuclear polarization III (anomalous multiplets of radical coupling and disproportionation products). *Chem. Phys. Lett.* 4:214–216.

Kaune W.T. and Gillis M.F. 1981. General properties of the interaction between animals and ELF electric fields. *Bioelectromagnetics* 2:1–11.

Kaune W.T., Guttman J.L., and Kavet R. 1997. Comparison of coupling of humans to electric and magnetic fields with frequencies between 100 Hz and 100 kHz. *Bioelectromagnetics* 18:67–76.

Katsir G., Baram S.C., and Parola A.H. 1998. Effect of sinusoidally varying magnetic fields on cell proliferation and adenosine deaminase specific activity. *Bioelectromagnetics* 19:46–52.

Katsir G. and Parola A.H. 1998. Enhanced proliferation caused by a low frequency weak magnetic field in chick embryo fibroblasts is suppressed by radical scavengers. *Biochem. Biophy. Res. Comm.* 252:753–756.

Kirschvink J.L., Walker M.M., and Diebel C.E. 2001. Magnetite-based magnetoreception. *Curr Opin Neurobiol.* 11(4):462–467.

Kitahama Y., Wakasa M., and Sakaguchi Y. 2004. Viscosity dependence of the magnetic field effect due to the delta g mechanism. *J. Phys. Chem. A* 108:754–757.

Krissinel E.B., Burshtein A.I., Lukzen N.N., and Steiner U.E. 1999. Magnetic field effect as a probe of distance-dependent electron transfer in systems undergoing free diffusion. *Mol. Phys.* 96:1083–1097.

Lander H.M. 1997. An essential role for free radicals and derived species in signal transduction. *FASEB J.* 11:118–124.

Lednev V.V. 1991. Possible mechanism for the influence of weak magnetic fields on biological systems. *Bioelectromagnetics* 12:71–75.

Letuta U.G., Berdinskiy V.L., Udagawa C. and Tanimoto Y. 2017. Enzymatic mechanisms of biological magnetic sensitivity. *Bioelectromagnetics* 38:511–521. doi:10.1002/bem.22071.

Levin M. 2011. Endogenous bioelectric signals as morphogenetic controls of development, regeneration, and neoplasm. In Pullar C.E., ed., *The Physiology of Bioelectricity in Development, Tissue Regeneration, and Cancer.* Boca Raton, FL: CRC Press, pp. 39–90.

Liboff A.R. 2005. The charge-to-mass ICR signature in weak elf bioelectromagnetic effects. In Lin J.C., ed., *Advances in Electromagnetic Fields in Living Systems,* vol. 4. New York: Springer, pp. 189–218.

Liboff A.R. 2007. The ion cyclotron resonance hypothesis. In Barnes F.S. and Greenebaum B., eds. *Bioengineering and Biophysical Aspects of Electromagnetic Fields.* Boca Raton, FL: CRC Press, pp. 261–292.

Marechal Y. 2007. *The Hydrogen Bond and the Water Molecule: The Physics and Chemistry of Water, Aqueous and Bio-media.* Amsterdam: Elsevier, 332 pp.

Markov M.S. and Pilla A.A. 1994. Static magnetic-field modulation of myosin phosphorylation—calcium-dependence in 2 enzyme preparations. *Bioelectrochem. Bioenerget.* 35(1–2):57–61.

Markov M.S., Wang S., and Pilla A.A. 1993. Effects of weak low frequency sinusoidal and DC magnetic fields on myosin phosphorylation in a cell-free preparation. *Bioelectrochem. Bioenerget.* 30:119–125.

McLauchlan K.A. and Steiner U.E. 1991. The spin-correlated radical pair as a reaction intermediate. *Molec. Phys.* 73:241–263.

Moller A.C. and Olsen L.F. 1999. Effect of magnetic fields on an oscillating enzyme reaction. *J. Am. Chem. Soc.* 121:6351–6354.

Moller A.C. and Olsen L.F. 2000. Perturbations of simple oscillations and complex dynamics in the peroxidase–oxidase reaction using magnetic fields. *J. Phys. Chem. B* 104:140–146.

Moller A.C., Lunding A., and Olsen L.F. 2000. Further studies of the effect of magnetic fields on the oscillating peroxidase–oxidase reaction. *Phys. Chem. Chem. Phys.* 2:3443–3446.

Musewald C., Gilch P., Hartwich G., Pollinger-Dammer F., Scheer H., and Michel-Beyerle M.E. 1999. Magnetic field dependence of ultrafast intersystem-crossing: A triplet mechanism on the picosecond time scale? *J. Am. Chem. Soc.* 121:8876–8881.

Nathan C. 1992. Nitric-oxide as a secretory product of mammalian-cells. *FASEB J.* 6:3051–3064.

Nelson M.E. and Maciver M.A. 1999. Prey capture in the weakly electric fish Apteronotus albifrons: sensory acquisition strategies and electrosensory consequences. *J Exp Biol.* 202(Pt 10):1195–1203

Neumann E. 1986. Chemical electric field effects in biological macromolecules. *Prog. Biophys. Molec. Biol.* 47:197–231.

Peckham P.H. and Knutson J.S. 2005. Functional electrical stimulation for neuromuscular applications. *Ann. Rev. Biomed. Eng.* 7:327–360.

Pedersen J.B. and Christensen M. 2004. The backward stochastic Liouville equation. *J. Phys. Chem. B* 108:9516–9523.

Phelan A.M., Lange D.G., Kues H.A., and Lutty G.A. 1992. Modification of membrane fluidity in melanin-containing cells by low-level microwave radiation. *Bioelectromagnetics* 13:131–146.

Potenza L., Cucchiarini L., Piatti E., Angelini U., and Dacha M. 2004. Effects of high static magnetic field exposure on different DNAs. *Bioelectromagnetics* 25:352–355.

Prato F.S., Kavaliers M., Cullen A.P., and Thomas A.W. 1997. Light-dependent and -independent behavioral effects of extremely low frequency magnetic fields in a land snail are consistent with a parametric resonance mechanism. *Bioelectromagnetics* 18:284–291.

Prato F.S., Kavaliers M., Thomas A.W., and Ossenkopp K.P. 1998. Modulatory actions of light on the behavioural responses to magnetic fields by land snails probably occur at the magnetic field detection stage. *Proc. Royal Soc. B* 265:367–373.

Qin S., Yin H., Yang C., et al. 2016. A magnetic protein biocompass. *Nat. Mater.* 15:217–226.

Ritz T., Adem S., and Schulten K. 2000. A model for photoreceptor-based magnetoreception in birds. *Biophys. J.* 78:707–718.

Ritz T., Dommer D.H., and Phillips J.B. 2002. Shedding light on vertebrate magnetoreception. *Neuron* 34:503–506.

Ritz T., Thalau P., Phillips J.B., Wiltschko R., and Wiltschko W. 2004. Resonance effects indicate a radical-pair mechanism for avian magnetic compass. *Nature* 429:177–180.

Rodgers C.T. and Hore P.J. 2009. Chemical magnetoreception in birds: the radical pair mechanism. *Proc Natl Acad Sci U S A.* 106(2):353–360.

Roy S., Noda Y., Eckert V., Traber M.G., Mori A., Liburdy R., and Packer L. 1995. The phorbol 12-myristate 13-acetate (PMA)-induced oxidative burst in rat peritoneal neutrophils is increased by a 0.1 mT (60 Hz) magnetic-field. *FEBS Lett.* 376:164–166.

Salikhov K.M., Moulin Yu.N., Sagdeev R.Z., and Buchachenko A.L. 1984. *Spin Polarization and Magnetic Effects in Radical Reactions.* Amsterdam: Elsevier, 244 pp.

Saunders R.D. and Jefferys J.G. 2002. Weak electric field interactions in the central nervous system. *Health Phys.* 83:366–75.

Scaiano J.C., Cozens F.L., and Mohtat N. 1995. Influence of combined AC-DC magnetic-fields on free-radicals in organized and biological-systems—Development of a model and application of the radical pair mechanism to radicals in micelles. *Photochem. Photobiol.* 62:818–829.

Scheeline A., Olson D.L., Williksen E.P., Horras G.A., Klein M.L., and Larter R. 1997. The peroxidase–oxidase oscillator and its constituent chemistries. *Chem. Rev.* 97:739–756.

Schulten K. 1982. Magnetic field effects in chemistry and biology. In Treusch J., ed., *Festkörperprobleme*, Vol. 22. Braunschweig: Vieweg, pp. 61–83.

Schulten K., Swenberg C.E., and Weller A. 1978. Biomagnetic sensory mechanism based on magnetic-field modulated coherent electron-spin motion. *Zeitsch. f. Physikal. Chem.-Frankfurt* 111:1–5.

Seto Y.J. and Hsieh S.T. 1981. Electric field induced rate effects in pharmacokinetic systems. *Proceedings of 1981 IEEE Antennas and Propagation Society International Symposium*, pp. 175–178.

Simko M., Droste S., Kriehuber R., and Weiss D.G. 2001. Stimulation of phagocytosis and free radical production in murine macrophages by 50 Hz electromagnetic fields. *Eur. J. Cell Biol.* 80:562–566.

Stell M., Sheppard A.R., and Adey W.R. 1993. The effect of moving air on detection of a 60-Hz electric field. *Bioelectromagnetics* 14:67–78.

Steiner U.E. and Ulrich T. 1989. Magnetic-field effects in chemical-kinetics and related phenomena. *Chem. Rev.* 89:51–147.

Taoka S., Padmakumar R., Grissom C.B., and Banerjee R. 1997. Magnetic field effects on coenzyme B-12-dependent enzymes: Validation of ethanolamine ammonia lyase results and extension to human methylmalonyl CoA mutase. *Bioelectromagnetics* 18:506–513.

Thannickal V.J. and Fanburg B.L. 2000. Reactive oxygen species in cell signaling. *Am. J. Physiol.— Lung Cell. Mol. Physiol.* 279:L1005–L1028.

Tigrek S. and Barnes F. 2010. Water structures and effects of electric and magnetic fields. In Giuliani L. and Soffritti M., eds., Non-thermal Effects and Mechanisms of Interaction between Electromagnetic Fields and Living Matter. *Eur. J. Oncol. Library* Vol. 5, pp. 25–50.

Till U., Timmel C.R., Brocklehurst B., and Hore P.J. 1998. The influence of very small magnetic fields on radical recombination reactions in the limit of slow recombination. *Chem. Phys. Lett.* 298:7–14.

Timmel C.R. and Henbest K.B. 2004. A study of spin chemistry in weak magnetic fields. *Phil. Trans. R. Soc. Lond. A* 362:2573–2589.

Timmel C.R. and Hore P.J. 1996. Oscillating magnetic field effects on the yields of radical pair reactions. *Chem. Phys. Lett.* 257:401–408.

Timmel C.R., Cintolesi F., Brocklehurst B., and Hore P.J. 2001. Model calculations of magnetic field effects on the recombination reactions of radicals with anisotropic hyperfine interactions. *Chem. Phys. Lett.* 334:387–395.

Timmel C.R., Till U., Brocklehurst B., McLauchlan K.A., and Hore P.J. 1998. Effects of weak magnetic fields on free radical recombination reactions. *Molec. Phys.* 95:71–89.

Townes C. and Schawlow A. 1955. *Microwave Spectroscopy*. New York: McGraw Hill, p. 290.

Walker M.M. and Bitterman M.E. 1989. Conditioning analysis of magnetoreception in honeybees. *Bioelectromagnetics* 10:261–275.

Walleczek J. 1995. Magnetokinetic effects on radical pairs: a paradigm for magnetic field interactions with biological systems at lower than thermal energy. *Electromagnetic Fields* 250:395–420.

Werber H.-J., Schulter K., and Weller A. 1978. Electron transfer and spin exchange contributing to the magnetic field dependence of the primary photochemical reaction of bacterial photosynthesis. *Biochim. Biophys. Acta* 502:255–268.

Werner U., Kuhnle W., and Staerk H. 1993. Magnetic-field dependent reaction yields from radical-ion pairs linked by a partially rigid aliphatic chain. *J. Phys. Chem.* 97:9280–9287.

Wiltschko W., Gesson M., Stapput K., and Wiltschko R. 2004a. Light-dependent magnetoreception in birds: Interaction of at least two different receptors. *Naturwiss.* 91:130–134.

Wiltschko W., Moller A., Gesson M., Noll C., and Wiltschko R. 2004b. Light-dependent magnetoreception in birds: Analysis of the behaviour under red light after pre-exposure to red light. *J. Exper. Biol.* 207:1193–1202.

Wood A.W. 2008. Extremely low frequency (elf) electric and magnetic field exposure limits: Rationale for basic restrictions used in the development of an Australian standard. *Bioelectromagnetics* 29:414–428.

Woodward J.R. 2002. Radical pairs in solution. *Prog. React. Kinet. Mec.* 27:165–207.

Yu B.P. 1994. Cellular defenses against damage from reactive oxygen species. *Physiol. Rev.* 74:139–162.

Zhadin M.N. 1998. Combined action of static and alternating magnetic fields on ion motion in a macromolecule: Theoretical aspects. *Bioelectromagnetics* 19:279–292.

Zaghi S., Acar M., Hultgren B., Boggio P.S., and Fregni F. 2010. Noninvasive brain stimulation with low-intensity electrical currents: Putative mechanisms of action for direct and alternating current stimulation. *Neuroscientist* 16:285–307.

Zhadin M. and Giuliani L. 2006. Some problems in modern bioelectromagnetics. *Electromag. Biol. Med.* 25:227–243.

8

Signals, Noise, and Thresholds

Martin Bier
East Carolina University

James C. Weaver
Massachusetts Institute of Technology

CONTENTS

8.1 Signals, Detection, and Measurement 261
8.2 Specificity 262
8.3 Signal-to-Noise Ratio 263
8.4 Detection Criteria 265
8.5 Equilibrium Noise 265
8.6 Nonequilibrium Noise 272
8.7 Quantum Noise 284
8.8 Chemical Noise 286
8.9 Interpretation of Experiments 290
Acknowledgments 291
References 292

8.1 Signals, Detection, and Measurement

Measurement is quantitative observation and well known to be of great importance to science. However, measurements involving biological systems are complicated by the complexity of cells and tissues, particularly if fields are expected to interact weakly and if field-induced changes are found to be small. Some key parameters, like the temperature coefficient of a measured quantity, may easily be inadequately characterized, and related quantities may thus be determined incompletely. Detection is a special case of measurement, where the measurement is so coarse that an observer can only distinguish between "signal" and "no signal."

Generally speaking, the smaller the change in an observed quantity (e.g., cell biomass) because of a stimulus (e.g., an applied electromagnetic (EM) field) the more difficult the experimental interpretation. There may be multiple candidate causes if small changes in biomass are found. It could be due to any of many growth-altering biochemical changes, unnoticed and uncharacterized temperature variations, or even changes in ambient light or mechanical vibration. In physical science, a model can often be made of the experiment. This allows for estimates of the influence of various quantities and parameters on the expected experimental outcome (change in observed quantity in response to a stimulus), and is valuable in interpretation of experiments. Similar approaches to bioelectromagnetics should also be valuable.

Consider an illustrative measurement on a biological system: a population of microorganisms contained within a glass toroid. Through the application of an alternating magnetic field by means of a primary coil, an alternating voltage in the toroid can be induced. The induced current can next be measured with another coil. The induced current is related to the electrical conductivity of the aqueous electrolyte. The electrical conductivity of the extracellular medium changes when small, charged metabolites are excreted and measurement of microbial metabolic activity can thus be accomplished electrically. First observed in 1899 by a nulling technique,[1] electrical impedance detection of microorganisms has received significant attention as a measurement method.[2,3] A toroidal device has actually been explored as the basis for determining microbial activity[4] with metabolic acid production causing a change in extracellular ion concentration (activity), and therefore creating a change in the electrical conductivity of the extracellular medium. But complications may arise. If cytotoxic chemicals leach from the glass there can be a time-dependent poisoning of microbial activity. Ambient temperature changes couple through the glass to create internal temperature variations that alter the conductivity. In short, because electrical conductivity change has more than one candidate cause, this measurement system lacks specificity. This also illustrates a basic challenge to measurement of effects of EM fields on biological systems. That challenge consists in demonstrating both a statistically significant change and convincing evidence that it is the field interaction with the biological system, not an associated competing influence that is responsible for the observation.

8.2 Specificity

Specificity is a hallmark of biological interactions involving biochemicals. A cell contains a large number of coexisting molecules whose interactions are not spontaneous, but instead highly regulated. Enzymes can be highly specific in the reactions they catalyze. Antibodies and receptor/ligand binding are also often specific. However, interactions of EM fields with a biological system are rather general. Magnetic fields interact indirectly by inducing electric fields and directly through magnetically sensitive reactions[5] and through interactions with magnetic material. Such magnetic materials may be contaminant ferromagnetic particles in the human body[6] or they may be biologically synthesized magnetite granules.[7,8] Electric fields interact nonspecifically with charge and polarizable material. Thus, unlike ligand/receptor biochemical interactions, there are no molecular receptors that are highly specific for EM fields. Instead, magnetic and electric sensory systems interact broadly and can be regarded as nonspecific. Evolved sensory systems are rather special. To date, it appears that biological electric and magnetic field reception is indeed accomplished by organized systems.

Lack of EM field specificity has important implications for interpreting experiments. If an experiment quantifies a change in an observed parameter, the cause of the change is not automatically known. Continuing the example of cell growth determination based on biomass measurement, if an increase in biomass (or cell number) is associated with a field exposure, then additional analysis is needed to determine whether this change is due directly to the field, or is instead due to interfering influences such as temperature change or biochemical concentration changes.

The challenge of specificity is not limited to weakly interacting fields. Consider the case of strong, electroporating fields *in vivo*, for which the motivation is local tumor treatment

Signals, Noise, and Thresholds

263

or gene therapy. Strong fields can generate tissue movement by stimulating muscles and possibly also by bulk tissue polarization forces. Tissue motion can itself create membrane openings, and these can lead to biochemical transport.[9–11] Thus, observation of molecular uptake associated with electrical pulsing does not by itself show that electroporation is responsible. Specificity is an issue.

8.3 Signal-to-Noise Ratio

We adopt a recent discussion of the signal-to-noise ratio, (S/N), for experiments with biological systems exposed to weakly interacting EM fields.[12] The observed quantity is x. For bioelectromagnetics experiments, examples of x include a local or spatially averaged transmembrane voltage change, temperature rise at a particular site, radioactivity of an incorporated unstable isotope, specific enzyme activity, intracellular calcium ion concentration, cell biomass, etc. Typically experiments obtain data which can be characterized by their means and standard deviations, often presented as a bar chart. One bar of each bar pair represents the control result, and the other bar represents the exposed result. Each bar height represents the mean value and the error bar is usually the standard deviation. (In some cases, the error bars instead represent the standard error, i.e., the uncertainty in the mean, rather than the standard deviation, but generally a report states which is being used.) Bar charts present a concise summary of an investigator's knowledge of the underlying natural distributions. The measured mean and standard deviation of the control distribution can be defined to be $\bar{x}_{con}$ and σ_{con}, respectively. Similarly, $\bar{x}_{exp}$ and σ_{exp} are the observed mean and standard deviation of the exposed distribution.

When repeating the same experiment and doing the same measurement many times over, one generally finds a Gaussian distribution of outcomes. This is because in a complex system there are many variables and sources of inaccuracy that are not under the control of the experimentalist. For the cumulative effect of all these imprecisions, the Central Limit Theorem becomes applicable. This theorem says that with many independent stochasticities involved, the outcome will be a Gaussian distribution.[13] As an example of this theorem in practice, do 100 coin tosses and record the number N of "heads." Repeat this experiment many times. The result will converge to a Gaussian distribution of N that is centered around 50.

The threshold for a field exposure effect occurs under conditions of detection, i.e., the minimum change of x that is discernable using generally accepted statistical criteria. This is equivalent to determining whether or not the control statistical distribution and the exposed distribution are distinguishable (significantly different by accepted criteria). This requires sufficiently precise knowledge of the statistical distribution parameters. Increasing the number of determinations of the natural distribution generates more precise knowledge of its parameters. For example, if an investigator carries out a number, m_{con}, of determinations of x_{con} and another number, m_{exp}, of determinations of x_{exp}, then the empirically determined values can be reported as

$$x_{con} = \bar{x}_{con} \pm \frac{\sigma_{con}}{\sqrt{m_{con}}} \text{ and } x_{exp} = \bar{x}_{exp} \pm \frac{\sigma_{exp}}{\sqrt{m_{exp}}}. \tag{8.1}$$

The ratio $\sigma/\sqrt{m}$ actually represents the aforementioned standard error. Increasing the number of determinations reduces the standard error and the ensuing uncertainty in the mean. However, it does not decrease the standard deviation, σ_{exp}, of the underlying distribution, which is assumed unperturbed by the measurement process.

As the means $\bar{x}_{con}$ and $\bar{x}_{exp}$ become better known through more determinations, the potential distinguishability of the two distributions increases. The "p-value" of the experiment is often reported as a measure of this distinguishability. The p-value is the probability that the two means would be found to be as different as observed (or even more different) purely due to random variability. For example, $p=0.01$ indicates that there is only a 1% chance that the difference (or a larger difference) between the control mean and the exposed mean would be due to the (assumed) random variability, i.e., the standard deviation, of the measured quantity.[14] After an investigator completes an experiment and finds a reasonably small p-value (0.01 and 0.05 are widely used values), then it is common practice for the investigator to report that an effect due to the field exposure has occurred. However, this assumes specificity, viz. that the field exposure rather than an associated competing influence is responsible. Indeed, a small p-value supports an effect of some sort, but not necessarily one due to the field during the exposure. Additional analysis that considers other competing influences such as temperature variations, vibrations, chemical concentration variations[15,16] is required for that conclusion.

Bioelectromagnetics experiments with weakly interacting fields typically involve determination of changes with respect to background values of, for instance, transmembrane voltage, fluorescence intensity, enzyme activity or cell number. Observed changes in "exposed" relative to "control" are generally small. At the other extreme, strongly interacting fields create large changes with respect to background, e.g., molecular uptake by electroporation [see Electroporation chapter, Chapter 7 of BMA]. For the "weakly interacting" situation the uncertainties (error bars) are about the same for "exposed" and "control." However, there is another figure of merit, distinct from the p-value, namely, an empirically determined signal-to-noise ratio, $(S/N)_{obs}$, which is associated with the observation and which is presumed due to the underlying statistical distributions for the control and exposed cases. Classical detection theory shows that the associated distributions are expected to be Gaussians.[17]

Continuing a recent discussion,[12] we consider the "observed signal" (S_{obs}) to be the difference between the control and the exposed means, and the "observed noise" (N_{obs}) as the standard deviation of the control distribution.[17] This yields

$$S_{obs} = \bar{x}_{exp} - \bar{x}_{con} \text{ and } N_{obs} = \sigma_{con}, \tag{8.2}$$

so that the empirically determined signal-to-noise ratio is the magnitude of

$$(S/N)_{obs} = \frac{\bar{x}_{exp} - \bar{x}_{con}}{\sigma_{con}}. \tag{8.3}$$

Like the p-value, $(S/N)_{obs}$ is a measure of the distinguishability of the two distributions. However, unlike the p-value, the signal-to-noise ratio is an inherent characteristic of the biological system, its environment and a particular field exposure, and does not depend on the number of determinations. In this view, S_{obs} is the observed change and is assumed to be a measure of the strength of the perturbation to the biological system by the field exposure. N_{obs} is a measure of the natural variability in the system for the conditions of the experiment. In the absence of an exposure, N_{obs} provides the appropriate scale to gauge the strength of S_{obs}.

$(S/N)_{obs}$ is based only on experimental determinations of x. However, in many cases the field exposure is believed to *indirectly* alter x. According to this general hypothesis, the

Signals, Noise, and Thresholds 265

field exposure affects one or more molecular-level biochemical processes through physical interactions. In this sense, the exposure is creating a "primary" molecular change that is then amplified through a biochemical cascade that creates a downstream change. It is this downstream change that is eventually measured. The signal-to-noise ratio cannot be increased by the amplification process. Later in this chapter, we will describe how amplification generally adds noise to a signal.

8.4 Detection Criteria

The criterion $(S/N) \leq 0.1$ is a very conservative basis for ruling out a particular class of biophysical mechanism for a given field exposure. Similarly, the criterion $(S/N) \geq 10$ is a conservative basis for ruling in a candidate biophysical mechanism for a given exposure, retaining that biophysical mechanism hypothesis for further evaluation. This approach provides a quantitative basis for rejecting or accepting hypothetical biophysical mechanisms as candidate explanations for an experimental measurement. The traditional choice $(S/N) \approx 1$ is a useful but somewhat arbitrary dividing line, which indicates conditions for which an effect might appear. The $(S/N) \leq 0.1$ and $(S/N) \geq 10$ provide criteria for stronger conclusions, allowing rejection or provisional retention of a biophysical mechanism hypothesis.

We should recognize that thresholds are defined by generally accepted statistical criteria. The widely used p-values of 0.01 and 0.05 are examples of such generally accepted statistical values. In the case of signal-to-noise ratios a commonly accepted value is $(S/N) \approx 1$, where the "approximately equal" symbol denotes the imprecision. Specifically, if (S/N) (empirical or theoretical) exceeds one, then the threshold is viewed as being exceeded. Similarly, if (S/N) is less than one, the response is interpreted as sub-threshold. Clearly, it makes little sense to take a strong position if (S/N) is close to one. But, as noted above, if the signal-to-noise ratio is significantly greater or less than one, then some confidence can be attached to the result. In short, a threshold is imprecise, but nevertheless a useful guide.

8.5 Equilibrium Noise

In this section, we will examine how Brownian noise, the simple random motion of molecules due to thermal agitation, interferes with the coupling of an EM field to a biochemical system. Some organisms have evolved an ability to sense and effectively "measure" electric and magnetic fields. We will see that the thermal noise that a signal has to compete against sets fundamental limits on detectability. We will also see how evolution has come up with structures to optimize the signal-to-noise ratio in sensory perception.

Fish generally carry a small dipolar electric field relative to the water that they swim in. Sharks, skates, and rays have developed special organs to detect such fields[18–20] and they use this ability to pinpoint the prey's position when they get close and the water is too turbulent to rely on smell. To be effective, the shark should be able to sense its prey instantaneously. So, in order for the signal not to be mistaken for Brownian noise and for Brownian noise not to be mistaken as a signal, a signal should carry an energy that is significantly larger than $k_B T$. Here k_B is Boltzmann's constant (1.4×10^{-23} J/K) and T represents the absolute temperature. $k_B T$ constitutes the average energy in the thermal noise band and can be considered to be the "quantum" of thermal energy.[21] This baseline criterion already works to explain some of the physiology of the electric sensing organs. The shark picks up electric fields through the so-called ampullae of Lorenzini. These ampullae terminate at pores in the skin around the fish's head. They are enclosed in a highly resistive material and are filled with a very conductive gel. The eventual setup is equivalent to an electrical wire with no voltage drop inside. These ampullae are, furthermore, well insulated against electrical noise that originates from the fish's own physiology. Two pores that are about 10 cm apart on the surface of the fish's head can, on the inside ends, be separated by a membrane that is only a few nanometers thick. A field of 1.0 μV/m in the water can now be detected; two pores that are 10 cm apart on the skin surface can transfer 0.1 μV to a transmembrane potential.

By having lots of ion channels whose open-closed probabilities depend sensitively on the transmembrane voltage, the thermal noise can be effectively averaged out. With N ion channels instead of just one, N times as much signal strength is picked up. The thermal noise at each channel is independent of that at any other channel. The noise is zero-average and the noise variances are added up for N channels. So the average noise amplitude will only be $\sqrt{N}$ times as large if N channels are involved instead of one (remember that the noise amplitude is a standard deviation and that the standard deviation is the square-root of the variance). After detection the fish has to amplify the submicrovolt signal to the millivolt range that the nervous system operates with. Amplifier noise constitutes a problem that builders of electric circuits have dealt with for decades. Amplifier noise is nonequilibrium noise and we will discuss it in a next section. Over the past decade researchers have built up a good and detailed understanding of the physiology[22] and physics[23,24] of the fishes' amplification system

Many animal species have the ability to detect the geomagnetic field. Two mechanisms have been proposed for magnetosensitivity. The first mechanism is a "radical pair mechanism" and it involves chemical transitions that are sensitive to external magnetic fields.[25,26] Upon excitation by light, many polyatomic molecules will start transiting between the singlet ground state, the singlet excited state, and the triplet excited state. The energy difference between a singlet ($\uparrow\downarrow$) state and a triplet ($\uparrow\uparrow$) state is affected by an external magnetic field. This energy difference is generally small for fields of the magnitude of the Earth's magnetic field. But the magnetism that living cells generate is even smaller. A magnetically sensitive reaction of this type is therefore not subject to significant thermal noise. However, a detection limit can be established by considering a model in which reacting product molecules can bind to receptors. There is an innate stochasticity in chemical reactions; rates represent an average behavior and there is a Gaussian distribution around this average. This is called fundamental chemical noise and we will come back to it later in this chapter. In this model, the average number of occupied receptors varies with the magnetic field and the detection limits are set by the fundamental chemical noise.[27] The fact that many bird species actually need light for their magnetic compass to work is a strong indication that singlet-triplet transitions are involved in the navigation. Additional evidence was found when it turned out that robins get disoriented when they are subjected to an RF (MHz) EM field that oscillates at the singlet-triplet resonance frequency[5] (for more details, see the chapter on free radical models).

The second mechanism that has been proposed to explain magnetosensitivity involves small (<100 nm in diameter) granules of magnetite (Fe_3O_4). This material, also known as lodestone, is biochemically formed and has about 30% of the magnetic strength of pure Fe.

Signals, Noise, and Thresholds

In the 1970s, it was discovered that certain microbes use arrays of biopolymer-embedded, single-domain magnetite granules, also called magnetosomes, as a kind of rudder to help them stay under water right at the interface between the water and the mud at the bottom. There is a force trying to align the array of magnetic granule(s) with the Earth's magnetic field and the microbe thus "finds out" what its own orientation is relative to the inclination of the Earth's magnetic field.[28,29] For a single-domain magnetite granule of about 100 nm in diameter the product μB of the magnetic moment μ and the Earth's magnetic field B amounts to about $5\,k_B T$. This $5\,k_B T$ alignment energy is sufficient to exceed the $k_B T$ random thermal agitation in the granule's rotation. It appears that the granules are generally embedded in biopolymers and lined up to form a rigid linear rod. Such an alignment effectively increases the magnetic moment and in this way a system can be constructed that is sensitive to small variations in the magnetic field.[30,31] Indications are that there can be up to a million magnetite-containing cells in the brain of almost any animal. Even humans, who exhibit no apparent magnetosensitivity, have magnetite in the brain tissue.[7,8]

The intensity of the Earth's magnetic field varies from 25 to 65 μT and the direction varies from parallel to perpendicular to the Earth's surface. The magnetic sensitivity of, for instance, homing pigeons has been shown to be such that field variations smaller than 10 nT can be detected. With such a sensitivity, the pigeon can use the change of the magnetic field vector to furnish itself a kind of GPS system.[32] Data indicate that some birds incorporate both magnetite and singlet-triplet chemistry in their magnetosense.[5]

It is tempting to hypothesize that extremely low-frequency (ELF) radiation or microwave radiation could have a physiological effect through the interactions with magnetosomes. Cells produce their own electricity and concurrent electric noise. But there is no significant endogenous magnetic field noise. So the magnetic part of ELF radiation or microwave radiation would not have to compete against such endogenous biological noise. The 24-h average of the 60 Hz magnetic field due to house wiring, distribution lines, electric motors etc., for individuals in the U.S. population is about 10^{-7} T,[33] i.e., orders of magnitude smaller than the earth's stationary magnetic field. Starting from this premise the magnetosome in the cytoplasm was modeled as a damped harmonic oscillator with an external 60 Hz modulation.[34] The restoring force is the force pushing to align the magnetosome's moment with the earth's magnetic field and the damping is due to the viscosity of the cytoplasm. The associated equation is easily solved. Using reasonable values for the involved parameters, it was found that even with exposure to a 60 Hz field with an amplitude of 5 μT, the alternating field transfers an amount of energy to the magnetosome that is orders of magnitude smaller than $k_B T$. In other words, the thermal agitations in the rotation far overwhelm any "signal" from an ambient 60 Hz field. But subsequently, the legitimacy of a simple linear approximation was questioned.[35] It was pointed out that there are intricacies that make the viscosity of the cytoplasm, which determines the damping coefficient in the model, hard to specify. Most importantly, the possibility of many individual magnetosomes in a cell acting in concert should be considered. With N magnetosomes in a cell instead of just one, the signal-to-noise ratio is $\sqrt{N}$ times larger. The explanation for this apparent amplification is the same as with the aforementioned N ion channels in the shark's electroreception. An alternative model that includes such cooperativity leads to a signal-to-noise ratio that is well over unity with a 2 μT amplitude 60 Hz magnetic field.[35] However, little is known about how forces on magnetosomes are transduced into physiological signals. More solid estimates of detection thresholds can probably only be derived after such biophysical mechanisms are revealed.

Electric fields are also of interest. Close to a power line, a human can be exposed to an electric field of about 10 kV/m. Two steps have to be taken to get to an assessment of the transmembrane voltage that such an exposure leads to. First of all, living tissue is much more conducting than air. Charge in the tissue will move - it will follow the external field and "try to compensate" for it. But different tissues have different resistivities. An approximation has been derived for the ratio between the internal field and the field in the air:[36,37]

$$\frac{E_i}{E_0} \approx \varepsilon_0 \omega \rho_t.$$

(8.4)

Here, $\varepsilon_0 = 8.8 \times 10^{-12}$ C^2/N m^2 represents the dielectric permittivity of a vacuum, ω is the angular frequency ($2\pi f$), and ρ_t is the resistivity of the tissue. So for, a frequency of about 100 Hz and with a typical tissue resistivity of about 1–2 Ωm, the attenuation factor for the field entering the body is found to be in a range of 10^{-8}–10^{-7}. Once inside the tissue, an amplification at the cell membranes occurs. This is because the intracellular and extracellular fluid are conducting and do not allow for the presence of an electric field. So eventually all of the voltage drop occurs at the nonconducting cell membranes. We will come back to this in the next paragraph. For a spherical cell with a diameter of about $d = 10$ μm in a field E, the voltage across the diameter will be $\Delta V = Ed$. The eventual field in the membrane will thus be of the order of $E_{mem} \approx E(d/h)$, where h is the thickness of the membrane. With $h \approx 5$ nm we find an amplification factor of about a 1000. All in all, we find a net conversion factor of 10^{-5}–10^{-4} and an electric field of about 0.1–1.0 V/m across a membrane as a result of the 10 kV/m power line exposure. This leads to an ELF-induced potential difference of at most 10^{-8} V across the membrane. It should, however, be noted that muscle cells or nerve cells are cylindrically shaped and may have lengths in the millimeter of even centimeter range. When the imposed field is along the axis of the cylinder, there may be a conversion factor at the caps of the cylinder that is 2 to 3 orders of magnitude higher.

When a living cell is suddenly exposed to an external electric field, ions will start flowing in the conducting interior to compensate for this field. In a typical mammalian cell, it is generally within microseconds that ions have accumulated near the membrane to achieve a zero intracellular electric field. This means that stationary electric fields and ELF (<300 Hz) AC fields distribute over cell membranes. Power lines and high-voltage distribution stations have been the subject of a lot of public anxiety. The power grid operates at 60 Hz in the USA and at 50 Hz in most other countries, i.e. well within the ELF regime.

This 10^{-8} V may appear small relative to, for instance, the transmembrane potential of about 0.1 V that is present in about every living cell. However, when we talk about detectability, this 10^{-8} V should first be compared to the transmembrane voltages due to Brownian motion. The thermal noise voltage across standard resistors was already detected in the 1920s.[38] A formula was subsequently derived by Nyquist:[39]

$$\langle dV^2 \rangle = 4 k_B TR df.$$

(8.5)

This equation gives the average square voltage in a frequency window of width df. The noise is white, i.e., it has the same intensity at all frequencies. Technically, this would lead to an absurdity. It would imply that the noise carries an infinite amount of energy. However, as Nyquist already pointed out, $\langle dV^2 \rangle$ starts vanishing when we get to high frequencies f such that $hf \approx k_B T$. Here h represents Planck's constant $h = 6.6 \times 10^{-34}$ J sec. At these high frequencies quantum physics takes over and makes $\langle dV^2 \rangle$ go to zero. Such high frequencies are not in our realm of interest.

What Nyquist had in mind for a resistor in his derivation was a Brownian gas of frequently colliding charge carriers. With a 5-nm-cell membrane that consists of a lipid bilayer

Signals, Noise, and Thresholds 269

with embedded proteins, the charge carriers are small ions (Na^+, K^+, Cl^-, etc.). The ions do not form a "gas" inside the membrane and it is not a priori obvious that Nyquist's formalism would apply. The equilibrium noise current through a membrane that separates two ionic solutions is due to two-sided shot noise. Shot noise was first described by Schottky[40] in the context of vacuum amplifier tubes. It is due to the elementary charge being finite and the charge carriers making random "jumps." It can be shown that two-sided shot noise ultimately leads back again to Nyquist's Equation (8.5).[41,42] Ultimately, Equation (8.5) is a manifestation of something much more general than Nyquist may have had in mind. What underlies Equation (8.5) is Einstein's Fluctuation–Dissipation Theorem. That theorem says that the same random collisions that cause diffusion, thermal noise, or shot noise also cause dissipation, friction, or resistance. The theorem, moreover, makes this connection quantitative:

$$\beta = \frac{k_\mathrm{B}T}{D}. \tag{8.6}$$

For the motion of a macromolecule in a liquid, D is the diffusion coefficient and β is the coefficient of friction, i.e., the ratio $\beta = F/v$ where F represents the pulling force and v represents the resulting average speed. But in the context of the current through a membrane, β represents the electrical resistance ($R = V/I$). For D we then find $D = e^2 P_\mathrm{S}c$ in the membrane electrical case. Here P_S is the membrane permeability to the monovalent ion S that is responsible for the current, c represents the concentration of this ion on both sides of the membrane, and e is the elementary charge.

Electrically a cell membrane can be modeled as in the sketch in Figure 8.1a. A pure lipid bilayer membrane has a capacitance of about 1 μF/cm^2. The capacitance of an actual cell membrane is generally not much different. The resistance of a pure lipid bilayer depends on the ionic concentrations of the solutions on either side of the membrane. With these concentrations at biological levels the resistance of a lipid bilayer membrane can be as high as 10^9 Ω cm^2. Due to the presence of ion channels, ion transporters, and ion pumps,[43,44] an actual cell membrane has a resistance that is orders of magnitude smaller (typically about 10^3 Ω cm^2). The resistance of a patch of membrane is inversely proportional to the area of that patch. So, in order to characterize a membrane, the approach is to measure the resistance through an actual patch and then next multiply with the surface area of that patch. This is why we give the resistance of a membrane in terms of Ω cm^2.

The setup in Figure 8.1a is equivalent to the one in Figure 8.1b, i.e., an ordinary RC circuit. When calculating the characteristic time, RC, of the circuit, the surface area cancels out. For a pure lipid bilayer, the RC-time constant can be of the order of minutes. But for a cell membrane it is of the order of milliseconds.

In our context, the resistor in Figure 8.1 is not just a resistor, but, following Nyquist (cf. Equation (8.5)), it is also a white noise generator. At each frequency the resistor generates a harmonic oscillation. All these harmonic oscillations have the same amplitude, but the noise ultimately looks random because the phases are randomized. To evaluate the voltage across the capacitor, we have to analyze a simple RC-circuit with an AC source. The high frequencies ($f > (RC)^{-1}$) that are generated in the resistor do not have enough time to build up across the capacitor.[45] However, for low frequencies ($f < (RC)^{-1}$) changes are sufficiently slow for the capacitor to keep up and follow the voltage in the resistor. Ultimately, the transmembrane voltage is the voltage across the capacitor and the equilibrium noise is thus expected to occur mostly at low frequencies. As was mentioned before, the RC-time of a cell membrane is of the order of milliseconds and external ELF fields thus operate in the

$f < (RC)^{-1}$ regime where the noise is largest. A straightforward quantitative analysis shows that the low frequency equilibrium noise far overwhelms any reasonable ambient power frequency field.[45] There would be no way to ever instantaneously detect such a field.

It was later put forward that everything that is happening in the cell membrane should, in the model of Figure 8.1, be imagined to happen inside the resistor.[46] Membrane proteins go through their catalytic cycle against a background of intramembrane noise. Inside the membrane means, in the context of Figure 8.1a, inside the resistor. In this picture, the thermal noise voltage (cf. Equation (8.5)) derives from a net electric field that results from inhomogeneities in the distribution of the charge carriers. Now at low frequencies the capacitor will be able to follow the imposed oscillation and effectively produce a field to counter the field generated inside the resistor (Figure 8.1a). This model thus leads to a vanishing net potential inside the membrane at low frequency. At high frequency the voltage changes in the resistor are too fast for the capacitor to keep up. In this view, the noise spectrum is the reverse of what was described in the previous paragraph: no noise at the low frequencies where and a flat spectrum at the high frequencies. In this situation, signals from ambient ELF fields would be detectable.

The above-described controversy can be resolved after the realization that Figure 8.1 is actually not the appropriate model when we try to derive the intramembrane electric fields. For a cell of about 20 μm in diameter, the surface area amounts to about a billion square nanometers. The membrane is only about 5 nm thick, so the resistor resembles a very thin sheet. The lateral conductivity, i.e., the conductivity form one place in the sheet to another, is very low. So at different spots on the sheet, different unrelated noise fields are generated. The more sensible model would therefore be one where the resistor in Figure 8.1 is cut up into millions of independent parallel resistors. Each of these resistors creates its own field. The capacitor plate corresponds to the conducting liquid on either side of the membrane and it can be conceived of as having perfect lateral conductivity. So each resistor generates its own particular field, but they all experience the same field from the capacitor. With this model the noise gets very large. First of all, there are more, say N, resistors that are producing noise. But on top of that, each of these resistors has a resistance NR (N parallel resistors of resistance NR lead to a net resistance of R) and, according to Equation (8.5), thus produces more noise. Because the N parallel resistors that make up the resistance R are independent, they oscillate out of phase at each frequency f. As a result the parallel resistors end up pushing a lot of current in and out of each other. Most of the generated noise current thus remains intramembrane and never reaches the capacitor. The mathematics associated with this parallel setup is challenging, but an exact solution can be derived.[42,47]

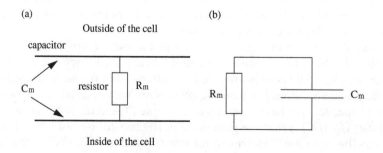

FIGURE 8.1
The electrical structure of the membrane is shown on the left. R_m and C_m are the resistance and capacitance between the inside and outside of the cell. The Brownian motion of charge carriers in the resistor leads to a fluctuating electromotive force (cf. Equation (8.5)). The equivalent circuit is shown on the right.

The capacitor, and therefore the *RC*-time, plays no role in the intramembrane noise. The intramembrane noise is white and it has an intensity that is many orders of magnitude larger than the noise that reaches the capacitor. What matters for biological function is actually the intramembrane noise. This, after all, is the noise that a membrane-embedded protein would "feel." The protein's catalytic cycle takes place against the background of such noise. The parallel setup model leads to a noise intensity that is much larger than that of the earlier models.

At first sight, all this extensive treatment of intramembrane noise may seem to have little to do with the two-sided shot noise that a membrane is subject to. However, when rigorously modeling the membrane as a thin sheet in an ionic solution, something similar to the overwhelming intramembrane noise is found. The ions that constitute the net charge on the membrane in Figure 8.1a move across the membrane-solution interface with an average speed of about 100 m/s. This is just their thermal motion and it is easily derived from $\frac{1}{2}mv^2 \approx k_B T$. This motion effectively causes laterally traveling electric pulses in the membrane. The noise intensity that is associated with these traveling electric pulses appears to be many orders of magnitude higher than the noise that is due to the shot-noise-like membrane passages by the ions.[42]

Current models of membrane noise thus lead to transmembrane voltage noise estimates that far exceed the strength of any reasonable magnitude ELF field-induced "signal." What the previous paragraphs lead up to is the conclusion that an ELF signal cannot be detected instantaneously in a cell membrane.

However, under certain conditions and given enough time, even the smallest signal can get out of the noise band. The following example is meant to illustrate this. Consider the system depicted in Figure 8.2. Let the resistance *R* represent a membrane patch. For simplicity, imagine that on either side of the resistor there is an infinite reservoir (i.e., a capacitor with infinite capacitance), so no net voltage can develop across the resistor. The average square charge $\langle q^2(t) \rangle$ that accumulates during a time *t* on either side of the membrane can be easily derived from Equation (8.5) and amounts to

$$\langle q^2(t) \rangle = \frac{2k_B T}{R} t. \tag{8.7}$$

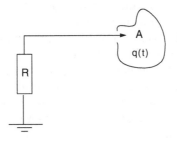

FIGURE 8.2
A resistor is connected to the ground and to an infinite reservoir A. The net voltage between the reservoirs remains zero. The situation is like the one in Figure 1 with the capacitor that has infinite capacitance. Due to Brownian motion of electrons in the conduction band, there is a zero-average fluctuating current through the resistor. The net charge accumulating in the reservoir A is the result of these fluctuations in the same way that diffusive displacement is the result of random Brownian kicks. We have $\langle q^2(t) \rangle = 2(k_B T/R)t$ for the average square charge accumulation in time *t*.

Again, there is an obvious analogy between Equation (8.7) and the well-known diffusion formula $\langle x^2(t) \rangle = 2Dt$, which describes the average square displacement of a particle with a diffusion coefficient D during a time interval of length t. The above formula clearly shows how, in an electrical context, $k_B T/R$ plays the role of the diffusion coefficient D.

From Equation (8.7) we infer that for the accumulated charge as a function of time, we have $|q_{Br}(t)| \approx \sqrt{\langle q^2(t) \rangle} \propto \sqrt{t}$. Here the subscript "Br" indicates that it is a Brownian-noise effect. For any charged or uncharged molecule on either side of the membrane, the thermal noise-driven accumulation carries this $\sqrt{t}$ proportionality. The coupling of ELF EM fields to biochemical activity occurs mostly through membrane proteins. Membrane proteins whose conformational changes involve significant changes of the dipole moment are particularly sensitive. ELF fields can affect the catalytic rates of such proteins. So, for instance, electrogenic ion pumps,[44] but also transporters or pumps that have a dipole, may have a slightly altered throughput in the presence of an ELF field. If there is no restoring force for a transported or pumped molecule, the accumulation will continue. The cumulative effect of the altered throughput will be a linear function of time. The excess charge that accumulates due to an ELF field thus follows $q_{ELF} \propto t$.

Consequently, we see that on a small timescale, the Brownian noise ($\propto \sqrt{t}$) will be stronger than the signal ($\propto t$). But there will always come a time $t = t_*$ when $|q_{Br}(t_*)| = |q_{ELF}(t_*)|$ and we then achieve $S/N = 1$ for the signal-to-noise ratio. It depends on the values of the proportionality constants when t_* occurs. If molecular change is the measurement criterion, then it is only on timescales of the order of t_* that the effect becomes measurable. Estimates for t_* with realistic ELF exposure have been made[48] and have led to a timescale larger than the age of the universe.

8.6 Nonequilibrium Noise

In the previous section we considered equilibrium noise. A living cell, however, constitutes a system that is far from equilibrium. Between the intracellular and extracellular solution there is an electric potential difference of about 100 mV. For ions like Na^+, K^+, Cl^-, and Ca^{2+} there is a more than tenfold difference between intra- and extracellular concentration. The 100 mV transmembrane electric voltage over a width of about 5 nm implies a very strong field of tens of megavolts per meter.

The electrochemical potential across the cell membrane is an energy source for many processes.[44] The Na,Ca-exchanger, for instance, is a membrane protein that picks up a sodium ion on the outside and then goes through a cycle in the course of which it drops the sodium ion off on the inside. The protein couples the energetically downhill movement of sodium to uphill transport of calcium. In the course of the cycle, a calcium ion is picked up on the inside and pumped, against the electrochemical potential, to the outside. The membrane potential is maintained by ATP-driven ion pumps. The most common of these is Na,K-ATPase. This is a membrane protein that, in the course of its catalytic cycle, hydrolyzes one ATP and uses the released energy to transport three sodium ions out of the cell and bring two potassium ions in.

Each working protein is like a small engine. A living cell contains millions of these engines: they are continuously converting energy from one form to another and, in the process, they are also generating heat, i.e., dissipating energy. A living cell constitutes a

Signals, Noise, and Thresholds

far from equilibrium system and the continuous transduction and dissipation of energy generates noise that adds to the thermal, Brownian noise that was discussed in the previous section.

It would not be against the First Law of Thermodynamics (i.e., conservation of energy) if ion pumps were to extract heat from the environment and use it to power the maintenance of the transmembrane potential. This would, however, be in gross violation of the Second Law of Thermodynamics. There are many equivalent formulations of the Second Law. The most common formulation is the proposition that every isolated system strives to increase and maximize its entropy. The teleological form of this formulation is somewhat bewildering. After all, most laws in science are formulated as conservation laws (e.g., conservation of energy) or as causal laws (e.g., Newton's Second Law, $F=ma$, which relates a causing force to an ensuing acceleration). However, after properly defining entropy, entropy maximization is often the easiest form of the Second Law to work with when dealing with macroscopic systems.

When going to the molecular realm, the Second Law can pose some challenging paradoxes. Consider, for instance, an ion channel in a cell membrane. Many ion channels rectify, i.e., they pass current more easily in one direction than in the other. So, the $I–V$ characteristic is not a straight line through the origin, but also has a curvature. Any frequency from the white spectrum of equilibrium noise should, in principle, be rectified. It thus might look like a rectifying ion channel could use zero-average, thermal, equilibrium Nyquist noise to charge a battery. Of course it would not work. As pointed out above, it would be in violation of the Second Law. Thinking in the context of rectifying $p–n$ junctions, solid state physicists ran into this paradox long before ion channels were discovered. In 1950, L. Brillouin wrote a paper "Can the Rectifier Become a Thermodynamic Demon?"[49] In it he presents a short derivation to show that, in a circuit with all components at the same temperature, no diode can rectify. He is aware that his case represents a special case of the so-called Principle of Detailed Balance: "No system in thermal equilibrium in an environment at constant temperature spontaneously and of itself arrives in such a condition that any of the processes taking place in the system by which energy may be extracted, run in a preferred direction, without a compensating reverse process." The principle is a consequence of the Second Law[50,51] and, for our rectifier, basically states that there must, on average, be as much current in one direction as there is in the opposite direction.

In the "Feynman Lectures on Physics"[53] a ratchet and pawl system, originally thought up by Smoluchowski,[52] is considered and eloquently discussed. The device operates as a mechanical rectifier (Figure 8.3) and essentially establishes the mechanical equivalent of Brillouin's paradox. The paradox is solved with the realization that also the pawl must be subject to thermal noise. The pawl involves a spring and the spring will, at thermal equilibrium, exhibit a Boltzmann distribution over the accessible energy range. Even here the Second Law is involved, though on a deeper level. Given the macroscopic variables (like temperature, concentration, pressure, etc.) there are many possible molecular arrangements, i.e., microstates, that correspond to that macrostate. For a fixed amount of energy, the Boltzmann distribution is the energy distribution that has the most permutations.[21] It is therefore the most likely distribution. On the level of statistical mechanics, the Second Law can be formulated as the rule that, given a macrostate, every microstate that corresponds to that macrostate has equal probability.

Second Law issues can be subtle. The connection between statistics, entropy, information, and physical work still poses paradoxes that can be hard to fathom. Books and articles still appear in which researchers are attempting to come to a fuller understanding and a better intuition.[54,55] At the scale of ion channels, the simple invocation of detailed

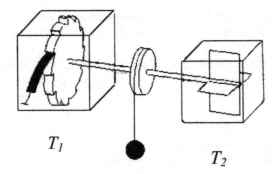

FIGURE 8.3
The mechanical thermal ratchet as it was originally conceived by Smoluchwski[52] and later discussed by Feynman et al.[53] The device is small and the paddle wheel in the right reservoir is moved by collisions of the molecules from the surrounding medium against the paddles. Because of the asymmetry of the teeth, the ratchet and pawl in the left reservoir allow motion in one direction and block it in the opposite direction. With the resulting net rotation, it should be possible, in principle, to lift a weight. However, it would be in violation of the Second Law of Thermodynamics to extract work from thermal fluctuations in the equilibrium situation, i.e., $T_1 = T_2$. The solution of the paradox lies in the realization that the ratchet and pawl are also subject to thermal fluctuations if the system is small.

balance reveals little. An appropriate description is like the one Feynman gave for his mechanical ratchet and pawl: it involves Boltzmann distributions and Brownian motion. So, it would simply be wrong to take any frequency from the white spectrum of equilibrium noise and model a rectifying ion channel as subject to this oscillation. The ion channel itself and its Brownian fluctuations have to be included in the description. At equilibrium, no part of a system can be "subject" to any other part. This is what detailed balance can be interpreted to mean.

However, when energy is dissipated, it is possible for one part of the system to impose its fluctuations on another part. When a rectifying ion channel is subject to nonequilibrium fluctuations, it will actually rectify the fluctuations and drive a net current. Consider, for instance, an electrogenic ion pump like Na,K-ATPase. As was mentioned before, this pump utilizes the energy of the hydrolysis of one ATP to pump three sodium ions out of the cell and pump two potassium ions into the cell. The ion transport is against the electrochemical potential and, all together, requires about 15 k_BT units of energy under physiological conditions. The hydrolysis of one ATP releases about 20 k_BT units of energy under physiological conditions. It is the remaining 5 k_BT that drives the process forward and that is ultimately released as heat. Na,K-ATPase is binding and releasing ions and thus generates fluctuating electric fields in its direct vicinity. For a nearby ion channel, these fields can be conceived of as imposed because the 5 k_BT that drives the Na,K-ATPase cycle is enough to overwhelm the small amount of energy (<1 k_BT[56]) necessary for the opening or closing of a channel. There is no feedback from the channel to the pump. The channel will rectify the fluctuations as a result and a zero-average field can thus lead to net charge transport. In essence, the nonequilibrium fluctuations generated by the pump and imposed on the channel are part of the conversion of chemical energy, i.e., the energy in ATP, to an electrochemical potential across the membrane.

So energy-dissipating, nonequilibrium oscillations and fluctuations are able to do work. ELF radiation from outside the organism can impose a varying field on an ion channel in much the same way that the nearby ion pump from the previous paragraph can impose a field on an ion channel. ELF radiation brings energy into the organism. Part of this energy

Signals, Noise, and Thresholds

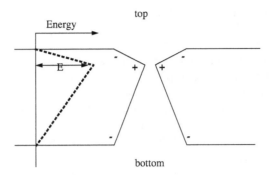

FIGURE 8.4
A simple continuum model of an ion channel imagined to be shaped like an asymmetric double cone. The energy profile on the left depicts the activation barrier that a positive ion going through the channel has to pass. The barrier has an obvious anisotropy.

will be dissipated to become heat and part of it may be converted into chemical and/or electrical work. There is obviously no feedback from an ion channel back to the ELF source.

The selectivity of ion channels for the different kinds of ions is still hard to understand and model. But the rectification property is much easier to intuit. Consider Figure 8.4. The channel is shaped like an asymmetric double cone and charges in the lining of the channel are indicated in the figure. A sodium or potassium ion that is going from the top to the bottom of the channel faces a rapid increase of the potential and then a slow decrease. A sodium or potassium ion that goes through in the opposite direction faces a slow increase and a fast subsequent decrease. A positive ion thus has a larger force to overcome when going top to bottom than when going bottom to top. Because of this, an imposed zero-average oscillation will lead to a net current.[57] As a matter of fact, any anisotropic potential shape along the length of the channel will rectify a zero-average harmonic field to lead to a net current.[58] Ion channels are proteins consisting of many amino acids and anisotropy along the inside lining will be the rule rather than the exception.

The plethora of ratchet research in the late 1990s has made clear that almost any zero-average oscillation or fluctuation imposed on a ratchet-like structure like in Figure 8.4 leads to a net current. Imagine, for instance, a temperature oscillation. With energy expressed in units of $k_B T$, a variation of temperature implies an oscillation of the barrier height E. Because of the difference in relaxation times on the slopes on either side of the barrier, a net current will result.[58-61] Ever more examples are found of nature exploiting ratchet effects for the purpose of regulation.[62]

Researchers have meanwhile also succeeded in making artificial channels. Cone shaped (and therefore anisotropic) channels form when a heavy ion is shot through an artificial membrane.[63,64] The I–V characteristic for the current of different types of ions has subsequently been recorded. It has even been experimentally shown that net charge transfer results when a zero average field is imposed on such an artificial channel. The channel is thus made to behave like a kind of pump that converts an AC input into a DC output.[65]

Imagine a number of identical anisotropic channels in a vesicle with an otherwise impermeable membrane. Next, put a large number of such vesicles in a beaker with an ionic solution. Any nonequilibrium fluctuation from the environment, or any "signal" for that matter, will now be picked up and converted into an electrochemical potential. The convection caused by a temperature gradient will heat up and cool down the vesicles and lead to their electrically charging up. The electric component of an ELF EM field will do the same thing. The beaker could thus be a battery that recharges by harnessing any incoming nonequilibrium fluctuation. This mechanism may, moreover, have played a role in the emergence of early prokaryotic life.

The Fourier spectrum of the noise that is associated with processes that dissipate energy is not white. Nonequilibrium noise appears to have higher amplitudes at lower frequencies, in other words, it exhibits an intensity that decreases with frequency. The so-called $1/f$ noise was first studied in the 1920s in the very nonequilibrium context of thermionic vacuum tube amplifiers.[40] In current scientific discourse, the term "$1/f$ noise" actually applies to all noises that have spectral densities behaving like $1/f^\alpha$, where α ranges from about 0.5 to about 1.5. Especially in electrical devices, such noise is very commonly and easily observed. It is also known as "excess noise" or "flicker noise." In a log-log plot the $1/f^\alpha$ behavior is usually seen to extend over several frequency decades.

In the 1930s, it was proposed that $1/f$ noise originated from a variable number of electrons being present in the conduction band. Electrons would shuttle between a free state and a bound state as in a chemical reaction. Let the relaxation time of that reaction be $1/\lambda$. This leads to a simple exponential relaxation $N(t) = N_0 \exp[-\lambda t]$ after any kind of fluctuation that has a magnitude N_0. The Fourier transform of the exponential decay is easily found:

$$F(\omega) = N_0 \int_{t=0}^{\infty} \exp\left[-(\lambda + i\omega)t\right] dt = \frac{N_0}{\lambda + i\omega}. \tag{8.8}$$

For the power spectral density, $S(\omega) = ||F(\omega)||^2$, we find:

$$S(\omega) \propto \frac{1}{\lambda^2 + \omega^2}, \tag{8.9}$$

where the proportionality constant involves the magnitudes of the fluctuations as well as the rates at which fluctuations occur. The power spectral density is a useful quantity as it describes how the energy in the noise is distributed over the different frequencies. $S(\omega)d\omega$ is proportional to the amount of power that the noise carries between the frequencies ω and $\omega + d\omega$. Equations (8.8) and (8.9) describe a so-called Lorentzian power spectrum. With a log scale for the frequency, the resulting curve is a sigmoid: at low ω, $S(\omega)$ is constant and at high ω, $S(\omega)$ goes asymptotically to zero as $1/\omega^2$. A good fit to $1/f$ noise can be obtained when a distribution of relaxation times is assumed.[66] Take, for instance, a uniform distribution of inverse relaxation times between λ_1 and λ_2. With Equation (8.9) this leads to:

$$S(\omega) \propto \frac{1}{\lambda_2 - \lambda_1} \int_{\lambda_1}^{\lambda_2} \frac{1}{\lambda^2 + \omega^2} d\lambda = \frac{1}{\omega(\lambda_2 - \lambda_1)} \left\{ \arctan\frac{\lambda_2}{\omega} - \arctan\frac{\lambda_1}{\omega} \right\}. \tag{8.10}$$

It is easy to check that on $\lambda_1 < \omega < \lambda_2$ this $S(\omega)$ is approximately proportional to $1/\{\omega(\lambda_2 - \lambda_1)\}$, i.e., there is $1/f$ noise between λ_1 and λ_2. This $S(\omega)$ is, moreover, roughly constant for $\omega < \lambda_1$ and drops off like $1/\omega^2$ when $\omega > \lambda_2$.

If we let, between λ_1 and λ_2, the relaxation rates contribute proportionally to $\lambda^{-\beta}$, we can actually get any $1/f^\alpha$ dependence that we want, since

$$S(\omega) \propto \int_{\lambda_1}^{\lambda_2} \frac{1}{\lambda^\beta \left(\lambda^2 + \omega^2\right)} d\lambda \propto \frac{1}{\omega^{1+\beta}} \text{ for } \lambda_1 < \omega < \lambda_2. \tag{8.11}$$

At $\omega < \lambda_1$, this spectrum would again flatten out.

Signals, Noise, and Thresholds

In experimental practice with electrical resistors and amplifiers, the $1/f$ behavior has been observed to extend over more than six frequency decades with no noticeable flattening at low frequency.[67]

$1/f$ spectra have been observed in nature in a wide variety of systems: electrocardiac waves,[68] the variation of sea levels,[69] tardiness at work,[70] etc. An essential feature of $1/f$ noise is that it exhibits self-similarity, i.e., if one magnifies both time and space with the appropriate factor, the noise pattern is indistinguishable from the original one. So the noise does not have a characteristic timescale (like the Lorentzian spectrum, cf. Equation (8.9)) or characteristic length scale. $1/f$ noise is often seen as a signature of the fractal character of nature.

In 1987, Bak, Tang, and Wiesenfeld proposed a model for a universal mechanism behind $1/f$ noise. In their landmark paper, they illustrated the concept of "self-organized criticality" with a sandpile model.[71] When a sandpile has an inclination steeper than the critical angle, avalanches will occur that bring the pile back to the critical angle. When sand is added to the pile in a random fashion, these avalanches do not exhibit a characteristic size, nor do they appear after regular time intervals. Instead, there are bigger avalanches that are relatively rare and smaller avalanches that occur more frequently. The ensuing distribution of avalanche size follows a power law in the frequency f. For instance, in one day there can be 1 avalanche involving more than 1,000 grains, 10 involving more than 100 grains, 100 avalanches involving more than 10 grains, and so on. The picture that emerges is one of a system that is sitting on the critical edge between two phases and is "organizing" avalanches to stay there.[72] The most commonly cited real-life example of self-organized criticality is the Gutenberg–Richter power law for earthquakes. It appears that every year, on average, there is one earthquake larger than magnitude 8, 10 earthquakes larger than magnitude 7, and 100 earthquakes larger than magnitude 6. The Richter scale for earthquake magnitude is already logarithmic, so the same power law as for the sandpile is apparent. Self-organized criticality is an attractive theory. It proposes a simple mechanism and it predicts power laws that can be easily verified or falsified. It has been utilized in a wide variety of contexts.[72] It has, for instance, been applied to evolutionary theory[73] and it has been used to explain frequency-size distributions of forest fires.[74]

How truly universally applicable self-organized criticality is and to what extent its claims may be unwarranted is still much debated. The $1/f$ proportionality for earthquakes only applies between magnitudes 5 and 8. Even for the archetypal sandpile, things appear to be more involved upon close inspection. Accurate measurements[75–77] on real sandpiles showed that in many cases there is no $1/f$ pattern in the avalanches. It turns out that system parameters, like the grain size and the rate of sand addition, determine to a large extent what kind of spectrum eventually emerges. The entire concept of *self*-organized criticality collapses, of course, if fine tuning by the experimentalist is crucial for the $1/f$ spectrum to materialize. All in all, $1/f$ noise is not as universal as first thought, and the dynamics behind nonequilibrium noise are usually best unraveled with *ad hoc* models.

The node of Ranvier is where the action potential for myelinated nerve cells is generated.[78] There is a high concentration of ion channels in the node of Ranvier and, in the days before patch clamp, it was a good place to record membrane electrical activity. In the mid-1960s, Verveen and Derksen measured 5 to 10 minutes of cell membrane voltage noise at a Ranvier node of an unstimulated nerve cell.[79,80] The resulting power spectrum showed two decades, between 10 Hz and 1,000 Hz, of $1/f$ noise (see Figure 8.5). This $1/f$ noise, they found, was much larger in magnitude than what Nyquist's $4k_BTR$ formula (cf. Equation (8.5)) would predict. Following the explanation for $1/f$ noise in ordinary resistors (cf. Equations (8.10) and (8.11)), Verveen and Derksen suggested that an ion channel could,

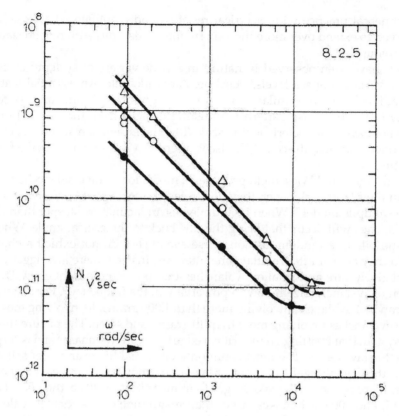

FIGURE 8.5
From the reference by Derksen. The voltage noise spectral densities from the frog node of Ranvier at room temperature at rest (open circles), at 10 mV depolarization (open triangles), and 10 mV hyperpolarization (filled circles). By copyright permission of the Dutch Physiological Society.

from time to time, get "clogged up." The wide distribution of waiting times (i.e., the λ's in Equations (8.8–8.11)) before getting unclogged would then give rise to the $1/f$ spectrum.[81]

In the last three decades, single channel recordings have shown how, even without stimulus, ion channels open and close repeatedly.[43,78] The kinetics behind the openings and closings is still very much a subject of debate. Modeling an ion channel as a two state molecule with an open and a closed state and chemical steps with constant rates connecting these states appears not to account for the data in many cases. Such a two-state model would lead to exponentially distributed open and closed times. However, nonexponential distributions have been commonly observed. Electrophysiologists have commonly resorted to explaining these nonexponential distributions with kinetic schemes that contain more than two states. With such an approach any distribution of open and closed times can always be fitted with a kinetic scheme.[82–84] It is just a matter of coming up with sufficiently many parameters (i.e., states and rates) to fit the data. In chemical kinetics, the transitions are always assumed to be Markov transitions, i.e., the probability to move from a state 1 to a state 2 is constant and does not depend on the time that the molecule has been in state 1. A channel that is making such Markov transitions between a finite number of states always exhibits a power density spectrum that is a sum of Lorentzians. The number of characteristic times in the spectrum will always be one less than the number of states. If the characteristic times are sufficiently far apart the power density

Signals, Noise, and Thresholds 279

spectrum will exhibit a number of identifiable plateaus when plotted on the customary logarithmic scale. The inflection points between the plateaus occur at the inverses of the characteristic times.

An alternative approach, foreshadowed by the aforementioned suggestion of Verveen and Derksen, has been to model the open to closed transition rates of an ion channel as time dependent, for instance $k(t) \propto t^{-\mu}$, where $0 < \mu < 1$.[85–88] The exponent μ is taken to be smaller than unity to make $\int_{\tau}^{\infty} k(t)\mathrm{d}t$ diverge for all $\tau > 0$ and thus guarantee the inevitability of an eventual transition. The proportionality $k(t) \propto t^{-\mu}$ leads to a decreasing transition probability, i.e., the channel is "stabilizing in its openness," as more time is spent in the open state. On the molecular scale, there is ample justification for the use of open-closed transition rates that vary in time. A protein has many degrees of freedom and is subject to many equilibrium and nonequilibrium fluctuations. If an intramolecular rearrangement, like a transition between an open and closed state, can be modeled as the crossing of an activation barrier, then that barrier will most likely not be fixed and stationary. A fluctuating barrier implies fluctuating open-closed transition rates. We could thus obtain the infinitely many relaxation rates that give rise to the $1/f$ power density spectra of Equations (8.10) and (8.11). Under physiological conditions an ion channel is trafficking ions in an electric field of tens of megavolts per meter and comparable chemical gradients. It is a very nonequilibrium setup and it has been conjectured that the channel operates as a self-organized critical structure. One authoritative textbook[68] states it as follows:

> A channel protein may be a self-organizing critical system. The channel protein consists of many pieces that interact with their neighbors. The energy added to the protein from the environment causes local strains that are spread throughout the structure. If these distortions spread faster than the time it takes for the structure to thermally relax, then the channel protein may be a self organizing critical system. If that is the case, then the fluctuations in the channel structure will be due to a global organization of the local interactions between many small interacting pieces of the channel protein. The fractal scaling would then be due to the fact that the channel structure is poised at a phase transition between its open and closed conformational shapes.

Over the past few years, increasing amounts of data have been gathered with ever more accurate technology. The $1/f$ power spectral density of a nerve cell that Verveen and Derksen discovered was more accurately rerecorded[89] in the early 2000s. But through careful subsequent experimentation and computer simulations these researchers were also able to show how the apparent $1/f$ result comes about as the sum of a number of Lorentzian contributions. Each type of channel has its own Lorentzian and because of close characteristic times the sum of the individual sigmoids appears like a smoothly decreasing $1/f$ curve.

For a single channel, things often turn out to be much more intricate than simple $1/f$ versus Markov kinetics. In single channel recordings of a bacterial ion channel it was found that actual channel openings and closings follow Markov kinetics and lead to Lorentzian contributions to the ultimate net power spectrum.[90] The $1/f$ noise that is present in the power spectrum originates from transitions between open states of a slightly different (about 1–5%) conductance. The rates of these mini-conductance transitions appeared to be independent of the transmembrane voltage. The small transitions in conductance have been conjectured to be due to small clusters within the channel's structure moving in and out of the lining of the pore.[90] A cluster can cause a partial flow constriction when it sticks out into the pore. Following this idea, the apparent $1/f$ behavior can be attributed to many different clusters moving in and out with equally many different relaxation times. The voltage independence comes about because these clusters are either uncharged or the external electric field is somehow screened. Noise in synthetic channels has also been studied.[91] There it was found that potassium currents through a one-state, permanently open channel exhibit $1/f^2$ noise. An artificial channel that can open and close, on the other hand, was found to exhibit $1/f$ noise when the externally applied voltage is in the right regime. With this latter artificial channel there is good ground to attribute the open-closed transitions to the movement of "dangling ends" of polymers in the pore's lining. So the result supports the "moving cluster" for the mechanism behind $1/f$ noise in biological channels.

There appears to be no simple theory that can convincingly bring all manifestations of $1/f$ noise under one common denominator. All the indications are that an *ad hoc* approach to nonequilibrium noise phenomena is still the most fruitful one.

In ordinary resistors the amount of $1/f$ noise grows linearly with the dissipated power W. The quantity $S(f)df$ represents the power (energy per unit of time, i.e., watts) within a frequency interval. For the power spectral density, the dimension is power per frequency and we thus have:

$$S(f) = \frac{gW}{f}. \tag{8.12}$$

Here g is a dimensionless constant the value of which depends on the type of resistor.

Nyquist noise is simple in that the net value of the resistance R fully determines the noise amplitude. With $1/f$ noise a more complex situation arises. Experimentally the constant g (cf. Equation (8.12)) turns out to be proportional to the power-to-volume ratio.[92] In Figure 8.6, the four resistors in design (b) are equivalent to the one resistor in design (a) in that they both lead to the same net resistance R. It is obvious that (a) and (b) will therefore exhibit the same amount of Nyquist noise. Design (a), however, will exhibit four times as much $1/f$ noise as design (b). Design (b) is quieter because the energy dissipation is distributed over a larger volume. Generally, we have $g \propto 1/V$, where V denotes the resistor's volume. The "gW" in Equation (8.12) can be expressed as "$g_e w$," where g_e is the g-value for a single elementary charge carrier in the resistor and w is the energy dissipated in the volume of such a single, independent charge carrier.

Pumps and carriers move ions one by one. Imagine a single pump or carrier that moves ions across the membrane at a rate v. During a small time interval dt there is a probability $p=vdt$ that an ion is transported. We take dt sufficiently small that the probability of more than one ion being transported during dt is negligible. We also take the duration of the catalytic cycle, i.e., the "processing" time for an ion going through the membrane, to be negligible in comparison to the time between catalytic cycles. If we were not to make the latter assumption, we would simply have to multiply by the probability that an average channel is available for transport when we want to express the transport rate. For the average number of ions $\langle n \rangle_{dt}$ transported by the channel in time dt we now have $\langle n \rangle_{dt} = 1 \cdot p + 0 \cdot (1-p) = p$. For the variance, we have $\sigma_{dt}^2 = \langle n^2 \rangle - \langle n \rangle^2 = 1^2 \cdot p - (1 \cdot p)^2 = p(1-p)$. For M subsequent timesteps and $Mdt=T$, the variances add up and we have $\langle n \rangle_T = Mp$ and $\sigma_T = Mp(1-p)$. So the standard deviation, i.e., σ_T, works out to be proportional to $\sqrt{M}$. Over time, the standard deviation becomes more and more negligible compared to the average. For sufficiently small dt we can take $1-p$ to be equal to 1 and we then have a variance that equals the average.

In the textbook by DeFelice,[92] it is shown how the power spectral density of the above process amounts to $S(f)=2\sigma_T/T=2v$. The flat frequency-independent power spectrum can be intuited as follows. If the actual transport time through the membrane is small, then we can conceive of the transmembrane current as delta function-like pulses occurring at

Signals, Noise, and Thresholds

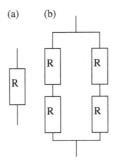

FIGURE 8.6
Design (a) and design (b) both have a net resistance R. They are different in that design (b) actually consists of two parallel resistors of 2R. Designs (a) and (b) will exhibit the same amount of equilibrium noise, as it is only the net resistance (cf. Equation (8.5)) that determines the equilibrium noise amplitude. It appears, however, that design (a) has four times as much power spectral density as design (b). The amount of nonequilibrium noise is proportional to the current density.

a rate v. The Fourier transform of a Dirac delta function is a flat spectrum. In order to go from particle current to electrical current we must, to obtain the current power spectral density, multiply with the square of the charge of the involved ion. Taking this to be the elementary charge e, we find

$$S_i(f) = 2ve^2 = 2e\langle i \rangle. \tag{8.13}$$

Here $\langle i \rangle = ev$ denotes the average current through one pump.

Next we let $\langle I \rangle$ denote the total transmembrane current due to pumps of a particular ion through the entire cell surface. We then have for the total current power spectral density due to pump activity:

$$S_I^{pu}(f) = 2e\langle I \rangle. \tag{8.14}$$

For a living cell in a steady state, for each kind of ion, there are just as many ions going in as there are going out, i.e., there is just as much uphill transport through pumps as there is downhill flow through ion channels. So we have the same current $\langle I \rangle$, uphill as well as downhill. Below we will first show that the downhill flow through the channels generates much more nonequilibrium noise than the uphill flow through the pumps. We will then show how the channel noise far exceeds the Johnson–Nyquist equilibrium noise.

Ion channels open for an average time of about $\tau_{op} = 10^{-3}$ sec. This is, for instance, the case for voltage-gated sodium channels that are involved in the propagation of an action potential in a nerve cell.[43,78] During that millisecond there is a current of about 10^7 ions per second (i.e., about 1 pA). So the equivalent of the previous paragraph's elementary charge is now $N = 10^4$ ions.

However, before we blindly substitute Ne for e in Equation (8.14) to obtain the current power spectral density generated by the channel population of a cell, we have to take another source of variance into account. The channel-open-time of about a millisecond is an average. If we view opening and closing of a channel as simple chemical steps between an open and a closed state, then the millisecond is the average of an exponential distribution of open times. For an exponential distribution the average open time equals the standard deviation in the open time. So the standard deviation ΔN equals N itself. The associated variance has to be added in. So, we have $S_I^{ch}(f) \approx 2ve^2\{N^2 + (\Delta N)^2\}$. The rate v

now represents the number of channel openings per unit of time. We thus get so we get for the current power spectral density produced by the channels:

$$S_I^{\mathrm{ch}} \approx 4Ne\langle I\rangle. \tag{8.15}$$

So the channel contribution to the total nonequilibrium current noise is about 10^4 times as large as the contribution of the pumps. For the total current power spectral density S_I^{noneq} due to nonequilibrum currents, we thus neglect the pump contribution.

The above Equation (8.15) constitutes $S_I^{\mathrm{ch}}(0)$. At higher frequencies, when f approaches $1/\tau_{\mathrm{op}}$, i.e., the inverse of the average open time of the channel, $S_I^{\mathrm{ch}}(f)$ will decrease. The characteristic inverse time for a channel is $f_* = \tau_{\mathrm{op}}^{-1} + \tau_{\mathrm{cl}}^{-1}$, where τ_{cl} is the average closed time of the channel. But since *in vivo* the closed time τ_{c} is generally much larger than the open time τ_{op}, we have $f_* \approx \tau_{\mathrm{op}}$. With only one type of channel present in a cell, there will be a sigmoidally shaped, Lorentzian noise spectrum with an inflection point at $f = f_*$. With many types of channels for different kinds of ions present it is indeed possible to obtain a $1/f$ spectrum over several decades as the sum of Lorentzians.[89]

To obtain the voltage power spectral density we have to multiply $S_I^{\mathrm{noneq}}(f)$ by R^2, where R represents the electrical resistance of the entire cell membrane. We then have $S_V^{\mathrm{noneq}}(0) \approx 4Ne\langle I\rangle R^2$. The equilibrium Nyquist voltage noise across the same cell membrane is $S_V^{\mathrm{eq}}(f) \approx 4k_{\mathrm{B}}TR$. This is white noise and has the same strength at all frequencies. We thus obtain the following formula at $f = 0$ for the ratio $\theta(0)$ of the nonequilibrium noise and the equilibrium noise:

$$\theta(0) \approx \frac{Ne\langle I\rangle R}{k_{\mathrm{B}}T}. \tag{8.16}$$

The transmembrane current $\langle I\rangle$ is proportional to the cell surface area A. The resistance R is inversely proportional to A. So eventually, the cell surface area and the cell geometry in general, cancel out of the equation.

Data for the steady state Na^+ flux through several types of cell membranes (rat soleus, sheep purkinje, squid axon, guinea pig auricles, frog sartorius) are available.[93] That flux is about 50 pmol/(cm^{2}s). The vast majority of transmembrane ion transport is carried out by Na,K-ATPase which transports 2 K^+ ions for every 3 Na^+ ions. We assume Na^+ and K^+ transport to therefore be about equal. After multiplication by Faraday's constant (the number of Coulombs in a mol, i.e., about 10^5), we get a total current of about $\langle I\rangle \approx 10\ \mu\mathrm{A/cm}^2$. The resistance of a cell membrane varies from $10^3\ \Omega\ \mathrm{cm}^2$ (squid axon) to $7 \times 10^3\ \mathrm{cm}^2$ (mammalian cardiac cell). We thus find for $\theta(0)$ a value of about 5,000.

Based on experimental data, it has been estimated that at 1 Hz the $1/f$ noise in the frog node of Ranvier is about a thousand times larger than thermal noise.[94] This is consistent with our estimate. Experimentally, it turns out that the power spectral density is constant from $f = 0$ up to about somewhere between 1 and 10 Hz.[89,92] At that point the power spectral density starts to fall off as $1/f$. This means that we reach $\theta(f) = 1$, i.e., the equilibrium and nonequilibrium noise being equal, somewhere near 10^4 Hz. Figure 8.5, where the horizontal axis is in radians per second, indeed shows flattening between 10^3 and 10^4 Hz. At the 50- and 60-Hz power line frequencies, the nonequilibrium voltage noise is expected to exceed the equilibrium voltage noise by a factor of at least 10^2.

However, we should pause before taking the value of θ and employ it to incorporate nonequilibrium noise in the evaluation of a signal-to-noise ratio. As we saw earlier in this

Signals, Noise, and Thresholds

section, nonequilibrium noise may be a way to transduce energy from one stored form to another. So a signal can come in the form of a piece of nonequilibrium noise. With this gray area between signal and noise, it may no longer be straightforward to calculate a signal-to-noise ratio.[95] There has been a natural selection toward high signal-to-noise ratios for signals whose detection has been important for the survival of the organism. But what the signal-to-noise ratios and detection thresholds are for ELF and microwave radiation, which are relatively new phenomena in the environment, and how nonequilibrium noise figures in all of this is still open to conjecture and debate.

With the white, Gaussian noise that is associated with equilibrium, the "white" part refers to the power spectrum, i.e., the distribution of the energies over the noise spectrum. Whatever the system is, with white noise and its flat frequency spectrum, most of the noise's energy will be in frequencies that are much larger than the highest characteristic frequency of the system. Because of this, we find that for any timescale Δt that is significant for the system, a noise term $\xi(t)$ at time t is not correlated with $\xi(t + \Delta t)$. With non-white noise this is no longer necessarily the case and correlations do arise.

By looking at non-white noise we did not interfere with the "Gaussian" part, i.e., the noise term $\xi(t)$ at time t still had a Gaussian distribution. Gaussians are natural. The aforementioned Central Limit Theorem[13] guarantees that if X is the cumulative result of many independent stochastic inputs, the distribution for X will be Gaussian. For noise in a bath there generally are many independent stochastic inputs.

As an illustration of the Central Limit Theorem, consider throwing N dice and adding the results. As N gets larger, the resulting distribution will be ever better approximated by a Gaussian centered around $7N/2$. The Gaussian distribution is an attractor and convergence to the Gaussian as N increases is generally fast.

In discussions of the Central Limit Theorem, it is often not mentioned that it only applies when all stochastic inputs have *finite* variance. For many examples in practice this is not the case. Take, for instance, the Gambler's Ruin that was first formulated in the 17th century by Christiaan Huygens. Here we play a simple iterated "heads or tails" game with a fair coin. If the outcome is "heads," you pay one dollar the bank and if the outcome is "tails," the bank pays one dollar to you. The average time after which you have one dollar more in your pocket that you started with is infinite and so is the associated variance. It is effectively because of this that casinos cannot be outsmarted and are guaranteed a profit. Another example is the zero-average Cauchy distribution: $f(x) = 1/(\pi(1 + x^2))$. It is easily verified that this distribution has an infinite variance.

In the early 20th century, mathematicians started to wonder what the equivalent of the attracting Gaussian would be for distributions with an *infinite* variance. The derivations are not trivial, but a result was ultimately derived.[96,97] It is the Lévy distribution, which is also often called the α-stable distribution, that is the attractor for distributions with an infinite variance. There is an analytic formula for this distribution,[98] but it is a complicated expression that involves generalized hypergeometric functions. The associated characteristic function, $\tilde{p}_\alpha(k)$, has a much easier and more intuitive form. For a symmetric, zero-average distribution the result is:

$$\tilde{p}_\alpha(k) \equiv \int p_\alpha(\xi) \exp[ik\xi] \mathrm{d}\xi = \exp\left[-\sigma^\alpha \, |k|^\alpha\right]. \tag{8.17}$$

As is obvious from the formula, the characteristic function strongly resembles a Fourier Transform. In the above formula, σ is a scale parameter and α is the so-called stability index, where $0 < \alpha < 2$. It is readily verified that for $\alpha = 2$ the Gaussian distribution is retrieved and that for $\alpha=1$ we have a Cauchy distribution. An essential feature of the Lévy distribution is the power-law tail, i.e., $p_\alpha(\xi) \propto |\xi|^{-(1+\alpha)}$ for $\xi \to \pm\infty$. The power-law tail contrasts sharply with the exponential tail of the Gaussian. It is commonly referred to as a "fat" tail and it leads to the infinite variance as $\int^\infty p_\alpha(\xi)\xi^2\,d\xi$ diverges for $0 < \alpha < 2$.

The mathematical work of Lévy, Kolmogorov, and many others took on practical significance when, in 1963, Mandelbrot discovered that the day-to-day increments of certain stock prices constitute a Lévy distribution instead of the Gaussian that many had expected.[99] It requires much data and much data processing to discriminate between a Lévy distribution and a Gaussian distribution. It is therefore that the research community did not pick up again on Mandelbrot's approach until the 1990s when desktop computers made storing and processing data easy and fast.

Over the past two decades, it has become clear that Lévy distributions are a signature of nonequilibrium and that they are ubiquitous. Biological systems are by their very nature nonequilibrium and commonly exhibit Lévy noise. It was, for instance, discovered in 1993 that the intervals between subsequent heartbeats are Lévy distributed.[100] Recently, experimentalists have developed the ability to follow displacements of biomolecules in a living cell with the use of quantum dots. Connecting a quantum dot to the cytoskeleton it was shown that such displacements are Lévy distributed and that the Lévy distribution evolved to become a Gaussian as the cell was slowly dying.[101,102]

As is the case for $1/f$ noise, there is no rigorous proof that a system that is out of equilibrium, i.e., an open system that is transferring or transducing energy, exhibits Lévy noise. However, it can be mathematically shown that Lévy noise breaks the essential equilibrium characteristic of microscopic reversibility[103] (microscopic reversibility is the property that every trajectory in the available phase space is traversed as much in the forward as in the backward direction). As a result the aforementioned detailed balance property can be broken. A plethora of experimental results suggests that Lévy noise and the accompanying fat, power-law tails are present whenever a system is out of equilibrium.

The fat, power-law tail of the Lévy distribution implies that "extreme events" (also called "Lévy jumps") are much more likely as compared to the Gaussian distribution with its exponential tail. The infinite variance and the frequency of the extreme events constitute a problem to the experimentalist who is trying to detect or measure the effect of an EM exposure on a biological system. The more "unruly" Lévy noiseband will make it harder to discriminate between biological signal and noise.

8.7 Quantum Noise

The noise that was discussed so far occurs because of an incomplete characterization of the system. Variations in temperature, concentration, etc. are unknown and lead to a margin of error in a measurement. Equilibrium thermal noise happens because most of biology takes place in a liquid environment. It is not computationally practical to characterize all the Brownian trajectories of all the involved particles. However, the effect of a bath that provides a temperature can be well described with averages and distributions. Temperature is simply a measure for the average thermal energy of a particle. Activation barriers of chemical transitions are crossed when an event from the high-energy tail of the Boltzmann distribution delivers sufficient energy.

Signals, Noise, and Thresholds

There is, however, another way to cross an activation barrier. A particle that does not have enough kinetic energy to overcome a potential barrier can nevertheless get across the barrier through the process of "quantum tunneling."[104] Tunneling explains many natural phenomena and has technological applications. The Scanning Tunneling Microscope, for instance, has a sharp conducting tip that scans a surface and records the current of electrons that tunnel through the vacuum between the tip and the surface. Such microscopes allow for the characterization of a surface on a subnanometer scale.[105]

Stochasticity is innate in the theory of quantum mechanics. The state of a system before measurement is represented by a state vector in a Hilbert space. Measurement of a variable A involves the collapse of the state vector onto a vector that is part of the orthogonal basis that corresponds to A. Each vector in the basis corresponds to a different value of A, i.e., a different outcome of the measurement. Only probabilities can be given for what outcome the measurement will yield. Generally, quantum mechanics applies on an atomic scale in a vacuum. The macroscopic scale is a limit where the stochasticity disappears and classical mechanics emerges.

There has been speculation about the extent to which biochemical processes should be described by quantum mechanics. Could an enzyme mediated conversion be more adequately accounted for through quantum mechanics? For a description in terms of quantum mechanics, the enzyme and reactant(s) together would have to be described by a state vector. Going to the product state would involve tunneling through the activation barrier. There is an obvious problem with this picture. In an aqueous bath at room temperature, water and dissolved ions move with speeds of the order of hundreds of meters per second. Molecules, moreover, are tightly packed in such an environment and the mean free path for a moving water molecule is about as large as the molecule itself. Consequently, a water molecule collides about 10^{12} times per second with other molecules. For a complete description, all molecules that enzyme and reactant(s) collide with in the course of a transition should be included in the formulation of a state vector. Next, molecules that collide with molecules that collide with enzyme and reactant(s) need to also be taken into account, etc. In other words, the only valid quantum description would be one of the entire biological system under consideration. There is wide agreement that biology is too wet and too hot for quantum mechanics to apply.[106] It has also been argued that a collision between two molecules implies a collapse of the state vector onto a vector of the basis that corresponds to the variable "position." After all, a collision is only possible if two molecules hit the same position at the same time.[107,108] In this view, a quantum state that entangles biomolecules with each other into one quantum mechanical state vector could never develop and each molecule keeps having a separate position of its own.

Only for a very fast transition where the involved distance is very small is there a possibility of a quantum process. It is in biochemical hydrogen transfer reactions that it has been demonstrated that tunneling is the underlying mechanism. H-transfers occur commonly in biochemical reactions. Calculations indicate that in many such transfers donor and receptor are brought into sufficiently close proximity for the initial and final hydrogen probability density functions to significantly overlap. In such a situation tunneling is likely to occur. Phosphate groups (PO_3) and methyl groups (CH_3) are also commonly transferred in biochemistry, but because of their larger size tunneling has negligible likelihood compared to thermal activation. Through measurement of the kinetic isotope effect, i.e., the ratio of the rate constants for hydrogen and deuterium transfer, experimental validation for tunneling was found.[109–111] Tunneling and thermal agitation predict different values for this ratio.[112] However, in this catalyzed hydrogen transfer, the tunneling, for both hydrogen and deuterium, is a very fast intermediate step. This actual transfer time is much shorter than the time it takes for the biomolecules to thermally sample the conformational space until the active sites arrive at the required proximity.[113] The thermal search is ultimately the rate limiting process for the transfer reaction.

All in all, an approach to biology where chemical activation is thermal and where stochasticity is Brownian in origin has generally been successful.

8.8 Chemical Noise

Chemical noise consists of both fundamental chemical noise (stochastic variations in net or accumulated amounts of a particular ion or molecule) and nonfundamental changes in chemical amount (molecular number) due to influences other than the applied field. We again adopt a recent discussion[12] in which an arbitrary biological system is considered. In the discussion, attention focuses on weakly interacting fields that can create small chemical changes, but much of the approach is also relevant to strongly interacting fields, e.g. those causing cell membrane electroporation (see the Electroporation chapter in this volume). To begin, consider a small physical perturbation of the biological system due to the interaction of a local EM field, $\vec{F}_{local}(\vec{r},t)$, that may vary from site to site within the volume of the biological system. In general, $\vec{F}_{local}$ may have a complicated dependence of its magnitude and direction on time and position, such that a formal prescription for calculating the field-induced molecular change due to an exposure is

$$\bar{n}_S = \int_{t=0}^{t=t_{exp}} \int_{system\ volume} J_0(t') f_{bpm}\left(\vec{F}_{local}(\vec{r},t')\right) dV\, dt'. \tag{8.18}$$

We regard $\bar{n}_S$ as a molecular change signal. It is the primary consequence of the field exposure for the case that only one process, or one step in a cascade, is altered. Integration is carried out over the entire biological system volume and over the time comprising the exposure, t_{exp} (or control). This yields the accumulated, total chemical (molecular) change due to the applied field during the exposure. Other changes in the same ionic or molecular species may result from competing influences, e.g. temperature variations, during t_{exp}.

The applied field interacts through one or more of a limited class of biophysical mechanisms. Here "biophysical mechanism" means a class of interactions by which the field alters an ongoing biochemical rate (transport or reaction), with the rate arising from nonequilibrium processes dependent on metabolism. Examples of known biophysical mechanisms involving electric fields are heating (most biochemical processes have a nonzero temperature dependence), voltage-gated channels, electroconformational coupling of membrane enzymes, electroporation, and iontophoresis (mainly electrophoresis, but in some cases also electroosmosis). Examples involving magnetic fields are radical-pair reactions and twisting of magnetic material (magnetite or contaminant magnetic particles). As used here, a biophysical mechanism modulates an ongoing biochemical process, and both the coupling strength and the magnitude of the basal rate are important.

For a particular type of biophysical mechanism ("bpm"), the function $f_{bpm}\left(\vec{F}_{local}(t)\right)$ describes the instantaneous alteration of the basal rate, J_0, which itself can vary in time.[114] The local field can be computed numerically at the tissue level (mm scale; see Dosimetry chapter in this volume)[115–121] and at the cellular level.[122,123] The time and position dependence of $\vec{F}_{local}(\vec{r},t)$ is often simple, viz. either a constant magnitude (steady or DC field),

Signals, Noise, and Thresholds

a constant amplitude periodic (AC) field, or at high frequencies a spatially decaying-amplitude field due to power absorption. Environmental and occupational fields can be much more complicated, such that piecewise continuous representations may be needed.

If a weakly coupled physical perturbation alters the basal rate of a biochemical process (transport or reaction), the total chemical (molecular) change, expressed as the number of molecules, is

$$\bar{n} = \bar{n}_0 + \bar{n}_S, \tag{8.19}$$

where $\bar{n}_0$ is the basal change during an exposure (sensing) time t_{exp}, and $\bar{n}_S$ is the (much smaller) molecular change due to the field exposure.[23,27,48,114] As noted above, $\bar{n}_S$ can be regarded as a molecular change signal. The basal process is far from equilibrium, driven by free energy differences associated with metabolism. The largest field-induced molecular change occurs for a steady (DC) field exposure,[23,124]

$$\bar{n}_S = K_{bpm,dc} F_0 J_0 t_{exp}, \tag{8.20}$$

where $K_{bpm,dc}$ describes the alteration of the basal rate by the steady field, here of magnitude F_0. Equation (8.20) is the DC version of the case of a weakly coupled periodic perturbation, previously described for the case of an extracellular electric field,[48,114] namely,

$$\bar{n}_S = K_{bpm,ac} F_0^2 J_0 t_{exp}, \tag{8.21}$$

where $K_{bpm,ac}$ describes the coupling that leads to rectification of the ongoing rate.[48] For basal rates with more complicated time dependence Equation (8.18) may need to be evaluated numerically, but the same basic ideas apply. Equation (8.21) is valid for long exposures, involving a large number of cycles of the periodic field. Basal rates that can be altered by weakly interacting EM fields by definition involve small interaction energies, so that thermal fluctuations and chemical free energy differences result in nonzero basal rates. A zero basal rate with an extremely large activation or interaction energy cannot, therefore, be expected to be changed to a measurable nonzero rate by a weakly interacting field.

A generalized, molecular-change-based signal-to-noise ratio can be constructed by estimating the ratio of primary molecular change to the combined competing changes for the same molecular (ionic) species. We consider the simplest case of the field altering the rate at one step in a single pathway, but note that in principle the present analysis can be extended to include multiple steps involving more than one biochemical pathway. We further assume that this biochemical has its rate through the pathway altered slightly by a physical perturbation, here an EM field. But competing influences can also alter the rate. Such influences include temperature variations, normal physiological concentration variations, changes in hormones and other regulating biochemicals, and mechanical perturbations of cells and tissues. Competing molecular changes can also be created by a background EM field, e.g., normal electrical activity within the human body or by movement in the earth's magnetic field, interacting through the same biophysical mechanism. Such competition goes beyond fundamental chemical noise (molecular shot noise). Non-ionizing influences can only modulate ongoing processes, and therefore such influences cannot (essentially by definition) introduce foreign molecules. This has the important consequence that competing molecular changes may arise from several sources (Table 8.1).

TABLE 8.1

Types of Molecular Changes

Symbol	Molecular Change	Source
S	$\bar{n}_S$	Field-induced molecular change signal
N	$\sqrt{\bar{n}} \approx \sqrt{\bar{n}_0}$	Molecular shot noise (fundamental)
V	$\bar{n}_V$	Molecular change due to temperature variations
C	$\bar{n}_C$	Molecular change due to concentration variations
I	$\bar{n}_M$	Molecular change due to mechanical interference
B	$\bar{n}_B$	Molecular change due to background fields

A generalized signal-to-noise ratio, $(S/N)_{gen}$, can thus be considered. The field-induced molecular change signal, S, is thereby quantitatively compared to the several sources of competing molecular changes for the same biochemical (molecule or ion), yielding

$$(S/N)_{gen} = \frac{S}{f_{com}(N,V,C,I,B)}. \tag{8.22}$$

The various competing molecular changes, which may or may not be independent, are combined to give the total competing molecular change, f_{com}. Important simplifications can be made if the various competing molecular changes can be approximated as independent and random around their mean values. In this case f_{com} can be approximated as

$$f_{com}(N,V,C,I,B) \approx [N^2 + V^2 + C^2 + I^2 + B^2]^{\frac{1}{2}}. \tag{8.23}$$

Alternatively, emphasizing the changes in terms of numbers of molecules,

$$f_{com}(N,V,C,I,B) \approx [\bar{n}_0 + (\Delta n_V)^2 + (\Delta n_C)^2 + (\Delta n_M)^2 + (\Delta n_B)^2]^{\frac{1}{2}}. \tag{8.24}$$

All significant sources of competing molecular change are directly relevant.

Consistent with experimental treatment of errors as random, here we consider the important special case that all of the important competing molecular changes can be approximated as independent and random variations around their mean value, as this allows the competing changes to be added in quadrature (Equation (8.23)). This leads to a general molecular-change-based signal-to-noise ratio that involves Gaussian distributions, viz.

$$(S/N)_{gen} \approx \frac{S}{[N^2 + V^2 + C^2 + I^2 + B^2]^{\frac{1}{2}}}. \tag{8.25}$$

Each of these competing molecular changes is discussed briefly below, with reference to Table 8.1.

As indicated in Table 8.1, $N = \sqrt{\bar{n}} \approx \sqrt{\bar{n}_0}$ is the competing molecular change due to fundamental stochastic variations in biochemical reaction and transport processes,[15,23,27,48,114] which provides a fundamental, minimum molecular change noise. Fundamental chemical noise is increasingly recognized as important to understanding other aspects of biological systems, such as the circadian clock,[125,126] control of genetic circuits[127,128] and bacterial chemotaxis.[129]

Signals, Noise, and Thresholds

Temperature variations within the volume of the biological system are generally expected to result in altered rates. When integrated over the system volume and over the exposure time a contribution to the endpoint molecular change is expected, because most biochemical processes have nonzero temperature dependence. Thus, $V = \bar{n}_V$ is the resulting, competing molecular change due to temperature variations.[15] Human core body temperature has daily variations more than 1°C,[130–135] and there are even larger variations in the extremities. Often *in vitro* electric and magnetic field experiments use feedback control, e.g., in temperature-regulated exposure chambers, but these typically have variations greater than about 0.01°C at one or a few temperature measurement sites. Temperature variations within the biological system itself are often inferred, preferably by numerical models that can reasonably predict the temperature through the biological system by first predicting the Specific Absorption Rate (SAR). During the exposure time, interfering temperature variation can be significant. To allow correction for temperature variations, the biological system should be characterized for its temperature sensitivity, and each particular apparatus should be characterized for its temperature variations for control and exposed conditions. As an example, an investigation first reporting a thermal effect[136] was subsequently found to have temperature variation ~0.1°C at temperature measurement sites.[137] Without thermal modeling of the exposure systems and the biological systems, however, larger temperature changes away from the measurement site cannot be ruled out. It is the temperature change and variation over the entire volume containing cells (or other specimens) that needs to be quantitatively understood. Temperature measurement at one site, typically somewhere along the perimeter or boundary of a temperature regulated apparatus, is generally insufficient. The measured biochemical quantity should also be characterized for its temperature sensitivity for the biological system studied, so that the expected V can be determined, to address the basic specificity question of whether an observed change is due to the field or to temperature changes.[138]

Changes in concentration of biochemicals involved in a process are well known to alter the rate of a process. Relevant chemical species include substrates, products, catalysts, inhibitors, etc. The competing molecular change due to one or more interfering concentration changes is $C = \bar{n}_C$. In this case, a significant difference may exist for *in vitro* and *in vivo* experiments. Usually only small, slow changes of chemical concentrations are expected *in vitro*, occurring, for example, through absorption or release of molecules (ions) from glass- and plasticware, spontaneous chemical decomposition, binding to cellular constituents, or through evaporation. Uptake or release of interfering biochemicals from a biological preparation could be the predominant source, particularly if cells grow (taking up molecules) or die (releasing molecules). *In vivo* concentration variations are relatively large, due to normal physiologic variations. For example, Ca^{2+} concentration varies in humans by more than 1% over a day.[139,140] Unless buffered, these normal biochemical variations also compete with the field-induced molecular change.

Movement of tissue *in vivo* and vibration of an experimental apparatus containing a biological system can also create mechanically induced molecular change, $I = \bar{n}_M$, that competes with a molecular change signal. In this case, the competing molecular change is due to interference of mechanical stress and strain,[141,142] often present at high levels in living humans,[11,143,144] but present also at low levels for *in vitro* experiments. *In vitro* apparatus can have quite different mechanical properties and isolation from ambient vibrations. Indeed, it has been found in some experiments that mechanical vibrations create effects larger than the field exposure.[145] Tissues *in vivo* experience significant mechanical deformation, but there is the least strain expected within bone marrow and the brain.[142] This may be relevant to the "contact current hypothesis" that suggests that currents in bone marrow may be important in exposures of children.[146–148]

290 *Electromagnetic Fields*

Background fields can, of course, also couple to biochemical processes through the same biophysical mechanisms as the applied field. Background field-induced molecular change competes, and is denoted by $B = \bar{n}_B$. Examples of background EM fields include the endogenous electrical fields generated within the body by cardiac, muscular, and neural activity, and the sampling of different field values (local anomalies) in the ambient magnetic field as mobile humans move about in their environment. *In vitro*, background fields will depend on the particular experimental environment, are usually small and constant, and are often measured.

8.9 Interpretation of Experiments

Specificity is fundamentally important to interpret experiments, as one wants to know what agent is responsible for the observed change(s). This is particularly relevant to experiments which find small changes in biological systems that are exposed to small EM fields. A basic challenge is to show that other influences are not responsible. Because it is well known that most biochemical processes have a significant temperature dependence, the approximate temperature sensitivity of the observed quantity should be determined or known, and some bound should be established for temperature drift or variations in the experiment. However, as already noted, even big changes can have more than one candidate cause. Both tissue electroporation and tissue movement can, for instance, underlie the changes in molecular uptake associated with large field pulses. For this reason, signal-to-noise ratio considerations should be preceded by establishing field specificity, which can be much more difficult than observing a change associated with a field exposure. To establish specificity, a number of issues must be considered, many of which will be discussed next.

Many experiments determine quantities related to biochemical change. Exceptions are experiments that determine physical quantities such as voltages and currents, temperature changes, and magnetic particle rotation. Electrical measurements are the most frequent physical measurement. These are incredibly important to systems of excitable cells, with experimental preparations ranging from isolated cells to electrophysiologic measurements on humans. Accumulation of charge might be measured, but then probably as a voltage on a capacitance. Signal-to-noise ratio issues are still important, of course, but usually there is an important distinction: voltages and currents (rarely charge) are readily measured continuously.

A further distinction is that most experiments involving exposures to small fields use long exposure times (many seconds to hours or even days). Such experiments commonly determine biochemical quantities directly, e.g., enzyme activity, or indirectly, e.g., fluorescence emission from fluorescent indicators of intracellular calcium concentration. In this broad case, consideration of generalized chemical noise is relevant. Following the discussion in a recent paper,[12] both the magnitude of the field perturbation, and the nature and magnitude of chemical competition need to be understood. Such analysis should explicitly estimate the coupling to ongoing, far from equilibrium, metabolically driven biochemical processes, and should quantitatively determine molecular changes due to competing influences. Only then can the analysis distinguish idealized conditions from *in vitro* conditions and *in vivo* conditions and then determine whether reported effects can be explained by known biophysical mechanisms.

In vivo there are several kinds of noise and it is important to distinguish between them. Equilibrium noise comes about as a consequence of Brownian motion, i.e., the random movement of molecules at finite temperature. At equilibrium every degree of freedom

Signals, Noise, and Thresholds

takes on the same amount of energy and equilibrium noise is therefore easy to evaluate. For a signal to exceed the equilibrium noise band, the quantitative criteria are often readily derived. Such baseline criteria can be useful when assessing the electroreception and magnetoreception that many organisms exhibit. But the nonequilibrium nature of life brings in nonequilibrium noise. When a primary molecular change is amplified through a biochemical cascade, "amplifier noise" is inevitable. Nonequilibrium noise appears whenever energy is dissipated, i.e., when work is done. In many biological contexts, the nonequilibrium noise is much more intense than the equilibrium noise. A serious complication is constituted by the fact that nonequilibrium noise, unlike equilibrium noise, is also able to perform work, i.e., be a power source for an energetically uphill process. Many biological processes may rely on the energy transduction that can be accomplished through nonequilibrium noise. The analysis of such situations poses challenges as the noise may be a signal and the signal may be noise. There is no easy general "common denominator" theory for nonequilibrium noise like there is for equilibrium $k_B T$-noise.

In a recent discussion,[12] it is argued that experimental measurements can be plausibly related quantitatively to an underlying primary molecular change due to a field exposure operating through a biophysical mechanism. It is further argued there that only the uncertainty in this change propagates through biochemical amplification and therefore dominates the measurement uncertainty. A more complete approach would involve traditional, independent determination of the instrumental or assay error (quantitative characterization of the experimental measurement system). After removal of the "instrumental noise," the generalized signal-to-noise ratio $(S/N)_{gen}$, could be revised upwards. This would allow interpretation (correction) of experimental error to estimate the uncertainty in the measured quantity itself. Assessment of combinations of biophysical mechanism models and particular exposure can then be carried out, using the most field-sensitive versions of theoretical models for the candidate biophysical mechanisms. The criterion $(S/N) \leq 0.1$ is a very conservative basis for ruling out a particular class of biophysical mechanism for a given field exposure. Similarly, the criterion $(S/N)_{gen} \geq 10$ is a conservative basis for ruling in a candidate biophysical mechanism for a given exposure, retaining that biophysical mechanism hypothesis for further evaluation. This approach provides a quantitative basis for rejecting or accepting hypothetical biophysical mechanisms as candidate explanations for an experimental measurement.

The traditional choice $(S/N)_{gen} \approx 1$ is a useful but somewhat arbitrary dividing line, which indicates conditions for which an effect might appear. The $(S/N)_{gen} \leq 0.1$ and $(S/N)_{gen} \geq 10$ provide criteria for stronger conclusions, allowing rejection or provisional retention of a biophysical mechanism hypothesis. This approach to interpreting experiments thus provides a general method for carrying out theoretical assessment of reported weak field exposures effects. This approach can distinguish relatively quiet *in vitro* conditions from *in vivo* conditions containing more and larger influences of competing molecular change. This in turn allows quantitative estimates of whether an *in vitro* result is relevant to *in vivo* conditions.

Acknowledgments

We wish to thank all of our many colleagues for numerous discussions. Due to space limitations we have been able to cite only some of their many published contributions. M. Bier is particularly grateful to Adam Offenbacher for the feedback on the section about quantum noise.

References

1. G.N. Stewart. The charges produced by the growth of bacteria in the molecular concentration and electrical conductivity of culture media. *J. Exp. Med.*, 4:235–243, 1899.
2. R. Firstenberg-Eden and G. Eden. *Impedance Microbiology*. Research Studies Press, Letchworth, Hertfordshire, UK, 1985.
3. M. Wawerla, A. Stolle, B. Schalch, and H. Eisgruber. Impedance microbiology: Applications in food hygiene. *J. Food Prot.*, 62:1488–1496, 1999.
4. J. McPhillips and N. Snow. Studies of milk with a new type of conductivity cell. *Aust. J. Dairy Technol.*, 3:192–196, 1958.
5. T. Ritz, P. Thalau, J.B. Phillips, R. Wiltschko, and W. Wiltschko. Resonance effects indicate a radical-pair mechanism for avian magnetic compass. *Nature*, 429:177–180, 2004.
6. D. Cohen. Ferromagnetic contaminants in the lungs and other organs of the body. *Science*, 180:745–748, 1973.
7. J. L. Kirschvink, A. K. Kirschvink, and B. J. Woodford. Magnetite biomineralization in the human brain. *Proc. Nat. Acad. Sci.*, 89:7683–7687, 1992.
8. J. R. Dunn, M. Fuller, J. Zoeger, J. Dobson, F. Heller, J. Hammann, E. Caine, and B. M. Moskowitz. Magnetic material in the human hippocampus. *Brain Res. Bull.*, 36:149–153, 1994.
9. P.L. McNeil and S. Ito. Molecular traffic through plasma membrane disruptions of cells. *In Vivo J. Cell Sci.*, 96:549–556, 1990.
10. P.L. McNeil and R.A. Steinhardt. Loss, restoration, and maintenance of plasma membrane integrity. *J. Cell Biol.*, 137:1–4, 1997.
11. P.L. McNeil and M. Terasaki. Coping with the inevitable: How cells repair a torn surface membrane. *Nat. Cell Biol.*, 3:124–129, 2001.
12. T.E. Vaughan and J.C. Weaver. Molecular change signal-to-noise criteria for interpreting experiments involving exposure of biological systems to weakly interacting electromagnetic fields. *Bioelectromagnetics*, 26:305–322, 2005.
13. N.G. van Kampen. *Stochastic Processes in Physics and Chemistry*. Elsevier, Amsterdam, 1992.
14. R.C. Duncan, R.G. Knapp, and M.C. Miller. *Introductory Biostatistics for the Health Sciences*. John Wiley & Sons, New York, 1983.
15. J. C. Weaver, T. E. Vaughan, and G. T. Martin. Biological effects due to weak electric and magnetic fields: The temperature variation threshold. *Biophys. J.*, 76:3026–3030, 1999.
16. J. C. Weaver. Understanding conditions for which biological effects of nonionizing electromagnetic fields can be expected. *Bioelectrochemistry*, 56:207–209, 2002.
17. C.W. Helstrom. *Statistical Theory of Signal Detection*. Pergamon Press, New York, 1968.
18. A.J. Kalmijn. Electro-perception in sharks and rays. *Nature*, 212:1232–1233, 1966.
19. A.J. Kalmijn. Electric and magnetic field detection in elasmobranch fishes. *Science*, 218:916–918, 1982.
20. R. Douglas Fields. The shark's electric sense. *Sci. Am*, 297(2):75–81, 2007.
21. W.J. Moore. *Physical Chemistry*. Longman, London, 1972.
22. A.J. Kalmijn. Graded positive feedback in elasmobranch ampullae of lorenzini. In S.M. Bezrukov, editor, *Unsolved problems of Noise and Fluctuations: UPoN 2002: Third International Conferenceroblems of noise and fluctuations: UPoN 2002: Third International Conference*, volume 665, pages 133–141, Melville, NY, 2003. American Institute of Physics.
23. R.K. Adair, R.D. Astumian, and J.C. Weaver. On the detection of weak electric fields by sharks, rays and skates. *Chaos*, 8:576–587, 1998.
24. S.M. Bezrukov. Sensing nature's electric fields: ion channels as active elements of linear amplification. In S.M. Bezrukov, editor, *Unsolved Problems of Noise and Fluctuations: UPoN 2002: Third International Conference*, volume 665, pages 142–149, Melville, NY, 2003. American Institute of Physics.
25. T. Ritz, S. Adem, and K. Schulten. A model for photoreceptor-based magnetoreception in birds. *Biophys. J.*, 78:707–718, 2000.

Signals, Noise, and Thresholds

26. R. Wiltschko and W. Wiltschko. Sensing magnetic directions in birds: Radical pair processes involving cryptochrome. *Biosensors*, 4:221–242, 2014.
27. J.C. Weaver, T.E. Vaughan, and R.D. Astumian. Biological sensing of small field differences by magnetically sensitive chemical reactions. *Nature*, 405:707–709, 2000.
28. R. Blakemore. Magnetotactic bacteria. *Science*, 190:377–379, 1975.
29. R.P. Blakemore. Magnetotactic bacteria. *Ann. Rev. Microbiol.*, 36:217–238, 1982.
30. J.L. Kirschvink, M.M. Walker, and C.E. Diebel. Magnetite-based magnetoreception. *Curr. Opin. Neurobiol.*, 11:462–467, 2001.
31. V.N. Binhi. Stochastic dynamics of magnetosomes and a mechanism of biological orientation in the geomagnetic field. *Bioelectromagnetics*, 27:58–63, 2006.
32. M.M. Walker, T.E. Dennis, and J.L. Kirschvink. The magnetic sense and its use in long-distance navigation by animals. *Curr. Opin. Neurobiol.*, 12:735– 744, 2002.
33. National Institute of Environmental Health Sciences (NIEHS). NIEHS report on health effects from exposure to power-line frequency electric and magnetic fields. Technical Report 99-4493, NIH, 1999.
34. R. K. Adair. Effects of ELF magnetic fields on biological magnetite. *Bioelectromagnetics*, 14:1–4, 1993.
35. C. Polk. Effects of ELF fields on biological magnetite: Limitations on physical models. *Bioelectromagnetics*, 15:261–270, 1994.
36. K.R. Foster and H.P. Schwan. Dielectric properties of tissues and biological materials: A critical review. *CRC Crit. Rev. Biomed. Eng.*, 17:25–104, 1989.
37. R.K. Adair. Constraints on biological effects of weak extremely-low-frequency electromagnetic fields. *Phys. Rev. A*, 43:1039–1048, 1991.
38. J.B. Johnson. Thermal agitation of electricity in conductors. *Phys. Rev.*, 32:97–109, 1928.
39. H. Nyquist. Thermal agitation of electric charge in conductors. *Phys. Rev.*, 32:110–113, 1928.
40. W. Schottky. Über spontane Stromschwankungen in verschiedenen Elektrizit¨atsleitern. *Ann. Phys. (Leipzig)*, 57:541–568, 1918.
41. R. Sarpeshkar, T. Delbru¨ck, and C.A. Mead. White noise in MOS transistors and resistors. *IEEE Circuits and Devices*, 9(6): 23–29, 1993.
42. M. Bier. Gauging the strength of power frequency electric fields against membrane electrical noise. *Bioelectromagnetics*, 26:595–609, 2005.
43. B. Hille. Ionic *Channels of Excitable Membranes*, 2nd Edition. Sinauer Associates, Sunderland, 1992.
44. P. Läuger. *Electrogenic Ion Pumps*. Sinauer Associates, Sunderland, MA, 1991.
45. J.C. Weaver and R.D. Astumian. The response of cells to very weak electric fields: The thermal noise limit. *Science*, 247:459–462, 1990.
46. W.T. Kaune. Thermal noises limit on the sensitivity of cellular membranes to power frequency electric and magnetic fields. *Bioelectromagnetics*, 23:622– 628, 2002.
47. G. Vincze, N. Szasz, and A. Szasz. On the thermal noise limit of cellular membranes. *Bioelectromagnetics*, 26:28–35, 2005.
48. R.D. Astumian, J.C. Weaver, and R.K. Adair. Rectification and signal averaging of weak electric fields by biological cells. *Proc. Nat. Acad. Sci.*, 92:3740–3743, 1995.
49. L. Brillouin. Can the rectifier become a thermodynamical demon? *Phys. Rev.*, 78:627–628, 1950.
50. P.W. Bridgman. Note on the principle of detailed balancing. *Phys. Rev.*, 31:101–102, 1928.
51. R.C. Tolman. The principle of microscopic reversibility. *Proc. Natl. Acad. Sci. USA*, 11:436–439, 1925.
52. M. von Smoluchowski. Experimentell nachweisbare, der üblichen Thermodynamik widersprechenden Molekularphänomene. *Physikalische Zeitschrift*, 13:1069–1080, 1912.
53. R.P. Feynman, R.B. Leighton, and M. Sands. *The Feynman Lectures on Physics*. Addison–Wesley, Reading, MA, 1966.
54. P.W. Atkins. *The Second Law*. Scientific American Books, New York, 1984.
55. H.S. Leff and A.F. Rex, editors. *Maxwell's Demon: Entropy, Information, Computing*. Princeton University Press, Princeton, NJ, 1990.

56. J. Howard and A.J. Hudspeth. Compliance of the hair bundle associated with gating of mechanoelectrical transduction channels in the bullfrog's saccular hair cell. *Neuron*, 1:189–199, 1988.

57. M. Magnasco. Forced thermal ratchets. *Phys. Rev. Lett.*, 71:1477–1480, 1993.

58. M. Bier. Brownian ratchets in physics and biology. *Contemp. Phys.*, 38:371–379, 1997.

59. R.D. Astumian and M. Bier. Fluctuation driven ratchets: Molecular motors. *Phys. Rev. Lett.*, 72:1766–1769, 1994.

60. R.D. Astumian. Thermodynamics and kinetics of a brownian motor. *Science*, 276:917–922, 1997.

61. M. Bier and R.D. Astumian. Biased brownian motion as the operating principle for microscopic engines. *Bioelectrochem. Bioenerget.*, 39:67–75, 1996.

62. I. Kosztin and K. Schulten. Fluctuation-driven molecular transport through an asymmetric membrane channel. *Phys. Rev. Lett.*, 93:238102, 2004.

63. Z. Siwy, I.D. Kosińska, and A. Fuliński. On the validity of continuous modelling of ion transport through nanochannels. *Europhys. Lett.*, 67:683–689, 2004.

64. Z. Siwy, I.D. Kosińska, A. Fuliński, and C.R. Martin. Asymmetric diffusion through synthetic nanopores. *Phys. Rev. Lett.*, 94:048102, 2005.

65. Z. Siwy and A. Fuliński. Fabrication of a synthetic nanopore ion pump. *Phys. Rev. Lett.*, 89:198103, 2002.

66. J. Bernamont. Fluctuations in the resistance of thin films. *Proc. Phys. Soc.*, 49:138–139, 1937.

67. B. Pellegrini, R. Saletti, P. Terreni, and M. Prudenziati. $1/f^\gamma$ noise in thick-film resistors as an effect of tunnel and thermally activated emissions, from measures versus frequency and temperature. *Phys. Rev. B*, 27:1233–1243, 1983.

68. J.B. Bassingthwaighte, L.S. Liebovitch, and B.J. West. *Fractal Physiology*. Oxford University Press, New York, 1994.

69. C. Wunsch. Bermuda sea level in relation to tides, weather, and baroclinic fluctuations. *Rev. Geophys.*, 10:1–49, 1972.

70. M. Dishon-Berkovits and R. Berkovits. Work-related tardiness: Lateness incident distribution and long-range correlations. *Fractals*, 5:321–324, 1997.

71. P. Bak, C. Tang, and K. Wiesenfeld. Self-organized criticality: An explanation of $1/f$ noise. *Phys. Rev. Lett.*, 59:381–384, 1987.

72. P. Bak. *How Nature Works*. Springer-Verlag, New York, 1996.

73. S. Kauffman. *Investigations*. Oxford University Press, 2000.

74. B.D. Malamud, G. Morein, and D.L. Turcotte. Forest fires: An example of self-organized critical behavior. *Science*, 281:1840–1842, 1998.

75. H.M. Jaeger, C. Liu, and S.R. Nagel. Relaxation at the angle of repose. *Phys. Rev. Lett.*, 62:40–43, 1989.

76. S.R. Nagel. Instabilities in a sandpile. *Rev. Mod. Phys.*, 64:321–325, 1992.

77. M. Bretz, J.B. Cunningham, P.L. Kurczynski, and F. Nori. Imaging of avalanches in granular materials. *Phys. Rev. Lett.*, 69:2431–2434, 1992.

78. J.G. Nicholls, A.R. Martin, and B.G. Wallace. *From Neuron to Brain*, 3rd edition. Sinauer Associates, Sunderland, MA, 1992.

79. H.E. Derksen and A.A. Verveen. Fluctuations of resting neural membrane potential. *Science*, 151:1388–1389, 1966.

80. H.E. Derksen. Axon membrane voltage fluctuations. *Acta Physiol. Pharmacol. Neerl.*, 12:373–466, 1965.

81. H.E. Derksen and A.A. Verveen. Fluctuations in membrane potential of axons and the problem of coding. *Kybernetik*, 2:152–160, 1965.

82. D. Colquhoun and A.G. Hawkes. On the stochastic properties of bursts of single ion channel openings and of clusters of bursts. *Philos. Trans. R. Soc. Lond. B Biol. Sci.*, 300:1–59, 1982.

83. S.B. Silberberg and K.L. Magleby. Preventing errors when estimating single channel properties from the analysis of current fluctuations. *Biophys. J.*, 65:1570–1584, 1993.

84. D. Colquhoun, C. Hatton, and A.G. Hawkes. The quality of maximum likelihood estimation of ion channel rate constants. *J. Physiol. (Lond.)*, 547:699–728, 2003.

85. L.S. Liebovitch, J. Fishbarg, and J.P. Koniarek. Ion channel kinetics: A model based on fractal scaling rather than multistate Markov processes. *Math. Biosci.*, 84:37–68, 1987.
86. L.S. Liebovitch. Analysis of fractal ion gating kinetics: kinetic rates, energy levels, and activation energies. *Math. Biosci.*, 93:97–115, 1989.
87. L.S. Liebovitch. Testing fractal and Markov models of ion channel kinetics. *Biophys. J.*, 55:373–385, 1989.
88. I. Goychuk and P. Hänggi. Fractional diffusion modeling of ion channel kinetics. *Phys. Rev. E*, 70:051915, 2004.
89. K. Diba, H.A. Lester, and C. Koch. Intrinsic noise in cultured hippocampal neurons: Experiment and modeling. *J. Neurosci.*, 24:9723–9733, 2004.
90. S. Bezrukov and M. Winterhalter. Examining noise sources at the single molecule level: $1/f$ noise of an open maltoporin channel. *Phys. Rev. Lett.*, 85:202–205, 2002.
91. Z. Siwy and A. Fulinński. Origin of $1/f^\alpha$ noise in membrane channel currents. *Phys. Rev. Lett.*, 89:158101, 2002.
92. L.J. DeFelice. *Introduction to Membrane Noise*. Plenum Press, New York, 1981.
93. O.M. Sejersted. Maintenance of Na,K-homeostasis by Na,K-pumps in striated muscle. *Prog. Clin. Biol. Res.*, 268(B):195–206, 1988.
94. F.S. Barnes. Interaction of DC and ELF electric fields with biological materials and systems. In C. Polk and E. Postow, editors, *Handbook of Biological Effects of Electromagnetic Fields*, pages 103–147. CRC Press, Boca Raton, FL, 1996.
95. M. Bier. How to evaluate the electric noise in a cell membrane? *Acta Phys. Pol. B*, 37(5): 1409–1424, 2006.
96. P. Lévy. *Calcul des Probabilités*. Gauthier-Vollars, Paris, 1925.
97. B.V. Gnedenko and A.N. Kolmogorov. *Limit Distributions for Sums of Random Variables*. Addison-Wesley, Cambridge, MA, 1954.
98. K. Górska and K.A. Penson. Lévy stable two-sided distributions: Exact and explicit densities for asymmetric case. *Phys. Rev. E*, 83:061125, 2011.
99. B. Mandelbrot. The variation of certain speculative prices. *J. Bus.*, 36:394–419, 1963.
100. C.-K. Peng, J. Mietus, J.M. Hausdorff, S. Havlin, H.E. Stanley, and A.L. Goldberger. Long-range anticorrelations and non-gaussian behavior of the heartbeat. *Phys. Rev. Lett.*, 70:1343–1346, 1993.
101. B. Stuhrmann, M. Soares e Silva, F.C. MacKintosh, and G.H. Koenderink. Nonequilibrium fluctuations of a remodeling in vitro cytoskeleton. *Phys. Rev. E*, 86:020901, 2012.
102. M. Soares e Silva, B. Stuhrmann, T. Betz, and G.H. Koenderink. Time-resolved microrheology of actively remodeling actomyosin networks. *New J. Phys*, 16:075010, 2014.
103. Ł. Kuśmierz, A. Chechkin, E. Gudowska-Nowak, and M. Bier. Breaking microscopic reversibility with Lévy flights. *Europhys. Lett.*, 114:60009, 2016.
104. S. Gasiorowicz. *Quantum Physics*, 3rd edition. Wiley & Sons, Hoboken, NJ, 2003.
105. C.J. Chen. *Introduction to Scanning Tunneling Microscopy*. Oxford University Press, New York, 1993.
106. M. Tegmark. Importance of quantum decoherence in brain processes. *Phys. Rev. E*, 61:4194–4206, 2000.
107. W.H. Zurek. Reduction of the wavepacket: How long does it take? In G.T. Moore and M.O. Scully, editors, *Frontiers of Nonequilibrium Statistical Physics*, volume 135 of *NATO ASI Series (Series B: Physics)*, pages 145–149. Springer, Boston, MA, 1986.
108. W.G. Unruh and W.H. Zurek. Reduction of a wave packet in quantum brownian motion. *Phys. Rev. D*, 40:1071–1049, 1989.
109. Y. Cha, C.J. Murray, and J.P. Klinman. Hydrogen tunneling in enzyme reactions. *Science*, 243:1325–1330, 1989.
110. J. Basran, M.J. Sucliffe, and N.S. Scrutton. Enzymatic H-transfer requires vibration-driven extreme tunneling. *Biochem.*, 38:3218–3222, 1999.
111. M.J. Knapp, K. Rickert, and J.P. Klinman. Temperature-dependent isotope effects in soybean lipoxygenase-1: correlating hydrogen tunneling with protein dynamics. *J. Am. Chem. Soc.*, 124:3865–3874, 2002.

112. A.V. Soudackov and S. Hammes-Schiffer. Proton-coupled electron transfer reactions: Analytical rate constants and case study of kinetic isotope effects in lipoxygenase. *Faraday Discuss.*, 195:171–189, 2016.
113. J.P. Klinman and A. Kohen. Hydrogen tunneling links protein dynamics to enzyme catalysis. *Annu. Rev. Biochem.*, 82:471–496, 2013.
114. J. C. Weaver, T. E. Vaughan, R. K. Adair, and R. D. Astumian. Theoretical limits on the threshold for the response of long cells to weak ELF electric fields due to ionic and molecular flux rectification. *Biophys. J.*, 75:2251–2254, 1998.
115. M. Stuchly and T. Dawson. Interaction of low-frequency electric and magnetic fields with the human body. *Proc. IEEE*, 88:643–662, 2000.
116. M. A. Stuchly and O. P. Gandhi. Inter-laboratory comparison of numerical dosimetry for human exposure to 60 Hz electric and magnetic fields. *Bioelectromagnetics*, 21:167–174, 2000.
117. P.A. Mason, W.D. Hurt, T.J. Walters, J.A. D'Andrea, P. Gajsek, K.I. Ryan, D.A. Nelson, K.I. Smith, and J.M. Ziriax. Effects of frequency, permittivity and voxel size on predicted specific absorption rate values in biological tissue during electromagnetic-field exposure. *IEEE Trans. Microwave Theory Technol.*, 48:2050–2058, 2000.
118. P. Gajsek, T. J. Walters, W. D. Hurt, D. A. Nelson, and P. A. Mason. Empirical validation of SAR values predicted by FDTD modeling. *Bioelectromagnetics*, 23:37–48, 2002.
119. M. Nadeem, T. Thorlin, O. P. Gandhi, and M. Persson. Computation of electric and magnetic stimulation in human head using the 3-D impedance method. *IEEE Trans. Biomed. Eng.*, 50:900–907, 2003.
120. T.W. Dawson, K. Caputa, M.A. Stuchly, and R. Kavet. Comparison of electric fields induced in humans and rodents by 60-Hz contact currents. *IEEE Trans. Biomed. Eng.*, 50:744–753, 2003.
121. S. J. Allen, E. R. Adair, K. S. Mylacraine, W. Hurt, and J. Ziriax. Empirical and theoretical dosimetry in support of whole body radio frequency (RF) exposure in seated human volunteers at 220 MHz. *Bioelectromagnetics*, 26:440–447, 2005.
122. T.R. Gowrishankar and J.C. Weaver. An approach to electrical modeling of single and multiple cells. *Proc. Nat. Acad. Sci.*, 100:3203–3208, 2003.
123. D.A. Stewart, T.R. Gowrishankar, and J.C. Weaver. Transport lattice approach to describing cell electroporation: Use of a local asymptotic model. *IEEE Trans. Plasma Sci.*, 32:1696–1708, 2004.
124. P.C. Gailey. Membrane potential and time required for detection of weak signals by voltage-gated ion channels. *Bioelectromagnetics*, 20:102–109, 1999.
125. N. Barkai and S. Leibler. Biological rhythms: Circadian clocks limited by noise. *Nature*, 403:267–268, 2000.
126. M.B. Elowitz and S. Leibler. A synthetic oscillatory network. *Nature*, 403:335–338, 2000.
127. T.S. Gardner, C.R. Cantor, and J.J. Collins. Construction of a genetic toggle switch in *Escherichia coli*. *Nature*, 403:339–342, 2000.
128. A. Becksei and L. Serrano. Engineering stability in gene networks by autoregulation. *Nature*, 405:590–593, 2000.
129. T.S. Shimizu, S.V. Aksenov, and D. Bray. A spatially extended stochastic model of the bacterial chemotaxis signalling pathway. *J. Mol. Biol.*, 329:291–309, 2003.
130. H.T. Hammel. Regulation of internal body temperature. *Ann. Rev. Physiol.*, 30:641–710, 1968.
131. S.A. Rubin. Core temperature regulation of heart rate during exercise in humans. *J. Appl. Physiol.*, 62:1997–2002, 1987.
132. W.R. Keatinge, A.C. Mason, C.E. Millard, and C.G. Newstead. Effects of fluctuating skin temperature on thermoregulatory responses in man. *J. Physiol.*, 378:241–252, 1986.
133. K. Shiraki, S. Sagawa, F. Tajima, A. Yokota, H. Hashimoto, and G.L. Brengelmann. Independence of brain and tympanic temperatures in an unanesthesized human. *J. Appl. Physiol.*, 65:482–486, 1988.
134. P. Webb. Temperatures of skin, subcutaneous tissue, muscle and core in resting men in cold, comfortable and hot conditions. *Eur. J. Appl. Physiol.*, 64:471–476, 1992.
135. R.K. Adair. Biophysical limits on athermal effects of RF and microwave radiation. *Bioelectromagnetics*, 24:39–48, 2003.

136. D. de Pomerai, C. Daniells, H. David, J. Allan, I. Duce, M. Mutwakil, D. Thomas, P. Sewell, J. Tattersall, D. Jones, and P. Candido. Non-thermal heat-shock response to microwaves. *Nature*, 405:417–418, 2000.

137. D.I. de Pomerai, B. Smith, A. Dawe, K. North, T. Smith, D.B. Archer, I.R. Duce, D. Jones, and E.P.M. Candido. Microwave radiation can alter protein conformation without bulk heating. *FEBS Lett.*, 543:93–97, 2003.

138. Y.L. Zhao, P.G. Johnson, G.P. Jahreis, and S.W. Hui. Increased DNA synthesis in INIT/10T$_{1/2}$ cells after exposure to a 60 Hz magnetic field: A magnetic-field or a thermal effect? *Radiat. Res.*, 151:201–208, 1999.

139. B. Morrison, A. Shenkin, A. McLelland, D.A. Robertson, M. Barrowman, S. Graham, G. Wuga, and K.J. Cunningham. Intra-individual variation in commonly analyzed serum constituents. *Clin. Chem.*, 25:1799–1805, 1979.

140. M.G. Weyer and H. Lommel. *LONG I: Eine Longitudinal-Studie über individuelle Normbereiche, individuelle Standardbereiche, statistische Normbereiche für Prävention und Früherkennung*. Verlag Kirchheim, Mainz, 1981.

141. T.E. Vaughan and J.C. Weaver. Energetic constraints on the creation of cell membrane pores by magnetic particles. *Biophys. J.*, 71:616–622, 1996.

142. T.E. Vaughan and J.C. Weaver. Molecular change due to biomagnetic stimulation and transient magnetic fields: Mechanical interference constraints on possible effects by cell membrane pore creation via magnetic particles. *Bioelectrochem. Bioenerget.*, 46:121–128, 1998.

143. P.L. McNeil. Cell wounding and healing. *Am. Sci.*, 79:222–235, 1991.

144. D. Bansal, K. Miyake, S.S. Vogel, S. Groh, C.C. Chen, R. Williamson, P.L. McNeil, and K.P. Campbell. Defective membrane repair in dysferlin-deficient muscular dystrophy. *Nature* 423: 168–172, 2003.

145. U. Valtersson, K. Hansson Mild, and M.-O. Mattsson. Uncharacterized physical parameters can contribute more than magnetic field exposure to ODC activity in vitro. In F. Bersani, editor, *Electricity and Magnetism in Biology and Medicine*, pages 449–452. Plenum Press, New York, 1999.

146. R. Kavet, L. Zaffanella, J. Gaigle, and K. Ebi. The possible role of contact current in cancer risk associated with residential magnetic fields. *Bioelectromagnetics*, 21:538–553, 2000.

147. R. Kavet, L.E. Zaffenella, R.L. Pearson, and J. Dallaplazza. Association of residential magnetic fields with contact voltages. *Bioelectromagnetics*, 25:530–536, 2004.

148. R. Kavet. Contact current hypothesis: Summary of results to date. *Bioelectromagnetics*, 26 Suppl. 7:S75–S85, 2005.

9

Computational Methods for Predicting Electromagnetic Fields and Temperature Increase in Biological Bodies

James C. Lin
University of Illinois

CONTENTS

9.1 Introduction 300
    9.1.1 Induced Field and Dosimetric Quantities 301
    9.1.2 Characterizing EMFs 302
9.2 Fundamental Interactions 304
    9.2.1 Thick Tissue Layers 304
    9.2.2 Multiple Layers of Tissue 306
    9.2.3 Spheroidal Models 310
9.3 Computation Algorithms 315
    9.3.1 The Quasi-Static Impedance Method 315
    9.3.2 The Volume Integral Equation MoM 316
    9.3.3 The SMoM 317
    9.3.4 The FEM 318
    9.3.5 The FDTD Method 319
        9.3.5.1 The Traditional FDTD Method 319
        9.3.5.2 Frequency-Dependent FDTD Formulation 321
9.4 Anatomically Realistic Body Models 322
    9.4.1 Cubic Cell Models 322
    9.4.2 Millimeter-Resolution Model Based on MRI Scans................................323
    9.4.3 The Visible Human Model 323
    9.4.4 Anatomical Family Computer Models 324
9.5 Applications of Anatomically Realistic Computer Models 325
    9.5.1 Currents Induced in the Human Body by Low-Frequency EMFs.................325
        9.5.1.1 Electric Blankets 325
        9.5.1.2 Power Transmission Lines 330
    9.5.2 Absorption in Human Bodies Exposed to Far-Field of RF Sources 333
        9.5.2.1 SAR Induced in Cubic Cell Models 333
        9.5.2.2 SAR in Fine Resolution Anatomical Models............................337
        9.5.2.3 Human Exposure to the Field Radiated by BTS Antennas................341
        9.5.2.4 Human Exposure to the Fields Produced By Coexisting Antenna Systems.................344
        9.5.2.5 Coupling of EM Pulses into the Human Body 345
        9.5.2.6 Absorption in the Head of Cell Phone Users...........................348

| | | 9.5.2.7 | Absorption in Human Body Exposed to Near-Field MRI Source ..... 353 |
9.6 | Temperature Elevations Induced in Biological Tissues by EM Power Deposition...... 359
    9.6.1   Introduction..359
    9.6.2   The Bio-Heat Equation 360
        9.6.2.1   Initial Conditions 361
        9.6.2.2   Boundary Conditions...362
    9.6.3   Thermoregulatory Responses..363
    9.6.4   Numerical Methods for Solving Thermal Problems 364
        9.6.4.1   Explicit FD Formulation..365
        9.6.4.2   Stability Criterion..366
        9.6.4.3   ADI Formulation 367
    9.6.5   Temperature Elevations in Subjects Exposed to EMFs 369
        9.6.5.1   Temperature Increments in the Human Body Exposed to the Far Field of Radiating RF Sources 369
        9.6.5.2   Temperature Increments in the Head of Cell Phone Users...............371
9.7 | Correlation between RF Absorption Metrics and Temperature Rise 374
    9.7.1   Near-Field RF Sources...374
    9.7.2   Far Field Plane Waves..380
    9.7.3   A Summary...383
        9.7.3.1   Short RF Exposures 383
        9.7.3.2   Prolonged RF Exposures Including Steady State 383
9.8 | Concluding Remarks..384
References..385

9.1 Introduction

Electromagnetic (EM) energy at both low and high frequencies can be transmitted into biological materials through the use of antennas or applicators. Antennas launch the EM energy into the medium. They serve to couple the generating source of EM energy into the medium, which surrounds it. The spatial distribution of EM energy from an antenna is directional and varies with distance from the antenna. At distances sufficiently far from an antenna, so that local field distribution changes predictably and varies mostly with distance, the region is called a far field or radiation zone. In the near field or near zone close to the antenna, the EM energy distribution varies as a function of both angle and distance. Moreover, the behavior of electromagnetic fields (EMFs) and their coupling and interaction with biological systems are very different, depending on whether they are in the near or far zone. In fact, these differences constitute the major variances between radio-frequency (RF) and low frequency energy deposition into biological systems. As shown in subsequent sections, the induction of electric and magnetic fields, deposition of EM power, absorption of EM energy, and their penetration into tissue, all are functions of the source and its frequency or wavelength. In general, when considering the interaction of EMFs with biological systems, it is necessary to account for the frequency or wavelength and its relationship to the physical dimensions of the body.

In addition, the interaction of EMFs with biological systems is characterized by the EM properties of tissue media, specifically, dielectric permittivity. Biological materials have magnetic permeability values close to that of free space, or vacuum and are independent of frequency. In a medium such as biological tissue with a finite electrical conductivity σ, a

Computational Methods and EM Fields

conduction current, $J = \sigma E$, can be induced to flow, giving rise to energy loss by Joule heating. Clearly, fields must be coupled into tissues and energy must be deposited or absorbed in the biological systems, regardless of the mechanism that is accountable for an effect, for the system to respond in some manner. Thus, to achieve any biological response, the electric, magnetic, or EMF that is exerting its influence must be quantified and correlated with the observed phenomenon.

The purpose of this chapter is to present an account of EM interactions in biological media, with special emphasis on the energy coupling and distribution characteristics in biological structures. Such Information is essential for analyzing the interrelationships among various observed biological effects, for separating known and substantiated effects from those that are speculative and unsubstantiated, for assessing therapeutic effectiveness of EM waves, and for extracting diagnostically useful information from field effects.

There exist a wide variety of methods for quantifying fields in biological bodies. The extent of computer usage varies, depending on specific information sought and the complexity of tissue geometry. This chapter outlines a number of techniques that have been successfully employed to analyze the propagation and absorption characteristics of EM energy in tissue structures. There are two general approaches: one involves extensive use of analytical development and the other relies more heavily on numerical formulation. Analytical computations are most suited for calculation of distribution of absorbed energy in simplified tissue geometries such as plane slabs, cylinders, and spheroids, whereas numerical methods offer the opportunity of analyzing the coupling of EM energy to animal and human bodies which is difficult, if not impossible, to approach analytically. The advantages and limitations of various methods for field computations, along with representative results, are provided in this chapter. In some case, for additional details, the reader is referred to previous editions of this handbook [1–3]. This chapter will begin with a brief introduction to the concepts of induced field and power deposition, and the characteristics of field strength, exposure intensity, and dosimetric quantities.

9.1.1 Induced Field and Dosimetric Quantities

The quantities of import to characterize coupling of EM energy into biological systems include the incident field, induced field, power deposition, and absorbed energy. The metrics of specific absorption rate (SAR) and specific absorption (SA) in biological systems or tissue models have been adopted as the dosimetric quantities, especially at RF frequencies. The metric SAR (in W/kg) is defined as the time derivative of the incremental energy absorbed by (or dissipated in) an incremental mass contained in a volume of a given density. SA (in J/kg) is the total amount of energy deposited or absorbed and is given by the integral of SAR over a finite interval of time. Information on SAR and SA is of interest because it may serve as an index for comparison and extrapolation of experimental results from tissue to tissue, from animal to animal, from animal to human, and from human to human exposures. It is also useful in analyzing relationships among various observed biological effects in different experimental models and subjects. This is in clear contrast to incident field or any other external measures of exposure, which often do not provide the same field inside biological systems of different size, shape, species, or constitutions.

Moreover, determination of the induced field would be preferred because it (1) relates the field to specific responses of the body, (2) facilitates understanding of biological phenomena, and (3) is independent of mechanisms of interaction. Once the induced field is known, quantities such as SAR (in W/kg) can be derived from it by a simple conversion formula. For example, from an induced electric field E (in V/m), the SAR can be derived as,

$$SAR = \frac{\sigma E^2}{\rho_m} \qquad (9.1)$$

where σ is the bulk electrical conductivity (S/m) and ρ_m is the mass density (kg/m^3) of tissue. However, when a small, isotropic, implantable electric field probe, with sufficient sensitivity, is unavailable for practical use, a common practice in experimental dosimetry relies on the use of temperature elevation produced under a short-duration (<30 s), high-intensity exposure condition. The short duration is not enough for significant convective or conductive heat contribution to tissue temperature rises. In this case, the time rate of initial rises in temperature (slope of transient temperature response curve) can be related to SAR through a secondary procedure, that is,

$$SAR = \frac{c\Delta T}{\Delta t} \qquad (9.2)$$

where ΔT is the temperature increment (°C), c is the specific heat capacity of tissue (J/kg°C), and Δt is the duration (sec) over which ΔT is measured. Thus, the rise in tissue temperature during the initial or a transient period of RF energy absorption is linearly proportional to the value of SAR. It is important to distinguish the use of SAR and its derivation from temperature measurement in the above equation. The quantity of SAR is merely a metric for energy deposition or absorption, and it should not be construed to imply any mechanism of interaction, thermal, or otherwise. It is noteworthy that the metric, SAR, is a unit that pertains to a macroscopic quantity by virtue of the use of bulk electrical conductivity or bulk specific heat capacity in its derivation (Equations 9.1 or 9.2).

It is of particular significance to emphasize the use of bulk electrical conductivity, the specific heat capacity, and the mass density (kg/m^3) of tissue in the derivation of SAR from electric field strength or temperature elevation. Their use in the definition means that a volume of tissue mass must be selected over which SAR is determined. It is self-evident that the numerical value of SAR would be the same, regardless of what volume is chosen if the induced field or power deposition is uniform in a selected issue medium. A difficulty arises when the absorption is not uniform, or when tissues with differing properties and conductivities are within the same volume. Thus, in general, a smaller averaging mass or volume would allow SAR—as a metric to provide a closer or more precise representation of its value and variation inside the body or tissue medium. This is especially important from its biological relevance.

9.1.2 Characterizing EMFs

The space surrounding a source antenna can be divided into near and far zones as a function of distance from the antenna [4–7]. The demarcating boundary occurs at a conservative distance of $R = 2D^2/\lambda$, where D is the largest dimension of the antenna. Furthermore, the near zone can be divided into two subregions: the radiative region and the reactive region. The vicinity of the antenna where the reactive components predominate is known as *the reactive region*. There is generally greater mutual interaction between the antenna and surrounding space. In *the radiative region*, the space that is further out and closer to $2D^2/\lambda$, the radiated power varies with distance from the antenna. The precise extent of these regions varies for different antennas. For most antennas, the transition point between reactive and radiative regions occurs from 0.2 to 0.4 D^2/λ. For a short dipole antenna, the reactive component predominates to a distance of approximately $\lambda/2\pi$, where the radiative and reactive components are equal to each other. However, the outer limit is on the order of a few wavelengths in most cases.

A typical wavelength in free space at extremely low frequencies (ELF, between 3 Hz and 3 kHz) is ~5000 km. The $\lambda/2\pi$ distance is about 800 km for the reactive and radiative fields to have equal amplitudes. Therefore, for most purposes, power transmission line fields are not radiative, but reactive and quasi-static in nature. This fact governs the coupling and induced field characteristics of ELF and other low-frequency electric and magnetic fields in biological tissue. In particular, (1) the electric field is enhanced at the surface of the biological body and is nearly perpendicular to the surface of the body, (2) electric and magnetic fields are decoupled inside a biological body, (3) the electric field applied through air is weakened by a large dielectric permittivity (by about 10^{-6}) upon penetration into biological tissues, (4) magnetic field remains the same inside and outside the body, but magnetically induced electric field inside the body encircles the magnetic field and produces an eddy current whose magnitude increases with distance from the center of the body, and (5) eddy currents appear in every region, inside the body, with a different conductivity and behave as a unit with its own body center and radius or an equivalent radius. These observations apply to all frequencies where the wavelength is long or the largest dimension of the body is small compared with a wavelength.

In contrast, the $2D^2/\lambda$ distance is approximately 6 cm for a 10-cm RF antenna operating at 900 MHz in free space. Clearly, both near-zone reactive and far-zone radiative interactions are encountered in the vicinity of wireless RF telecommunication systems. In the near zone, the coupling of RF energy to the human head is substantial. As much as 40%–50% of the radiated RF power is transferred back and forth between the radiating antenna and the head. SAR will vary with specific antenna configuration and its placement next to the head. The bulk of power deposition is in the side of the head nearest to the radiating structure of the cellular mobile telephone and follows an exponential trend away from the antenna. Anatomy of the head and tissue inhomogeneity can influence the maximum value and distribution of SAR in the head of a mobile telephone user. However, the integrated SAR in the head is similar for a homogeneous or inhomogeneous model. Some of the major features of near-zone field are that (1) RF electric and magnetic fields are decoupled and are not uniform, (2) wave impedance varies from point to point, (3) beam width from the antenna is divergent and is small compared with the head or human body, (4) electric field effect is weaker since dielectric permittivity of tissue is relatively high, and (5) inductive coupling of antenna-current-generated magnetic field dominates power deposition.

In the far field, coupling is characterized by plane wave RF field interaction and is independent of source configurations. Electric and magnetic fields are uniquely defined through the intrinsic impedance of the medium. Thus, determination of the electric field behavior is sufficient to characterize the interaction. The coupling of RF power from air into planar tissue ranges from 20% to 60%, at wireless communication frequencies. However, enhanced coupling can occur at greater depth in bodies with curved surfaces. In fact, RF energy is resonantly absorbed by the head at 400–1500 MHz, and SAR peaks or hot spots may occur near the center of the head. The interaction of RF energy with biological systems depends on electric field polarization for elongated bodies whose height-to-width ratio is large. It is significant to observe that the integrated SAR or total absorption in the biological body is similar for a homogeneous or inhomogeneous model.

9.2 Fundamental Interactions

When the radius of curvature of the body surface is large compared to the wavelength and the beam width of the impinging radiation, planar tissue models may be used to estimate the absorbed energy and its distribution inside the body. As a first-order approximation, the plane-wave configuration is often used for its simplicity to assess EMF interaction with planar biological tissues.

9.2.1 Thick Tissue Layers

For a linearly polarized plane wave impinging normally on a boundary separating two semi-infinite issue media, the reflection and transmission coefficients are given by

$$\Gamma = \frac{\eta_2 - \eta_1}{\eta_2 + \eta_1} \tag{9.3}$$

and

$$T = \frac{2\eta_2}{\eta_2 + \eta_1} \tag{9.4}$$

respectively, where η_1 and η_2 are the intrinsic impedance of media 1 and 2. If intrinsic impedances of the two media are approximately equal or if the dielectric permittivities are comparable, most of the energy is transmitted into the second medium and the reflected field is relatively small. Conversely, if intrinsic impedances differ greatly, or if the dielectric permittivities are very different, the transmitted field is small and the quantity of reflected energy is large.

Table 9.1 summarizes the magnitude of the reflection coefficient at the boundary separating various tissues. The fraction of normally incident power reflected by the discontinuity is given by Γ^2. Clearly, up to one half of the incident power is reflected at the air-skin boundary. The reflection coefficient for tissue–tissue interfaces generally is smaller than air–tissue interfaces. The percent reflected power for tissue–tissue interfaces range from a low of less than one for muscle–blood to a high of 30 for fat–biological fluid interfaces. This suggests that the closer are the dielectric properties on both sides of the interface, the smaller is the power reflection.

The fraction of power transmitted is related to the power transmission coefficient, $T^2 = 1 - \Gamma^2$. It is readily apparent from Table 9.1 that the power transmitted at air-tissue interfaces is quite substantial at RF and microwave frequencies. Moreover, the power transmission coefficient is highly frequency dependent.

As the transmitted wave propagates in the tissue medium, energy is extracted from the wave and absorbed by the medium. This absorption will result in a progressive reduction of the power density of the wave as it advances in the tissue. This reduction is quantified by the depth of penetration (skin depth), which is the distance in which the power density decreases by a factor of e^{-2}. Table 9.2 presents the calculated depth of penetration in selected tissues using typical dielectric constants and conductivities. It is seen that the penetration depth is frequency dependent and takes on different values for different tissues. In particular, the penetration depth for fat and bone is nearly five times greater than for higher-water-content tissues such as muscle.

Computational Methods and EM Fields

TABLE 9.1

Representative Reflection Coefficient (Magnitude in Percent) Between Biological Tissues at 37°C

| | Frequency | | Fat | | | Muscle | |
	(MHz)	Air	(bone)	Lung	(skin)	Blood	Saline
Air	433	0	46	76	82	81	83
	915	0	43	73	78	79	80
	2,450	0	41	71	76	77	79
	5,800	0	39	70	75	76	78
	10,000	0	37	70	74	76	78
Fat (bone)	433		0	46	56	56	60
	915		0	43	52	54	57
	2,450		0	42	50	53	57
	5,800		0	42	50	53	56
	10,000		0	45	52	54	58
Lung	433			0	14	13	19
	915			0	12	14	18
	2,450			0	10	15	19
	5,800			0	10	14	19
	10,000			0	10	13	18
Muscle (skin)	433				0	4	6
	915				0	4	7
	2,450				0	5	10
	5,800				0	4	9
	10,000				0	3	9
Blood	433					0	6
	915					0	4
	2,450					0	5
	5,800					0	5
	10,000					0	6
Saline	433						0
	915						0
	2,450						0
	5,800						0
	10,000						0

TABLE 9.2

Depth of Penetration of an EMF in Biological Tissues As a Function of Frequency

| | | Tissue | | |
| Frequency | | | Muscle | Fat | |
(MHz)	Saline	Blood	(skin)	Lung	(bone)
Depth of Penetration (cm)					
433	2.8	3.7	3.0	4.7	16.3
915	2.5	3.0	2.5	4.5	12.8
2,450	1.3	1.9	1.7	2.3	7.9
5,800	0.7	0.7	0.8	0.7	4.7
10,000	0.2	0.3	0.3	0.3	2.5

A wave of unspecified polarization usually is decomposed into its orthogonal linearly polarized components whose electric or magnetic field parallels the interface. These components can be treated separately and combined afterward. Figures 9.1 and 9.2 illustrate the magnitude and phase of the reflection coefficients of representative tissue interfaces at a temperature of 37°C for irradiation at 2450 MHz. The figures clearly show the difference between *E* and *H* polarization. *E* polarization, also called perpendicular polarization and *H* polarization, also referred to as parallel polarization. For *E* polarization, there is only a slight variation in magnitude and phase of the reflection coefficient with incidence angle. For *H* polarization, however, there is a pronounced dependence on incidence angle. The reflection coefficient reaches a minimum magnitude and has a phase angle of 90° at Brewster's angle. Thus, the *H* polarized wave is totally transmitted into the muscle medium at Brewster's angle.

9.2.2 Multiple Layers of Tissue

When there are several layers of different tissues, the reflection and transmission characteristics become more complicated. Multiple reflections can occur between the skin and subcutaneous tissue boundaries, with a resulting modification of the reflection and transmission coefficients [8–11]. In general, the transmitted wave or field will combine with the reflected field to form standing waves in each layer. This phenomenon becomes especially pronounced if the thickness of each layer is less than the penetration depth for that tissue. Plane waves impinging on the human body considered as consisting of parallel layers of subcutaneous fat and more deeply lying muscle have been studied in detail by Schwan and Li [9,10].

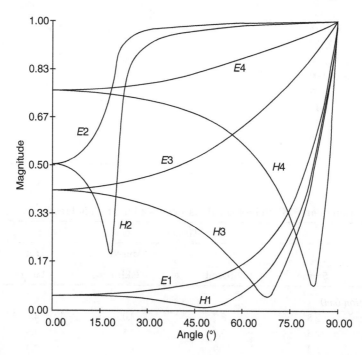

FIGURE 9.1
Magnitudes of reflection coefficients for *E* and *H* polarized plane waves at 2450 MHz as a function of incidence angle.

Computational Methods and EM Fields

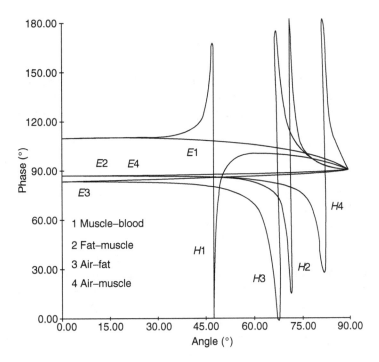

FIGURE 9.2
Phase values of reflection coefficients for E and H polarized 2450 MHz plane waves as a function incidence angle.

For the tissue model depicted in Figure 9.3, the electric field strength in the fat layer is given by

$$E_f = F_l E_0 \left[e^{-(\alpha_2 + j\beta_2)z} + \Gamma_{32} e^{(\alpha_2 + j\beta_2)z} \right] \quad (9.5)$$

and the electric field in the underlying muscular tissue is given by

$$E_m = F_t E_0 e^{-(\alpha_3 + j\beta_3)z} \quad (9.6)$$

where $\alpha_2, \beta_2,$ and $\alpha_3, \beta_3,$ are the attenuation and propagation coefficients in fat and muscle, respectively. The layer function F_l and the transmission function F_t, are given by

$$F_l = \frac{T_{12}}{e^{(\alpha_2 + j\beta_2)l} + \Gamma_{21}\Gamma_{32} e^{-(\alpha_2 + j\beta_2)l}} \quad (9.7)$$

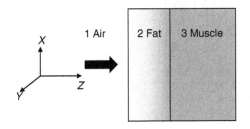

FIGURE 9.3
Plane wave in air impinging on a composite fat-muscle layer.

$$F_t = \frac{T_{12}T_{23}}{e^{(\alpha_2+j\beta_2)l} + \Gamma_{21}\Gamma_{32}e^{-(\alpha_2+j\beta_2)l}} \quad (9.8)$$

where T_{12} and T_{23} are the transmission coefficients at the air–fat and fat–muscle boundaries, respectively. Γ_{21} and Γ_{32} denote the reflection coefficients at these boundaries, respectively, and l is the thickness of the fat layer. The power deposition in a given layer can be obtained from Equation 9.1.

Figure 9.4 shows computed results of SAR distribution in fat–muscle layers for four different frequencies. The values are normalized to the SAR in muscle at the fat-muscle boundary. Note the absorbed energy is much lower in fat than in muscle. The standing wave maximum becomes bigger in fat and the penetration into muscle becomes less as the frequency increases.

The EM energy absorbed in models composed of planar layers of skin, fat, and muscle can be analyzed in a similar manner [9–12], except the distribution of absorbed energy becomes more complex. Figure 9.5 shows that in addition to frequency dependence, the peak SAR exhibits considerable fluctuation with thickness of the subcutaneous fatty layer. The incident power density is, in this case, $10\,W/m^2$ and the skin layer is 0.2 cm thick. Note that the peak SAR is always higher in the skin layer for planar models at microwave frequencies. The depth of penetration for 10 GHz radiation in skin is less than 0.5 mm— the transmitted energy is almost completely absorbed in the skin and the SAR is rather unaffected by changing fatty layer thickness. The fact that SAR is highest in the skin is significant, since skin is populated with thermo-sensitive free nerve endings which may be excited along with cutaneous pain receptors when the absorbed energy exceeds the normal range that can be handled by thermoregulation.

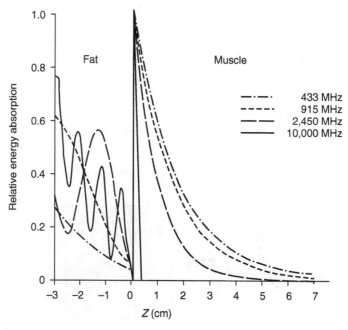

FIGURE 9.4
SAR expressed as absorbed power density in planar fat-muscle layers.

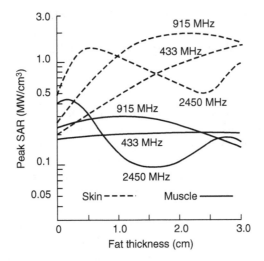

FIGURE 9.5
Peak SAR expressed as absorbed power density in models composed of fat–skin–muscle layers.

Figure 9.6 shows the distribution of induced electric field strength in a layer of muscle beneath layers of fat, muscle, and bone for two frequencies [9–12]. It is seen that in addition to frequency dependence, the electric fields exhibit considerable fluctuation within each tissue layer. While the standing-wave oscillations are larger at 2450 than at 915 MHz, microwave energy at both frequencies penetrates to deeper tissues. This result, together with Figures 9.4 and 9.5, implies that at frequencies between 300 and 3000 MHz, sufficient energy may be transmitted and reflected to allow interrogation of organs within the body. Furthermore, at these frequencies, EM energy can penetrate into more deeply situated

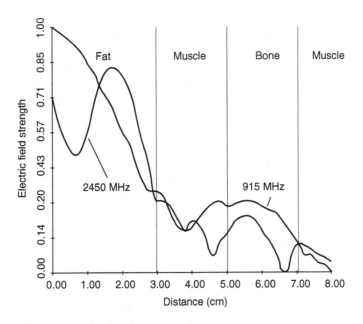

FIGURE 9.6
Distribution of electric field strength in planar layer of fat–muscle–bone–muscle tissue model.

tissues, making it especially desirable for therapeutic applications. They also call for special attention for safety considerations since EM energy in this frequency range can produce higher SAR at greater depth compared to superficial tissues.

9.2.3 Spheroidal Models

Although depth of penetration and reflection and transmission characteristics in planar tissue models provide considerable insights into coupling and distribution of EM energy, biological structures generally are more complex in form and exhibit substantial curvature that can modify EM energy transmission, reflection, and distribution. For bodies with complex shapes, the propagation characteristics depend critically on polarization and on orientation of the incident wave with respect to the body, as well as on the ratio of body size to wavelength. These complications place severe limitations on calculations of reflected and transmitted RF energy for bodies of arbitrary shape and complex permittivity. Nevertheless, analytic calculations can yield sights into their fundamental interactions. This section presents a summary of results for homogeneous and multilayered spheroidal models that approximate certain mammalian tissue structures [11–21].

For example, at 918 and 2450 MHz—two of the most popular frequencies used in cellular mobile systems, SAR calculations approximating a rhesus monkey, a human child, or adult head show maximum absorption occurring near the center and inside of all the brain spheres for 915 MHz. When the frequency is increased to 2450 MHz, the location of peak SAR for the smaller brain sphere remains near the center, whereas that for an adult-size brain sphere moves to an anterior location. In general, standing-wave SAR patterns with many oscillations are observed. The peak absorption may be several times greater than the average, and the enhanced absorptions near the center of these brain models may be significantly greater than that expected from the planar tissue models. The increased absorptions are due to a combination of high dielectric constant and curvature of the model, which produces a strong focusing of energy toward the interior of the sphere that more than compensates for the transmission losses through the tissue.

The absorbed energy varies widely with sphere size and frequency. In general, the absorption increases rapidly with increasing radius and is then followed by some geometrical resonant behavior. The peaks of these resonant oscillations are related to the maxima, or hot spots, in the distribution of absorbed energy inside the head model. For $(2\pi a/\lambda_0) < 0.4$, where a is the sphere radius and λ_0 is the wavelength in vacuum, hot spots do not occur inside the sphere. However, for some combinations of exposure frequency and radius hot spots will occur, e.g., in brain spheres with radii between 2 and 8 cm at 915 MHz and between 0.9 and 5 cm at 2450 MHz. For larger brain spheres, the maximum absorption appears at the anterior portion (exposed surface) of the brain sphere, and the penetration depth at the surface becomes a dominating factor for exposures at frequencies in this range. The planar model discussed previously may be applied to obtain a theoretical estimation of the absorbed energy in this case.

The frequency dependence of energy absorption by head-size spheres is typified by occurrence of resonant peaks. However, with increasing frequency, energy is absorbed in a decreasingly smaller volume as result of shortened penetration depth.

The effects of skin, fat, bone, dura, and cerebrospinal fluid on the absorption of radiofrequency radiation by the brain have been investigated using structures where the spherical core of brain is surrounded by five concentric shells of tissues [13,17,18]. It is interesting to note that if brain sizes remain unchanged, but the overall sphere diameter is increased to account for the outer tissue layers, absorption in brain tissues may be increased by 25%

Computational Methods and EM Fields

for human- and cat-sized heads at 915 MHz or decreased by 70% or more in the case of 2450 MHz. Moreover, surface absorption is greatly increased in the case of layered models, while fat and bone always absorb the least amount of energy.

If the outer diameter of the sphere remains the same, while the tissue layers are allowed to be either layered or homogeneous, the peak and average SARs show very little change except when the radius of the spherical head is between 0.1 and 1.0 times the wavelength in air. The peak and average SARs for layered models may be several times greater than for homogeneous models. Enhancement is apparently the result of resonant coupling of energy into the sphere by the outer tissue layers.

A study also has been made of the interaction of circularly polarized plane waves [19]. Results showed distribution of absorbed energy for circularly polarized waves is more uniform compared with the linearly polarized case. In fact, the absorbed energy distribution in the planes transverse to the direction of propagation is rotationally symmetric, that is, it is independent of angular variation.

Spherical models of muscle [20,21] have been used as a first-order approximation for the extrapolation to human beings of results obtained from laboratory animals and as an index of whole-body absorption of EM energy as a function of frequency. The spherical model is attractive since exact solutions for absorbed energy can be obtained for all frequencies and body sizes. While in this case the peak absorption is of very limited utility, the average absorption per unit surface area is related to the time and power required to overload the thermoregulatory capacity of an exposed subject. The absorptions for homogeneous muscle spheres, whose volumes correspond to small animals, such as a rat, and standard man, computed as functions of frequency showed that the average absorption for the rat model is at least ten times higher than for a muscle sphere representing a human body at frequencies greater than 500 MHz. The absorption increased rapidly with frequency until the free space wavelength of the impinging radiation approaches the diameter of the sphere. A number of resonant oscillations appear which tend to increase the amount and nonuniformity of absorbed energy. Above this range the absorption falls off slowly, indicating that details of body surface curvature are of little significance.

It is interesting to note that when the sphere size is small compared with the wavelength, the absorbed energy distribution varies almost as the square of the radius or distance from the axis parallel to the direction of magnetic field vector. If the sphere is extremely small compared with the wavelength, the absorbed energy distribution becomes nearly uniform in the transverse directions, but decreases continuously with distance from the exposed surface. This behavior can be explained by a quasi-static field theory [4,20]. The electric component of the incident field couples to the object in the same fashion as an electrostatic field. This gives rise to a constant induced electric field inside the sphere which has the same direction but is reduced by $3/\varepsilon$ from the applied electric field for biological materials and is independent of sphere size. Similarly, the magnetically induced electric field inside the body is identical to the quasi-static solution whose magnitude is given by $E = \pi f \mu r H$, where f is the frequency, μ is the permeability, r is the radius, and H is the magnetic field strength. Thus, the magnetic component of the incident field, which remains unchanged inside the body, produces an internal electric field that varies directly with distance away from the axis and in proportion to the frequency. This magnetically induced electric field encircles the magnetic axis and gives rise to an eddy current whose magnitude increases with distance from the magnetic axis. It indicates that while the H-induced energy absorption in a mouse or larger animal is much greater than the E-induced component, electrically and magnetically induced absorption may be equally significant in smaller animals at lower frequencies (below 30–40 MHz). Moreover, for a small insect or pupae the electric field will be the predominant factor.

The variation of average and maximum energy absorption with frequency for a human-size sphere is illustrated in Figure 9.7. In the frequency range from 1 to 20 MHz, the maximum absorption rate is only 10^{-6} to 10^{-3} W/kg per watt per meter squared of incident power. Inspection of the maximum absorption rate induced by a plane wave, a quasi-static electric field, and a quasi-static magnetic field shows that absorption at frequencies below 20 MHz is primarily due to the magnetically induced eddy current and is characterized by a square-of-frequency dependence. The approximate frequency dependence of average or total energy absorption throughout the frequency range from 1 MHz to 10 GHz is indicated by the dashed line. For frequencies below 20 MHz the average absorption varies as the square of the frequency. In the frequency range of 20–200 MHz, the average absorption increases directly in proportion to frequency and attains a maximum of about 2×10^{-3} W/kg per watt per meter squared of incident power at 200 MHz. The average absorption rate remains fairly constant with increasing frequency. (Its slow variation is inversely proportional to frequency for higher frequencies.) Thus, EM energy absorption varies both with frequency and body size, and in a predictable manner.

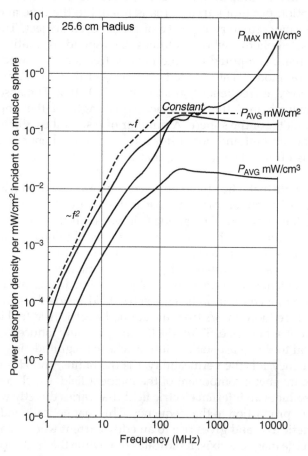

FIGURE 9.7
Frequency dependence of absorption in a spherical model of the human body.

Also, the canonical model of a prolate spheroid can emulate more closely the body shape of humans and experimental animals [22–24]. As in the case of spherical models, for frequencies below resonance absorption, long-wavelength formulations and quasi-static approximations have been used to obtain absorption information.

Three orientations of the impinging plane wave with respect to the body must be distinguished: E-polarization in which the electric field is parallel to the major axis of the spheroid, H-polarization in which the magnetic field vector is parallel to the major axis, and K-polarization in which both electric and magnetic field vectors are perpendicular to the major axis of the spheroid. In general, E-polarization produces the highest energy absorption for frequencies up to and slightly beyond the resonance region.

For a plane wave with long wavelength, i.e., $\lambda > a$, where a is the semi-major axis of the prolate spheroid, the induced fields within the spheroid are uniform and independent of size when the external field is uniform. For $\varepsilon_r > 1$, the field inside the spheroid is weaker than the applied field. Moreover, the whole-body energy absorption depends not only on the strength of applied fields, but also on the orientation of the field with respect to the major axis of the body. As in the case of spherical models, the absorption is produced by an electrically induced current in the direction of the applied E-field vector, combined with a circulating eddy current induced by the incident magnetic field [20]. One would, therefore, expect the electrically induced absorption to be uniform, whereas the absorption due to the circulating eddy current would be zero at the center of the body and increase as square of the distance from the center.

For a given incident field orientation, the average SAR for humans may be either higher or lower than for rats, depending on the frequency. For example, at 70 MHz, the average SAR is the highest for humans, having a value of 0.25 W/kg for an incident power density of 10 W/m², the average SAR for a rat is only 0.0125 W/kg. In contrast, the average SAR of 0.8 W/kg at 700 MHz is the highest for rats; the corresponding value for humans is less than 1/25. It is thus extremely important to take into account the body size and operating frequency to draw any relationship between the biological effects that arise in the laboratory and corresponding effects that might occur in humans at a given incident power density [1,2].

The frequency for maximal absorption (resonance frequency) depends on the subject and its orientation with respect to the incident field. In general, the shorter the subject, the higher the resonance frequency and vice versa. Further, the frequency dependence of whole-body or average absorption may be partitioned into three regions (Figure 9.8). This may be illustrated using the orientation that is most efficient in energy coupling, E-polarization. For frequencies well below resonance such that the ratio of the longest body dimension (L) to free space wavelength (λ) is less than 0.2, the average SAR is characterized by an f^2 dependence. The average absorption goes through a resonance in the region where $0.2 < L/\lambda < 1.0$. In this case, the average SAR rapidly increases to a maximum near $L/\lambda = 0.4$ and then falls off as $1/f$. At frequencies for which $L/\lambda > 1.0$, the whole-body absorption decreases slightly, but approaches asymptotically one half of the incident power (1-power reflection coefficient).

It should be noted that the resonant absorption length of $0.4\,\lambda$ is in good agreement with results from antenna analysis. In addition, whole-body absorptions for H- and K-polarizations are totally different. The resonances are not nearly as well defined as for E-polarization. In fact, the whole-body absorption curve for H-polarization gradually reaches a plateau and stays at that plateau for higher frequencies.

At 10 MHz, the size of the spheroidal model approximating an average human body—height equals 1.75 m with a major-to-minor axis ratio of 6.34 and a 70-kg mass—is small

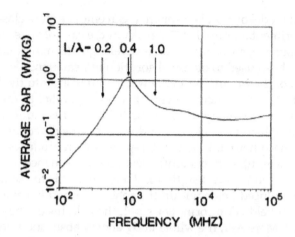

FIGURE 9.8
Frequency dependence of whole-body or average absorption may be partitioned into three regions for E polarization.

compared with a wavelength. The distribution of absorbed energy in the spheroidal model is qualitatively similar to those for spherical models. But quantitatively, the difference could be as much as one order of magnitude. As expected, the absorbed energy is highest for E-polarization—there is a strong coupling of the applied electric field into the interior of the prolate spheroid, and a relatively weak eddy-current contribution due to a smaller cross-section for intercepting the magnetic flux. The absorption along the direction of incident field indicates that the electrically and magnetically induced field components are nearly equal. The electric polarization field and the circulating eddy current add at the front side and subtract on the back side of the spheroid to render an absorption pattern that peaks at the front surface and is reduced to almost zero deeper inside the spheroid.

For H-polarization, the electrically induced current flows along the axial direction of incident E field and the eddy current field encircles the axial direction of incident H field. The relatively low power along the H-field axis comes solely from the incident electric field. The combination of E- and H-induced components generates a displaced parabolic energy absorption pattern along both the E-field and H-field axes. Clearly, the magnetically induced eddy current predominates in this case and the absorption is highest along the transverse circumference at the middle of the prolate spheroid. For K-polarization, both the electric and magnetic components of the incident field are along the minor axes of the spheroid: the electrically induced current flows along one axis, and the incident magnetic field induces an eddy current electric field that encircles another axis. The absorption is lowest at the center. Whereas in both E- and H-polarization cases, the peak absorption occurs at the front surface of the spheroid irradiated by the incident field, this is not the case for K-polarization. Maximum absorption appears at the surface of the narrow cross-section, and the absorbed energy varies parabolically. This is the result of the large quantity of magnetic flux intercepted by the broad cross-section (and resulting concentration of eddy current). The results match well with experimental measurements [25]. Moreover, the peak absorptions may be two orders of magnitude higher than those for spherical biological bodies of equal mass.

We have summarized above some of the computational approaches to calculate absorbed energy in simple models of biological objects. It should be recognized that while spheroids are good models for understanding fundamental interactions and for indexing EM energy

Computational Methods and EM Fields

absorption by animal bodies or for certain body parts, they are not exact and may not be adequate for humans and experimental animals under various exposure situations. More convincing models, formed from small-sized, computational-cell volumes were initially created to account for the differing tissue compositions and irregular body shapes [26–30]. Since then more realistic anatomical models of human and animal bodies have been developed to mimic inhomogeneous tissue compositions and variable organ and body shapes. These models, based on numerical techniques have been a great asset in efforts to accurately predict power deposition and its distribution in biological objects exposed to EMFs and RF radiation. In what follows, we shall summarize a number of computer techniques that have been applied with great success in solving EM energy absorption and SAR distribution problems. We shall also describe some results obtained using these computational methods.

9.3 Computation Algorithms

The computational algorithms based on numerical techniques applied to predict EMF strengthens and SAR distributions in anatomically realistic models of human and animal bodies are presented in this section. However, the use of a given methodological algorithm and the number of computational cells involved in the models typically dictate the domain of applicability of the techniques.

The numerical methods used to predict induced fields in biological bodies of realistic shape and composition include the quasi-static impedance method, the method of moments (MoMs), the finite element method (FEM), and the finite difference time domain (FDTD) methods. Note that the quasi-static impedance method is restricted to lower frequencies (<30–40 MHz for the human body), but the MoM, the FEM, and the FDTD methods may be used for any frequency of interest. In addition, both the finite element and FDTD methods involve solving Maxwell's equations in the differential form for the computation of induced fields.

9.3.1 The Quasi-Static Impedance Method

For low-frequency situations, where the dimensions of the biological body are small compared to the wavelength, the impedance method has been found to be highly efficient as a numerical procedure for calculating internal current densities and induced electric fields [31–35]. In this method, the biological body or the exposed part thereof is represented by a three-dimensional (3-D) network of impedances whose individual values are obtained from the complex conductivities $\sigma + j\omega\varepsilon$ for the various locations of the body. The impedances for various directions for the 3-D network can be written as:

$$Z_m^{i,j,k} = \frac{\delta_m}{\delta_n \delta_p (\sigma_m^{i,j,k} + j\omega\varepsilon_m^{i,j,k})} \tag{9.9}$$

where i, j, k indicate the cell index; m is the direction in x, y, or z for which the impedance is calculated; and σ_m and $j\omega\varepsilon_m$ are the conductivities and the dielectric permittivities for the cell (i, j, k). δ_m is the thickness of the cell in the m-th direction, and δ_n and δ_p are the widths of the cell in directions at right angles to the m-th direction.

In the impedance method formulation, it can be seen that the cells need not be identical so that fairly thin features of the body can be modeled as well as the interfaces between the various tissues and organs. Also, the conductivity for a given cell can be directionally dependent. This feature will be useful in allowing for the highly anisotropic conductivities of the tissues that have been reported for low frequencies including the power-line frequencies [36,37].

Employing anatomically based models of the human body, the impedance method has been used for the following applications:

a. Calculation of SAR distributions for operator exposure to spatially variable fields of induction heaters [33].

b. SAR distributions for linearly or circularly polarized RF magnetic fields representative of magnetic resonance imagers [34].

c. SAR distributions due to capacitive-type electrodes used for hyperthermia [35].

d. SAR distributions for interstitial RF needle applicators for hyperthermia [38].

Some calculations using the impedance method are listed below:

a. Internal electric fields and current densities induced in the human body for exposure to magnetic fields of high-voltage power transmission lines [39].

b. Electric fields and current densities induced in the human head by magnetic fields of a hair dryer [40].

In the section that follows, the use of the impedance method is described below for calculating currents in models of the human body exposed to electric and magnetic fields of both the conventional (pre-1990) electric blanket and the new low-magnetic-field electric blanket.

9.3.2 The Volume Integral Equation MoM

The MoM [41] is used either in conjunction with the volume integral equation method or the surface integral equation method for finding solutions to the unknown fields inside the body. The approaches differ, however, in specifics, in that the surface integral equation MoM (SMoM) finds the unknown currents on the body surface and calculates the interior fields from the surface currents, the reciprocity theorem, and a "measurement matrix." In contrast, the volume integral equation MoM (VMoM) requires determination of unknown fields throughout the volume of the body using the volume equivalence principle [42] and the MoM.

The numerical technique that has been adopted for most of the early EMF computations is the VMoM, employing the volume equivalence principle [28,29,43]. The MoM is used to transform the integral equation into a matrix equation by subdividing the body into N simply shaped cells. This is accomplished with the aid of an appropriate set of expansion functions, chosen to satisfy the boundary conditions, and a set of weighting (testing) functions to reduce the matrix fill-in time. The total electric field in each of the N cells is given by matrix inversion. A more detailed description of the volume integral equation method is included in the next section.

However, it should be noted that a fundamental limitation of this method is the use of full or nearly full matrices and therefore, the requirement of extensive computer storage

Computational Methods and EM Fields 317

and long running time. Even with the availability of larger and faster computers, this difficulty is not completely obviated. The need for excessively large numbers of mathematical cells to render a more accurate representation of the body will give rise to an equally large and full matrix. The inversion of large, full matrices often leads to numerical instabilities in the solution. Nevertheless, the method does allow the use of inhomogeneous models with 1000 cells or more. In fact, this method has been employed, successfully, to calculate whole-body averaged absorption and to obtain regional distribution of absorbed RF energy using inhomogeneous block models composed of rectangular cells [28,29,30,44]. This method also has been used to study the interaction of the near-zone field of an antenna with biological bodies [45,46].

9.3.3 The SMoM

Another approach for predicting the distribution of absorbed EM energy is the SMoM [47–49]. This method makes use of two coupled integral equations, that is, the electric field and magnetic field integral equations for the tangential components of the field on the surface separating the biological body from air. The unknown surface currents are found by Fourier decomposition and the moment method. The fields inside the biological body are calculated using the previously computed surface currents, the reciprocity theorem, and the concept of measurement matrix [48,50–53].

The method begins with the matrix representation of the coupled integral equations. If the body is assumed to be rotationally symmetric, the incident wave and the induced current could then be expanded in a Fourier series expansion in the angle of rotation. This reduces the problem to that of solving a system of orthogonal modes. The method further expands the surface components in terms of triangular expansion or basis functions and allows the testing functions to be the complex conjugate of the basis functions taking advantage of the orthogonality property. Thus, the major advantage of introducing the Fourier series is to enable each mode to be treated completely independently of all other modes. This results in a much smaller size, manageable matrix equation to be evaluated for the unknown expansion coefficients which determine the surface currents. It should be noted that for biological bodies, triangular expansion and testing functions are preferred over flat pulse expansion functions [47,48]. In fact, an expansion function with a continuous first derivation may constitute an even better choice for the expansion basis function. In any event, once the surface currents are obtained, the fields everywhere, or SAR at each point inside the body, can be calculated using the reciprocity theorem [52,53]. The total absorption can be found by integrating the surface Poynting vector.

The validity of SMoM has been substantiated by using a dielectric sphere [47]. Calculations for a human torso modeled by a homogeneous muscle body of revolution with a height of 1.78 m at 30, 80, and 300 MHz showed enhanced absorption in the neck region for all three frequencies and both vertical and horizontal polarizations [48]. Note that the vertical direction is aligned with the long dimension of the torso and serves as the axis of symmetry. The strongest absorption in the torso model was found to occur with vertical polarization and near the first resonance frequency of the torso (80 MHz). In general, the surface integral equation method is applicable to any arbitrarily shaped homogeneous body of revolution. The method can be used not only with incident plane waves, but also with a wide variety of other field exposure conditions, including direct contact situations and near-zone sources.

Since both the surface and volume integral equation methods for EMF prediction rely on the MoM for implementation, it is instructive to compare the relative advantages of these two techniques. For simplicity, consider a homogeneous cube with N samples on each side: the computer storage requirements are N^2 and N^3 for the surface and volume integral methods, respectively [48]. For sufficient sampling to ensure accurate description of field variations, N is usually a large number. Thus, the surface integral equation method requires significantly fewer unknowns for homogeneous models. Moreover, in cases where permittivity and conductivity values are large, such as in biological bodies, the wavelength becomes contracted inside the body, and a much larger number of cells than that indicated above may actually be needed. If the model is inhomogeneous, then the volume integral equation would prove to be more suitable. It is possible, however, to generalize the surface integral equation technique to account for inhomogeneities by employing the invariant imbedding procedure.

9.3.4 The FEM

The FEM has been a preferred numerical algorithm in many fields of application. However, its use and popularity in predicting EMF in biological systems have been modest until recent progress in mesh generation, boundary conditioning, and large matrix solvers. The FEM method is a near-neighbor, volume method for solving Maxwell's differential equations and is associated with a sparse system of equations [54,55]. Aside from the low memory requirement (on the order of N), an inherent attraction of FEM is its adaptability in modeling inhomogeneities and complex geometries. The feature of conforming and variable-sized cell elements of the computational volume is extremely important in bioelectromagnetics.

The basic approach of the FEM method for predicting EMF distributions inside biological bodies starts by subdividing the physical space and biological body of interest into meshes of small volumes or cells of tetrahedral elements. This step is very important since the manner in which the volume is subdivided will dictate the computational resources required and the speed of the computation and accuracy of the results. Each cell element and node location will have to be systematically numbered and described. Once the volume has been subdivided, labelled, and appropriate property values ascribed, the unknown field within each element is then approximated using linear extrapolation. A major step in FEM is the formulation of the system of linear equations using either the Ritz or Galerkin algorithm with proper boundary conditions. There are two approaches to solving the system of linear algebraic equations: the direct method of Gaussian elimination or the iterative method that starts with an initial guess. In practice, either method can produce an approximate solution to the unknown field intensity with a prescribed accuracy.

It should be noted that a large region exterior to the biological body is often encountered in bioelectromagnetic situations, where the biological body or portion of it, is part of a region into which EM energy is radiated and scattered. The region of space exterior to the biological body and applicator must be truncated with an artificial boundary to limit the volume elements and the number of unknowns. Consequently, an appropriate boundary condition needs to be established at this artificial boundary for a unique finite element determination of the induced fields inside the body. The most common boundary conditions selected for this purpose are the absorbing boundary conditions which minimize the nonphysical reflections from the artificial boundaries by making boundaries transparent to the scattered field.

Fairly large-scale calculations, on the order of 200,000 elements, have been conducted effectively in the workstation computing environment. Specifically, detailed power

Computational Methods and EM Fields　　　　　　　　　　　　　　　　　　319

deposition patterns have been simulated in full and partial models of the human body undergoing EM hyperthermia treatment for cancer [56]. In this case, the cell elements were generated from computerized tomographic data obtained on human patients.

9.3.5 The FDTD Method

The FDTD approach is an attempt to solve Maxwell's curl equations by directly modeling propagation of waves into a volume of space containing the biological body. By repeatedly implementing a finite difference (FD) representation of the curl equations at each cell of the corresponding space lattice, the incident wave is tracked as it first propagates to the body and then interacts with it through surface current excitation, transmission, and diffraction. This wave-tracking process is completed when the steady-state behavior is observed at each lattice cell. Considerable simplification is achieved by analyzing the interaction of the wavefront with a part of the body surface at a time, rather than attempting a simultaneous solution of the entire problem.

The FDTD method has become one of the most successful methods for SAR calculations. The method was first proposed by Yee [57] and later developed by Taflove [58–60], Holland [61], and Kunz and Lee [62]. Several books are devoted to the FDTD method and some of its applications [63–65]. For bioelectromagnetic applications the FDTD method has been found to be extremely versatile and has been used for whole-body or partial-body exposures due to spatially uniform or nonuniform fields (far- or near-fields), sinusoidal time-varying EMFs, and for transient fields such as those of ultra-wide-band (UWB) and electromagnetic pulses (EMPs) [66–70]. Accordingly, some details of FDTD are included in this section.

9.3.5.1 The Traditional FDTD Method

In this method, the time-dependent Maxwell's curl equations

$$\nabla \times E = -\mu \frac{\partial H}{\partial t} \tag{9.10}$$

$$\nabla \times H = \sigma E + \varepsilon \frac{\partial E}{\partial t} \tag{9.11}$$

are implemented for a lattice of subvolumes or "Yee cells" that may be cubical or parallelepiped with different dimensions δ_x, δ_y, and δ_z in x-, y-, or z-directions, respectively. The components of $\mathbf{E}$ and $\mathbf{H}$ are positioned about each of the cells as shown in Figure 9.9 and calculated alternately with half-time steps where the time step $\delta t = \delta/2c$. Here, δ is the smallest of the dimensions used for any of the cells and c is the maximum phase velocity of the fields in the modeled space. Since some of the modeled volume is air, c corresponds to the velocity of EM waves in air.

In the FDTD method, it is necessary to represent not only the scatterer or absorber, such as the human body or a part thereof, but also the sources, including their shapes, excitations, etc., if these sources are in the near-field region. The far-field sources, on the other hand, are described by means of incident plane-wave fields prescribed for a "source" plane, typically six to ten cells away from the exposed body. The source-body interaction volume is subdivided into Yee cells of the type shown in Figure 9.9. The interaction space consisting of several hundred thousand to a few million cells is truncated by means of

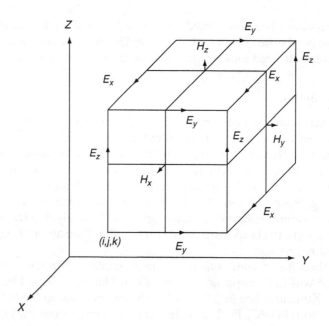

FIGURE 9.9
Unit cell of Yee lattice showing positions for various field components.

absorbing boundaries. The prescribed incident fields are tracked in time for all cells of the interaction space. The solution is considered completed when either the fields have died off or, for sinusoidal excitation, when a sinusoidal steady-state behavior for **E** and **H** is observed for the interaction space.

The body of interest is mapped into the lattice space by first choosing the lattice increment and then assigning values of permittivity and conductivity to each cell. The boundary conditions at media interfaces are inherently generated by the curl equations. Thus, once a computer program is developed, the basic routines need not be changed for different model geometries. In fact, inhomogeneities and fine structural details could be modeled with a maximum resolution of one unit cell.

Time-stepping for the FDTD method is accomplished by an explicit FD procedure [57,63]. For a cubic cell lattice space, this procedure involves positioning the electric and magnetic field components about a unit cell of the lattice and then evaluating the components at alternate half-time steps. In this manner, centered difference expression can be used for both the space and time increments without solving simultaneous equations to compute the fields at the latest time step.

The explicit formulation of the FDTD method is particularly suited for execution with minimum computer storage and run-time using current array-processing computers. The required computer storage and run-time increase only linearly with N, the numbers of cells. In fact, it has been shown that the FDTD method is capable of solving for more than 1 million unknown field components within a few minutes on an array-processing computer. Field intensities have been predicted to within 2.5% accuracy relative to known analytical and experimental bench marks. Recently, the FDTD technique has been constructed to allow solutions for field penetration and absorption in large, complex, inhomogeneous, and irregularly shaped biological bodies in three dimensions, with submillimeter range spatial resolution. With the exception of a few early attempts with lossy

Computational Methods and EM Fields

biological objects [58,66], a majority of early efforts have been directed toward application of the FDTD method to EM interaction in time-varying inhomogeneous media [59], and with metallic bodies of revolution [60]. However, during the past two decades, the FDTD method has become the most extensively used numerical procedure for bioelectromagnetic computations.

9.3.5.2 Frequency-Dependent FDTD Formulation

For short pulses where wider bandwidths are generally involved, a frequency-dependent FDTD or (FD)²TD method is needed. There are two general approaches to the (FD)²TD method. One approach is to convert the complex permittivity from the frequency domain to the time domain and convolve this with the time-domain electric fields to obtain time-domain fields for the dispersive material. This discrete time-domain method may be updated recursively for some rational forms of complex permittivity, which removes the need to store the time history of the fields and makes the method feasible. This method has been applied to materials such as water for which the permittivity may be described by a first-order Debye equation [71–73] or more complex materials with dielectric properties given by a second-order Lorentz equation with multiple poles [74].

A second approach is to add a differential equation relating the electric flux density $\mathbf{D}$ to the electric field $\mathbf{E}$ and solve this equation simultaneously with the standard FDTD equations. This method has been applied to 1-D and 2-D examples with materials described by a first-order Debye equation or second-order single-pole Lorentz equation [75], and to 3-D spherical models and homogeneous two-thirds muscle-equivalent man model with properties described by a second-order Debye equation [76,77]. The following is a description of this differential equation approach, which has been used for induced current and SAR calculations for a heterogeneous model of the human body [78].

The time-dependent Maxwell's curl equations used for the FDTD method have already been given as Equations 9.10 and 9.11. The curl $\mathbf{H}$ can also be written as follows:

$$\nabla \times H = \sigma E + \varepsilon \frac{\partial E}{\partial t} \tag{9.12}$$

where the electric flux density vector $\mathbf{D}$ is related to the electric field through the complex permittivity $\varepsilon^*(\omega)$ of the local tissue by the following equation:

$$D = \varepsilon^*(w)E \tag{9.13}$$

Since Equations 9.10 and 9.12 are to be solved iteratively in the time domain, Equation 9.13 must also be expressed in the time domain. This may be done by choosing a rational function for $\varepsilon^*(\omega)$, such as the Debye equation with two relaxation constants:

$$\varepsilon^*(\omega) = \varepsilon_0 \left[\varepsilon_\infty + \frac{\varepsilon_{s1} - \varepsilon_\infty}{1 + j\omega\tau_1} + \frac{\varepsilon_{s2} - \varepsilon_\infty}{1 + j\omega\tau_2} \right] \tag{9.14}$$

Rearranging Equation 9.14 and substituting in Equation 9.13 gives

$$D(\omega) = \varepsilon^*(\omega)E(\omega) = \varepsilon_0 \frac{\varepsilon_s + j\omega(\varepsilon_{s1}\tau_2 + \varepsilon_{s2}\tau_1) - \omega^2\tau_1\tau_2\varepsilon_\infty}{1 + j\omega(\tau_1 + \tau_2) - \omega^2\tau_1\tau_2} E(\omega) \tag{9.15}$$

where the static (zero frequency) dielectric constant is given by

$$\varepsilon_s = \varepsilon_{s1} + \varepsilon_{s2} - \varepsilon_\infty \tag{9.16}$$

Assuming $e^{j\omega t}$ time dependence, Equation 9.15 can be written as a differential equation in the time domain.

$$\tau_1\tau_2\frac{\partial^2 D}{\partial t^2} + (\tau_1 + \tau_2)\frac{\partial D}{\partial t} + D = \varepsilon_0\left[\varepsilon_s E + (\varepsilon_{s1}\tau_2 + \varepsilon_{s2}\tau_1)\frac{\partial E}{\partial t} + \varepsilon_\infty\tau_1\tau_2\frac{\partial^2 E}{\partial t^2}\right] \tag{9.17}$$

For the (FD)²TD method, Equations 9.10 and 9.12 need to be solved subject to Equation 9.17. These equations can be written in the difference form [76,77], and solved to find **E**, **H**, and **D** at each cell location. The **E** → **H** → **D** loop is then repeated until the pulse has died off.

9.4 Anatomically Realistic Body Models

Computational algorithms based on numerical techniques described in the previous section have been applied to calculate field intensities and SAR distributions in anatomically realistic models of human bodies. However, the use of a given numerical algorithm and the number of computational cells involved in the models typically dictate the applicability of the techniques, fidelity of the model, the degree of accuracy attainable, and its domain of application. In the following sections, a few of the models will be described, and they will be followed by results obtained using the models.

Models proposed as better representations of the complex geometry and composition of the human body include constructions using small-volume-cubic cells or cell meshes and anatomically realistic models generated from x-ray computerized tomography (CT) and magnetic resonance imaging (MRI) data.

9.4.1 Cubic Cell Models

Models of the human body consisting of 200–1000 cubic cells that account more realistically for the gross anatomic and biometric characteristics of human bodies have been used by several investigators [26,30]. The models are 1.75 m tall and can be made either homogeneous or inhomogeneous by choosing an equivalent or a volume-weighted complex permittivity for each cell. The cubic-cell model has been employed, successfully, to calculate whole-body averaged absorption. It is important to note that for subdivision with less than three cells per wavelength, the magnitude and phase resolutions would be such that even with convergence the reliability of the MoM computed SAR would be questionable. Therefore, if the interest is primarily in whole-body SAR, this model may provide quite adequate results for frequencies lower than 30 MHz. To achieve more accurate structural representation of the human body, anatomically based models should be used.

Computational Methods and EM Fields

9.4.2 Millimeter-Resolution Model Based on MRI Scans

Millimeter (mm), and in some cases, sub-mm resolution models of the human body have been developed from the MRI scans. For example, a male volunteer of height 176.4 cm and weight 64 kg [79,80]. The MRI scans were taken with a resolution of 3 mm along the height of the body and 1.875 mm for the orthogonal axes in the cross-sectional planes. Even though the height of the volunteer was quite appropriate for an average adult male, the mass was somewhat lower than an average of 71 kg, which is assumed for an average male. This problem can, to some extent, be ameliorated by assuming that the cell dimensions for the cross-sections are larger than 1.875 mm by the ratio of $(71/64)^{1/2} = 1.053$. By taking the larger cell dimensions of $1.053 \times 1.875 = 1.974$ mm for the cross-sectional axes, the volume of the model can be increased by $(1.053)^2 = 1.109$, that is, by about 10.9% which results in an increase of its mass by approximately the same percentage, that is to a new mass of approximately 71 kg. The MRI sections were converted into images involving 29 tissue types whose dielectric properties can then be prescribed at the exposure frequency. The tissue types are fat, muscle, bone, cartilage, skin, brain, nerve, cerebrospinal fluid (CSF), intestine, spleen, pancreas, heart, blood, eye, eye humor, eye sclera, eye lens, ear, liver, kidney, lung, bladder, stomach, ligament, compact bone, testicle, spermatic cord, prostate gland, and erectile tissue. This model has been used to calculate the EM absorption in the human head, neck, and shoulders for cellular telephones operating at frequencies of 800–900 MHz. Because of the localized nature of exposure fields, it was possible to use the model corresponding to the top 42 cm of the body for SAR calculations.

9.4.3 The Visible Human Model

The Visible Human (VH) Project, developed by the National Library of Medicine, is a 3-D digital image library representing an adult human male and female [81]. The VH data set for both the male and female includes photographic images obtained through cryosectioning of human cadavers, and digital images obtained through CT and MRI imaging of the same cadavers. In particular, the photographic images represent a highly accurate and realistic representation of the anatomical cross-sections contained in human anatomy atlases. The male data set, the first to be constructed (released in 1994), consists of 1871 digital axial images obtained at 1.0-mm intervals, with a pixel resolution of 1 mm; the female one contains 5189 digital axial images (released in 1995), obtained with a finer spatial step of 0.33 mm. While these digital data sets represent a unique tool to explore human anatomy, their direct use for computational EM dosimetry is limited by the fact that images cannot be directly used as an input for a numerical EM tool, but must be converted to a so-called "segmented" version. A segmented model is a model where every pixel, usually called in such models "voxel," does not contain information about the color (like in digital images) but rather a label which is uniquely associated to a given tissue. In such a way, it is possible to know which tissue fills each of the model voxels and hence assign the correct complex permittivity values to be used in numerical simulations.

Segmentation of the original image sets is a complex and time-consuming activity, which is difficult to be carried out making exclusive use of automatic procedures, such as contour recognition algorithms, but inevitably requires intervention by experts in human anatomy. The segmentation procedure has been carried out for the male model by researchers at the Air Force Research Laboratory, Brooks Air Force Base, TX [82]. The final segmented model, made freely available to the scientific community, comprises $586 \times 340 \times 1878$ voxels with a resolution of $1 \times 1 \times 1\,mm$, and is segmented in about 40 different tissue types [83]. The VH model has been widely used to study both whole-body and localized human exposure to EMFs generated by various types of sources. It has been included in several commercially available EM simulation tools with capabilities for dosimetric evaluation.

The original VH model has a height of 1.88 m and a mass of 103 kg. The VH model has often been scaled in its axial cross-sections (for example, with a 0.91 scaling factor in the shoulder-to-shoulder direction and 0.83 in the front-to-back direction) to arrive at a mass of about 80 kg, to mimic a more typical-mass for adult-male [84].

Also, two child-scale models were obtained using scaling factors along the three directions of the VH model to reproduce the 50% mass-for-age and stature-for-age percentiles for their age group [85]. The final 13-year-old child model (0.71 scaling factor in the axial sections and 0.83 in the vertical direction) has a height of 156 cm and mass of 44 kg, while the 7-year-old child (0.59 scaling factor in the axial sections and 0.67 in the vertical direction) is 125-cm tall, weighs 24 kg.

It should be mentioned that the scaling procedure, however, does not produce anatomically correct child (CL) models, particularly with reference to the proportion between the head and the trunk. Indeed, it is well known that children, proportionally, tend to have larger heads than adults. For this reason, two child-like models have also been derived, applying different scaling factors to different body segments. In particular, the body has been divided into four major segments: the trunk (T), going from the feet to the neck, lower face (LF), going from the chin to the center of the mouth, upper face (UF), spanning from the center of the mouth to the center of the eyes, and head (H), above the center of the eyes. The scaling factors for the trunk were kept the same as those adopted for the child-scale models, while scaling factors for the face and head were based on anthropometric data [86].

Even though the nonuniform scaling procedure adopted for the CL models can yield realistic body shapes, it does not ensure that the internal organ structure is accurate or realistic. However, the resulting models are suitable for considering the effect of body dimension on global or whole-body exposure parameters and for assessing whether increasing anatomical realism makes any difference for compliance assessment. It is also worth mentioning that most models are representative of a standing or laying postures, while it is clear that an individual spends many hours a day sitting. But the standing posture gives rise to higher SAR values and can therefore represent a worst-case scenario for compliance assessment [87,88].

9.4.4 Anatomical Family Computer Models

Lastly, several computer models with mm resolution have been developed to further improve the anatomical realism and fidelity of human models for various application scenarios. Some anatomically realistic human models developed for computer simulation are illustrated in Figure 9.10. They are mostly based on MR images of healthy adults and children, and have been segmented into more than 80 distinct tissue types. Examples are the Japanese voxel model [89,90], virtual family data set [91], Chinese anatomic models of adult and infants [92,93]. Developments have also included variable postures and two-body infant-and adult models with different skin-to-skin contact areas and positions [94].

Computational Methods and EM Fields 325

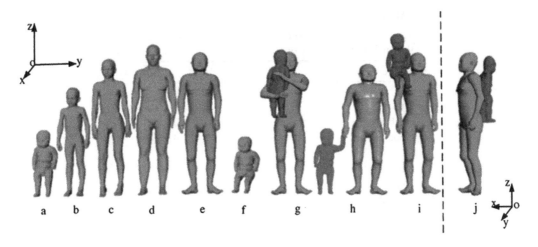

FIGURE 9.10
Anatomically realistic human models developed for computer simulation. From left, (a) infant model in standing posture, (b) Thelonius (6-years-old), (c) Billie (11-years-old), (d) Ella (26-years old), (e) Chinese adult female, (f) sitting infant model. (g-j) two-body, infant-and-adult models with different skin-to-skin contact areas and positions.

Source: From Li, C., and Wu, T., 2015 [94] with permission.

9.5 Applications of Anatomically Realistic Computer Models

This section describes applications of anatomically realistic computer models to study both whole-body and localized human exposure to EMFs generated by various types of sources.

9.5.1 Currents Induced in the Human Body by Low-Frequency EMFs

This discussion will begin with details on the use of the impedance method to calculate currents induced in the human body by the EMFs of electric blankets. It also includes the use of the FDTD method has been used for calculations of internal **E** and **H** fields and induced current densities for exposure to electric, magnetic, or combined electric and magnetic fields at power-line frequencies. The results given below were obtained using a 1.31-cm resolution, anatomically based model of the human body. Since the term $j\omega\varepsilon$ can be neglected as compared to σ for the various tissues at extremely low frequencies including electric power frequencies (50/60 Hz), the impedances for the various cells of the model given by Equation 9.9 can be replaced by resistances. It is recognized that the conductivities of various tissues, for example, skeletal muscle, heart, bone, etc., are anisotropic for power-line frequencies [36,37,95]. The anisotropy has been neglected in this case, however, and average values of conductivities given in Table 9.3 have been taken for the various tissues for the calculations.

9.5.1.1 Electric Blankets

To illustrate the use of the impedance method, currents induced in the human body by the EMFs of two types of electric blankets have been calculated [2]. The two models used

TABLE 9.3

Tissue Conductivity (s) Used for Calculations at the Power-line Frequency of 60 Hz

Tissue Type	s (S/m)
Air	0
Muscle	0.52 or 0.11
Fat, Bone	0.04
Blood	0.6
Intestine	0.11
Cartilage	0.04
Liver	0.13
Kidney	0.16
Pancreas	0.11
Spleen	0.18
Lung[a]	0.04
Heart	0.11
Nerve, Brain	0.12
Skin	0.11
Eye	0.11

[a] The dielectric properties of the lung consisting of 33% lung tissue and 67% air.

for the blanket are: (a) a low-magnetic-field blanket, and (b) a conventional (pre-1990) electric blanket. The low-magnetic-field blanket uses two parallel leads carrying equal and opposite currents to reduce the net magnetic field around the conductors. The two leads are separated typically by 1.5 mm and are embedded in a positive temperature coefficient (PTC) conductive polymer and insulated by polyvinyl chloride (PVC). The PTC conductive polymer surrounding the two leads may be represented by a set of distributed resistors which would result in linearly decreasing equal but opposite currents flowing through the two leads over the length of the wiring used for the blanket. By comparison, the conventional electric blanket uses a resistive alloy wire wrapped on a nylon cord and insulated with PVC. Because of the distributed resistance of the wire, this blanket would therefore have a linearly diminishing voltage and identical magnitude of current over the length of the wiring used for the blanket.

The validity of the calculated results has been established by comparing results obtained using the impedance algorithm and those reported by others. The calculated fields are in excellent agreement with the data given in [96,97]. Currents are induced in the body by the following sources:

1. Time and spatially varying magnetic fields of the blanket-induced voltages in the various resistance loops of the body.
2. Currents launched into different subareas at the body surface by means of the capacitively coupled currents from the various conductors of the blanket.

The spatial variations of the magnetic fields were calculated from the Biot–Savart's law for a short current-carrying conductor [2]. By integrating it over the entire length of the current-carrying conductors, one can obtain the vector magnetic fields at the centers of the cells representing the model of the human body or any of the other points in space. From

Computational Methods and EM Fields

the vector magnetic fields thus calculated for each of the cell centers for the impedance model of the human body, the induced voltages for each of the faces of the cells can be written [34]. This information is then used to calculate the induced currents for the various impedances, that is, resistances. The average current densities J_x, J_y, and J_z for each of the cell centers can be obtained by taking the average of the currents through the resistances representing the four edges each of the cell in the respective directions and dividing the same by the cross-sectional area δ^2 (= 1.31×1.31 cm²).

To calculate the electric-field distribution in air, a 3-D impedance model consisting of capacitors representing the space between the various faces of the cells was used. For cubic cells of dimension $\delta = 1.31$ cm, the capacitances used are $\varepsilon_0 \delta^2/\delta = 0.116$ pF.

For currents induced in the human body due to electric fields, it should be recognized that the energized conductors of the blanket are capacitively coupled to the body. The capacitance between a given conductor and the highly conducting human body can be obtained by using an expression similar to that for a conductor at a distance S from the ground plane. Capacitance per unit length C of a wire of diameter d parallel to but separated a distance S from the ground plane is given by

$$C = (2.73\varepsilon_{\text{eff}})/\left[\log_{10}(4S/d)\right], \text{pF/m} \tag{9.18}$$

For a spacing, $S = 5$ mm and a wire diameter, $d = 0.8$ mm, and for $\varepsilon_{\text{eff}} = 2.5\varepsilon_0$, which is a value intermediate between the permittivity ε_0 for air and $4\varepsilon_0$ for the material of the blanket, we can calculate $C = 43.1$ pF/m. For a cell length $d = 1.31 \times 10^{-2}$ m, the coupling capacitance C_c between the wire and the cell can be calculated to be 0.565 pF. Since the interconductor spacing of 1.5 mm for a PTC blanket is fairly small as compared to the cell size, a proportionately smaller resistance is taken for the tissue-equivalent cells immediately underneath the conductors for the direction parallel to the interconductor spacing. Capacitances of 0.565 pF are taken from each of the conductors of the PTC blanket to the appropriate points on the impedance model of the human body. In the presence of an electrical grounding surface, the space underneath the model is represented by a 3-D network of capacitors each of value 0.116 pF representing the air space between the various faces of the cubic cells of dimension $d = 1.31$ cm for each of the sides.

For the PTC low-magnetic field blanket, a constant voltage of 110 V ac is taken between the conductors of the twin-lead wiring for calculation of currents induced/injected into the human body due to electric fields. For calculating the magnetic fields, an input current of 1 A is taken. On account of the conductive polymer surrounding the parallel wires, this current diminishes linearly to zero at the end of the PTC wiring. This assumes a blanket input power of 110 W under normal operating conditions. If magnetic fields or induced current densities due to higher input powers are desired, the numbers calculated for 1 A input current may then be multiplied by the appropriate factor.

The conventional blanket, on the other hand, uses a resistive conductor for which the voltage diminishes linearly from 110 V to zero over the length of the wiring. For this blanket the current throughout the length of the wiring is the same as at the input, that is, 1 A, which is assumed for the calculation of magnetic fields.

The magnetically induced, section-averaged magnitudes of the total current densities, from head to feet for the two types of blankets are shown in Figures 9.11a and b, respectively. For these calculations, the wiring of the blanket was taken to be 0.5 cm from the surface of the body. Nearly identical current densities were also obtained for a grounding plate underneath the body at distances of 0.25, 0.5, and 1.0 m. It is interesting to note that

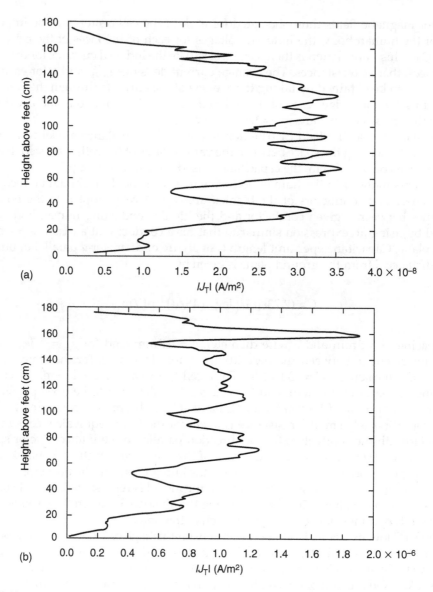

FIGURE 9.11
Section-averaged magnitudes of total current densities for the various sections of the body for magnetic fields of the blankets. Nearly identical current densities were obtained also for a grounding plate at distances of 0.25, 0.5, and 1.0 m underneath the body. Input current = 1 A.

the induced current densities are larger by a factor of about 500 for the conventional blanket *vis a vis* those for the low-magnetic-field blanket.

The calculated section-averaged magnitudes of the total current densities due to electric fields of both of the blankets in the absence of a grounded plane are shown in Figures 9.12a and b, respectively. It should be noted that while the current densities induced by the electric fields of a low-magnetic field blanket (Figure 9.12a) are considerably higher than those due to magnetic fields (Figure 9.11a), the converse is true for a conventional blanket. For this blanket, the current densities induced by the magnetic fields (Figure 9.11b) are higher

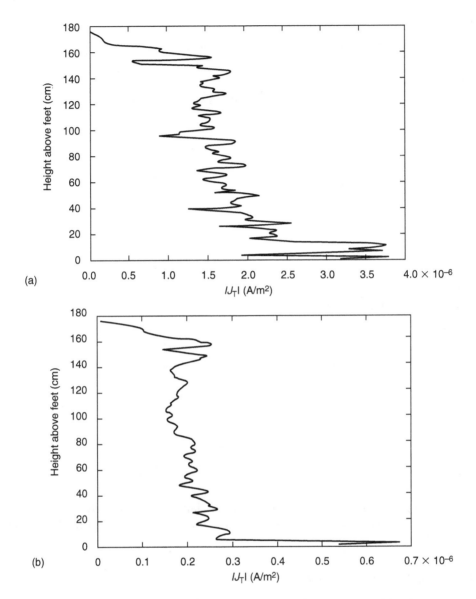

FIGURE 9.12
Section-averaged magnitudes of total current densities for the various sections of the body for electric fields of the blankets. No ground plane underneath the body.

than those due to electric fields (Figure 9.12b). In fact, while the current densities due to magnetic fields are fairly small for a low-magnetic field blanket as compared to those for a conventional blanket, the current densities due to electric fields of a low-magnetic field blanket are even higher than those for a conventional blanket (see Figures 9.12a and b). The reasons for these observations can be seen from the values of magnetic and electric fields given in Table 9.4 for the two types of blankets, respectively. While fairly small magnetic fields are calculated for the low-magnetic field blanket as compared to those for the conventional blanket, the converse is true for the electric fields created by these blankets. As seen in Table 9.5, somewhat higher electric fields are created by the low-magnetic-field

TABLE 9.4

Comparison of the Calculated and Measured Magnetic and Electric Fields Close to a Flat Electric Blanket

Low Magnetic Field Blanket

For this blanket, the magnetic-field results are normalized for a blanket input current of 1.227 A, i.e., a power input of 135 W.

Magnetic Field (μT)

	Grid Size (cm)	Calculated	Measured
Average	1.31 × 1.31	0.056	—
	10.5 × 10.5	0.072	0.09
Peak	—	0.20	0.26

Electric Field (V/m)

	Grid Size (cm)	Calculated	Measured
Average	1.31 × 1.31	103.7	—
	10.5 × 10.5	144.6	111.2
Peak		159.7	176.0

Conventional Electric Blanket

For this blanket, an input current of 1 A is assumed.

Magnetic Field (μT)

	Grid Size (cm)	Calculated	Measured
Average	1.31 × 1.31	2.16	—
	10.5 × 10.5	2.45	2.18
Peak	—	3.52	3.94

Electric Field (V/m)

	Grid Size (cm)	Calculated	Measured
Average	1.31 × 1.31	57.3	—
	10.5 × 10.5	70.1	95.4
Peak	—	176.1	167.2

blanket as compared to those for the conventional blanket. This is likely due to the higher potential difference between the twin-lead conductors that are used for the low-magnetic field blankets.

9.5.1.2 Power Transmission Lines

The FDTD method has been used for calculations of internal **E** and **H** fields and induced current densities for exposure to electric, magnetic, or combined electric and magnetic fields at power-line frequencies [39]. While recognizing that the conductivities of many biological tissues (skeletal muscle, bone, etc.) are highly anisotropic for power-line frequencies; however, the effect of anisotropy is neglected for simplicity. They could be included in more complex models by separately identifying these tissues.

Both sinusoidal and prescribed time-varying incident fields can be used with the FDTD procedure—hence, the method is well-suited also for transient exposures that are often of interest at power-line-related frequencies. For sinusoidal time varying fields, the solution is completed when a sinusoidal steady-state behavior for **E** and **H** fields is observed for each of the cells. For lossy biological bodies this typically takes a step time on the order of three to four time periods of oscillation. Since Δt is fixed for a given cell size, a larger number of iterations is therefore needed at lower frequencies. Because of the large number

Computational Methods and EM Fields

TABLE 9.5

Reported SAR Values, Averaged Over the Whole Body (SAR_{WB}), for Plane Wave Exposures

Frequency [MHz]	SAR (W/kg)					
	Grounded shoes [108]	Grounded [111]	Isolated [111]	Isolated (resol. 3 mm) [112]	Isolated (resol. 5 mm) [112]	Grounded[a] [113]
10	0.027	0.045				
20	0.102	0.182	0.021			
30	0.180	0.313	0.054			
40	0.291	0.348	0.114			
50	0.230	0.293	0.199			
60	0.177	0.231	0.288			
70	0.152	0.188	0.302	0.270	0.290	
80	0.130	0.162	0.251			
90	0.107		0.195			
100	0.092	0.118	0.155			0.123[b]
200	0.062	0.081	0.080	0.048	0.051	0.078[c]
300	0.054					
400	0.060	0.063	0.063	0.064	0.060	
500	0.058					0.060
600	0.057		0.063	0.067	0.066	
700	0.059					
800	0.061			0.064	0.063	
900	0.061	0.062	0.064			
1000				0.063	0.061	0.057
1400			0.063			
1800		0.057	0.058	0.056	0.060	
2000				0.055	0.060	

[a] the number in reference list.
[b] the frequency considered is 120 MHz.
[c] the frequency considered is 210 MHz.

of iterations, the FDTD procedure would be clearly inapplicable for calculations at power-line frequencies were it not for the quasi-static nature of the coupling at low frequencies [20,98,99]. Thus, the field outside the body does not depend on the internal tissue properties, but it depends only on the shape of the body so long as the quasi-static approximation holds, that is, the size of the body is a factor of ten or more smaller than the wavelength, and $|\sigma + j\omega\varepsilon| \gg \varepsilon_o$ where σ and ε are the conductivity and the permittivity of the tissues, respectively, $\omega = 2\pi f$ is the radian frequency, and ε_o is the permittivity of the free space outside the body. Under these conditions, the electric fields in air are normal to the body surface and the internal tissue electric fields can be obtained from the boundary conditions in terms of fields outside,

$$jw\varepsilon_o E_o = (\sigma + jw\varepsilon)E_{\text{tissue}} \tag{9.19}$$

A higher quasi-static frequency f', at 5–20 MHz, may therefore be used for exposure of the E model and the internal fields E thus calculated may be scaled back to frequency f of interest, e.g., 60 Hz. Since in the FDTD method, one needs to calculate in the time domain until convergence is obtained, this frequency scaling to 5–20 MHz for f reduces the needed number of iterations by over five orders of magnitude. From Equation 9.19 we can write

$$w'(\sigma + jw\varepsilon)\, E_{\text{tissue}}(f) = w(\sigma' + jw\varepsilon')\, E'_{\text{tissue}}(f') \tag{9.20}$$

or

$$E_{\text{tissue}}(f) = (f\sigma' / f'\sigma)\, E'_{\text{tissue}}(f') \tag{9.21}$$

assuming that $\sigma + jw\varepsilon \sim \sigma$ at both f' and f [2,100]. To validate the use of a higher frequency f to obtain induced E fields at ELF frequencies, test cases involving homogeneous and layered spheres have been used. Excellent agreement between the numerical and analytical results lends support to the validity of the FDTD method for calculating internal E fields and current densities at power-line-related frequencies. It should be noted that incident E and H fields of any orientation and relative magnitudes can be prescribed in the FDTD method allowing the possibility of calculations for realistic exposure conditions. Also the choice of a considerably higher frequency such as 5–20 MHz reduces the number of iterations needed to obtain converged results by five to six orders of magnitude as compared to those that would be needed at ELF frequencies of 10 Hz–1 kHz.

Some calculated results using a 16-tissue, 1.31-cm-resolution, anatomically based model of the human body are given in Figure 9.13. A frequency f' of 5–10 MHz was used to reduce the computation time. At the higher exposure frequency f', $\sigma' = \sigma$ was assumed, i.e., conductivities of the various tissues at 60 Hz. Furthermore, the incident E field $\mathbf{E}_i(f') = 60\, \mathbf{E}_i(f)/f'$ was used to obtain $\mathbf{E}_{\text{tissue}}(f)$ at say $\mathbf{E}_i(f) = 10$ kV/m. The incident magnetic field $\mathbf{H}i(f')$ has similarly been taken to be considerably lower ($= 60\, \mathbf{H}_i(f)/f'$) to account for the fact that the

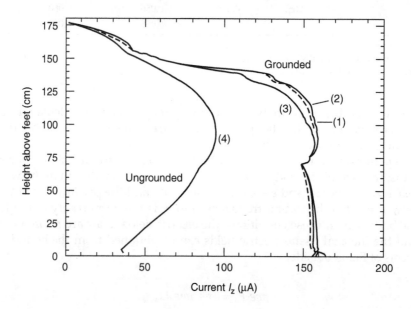

FIGURE 9.13
Calculated layer currents for anatomically based grounded and ungrounded models exposed to EMFs at 60 Hz. For curves (1) and (2) $s = 0.52$ S/m for skeletal muscle and $s = 0.11$ S/m for the interior muscle. For curves (3) and (4) $s = 0.11$ S/m for all of the muscle. $E = 10$ kV/m (vertical), $H = 26.5$ A/m from side to side for all of the curves except for (2) for which only E-field exposure is assumed.

Computational Methods and EM Fields

induced current densities and internal electric fields are proportional to the frequency of the incident fields and would therefore be higher at the assumed frequency f'. Recognizing the anisotropy in the conductivity of skeletal muscles, two different values of muscle conductivities are taken for curves (1) and (2). For these curves a higher conductivity of 0.52 S/m is taken for the skeletal muscle and an average value of 0.11 S/m is taken for the muscle in the interior of the body. For curves (3) and (4), however, a lower conductivity of 0.11 S/m is taken for all of the muscle, interior or skeletal. The results shown in Figure 9.13 curves (1), (3), and (4) are for $E_{inc} = 10$ kV/m (vertical) and $H_{inc} = 26.5$ A/m ($B_{inc} = 33.3$ μT) from side to side of the model. To point out the preponderance of the induced currents due to incident electric field, $H_{inc} = 0$ is assumed for the calculations shown in curve (2). It is interesting to note that the layer currents due to E-field exposure alone are almost 98%–99% of the currents calculated for the combined electric and magnetic fields. It is also interesting to note that the calculated foot currents of 155–160 μA are in good agreement with 165 μA that would be projected from measurements for the human body [101]. The variations of the induced currents calculated along the height of the body have been checked against measured results [102]. The agreement with the results of these two authors who had used a vertical electric field such as that under a high-voltage power line was found to be excellent [39].

9.5.2 Absorption in Human Bodies Exposed to Far-Field of RF Sources

As noted the configuration and frequency of the EM source, and the geometry and composition of the biological body will influence the induced field, and power deposition and distribution inside the body. Moreover, the field emitted from a source is dictated by the frequency, size, and configuration of the source. Near an antenna, the radiated energy is in the form of a spherical wave in which the wave-fronts are concentric shells. The spheroidal wave-front expands as the wave propagates outward from the source. At distances far from the source, the radius of curvature of the spherical shells becomes so large that the wave-front would essentially appear as a plane. They are therefore referred to as plane waves. Plane waves are important since their behavior is well quantified—the fields are uniform in planes normal to the direction of propagation and the power density varies only in the direction of propagation. In this case, both electric and magnetic fields of the propagating wave are orthogonal in space and lie in the plane of the wave front, and are related through the intrinsic impedance of the medium. In other words, in the far or radiation zone, the electric and magnetic fields have only transverse components.

In this section, we shall briefly summarize some of the efforts devoted to field computation using various models of the human body, which consists of large quantities of numerical cells, and present some results obtained for plane wave exposures. Note that some, especially the simpler models are of interest primarily for whole-body SAR, and can provide useful results for frequencies lower than 30 MHz. To achieve more accurate structural representation of the human body, anatomically based models are needed.

9.5.2.1 SAR Induced in Cubic Cell Models

The VMoM for field computation has been used for models of the human body consisting of 200–1000 cubic cells. These models account for the gross anatomic and biometric characteristics of human bodies, and have been used by several investigators [26–30]. The models are 1.75-m tall and can be made either homogeneous or inhomogeneous by choosing an equivalent or a volume-weighted complex permittivity for each cell. The cubic-cell model has been employed, successfully, to calculate whole-body averaged absorption. It is important to note that for subdivision with less than three cells per wavelength, the magnitude and phase resolutions would be such that even with convergence the reliability of the MoM computed SAR would be questionable.

According to the MoM method, the body may be partitioned into N cubic subvolumes or cells which are sufficiently small for the electric field and dielectric permittivity to be constant within each cell. The integral equation is then transformed into a system of $3N$ simultaneous linear equations for the three orthogonal components of the electric field at the center of each cell. The simultaneous equations may be written in matrix form as:

$$[G][E] = -[E^i] \tag{9.22}$$

where [G] is a $3N \times 3N$ matrix and $[E^i]$ and [E] are column matrices representing incident and induced electric field at the center of each cell. The elements of [G] are evaluated for each cell [26]. In particular, the diagonal elements of the [G] matrix may be evaluated exactly by approximating each subvolume with a sphere of equal volume centered at the position of an interior point. If the actual shape of the cell differs appreciably from that of a sphere, this approximation may lead to unsatisfactory numerical results [38]. In such cases, a small cylindrical volume may be created around an interior point. It may also be necessary to evaluate these terms by numerical integration throughout the cubic subvolume for increased accuracy. The evaluation of off-diagonal elements of the [G] matrix is considerably simplified since it does not involve principal value operations. Therefore, for a given applied field configuration, the induced electric fields inside the body are obtained by matrix inversion. That is,

$$[E] = -[G]^{-1}[E^i] \tag{9.23}$$

Factors that influence the computational accuracy include frequency, body size, cell dimensions, and computer memory. It has been found that reliable numerical results can be obtained if the linear dimensions of the cell do not exceed a quarter free-space wavelength [26]. For a computer with sufficient memory capacity to invert a 120×120 matrix, for example, the maximum number of cells is limited to 40. If we assume, for simplicity, symmetries between the right and the left half and the front and the back of 1.7-m-tall adult human body, this computer would handle approximately a cell size around $10^{-5}\,\mathrm{m}^3$. Once the $10^{-5}\,\mathrm{m}^3$ cell size is adopted, $750\,\mathrm{MHz}$ would be the highest frequency that can be considered for field intensity calculation without violating the criterion that the linear dimensions of the cell not exceed a quarter free-space wavelength.

The computational resources necessary to obtain even a regional SAR using this MoM approach can be extensive but does not constitute a challenge with today's computer technology. In any event, a relatively full complex matrix, $3N \times 3N$ in dimensions, is required for a model with N cells. The computation time required for a noniterative solution of the matrix equation is therefore pro1portional to between N^2 and N^3, which increases rapidly as N increases. The faithfulness with which a cubic cell model approximates the detailed structure of a biological body and the maximum usable frequency increases with the number of cells. In fact, substantial errors will occur if

$$N < (2\pi L)/(\lambda' 6^{1/2}) \tag{9.24}$$

where L/λ' is the ratio between the linear dimension of the body and the wavelength in the body.

Computational Methods and EM Fields

The accuracy of the numerical method can be verified by comparison with known results from exact analytic solutions based on well-characterized canonical geometric bodies, such as spheres. It should be noted that perfect agreement between the exact solution, based on Mie theory, and the numerical method, based on the volume integral equation, is not expected unless a large number of cubic cells are used to simulate the sphere. Figure 9.14 shows one-eighth of a sphere approximated by one-eighth of a "cubic model of a sphere," which is constructed from 73 cubic cells. Clearly, a better approximation can be achieved by a larger number of smaller cubic cells. Nevertheless, for a brain sphere constructed from 40 cubic cells at a frequency of 915 MHz, the computed maximum field intensity deviated from the exact solution by less than 9% [103].

A model of a human body consisting of 180 cubic cells that accounts for the anatomic and biometric characteristics of human beings is shown in Figure 9.15. The model is 1.75-m tall and can be made either homogeneous or inhomogeneous by using an equivalent or a volume-weighted complex permittivity for each cell [104]. The average absorption or whole-body SAR for the model of the human body shown in Figure 9.15 as a function of frequency is illustrated in Figure 9.16. The electric field vector is along the height of the body and the plane wave propagates from front to back of the model with an incident power density of 10 W/m². A homogeneous complex permittivity approximately two-thirds of that for muscle is used in the calculations. Note that the whole-body SAR increases with frequency until it reaches a maximum of about 0.23 W/kg at 77 MHz (resonance frequency) and then decreases by 1/frequency. The experimental data shown in Figure 9.17 are obtained from a saline-filled scale model of the human body. It can be seen that the calculated absorption is in good agreement with that found experimentally [29,105], except for the resonant

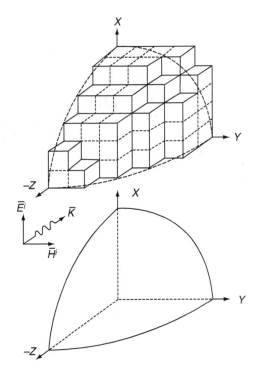

FIGURE 9.14
Approximation of one-eighth of a sphere by an equivalent cubic-cell-formed structure.

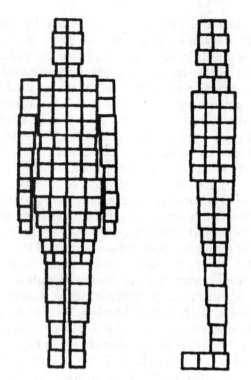

FIGURE 9.15
A model of a human body consisting of 180-cubic cells that accounts for anatomic and biometric characteristics.

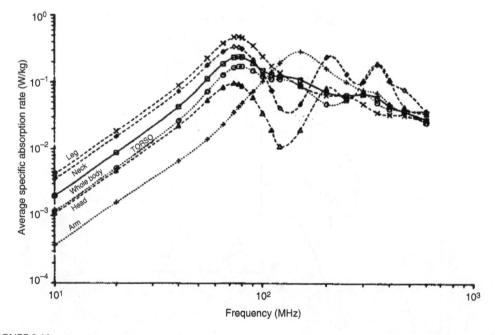

FIGURE 9.16
Average SARs for a homogeneous 180-cell model of the human body exposed to vertically polarized, 80 MHz plane wave. The incident power density is 10 W/m².

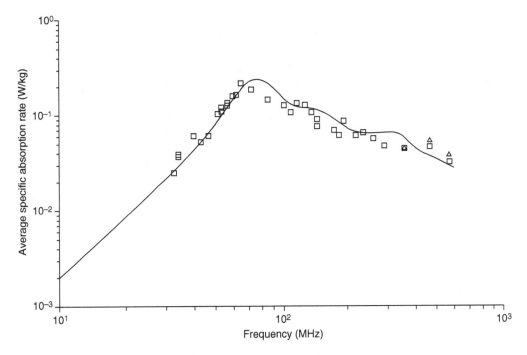

FIGURE 9.17
Whole-body averaged absorption for a homogeneous cubic-cell model of humans exposed to vertically polarized plane in free space. The incident power density is 10 W/m².

frequency which is somewhat lower (70 MHz) in the experimental case. It should be mentioned that whole-body SAR given in Figure 9.16 is typically within 10% of that estimated from prolate spheroidal models of the same height and dielectric property. Further, when inhomogeneous complex permittivities are used with the model, the whole-body SAR changes less than 2% from that depicted in Figure 9.16. Thus, if one is primarily concerned with average absorption over the body, a homogeneous prolate spheroidal model may be adequate.

While MoM methods based on the volume integral equation has been a useful numerical procedure for computation of average SAR and SAR distribution in complex tissue geometries, the requirement of a full $3N \times 3N$ matrix represents a limitation. However, this is easily surmounted by current generation of computational resources, so the limitation is no longer as severe. Nevertheless, the computation time required to provide SAR distribution of sufficient resolution to delineate the resonant frequency for the head region of 340 cells, increased the computation time by a factor of four over the 180-cell models [105,106]. Matrix inversion operations consume the largest block of time in MoM solutions for the cubic cell models.

9.5.2.2 SAR in Fine Resolution Anatomical Models

To accurately evaluate SARs induced in the human body, the FDTD method has been introduced in the late 1980s, when the memory requirements imposed limitations on the MoM. The capability of FDTD to take into account heterogeneities in models of the human body was first demonstrated using a model of the isolated human torso [68]. Later, a complete model of the human body was considered, and results for an isolated homogeneous man model standing in free space were compared with results for an inhomogeneous man model, under both isolated and grounded conditions [107]. The incident field was a plane wave propagating parallel to the ground plane and with the electric field vertically polarized (parallel to the height or long axis of the human body), at the frequencies of 100 and 350 MHz. The human-body model was obtained from cross-sectional diagrams and had a resolution of 2.62 cm at 100 MHz. The total occupied volume was $23 \times 12 \times 68$ cubic cells. At 350 MHz, the resolution was 1.31 cm for a total volume of $45 \times 24 \times 135$ cubic cells. The result, depicted as layer-averaged SAR or organ-averaged SAR, demonstrated the importance of considering inhomogeneous models of the human body. For example, the homogeneous model was not able to predict the peak SAR obtained in the eyes at 350 MHz, nor the difference in absorption among the different organs.

Since these first works on RF absorption, many papers have been published using anatomical models of the human body with finer resolutions.

The VH body model has been used to evaluate RF absorption and temperature increase as a function of frequency of the incident plane wave, by considering a grounded male, either barefoot or with shoes [108]. The model had a resolution of 5 mm, a total height of 180 cm, and a mass of 103 kg. The large mass was due to the use of the VH model which is far from the so called "reference man." The reference man weighs 73 kg and has a height of 176 cm [109]. In the referenced paper [108], for the frequency range between 10 and 900 MHz, SARs averaged over the whole body (SAR_{WB}) and locally, that is, averaged over 1.0 g (SAR_{1g}) and 10 g (SAR_{10g}) were evaluated. In particular, it has been found [108] that when the incident power density is equal to the reference levels set in the exposure standards, the basic restriction on SAR_{WB} and on local SARs are never exceeded. Moreover, it has been shown [108] that the ratio, SAR_{10g}/SAR_{WB} was about the same (either 25 or 50 according to the body part considered) as the value used in the safety guidelines to convert basic restrictions on SAR_{WB} to basic restriction on local peak SAR [110].

The influence of the human-body model on RF absorption is further illustrated in Figure 9.18, where a comparison among the SAR_{WB} obtained with the heterogeneous VH model and a homogeneous VH model consisting either of muscle or fat is presented. The frequencies considered are from 10 to 200 MHz to highlight the differences in RF absorption at resonance. It can be seen that a higher peak appeared at resonance in the homogeneous muscle model, and lower absorptions were obtained in the homogeneous fat model. Moreover, data from a lighter model (65.8 kg) obtained by reducing the cell dimension on the horizontal plane suggested that the lighter body absorbed more EM energy than the heavier one. The frequency dependence of RF absorption is clearly evident in Figure 9.18. Indeed, this frequency dependence was the basis of the different limits imposed on the reference levels for different frequencies in the safety guidelines [110].

Some literature data are summarized in Table 9.5 for the SAR_{WB} as a function of frequency (10 MHz–2 GHz) for a grounded and isolated man model exposed to an incident power density of 10 W/m². Note the resonant frequencies of 40 versus 70 MHz for grounded or isolated bodies. Moreover, it has been have shown that non-significant differences in SAR averaged over the whole body by changing the model resolution from 3 to 5 mm [112]. For the same reason, the cubic-cell model described in the previous section had been employed, successfully, to calculate whole-body averaged absorption. The SAR_{WB} has a weak dependence on model resolution.

Likewise, a study on the SAR dependence upon permittivity values [114] showed that uncertainty in permittivity values does not substantially affect the SAR as averaged over whole body, while the same uncertainties have a greater effect on local SAR. In particular, considerations of different frequencies and orientations of the incident plane wave,

Computational Methods and EM Fields

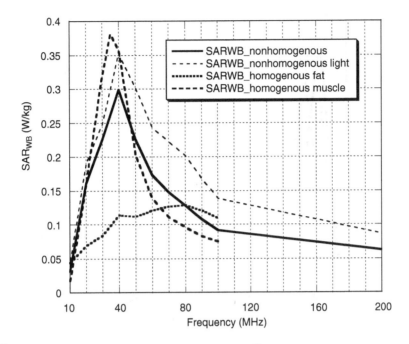

FIGURE 9.18

SAR$_{WB}$ as averaged over the whole body as a function of the frequency for different VH body model: non-homogeneous, non-homogeneous with a lighter weight (65.8 kg vs. 103 kg), homogeneous fat, homogeneous muscle.

or higher or lower permittivity values, showed that the maximum difference in SAR$_{WB}$ was within ±20% [112]. Larger differences were found in local SAR, particularly when the permittivity of muscle, representing about the 42% of the whole-body mass, was changed [112].

A high-resolution human body model (1.974 × 1.974 × 3.0 mm) and a coarser one (5.922 × 5.922 × 6.0 mm) both for isolated and grounded conditions, were employed to determine absorption in the head and neck region and to evaluate the frequencies at which the absorption may be maximized [115]. It was observed that under isolated conditions two resonant frequencies occurred for the head and neck, one associated with the whole-body resonance and the other with a local resonance of the head and neck. Under grounded conditions, three resonances were observed. The additional resonance was attributed to a torso resonance.

Some studies were conducted to evaluate power absorption in models of women and children. Specifically, a 10-year-old child and a 5-year-old child were considered by scaling the adult human body model [89]. It is noted that simply scaling the adult human body model to the children's dimensions does not produce an accurate model since the different organs scale differently; however, the general features in terms of height and mass are fulfilled thus allowing for the determination of general properties of EM energy absorption. In this way, resonant frequencies of 104 MHz for the isolated model and 65 MHz for the grounded 10-year-old child were obtained, while for the 5-year-old model, they were 126 and 73 MHz, respectively.

In a different study absorption in scaled versions of adult-human body model representing 10-, 5-, and 1-year old children were evaluated both for grounded and isolated conditions [111]. Figure 9.19 gives the SAR$_{WB}$ obtained for the three child models under isolated conditions, and an incident power density of 10 W/m². A shift in the resonant frequency

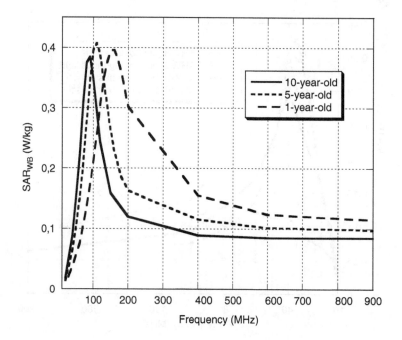

FIGURE 9.19

SAR$_{WB}$ as averaged over the whole body as a function of the frequency for different children body models: 10-, 5-, 1-year-old. Incident power: 10 W/m². Data taken from [103].

with the height of the model—the taller the model, the lower the resonance frequency—can be observed from the figure; note also the higher absorption in the smaller child body model [111].

The potential differences between SAR induced in man and woman have been explored using slightly different models [89,116]. In one study, 2-mm resolution models were developed for evaluating power absorption in Japanese males and females. Note that the use of the 2-mm resolution body models had led to an over-estimation of the skin mass by 50% or more than the average value for the Japanese reference body [89]. The calculated results showed that difference in SAR$_{WB}$ between male and female models was small, all within 1.1 dB. The authors concluded that gender does not affect SAR$_{WB}$. Similarly, they obtained no significant differences between the male and female models also with regard to local SARs. However, the over-estimation of the skin mass, and perhaps other tissues in the 2-mm resolution body models could have influenced their results and conclusions.

In contrast, a clear difference in absorption was reported between Caucasian male and female models [116]. The two Caucasian body models were developed using the semi-automated procedure previously cited [113]. In particular, considerably greater SAR$_{WB}$ was obtained in the female model than in the male one: about 40% higher in the frequency range between 500 MHz to 2.0 GHz, and 25% higher in the frequency range between 2.0 and 4.0 GHz. The difference in local SARs (both SAR$_{1g}$ and SAR$_{10g}$) were insignificant between genders for up to 3.0 GHz, while above this frequency, that is, up to 4 GHz, the SAR$_{1g}$ and SAR$_{10g}$ in the female model became larger than those in the male model. It was observed that this result could be explained by the difference in subcutaneous fat between man and woman. A better identification and modeling of the skin layer could potentially influence the results. Further studies are needed to assess the similarities and differences in absorption between male and female body models exposed to EMFs of radiating sources.

Computational Methods and EM Fields

In summary, available data on EM energy absorption in human body models exposed to plane wave fields show that the choice of the human body model affects the obtained results. The observed differences among the published data are usually more pronounced in local SAR values than in SAR values averaged over the whole body. The body height, mass, tissue distribution and composition, including fat and muscle are important factors in absorption and can explain some differences among the published data. Another fundamental aspect is the value assigned to the dielectric properties of different tissues or organs identified in the body model. In the case of children, the variation in tissue dielectric properties with age also may influence the computed results. It is noteworthy that the above publications have used dielectric properties from the same sources [117,118].

9.5.2.3 Human Exposure to the Field Radiated by BTS Antennas

The enormous growth in the number of users of mobile telecommunication systems in the past decades has pushed upward the system's capacity. As a result, more-and-more base stations have been installed nearly everywhere, including on the rooftop of existing buildings in densely populated areas, and many more are expected to be set up as the next-generation mobile networks are deployed. These installations are giving rise to widespread concerns among the population about possible deleterious effects on human health from exposure to the EMFs radiated by the base-station (BTS) antennas. Recently, increasing attention has been paid to the topic of numerical exposure and compliance assessment for base-station installations.

A great deal of work has been done in the area of field strength prediction in the vicinity of base-station antennas to determine the so-called free-space compliance boundary. The studies were aimed toward a direct comparison with reference levels suggested by international exposure guidelines. They generally have neglected both the influence of the environment in which the antennas operate and the dosimetric problem of SAR evaluation inside an exposed subject. In particular, considerable efforts have been spent on determining simplified and efficient analytical [119,120] and numerical [121,122] models to evaluate field levels near base-station antennas. Starting from the theory of collinear dipole arrays, typically employed in base-antennas, practical analytical formulas have been derived to predict average power density fall-off as a function of distance from the antenna. The space surrounding the antenna is often divided into a cylindrical wave region-closest to the antenna, and a spherical wave region, further away [119]. A complementary formulation also has been proposed, on the basis of an exact asymptotic solution for the radiated field, to derive approximate analytical formulas that allow a conservative prediction of equivalent peak power density as a function of the distance from the antenna [120].

Besides the above mentioned practical analytical formulations, simplified numerical models are often used, by subdividing the antenna into elementary radiators [121,122]. Under the hypothesis of weak coupling between the sub-elements, the near field can be quickly computed through a superposition of the fields independently radiated by the different elements. Once the radiation pattern of the sub-elements is known, the field is derived using the antenna-gain-based formula. For better accuracies in the vicinity of the antenna, a MoM simulation of the sub-element can be invoked [122]. These simplified approaches represent fast tools for field strength prediction, but they are limited by a minimum distance from the antenna where they can be applied in order to maintain an acceptable computational accuracy. On the other hand, when field computations within a distance of few wavelengths from the antenna have to be done, full-wave numerical techniques, such as FDTD, must be adopted. The accuracy of FDTD models for evaluating the near field of base-station antennas has been investigated and validated through comparison with measurements carried out in an anechoic chamber [123].

Full-wave approaches require knowledge of the internal structure of the antenna, which is not always available. Cylindrical and spherical-wave expansion techniques have been proposed to evaluate the near field starting from measurements performed on a surface enclosing the antenna [124–126]. The basic approach consists of performing field measurements on a spherical surface surrounding the antenna and describing the measured field as a superposition of spherical modes [124]. Once the spherical-wave expansion coefficients have been determined, the near field can be extrapolated for all points lying outside the minimum sphere enclosing the antenna. This technique also has been improved to allow extrapolation of the field inside the minimum sphere [125]. To this end, the spherical-wave expansion coefficients are derived for each of the antenna sub-elements. This approach extends the range of applicability of the formulation to all points outside the minimum sphere of a single sub-element, which is much closer to the antenna than the minimum sphere of the overall array. Recently, an alternative solution to extend field extrapolation close to the antenna was proposed, which consists of spherical-wave expansion outside the minimum sphere of the antenna, and cylindrical-wave expansion for the region close to the antenna, with an appropriate matching of the two expansions [126].

The effect of the surrounding environment must be taken into account to some extent in dealing with the problem of evaluating induced SAR in a subject exposed to the field radiated by BTS antennas, since the antenna is not operating in a free-space condition. A very interesting approach, applicable to on-site evaluations, consists of using mixed experimental/numerical procedures [127–129]. One procedure is based on on-site measurement of the amplitude and phase of the exposure field distribution over a surface surrounding the antenna. The measurement is then used to numerically evaluate induced SAR distributions inside a phantom. The measured fields are used to excite the FDTD domain via the equivalence principle [127]. A much faster and efficient procedure uses previously stored FDTD-computed E-field distributions inside a phantom exposed to spatially impulsive electric fields, the equivalent spatial impulsive responses of the phantom or Green's functions. The on-site measurement of amplitude and phase of the exposure field is made over an equally spaced grid of points placed on an appropriately chosen surface [128]. The procedure has also been enhanced and made faster by substituting the spatial impulse response with responses to spatial harmonic components [129]. In this way, good accuracy is achieved using only six to ten spatial harmonic components, as opposed to the 54 spatial impulse responses needed previously.

The aforementioned hybrid experimental/numerical procedures have the advantage of allowing easy characterization of environmental perturbations to the exposure field by directly including them in the measured field. On the other hand, they require the antenna to be already installed and operating at the time of measurement. The last point makes such procedures not suitable for a priori compliance assessment evaluations during the planning stage of a cellular network. For such evaluations, a thorough numerical dosimetric analysis is required. Once again, a possible approach, when the environment can be neglected and the antenna can be supposed to operate under free-space conditions, consists of performing full-wave FDTD simulations, and modeling both the BTS antenna and a numerical phantom of the exposed subject. The applicability of such an approach has been demonstrated, also through a comparison with SAR measurements, for exposure locations in close proximity to the antenna [130]. The main drawback of full-wave FDTD analysis is the large amount of memory required to discretize the simulation space for phantom locations not in the close proximity of the antenna. This problem

Computational Methods and EM Fields

can be faced by exploiting parallel computer architectures with parallelized versions of the FDTD code [131]. Parallel FDTD also allows SAR computations for large antenna-phantom distances.

More efficient techniques have been developed, that combine two different techniques, used to model BTS antenna and propagation in free space and SAR inside the phantom, respectively [132,133]. In particular, if the antenna-phantom distance is such that mutual coupling can be neglected, a hybrid ray-tracing (RT)/FDTD approach can be used [133]. RT is used to model field propagation from the BTS antenna to an equivalence surface surrounding the phantom, and FDTD is employed to study absorption inside the phantom, using RT-derived exposure fields for excitation. For closer antenna-phantom distances, where the mutual coupling cannot be neglected, a hybrid FEM-MoM technique has been proposed [133]. In this case, MoM is used to model the BTS antenna, while FEM is used to study absorption inside the phantom. The MoM and FEM formulations are coupled together and are solved iteratively. These hybrid approaches allow very efficient SAR computation for different antenna-phantom distances, and are well suited for evaluating free-space compliance distances, on the basis of SAR restrictions. They do not require the use of derived exposure field reference levels. For example, the RT/FDTD technique has been applied to a common 14-dBi gain GSM900 antenna, using the VH phantom. It was shown that for a total radiated power of 30W, typical for urban-area installations, SAR basic restrictions for the general population may be exceeded at distances of 2 m or less. Note that, at these distances, only occupational personnel are allowed [132].

The RT/FDTD hybrid technique also has been successfully employed to study human exposure to the field radiated by a BTS antenna in an urban scenario, including the effect of environmental perturbations to the exposure field [134]. In this case, image sources have been introduced to represent corner-reflector-like urban scenarios. Three different exposure conditions have been considered for a rooftop-mounted 14-dBi gain BTS antenna, radiating 30 W in the GSM900 frequency band: (1) A subject standing on the rooftop, near the antenna mast; (2) a subject standing on a balcony of building facing the antenna at a distance of 30 m, within the antenna main beam; and (3) a subject standing in the street below the 30-m tall building on which BTS antenna was mounted. The computed results for the incident electric field and SAR values, under these exposure conditions, are given in Table 9.6.

From Table 9.6, due to the high directivity over the vertical plane of BTS antennas, it appears that the highest field levels are not obtained on the rooftop of the building where the antenna is located. Instead, they are on the nearby building, in the direction of the maximum antenna radiation. As expected, the lowest field levels are experienced by a subject standing in the street, as a result of the large distance from the antenna and the off-axis position with respect to the antenna pointing direction. The 1-g SAR nearly doubles the value for 10-g SAR and is more than 20 times higher than whole body SAR. In all cases,

TABLE 9.6

Spatial Maximum (E_{iMAX}), and Spatial Average (E_{iAVE}), of the Incident Field (rms Value); Maximum SAR Values Averaged Over 1 g (SAR_{1g}), Over 10 g (SAR_{10g}), and SAR Value Averaged Over the Whole Body (SAR_{WB}) for Three Exposure Conditions

	E_{iMAX} (V/m)	E_{iAVE} (V/m)	SAR_{1g} (mW/kg)	SAR_{10g} (mW/kg)	SAR_{WB} (mW/kg)
Rooftop	4.2	2.8	5.3	3.0	0.12
Balcony	8.1	5.5	13.2	8.5	0.46
Street	1.3	1.1	0.26	0.17	0.01

the calculated SAR values are at least two orders of magnitude lower than the basic restrictions, confirming the expected low exposure levels for people living near a BTS installation in urban areas.

Some hybrid techniques have been developed, with enhanced capabilities in modeling complex urban environments, by taking into account diffraction phenomena [134,135]. One such technique uses FEM to model the BTS antenna, the uniform theory of diffraction (UTD) to model the effects of the environment on wave propagation, and FDTD to study absorption in the exposed subject [134]. The technique has been employed to study exposure of a subject standing inside a room, with a microcell BTS antenna mounted on the external wall. Another possible hybrid solution exploits time-domain physical-optics, instead of UTD to model field scattering from the environment, and FDTD to study absorption inside the exposed subject [135].

Finally, a hybrid UTD/FDTD technique has been developed to highlight some key-points related to compliance assessment procedures for BTS antennas, in a realistic urban environment [136]. The scenario analyzed consists of a room in one building where the field, radiated by a GSM900 or a UMTS BTS antenna installed on a facing building, penetrates through the room's external wall and window. The relation between SAR in an exposed subject and ambient field in the absence of the subject has been investigated for the complex scenario. As expected, the ambient field showed a highly nonuniform distribution resulting from the many reflections and diffractions that took place. The results showed that whole-body averaged SAR (SAR_{WB}) are closely correlated with the exposure field value averaged over the volume that would be occupied by the exposed subject. In particular, it has been estimated that assessing SAR_{WB} on the basis of volume-averaged field values yields an average error of approximately 6%. Peak 1-g and 10-g averaged SAR values, instead, show a rather complex and difficult-to-predict relation with reference to the exposure field. Analysis has revealed that the use of the volume-averaged exposure field value, in the absence of the subject, can lead to an underestimation of the peak local SAR values, up to 36%. On the contrary, using the maximum volumetric value yields an overestimation of peak local SAR (up to approximately four times). The conclusion was that peak local SAR showed a good correlation (15% average error) with the maximum average exposure field value obtained by varying the position of a vertical averaging plane, having a surface equivalent to the projected human body area, inside the volume occupied by the subject.

9.5.2.4 Human Exposure to the Fields Produced By Coexisting Antenna Systems

The discussions thus far have dealt with the problem of human exposure to fields radiated by a single BTS antenna from the cellular mobile communication systems (i.e., GSM, UMTS, etc.). However, as the development of communication systems making use of wireless technology expands, new exposure scenarios are encountered in everyday life. In addition to the huge growth in the number of BTS in densely populated areas, one of the most common systems is the Wi-Fi system, namely wireless LAN adopting the IEEE 802.11b communication standard. Wi-Fi is characterized by completely different coverage ranges. Unlike BTS antennas of cellular systems which are installed almost entirely in outdoor locations, access points (APs) of Wi-Fi systems operate principally inside buildings. Nonetheless, the EMFs radiated by the two systems will coexist in indoor environments, particularly if buildings located in front of a rooftop-mounted BTS antenna are considered. This poses new questions about human exposure in such environments. It becomes important to assess typical exposure levels attributable to each system.

Computational Methods and EM Fields

The problem has been addressed by considering exposure of a subject standing inside a room with a Wi-Fi AP, and is facing a dual-band GSM900/GSM1800 BTS antenna mounted on the rooftop of a nearby building [137]. The AP radiates a power of 100 mW at 2.44 GHz, while the GSM BTS employs an antenna with an 18-dBi gain, radiating a total power of 30 and 20 W in the GSM900 and GSM1800 frequency bands, respectively. The calculated results for exposure field and SAR are summarized in Tables 9.7 and 9.8. Specifically, the first two columns of Table 9.7 show the peak ($E_{\text{vol peak}}$) and average ($E_{\text{vol ave}}$) rms exposure fields over the entire parallelepiped volume where the subject will be placed, while the third column reports the average ($E_{\text{sup ave}}$) rms exposure field over vertical sections of the parallelepiped volume. In particular, the minimum and maximum field values are given because the averages depend on where exactly the surface is placed. Table 9.8 presents whole-body, peak 1-g and 10-g averaged SARs inside the exposed subject.

It can be seen from Table 9.7 that the highest contribution to the total field level inside the room is not due to the indoor source but to the outdoor one. In particular, the average E-field value attributable to the Wi-Fi system is as low as 1 V/m. The calculated data also demonstrate that coexistence of the two systems (GSM and Wi-Fi) is possible without exceeding reference levels for the exposure field, as averaged over the volume occupied by the body or over an equivalent surface, even if the particularly stringent limits issued by some national regulations (e.g., 6 V/m) are considered. Finally, the SARs presented in Table 9.8 suggest that a typical exposure scenario results in RF absorption that is two orders of magnitude below the basic restrictions, both for whole-body and for local-averaged SAR.

9.5.2.5 Coupling of EM Pulses into the Human Body

EM transient radiations are widely used for studying the susceptibility of test objects to broadband EMP, and increasingly, pulsed fields are being explored for telecommunication and sensing purposes. The main characteristics of these pulse fields are waveforms

TABLE 9.7

Exposure Field (rms values) for the Indoor Scenario (Coexisting Outdoor GSM BTS and Indoor Wi-Fi AP)

	$E_{\text{vol peak}}$ (V/m)	$E_{\text{vol ave}}$ (V/m)	$E_{\text{sup ave}}$ (V/m)
GSM900	5.57	3.13	2.73–3.44
GSM1800	3.61	1.70	1.62–1.91
Total GSM	6.18	3.56	3.19–3.93
Wi-Fi	2.51	1.13	1.05–1.19
Total	6.30	3.74	3.40–4.09

TABLE 9.8

SARs for the Indoor Scenario (Coexisting Outdoor GSM BTS and Indoor Wi-Fi AP)

	SAR_{WB} (mW/kg)	SAR_{1g} (mW/kg)	SAR_{10g} (mW/kg)
GSM900	0.109	2.41	1.08
GSM1800	0.027	1.31	0.58
Total GSM	0.136	3.07	1.46
Wi-Fi	0.014	0.79	0.35
Total	0.150	3.66	1.60

that include a high peak powers, fast rise times, and a narrow pulse width. The EMPs with electric fields ranging from 20 to 500 kV/m or higher and with frequency spectra of 0–80 MHz are produced by nuclear EMP simulators. They are used to assess the EM compatibility or immunity of electronic instruments and systems under the conditions of a nuclear burst such as EMP bombs. The biological effects of EMPs of varying durations have long been investigated in research laboratories. However, it is only during recent years that the benefit and capability of the large bandwidth provided by very short or ultra-wide-band (UWB) EM pulses have been considered for imaging, sensing, and communication applications [138–142].

Earlier investigations on pulse interaction with biological systems relied on mathematical analyses of canonical shapes of dielectric equivalent bodies, such as planar tissue layers and bodies of revolution [143–146]. The well-known effect of microwave hearing from pulse-induced thermoelastic pressure waves in the human head have been investigated both analytically [147–152] and numerically [153–156].

This section presents predictions of fields and power depositions, which have been obtained from the frequency-dependent FDTD formulations for various models of the biological body.

1.5.2.5.1 Modeling of Tissue Properties with the Debye Equation

For UWB calculations using the (FD)^{2}TD method, the measured properties for the various tissues may be fitted to the Debye equation (Equation 9.14) with two relaxation constants [76–78]. For the results shown here, the measured properties of biological tissues (muscle, fat, bone, blood, intestine, cartilage, lung, kidney, pancreas, spleen, lung, heart, brain/nerve, skin, and eye) were obtained from the literature. Optimized values for ε_{s1}, ε_{s2}, ε_4, τ_1, and τ_2 in Equation 9.14 were obtained by nonlinear least squares matching to the measured data for fat and muscle (Table 9.9), with τ_1 and τ_2 being the average of the optimized values for fat and muscle. All other tissues have properties falling roughly between these two types of tissues. This was done to facilitate volume averaging of the tissue properties in

TABLE 9.9

Debye constants for tissues.

$\tau_1 = 46.2 \text{ H } 10^{-9} \text{ s}$

$\tau_2 = 0.91 \text{ H } 10^{-10} \text{ s}$

(Average of optimum for fat and muscle)

Tissue	ε_4	ε_{s1}	ε_{s2}
Muscle	40.0	3948.	59.09
Bone/Cartilage	3.4	312.8	7.11
Blood	35.0	3563.	66.43
Intestine	39.0	4724.	66.09
Liver	36.3	2864.	57.12
Kidney	35.0	3332.	67.12
Pancreas/Spleen	10.0	3793.	73.91
1/3 Lung	10.0	1224.	13.06
Heart	38.5	4309.	54.58
Brain/Nerve	32.5	2064.	56.86
Skin	23.0	3399.	55.59
Eye	40.0	2191.	56.99

cells of the heterogeneous human model. Having τ_1 and τ_2 constant for all tissues, allowed linear (volume) averaging of the ε values for each tissue in a given cell to calculate ε values for that cell.

9.5.2.5.2 Induced Currents and SAs

The (FD)²TD formulation has been used to calculate coupling of an ultra-short pulse to the heterogeneous model of the human body. From the calculated internal fields, the vertical currents passing through the various layers of the body are calculated, by using the following equation:

$$I_z(t) = \delta^2 \sum_{i,j} \frac{\partial D_z}{\partial t} \tag{9.25}$$

where δ is the cell size (= 1.31 cm), and the summation is carried out for all cells in a given layer. The layer-averaged absorbed energy density or SA and the total energy W absorbed by the whole body can be calculated using the following relationships:

$$SA\big|_{\text{layer } k} = \frac{\delta t}{N_k} \sum_{i,j,t} \frac{E(i,j,k,t)}{\rho(i,j,k)} \cdot \frac{\partial D(i,j,k,t)}{\partial t} \tag{9.26}$$

$$W = \delta t \cdot \delta^3 \sum_{i,j,k,t} E(i,j,k,t) \cdot \frac{\partial D(i,j,k,t)}{\partial t} \tag{9.27}$$

In Equations 9.26 and 9.27, dt is the time step (= $\delta/2c$ = 0.02813 ns) used for the time-domain calculations, N_k is the number of cells in layer k of the body, and $\rho(i, j, k)$ is the mass density in kg/m³ for each of the cells in the corresponding layers.

A typical time domain, UWB pulse with a peak amplitude of 1.1 V/m is shown in Figure 9.20. It is interesting to note that the pulse has a rise time of about 0.2 ns and a total time duration of about 7–8 ns. The Fourier spectrum of the pulse is shown in Figure 9.21.

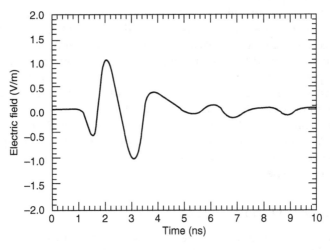

FIGURE 9.20
A representative UWB EMP. Peak incident electric field = 1.1 V/m.

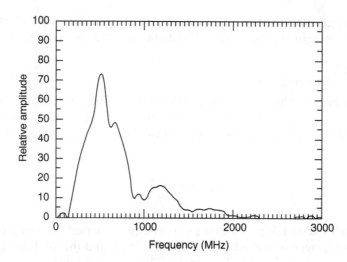

FIGURE 9.21
Fourier spectrum of the EMP of Figure 9.20.

Most of the energy in the pulse is concentrated in the 200–900 MHz band with the peak of the energy being at about 500 MHz.

For purposes of illustration, the results that follow assume the incident fields to be vertically polarized, since this polarization is known to result in the strongest coupling for standing individuals [157]. The $(FD)^2TD$ procedure is used to calculate the temporal variations of total vertical currents for the various sections of the body for both the shoe-wearing grounded and ungrounded exposure conditions of the model. The current variations for a couple of representative sections such as those through the eyes and the bladder are given in Figures 9.22a and b, respectively. The calculated peak currents for the various sections are on the order of 1.1 to 3.2 mA/(V/m). It is interesting to note that there is very little difference in the induced currents whether the model is grounded or not. This is due to the fact that most of the energy in the pulse is at frequencies in excess of 300 MHz, where the effect of the ground plane on the induced currents or the SARs is minimal.

In Figure 9.23, the peak current for each section of the body is plotted with a section resolution of 1.31 cm. The maximum peak sectional current of 3.5 mA, which is equal to 3.2 mA/(V/m), occurs at a height of 96.3 cm above the bottom of the feet. A very similar result also had been observed for calculations using isolated and grounded models of the human body for plane-wave exposures at frequencies of 350–700 MHz, where the highest induced currents on the order of 3.0–3.2 mA/(V/m) were calculated for sections of the body that are at heights of 85–100 cm relative to the feet.

The SA and the total absorbed energy for exposure to the UWB pulse can be calculated using Equations 9.26 and 9.27. The total energy absorbed by the body exposed to a single pulse of the type shown in Figure 9.20 is 2.0 and 1.91 pJ for isolated and shoe-wearing grounded conditions, respectively.

9.5.2.6 Absorption in the Head of Cell Phone Users

The wide-spread use of cellular mobile telephone systems has brought about an increased concern for possible adverse health effects from the RF field emitted by the handset. Indeed, exposure standards have been mandated by various national bodies to limit

Computational Methods and EM Fields

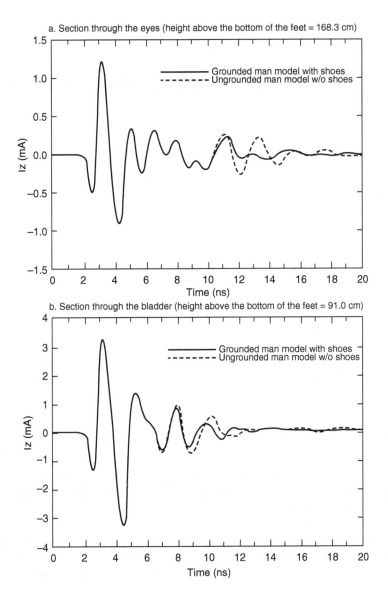

FIGURE 9.22
Currents induced for the various sections of the body for shoe-wearing grounded and ungrounded conditions of exposure. $E_{peak} = 1.1\,\text{V/m}$.

human exposure to cell phone radiations. These RF exposure standards provide specifications, in terms of power deposition per unit mass, i.e., SAR induced in the user's head to which cell phones must comply [158,159].

Laboratory procedures for compliance testing of mobile phones are based on experimental measurements, performed according to published protocols [158,159]. In these tests, real phones and phantom head models, shells filled with a material with dielectric properties equivalent to those of the brain tissue at the frequencies of interest, are used. Clearly, the phantom is a simplified model of the human head and is specifically designed for compliance testing. Consequently, it is not suited for an accurate analysis of the SAR

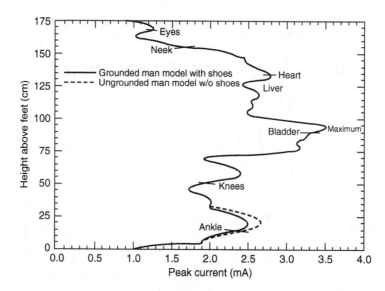

FIGURE 9.23
Peak currents induced for the various sections of the body for shoe-wearing grounded and ungrounded conditions of the model. $E_{peak} = 1.1$ V/m.

distribution in various tissues and organs of the head. A detailed analysis of the distribution of the absorption would be required to obtain a better understanding of SARs inside the head. Such information is needed for the necessary extrapolation of results from *in vivo* and *in vitro* experimental studies devoted to investigating the effects of RF radiation on humans. They would provide the exposure data needed in epidemiological studies aimed at evaluating any possible dose-effect relations.

Increasingly, advances in computational bioelectromagnetics have made detailed evaluation of SAR distribution inside the human head possible through the use of accurate and realistic models of the human head and the source, that is, the mobile phone, and the use of suitable numerical methods such as the FDTD technique.

The earlier numerical studies were performed by simulating the phone's radiating element as a half-wavelength dipole or a quarter-wavelength monopole mounted on a box [160–165]. These antenna models and the latter in particular, can only be used as a rough model of the retractable antenna, which at the beginning was in nearly all cell phone handsets. However, at present, the need for more and more compact terminals and for dual or multi-band operation has given rise to new antenna types. In particular, two types of antennas have been developed: planar integrated antennas and helical antennas. While half wavelength dipoles and monopoles can be easily implemented inside an FDTD code, modeling of helix or planar antennas can become a rather difficult task.

The difficulties in modeling helical structures with the FDTD method may be seen from the following examples. Initially, only rather large structures were studied employing a pure FDTD scheme [166,167]. For smaller structures, published reports had either employed equivalent sources [168] or a hybrid MoM/FDTD technique [169,170]. While these reports show some problems and drawbacks, investigations using FDTD, properly modified through the use of a graded mesh, have obtained good agreement with MoM and experimental results [171,172]. In these studies, both near-field and radiation patterns of dual-band cell phones equipped with a helical antenna were reproduced. The SAR distributions inside the VH model of the head were computed, showing a higher penetration depth at

Computational Methods and EM Fields 351

900 MHz and higher superficial SAR values at 1800 MHz. Moreover, approximately 80% and 50% of the radiated power was absorbed inside the head at 900 and 1800 MHz, respectively. For a phone in contact with the ear and tilted to bring its axis along the ear–mouth axis (the so-called cheek position), radiating an average power of 250 mW at 900 MHz and 125 mW at 1800 MHz, peak 1g SAR of 1.65 and 1.08 W/kg were obtained in the head at 900 and 1800 MHz, respectively. In the same examples, the peak 1g SAR in the brain was 0.13 and 0.06 W/kg at these two frequencies, respectively.

Planar antennas can be mounted on top, lateral, or back side of the phone [173–176]. Shorted patch antennas typically have a 10 dB bandwidth between 5% and 10% that can be increased to about 12% by parasitically coupling another printed radiator in the vertical direction (stacked patch). For comparison, the bandwidth is about 30% for the monopole antenna [174]. In this case, an important consideration is the influence of the hand wrapped around the handset. For a cell phone equipped with a planar antenna, the hand has a detuning effect on the antenna resonant frequency and causes a reduction of the bandwidth; both are evident where the hand masks the antenna. About 30% of the radiated power was absorbed by the hand, while for the monopole the hand absorption was only 15% [174]. For a radiated power of 250 mW at the frequency of 900 MHz and a head-handset separation of 2 cm, the computed peak 1g SAR was 0.95 W/kg for a laterally mounted PIFA and the result was 0.49 W/kg for a monopole antenna [174]. When a phone equipped with a side-mounted PIFA was kept in contact with the ear, the peak 1g SAR increased to 1.4 W/kg [175]. Note that the back mounting configuration gave rise to a substantial (up to three times) reduction in the peak SAR [173].

Another important task for an accurate evaluation of the absorption in the head is the model adopted for the phone case. The typical approach consists of representing the case as a box, that is, a plastic-coated metal parallelepiped [160–176]. In order to model the correct shape of cell phones, both CAD files [177] and topometric sensors [178] have been used. Also, in earlier studies, the internal structures of the phone were modeled simply as a homogeneous perfect conductor. Since then, CAD files have been used to model the internal structures (printed circuit board, battery, keypad, and buttons, etc.) of the phone [179].

An alternate approach to a suitable numerical model of the mobile phone starts with a simplified model, which includes only the main phone parts (antenna, keyboard, internal box, plastic coating, etc.) having "real" dimensions and electrical properties [180]. The "real" parameters are then tuned by using an optimization procedure, which minimizes a functional that depends on the differences between the measured and simulated electric and magnetic fields in front of the phone and on the SAR inside a cubic phantom. As an example for the applicability of the proposed optimization method, a numerical model of a commercial phone, operating at 900 MHz, was implemented and the power deposition in the VH model of the human head was computed for various phone-head distances. The results in terms of peak SAR in various head tissues and for various phone-head distances are presented in Table 9.10. The SAR_{1g} and SAR_{10g} show a monotonic decrease when the phone-head distance increases, while the peak SAR inside the head tissues reach their maxima when the phone was at a specific distances from the head. This behavior is due to the fact that with the telephone pressed against the head, the absorption was confined to a limited region in front of the antenna feed point, whereas by moving the handset away from the head, a greater portion of the head was exposed. When the distance was further increased, the SAR decreased monotonically as a result of the decay in field intensity. This study also showed that the use of inaccurate phone models (last row in Table 9.10) could give rise to SAR values, averaged over 1g, up to three times higher than those computed for the optimized model [180].

TABLE 9.10

Peak SAR Averaged Over 1 g (SAR_{1g}), 10 g (SAR_{10g}), and the Peak SAR as Averaged Over 1 g in Various Organs and Tissues, for Different Distances Between the Phone and the VH Phantom for a Radiated Power of 250 mW at 900 MHz

	SAR_{1g} (W/kg)	SAR_{10g} (W/kg)	$SAR_{1\,brain}$ (W/kg)	$SAR_{1\,eye}$ (W/kg)	SAR_{1skin} (W/kg)	$SAR_{1\,muscle}$ (W/kg)	$SAR_{1\,fat}$ (W/kg)	$SAR_{1\,gland}$ (W/kg)
$d = 0$ mm	1.450	0.600	0.125	0.0102	0.504	0.223	0.142	0.448
$d = 2$ mm	0.740	0.500	0.123	0.0101	0.504	0.244	0.162	0.493
$d = 6$ mm	0.670	0.470	0.174	0.0100	0.482	0.278	0.165	0.471
$d = 8$ mm	0.630	0.450	0.109	0.0103	0.460	0.280	0.160	0.445
Cheek position ($d = 0$ mm) Optimized	0.810	0.410	0.088	0.0360	0.171	0.447	0.301	0.420
Cheek position ($d = 0$ mm) non optimized	2.568	0.888	0.177	0.0578	0.315	0.721	0.400	0.664

Faced with a rapid saturation of the cellular phone market, many cell-phone manufacturers and service providers are turning their attention toward youths in promoting handsets that are cheap, with inexpensive service plans, or both [181]. An issue of particular interest is the possible difference in RF absorption between children and adult. To answer this question, the first problem to be addressed is the realization of an accurate numerical model of a child's head. Because of ethical concerns, the availability of anatomical models of children has been limited. An approach for obtaining a model of the child was to reduce the dimensions of the voxel size of adult models, for example, the CL model described before. However, the dielectric permittivity for children may be considerably higher than adults [182]. However, since the detailed data for the dielectric properties of tissues in children are scarce, they are usually assumed to be equal to those of adults or generically increased by a constant factor in most models. Nevertheless, using these models, some papers have reported increases up to 50% in the peak 1g SAR in children's head, compared to an adult head, for exposure to cell phones operating at frequencies around 835 and 1900 MHz [162,183]. A similar increase has been observed in the peak 1g SAR obtained in the brain. A possible explanation of these results is the larger depth of penetration of power for the child models as compared to the adult one [162,183]. Other papers devoted to the investigation of differences between child and adult exposure to cellular phones have shown no significant difference in peak 1g SAR between adults and children [184,185]. There are several possible explanations for the discrepancy. It has been suggested that the contradictory results may be due to the different phone excitation schemes used by different authors [186]. The disparity in distances of separation between the antenna and the head also was suggested as a pivotal factor in determining the reported discrepancies [181].

In an effort to help resolve the discrepancies, the SAR distributions induced in two children's head models: an isotropic scaling of the VH head (child sized—CS), and an anisotropic scaling of the VH head (CL), have been computed and compared with SAR distributions induced in the VH by a mobile phone equipped with a back-mounted dual-band patch antenna [187]. Some of the results are presented in Table 9.11. It can be seen that the peak SAR_{10g} showed an increase of about 50% and a reduction of about 25% for the child models compared to the adult model at 900 and 1800 MHz, respectively. Moreover, as the brain is nearer to the mobile phone in the case of CS and CL heads, the SAR_{1g} in the brain of children is slightly more significant than that for the adult.

Computational Methods and EM Fields

TABLE 9.11

Peak SAR Averaged Over 10 g (SAR_{10g}), and Peak SAR as Averaged Over 1 g in Various Organs and Tissues, for Radiated Powers of 250 mW at 900 MHz and 125 mW at 1800 MHz in Children and Adult

		SAR_{10g} (W/kg)	SAR_{1skin} (W/kg)	$SAR_{1muscle}$ (W/kg)	SAR_{1BONE} (W/kg)	SAR_{1CSF} (W/kg)	SAR_{1brain} (W/kg)
900 MHz	VH	0.67	2.00	0.67	0.20	0.34	0.16
	CS	1.18	4.02	1.03	0.31	0.45	0.25
	CL	1.03	1.15	0.41	0.14	0.23	0.20
1800 MHz	VH	0.39	0.99	0.30	0.08	0.12	0.08
	CS	0.29	0.87	0.30	0.08	0.13	0.09
	CL	0.27	0.91	0.30	0.06	0.15	0.10

Other exposure scenarios also have been investigated, including head exposure inside a car and for cell phones placed not in contact with the ear. In some studies, the influence of the metallic and dielectric structures of a car on SAR induced by a cellular phone inside an adult head was analyzed [166,188]. Studies performed by modeling the whole car have showed that the main influence on SAR distribution was due to structures that were very close to the head. In particular, the presence of a vertical glass wall in parallel with the antenna axis, did not significantly influence the SAR distribution, while a metallic wall can cause up to an 80% increase in the peak 1g SAR [166,188]. The presence of a reflecting wall placed horizontally over the head, simulating the roof of a car, rendered the SAR distribution more uniform, increasing the lower values and reducing the higher ones [167].

9.5.2.7 Absorption in Human Body Exposed to Near-Field MRI Source

MRI is widely regarded as the radiological modality of choice for medical diagnostic procedures. To form images, RF magnetic fields are used to excite and detect magnetic resonance (MR) signals from body tissues. For the commonly employed 1.5 tesla (T) and 3.0 T clinical magnetic resonance imaging (MRI) scanners, the associated RF frequencies for hydrogen proton imaging at 1.5 and 3.0 T are about 64 and 128 MHz, respectively. While MRI resolution is best under conditions of uniform magnetic field distributions, the distribution of applied RF fields are inherently nonuniform. Moreover, an optimized choice is often made in MRI scanner design to ensure that the RF energy absorbed by human subjects during MRI does not produce harmful health effects to the patient, including thermal damage to local tissue or whole-body thermoregulatory challenges. Indeed, regulatory entities have set limits on the maximum local, partial-body, and whole-body absorption of RF energy [189–191].

There are two basic methods that are commonly employed or recommended to determine SAR induced by MRI scanners: the power method and the calorimetry method [192]. In the power method of measuring whole-body SAR for a subject of a given mass, the total patient absorption is calculated by subtracting from the forward power, the reflected power and power lost to the MR coil antenna. For the calorimetric method, the increase in whole-body temperature over a given duration is measured. Partial-body SAR is estimated by a formula that accounts for the ratio between RF exposed partial-body mass and total-body mass. This curve-fitting routine is typically used by the MRI system as the SAR monitor in radiological imaging facilities. SAR values are obtained by entering the height and mass for the patient in each case. In principle, the same ratio methods may be used to calculate local SAR in smaller masses of RF exposed tissue. However, numerical methods combined with anatomical models would provide more realistic or dependable local SAR values. Although many authors have published numerical computations of SARs in anatomical models of the human body for MRI [193–196], there are few reports presenting comparisons between results derived from various methods used for SAR calculation.

The objective of this section is to examine partial-body and local SARs through numerical computations for anatomical models of male and female humans in 1.5 T (64 MHz) and 3.0 T (128 MHz) MRI systems and compare them to results obtained from mass ratio (curve-fitting) formulas used as SAR monitors in MRI scanners. In these computations, the birdcage coils are centered on the chest, umbilicus, and knee region of the model for partial-body exposures.

The male VH body model consists of 293 × 170 × 939 voxels with 39 tissue types at a 2 mm isometric resolution, and the female VH model is interpolated to 266 × 143 × 864 voxels at 2 mm resolution [197–199]. These models were adapted for commercially available SEMCAD FDTD) software (SPEAG; Zurich, Switzerland). The accuracy of the SEMCAD software was validated against published algorithms [155,200]. A four-parameter Cole–Cole extrapolation was used to determine values for the permittivity properties of various tissues [201,202].

A 16-rung, body size (610-mm coil diameter and 620 mm length with 660 mm shield diameter and 1.22 m length) high-pass birdcage coil antenna was modeled. For partial-body SAR calculations, the birdcage coils were centered on the chest; umbilicus and knees of the body models (see Figure 9.24 for the model and coil). With the support of acceleration hardware, the human models and the coil were meshed at an excess of 42 million voxels. The coils were driven with 32 current sources placed at the end-rings, and a 22.5° phase

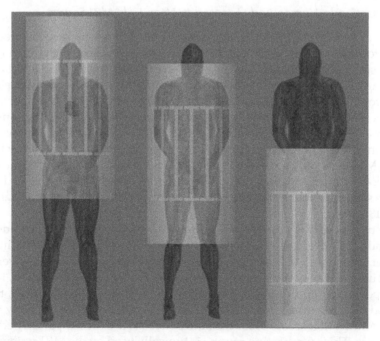

FIGURE 9.24
Geometry of coil and body model for partial body SAR: From left to right for coils centered on the chest, umbilicus, and knee regions, respectively, for partial-body exposure.

shift between adjacent rungs. This scheme gives practically identical results as driving the coils at resonance in quadrature for frequencies up to 128 MHz [203].

Local SARs in a body region surrounding a central voxel are averaged as the region was expanded by one voxel at a time until a specified mass of tissue (1 g, 10 g, partial body or whole body) is reached. The IEC scale was used to compute partial-body average SAR under normal operating mode. In particular,

$$\text{SAR} = 10\ \text{W/kg} - \left(8\ \text{W/kg} \times \text{exposed body mass/total body mass}\right) \qquad (9.28)$$

and for first-level-controlled operating mode:

$$\text{SAR} = 10\ \text{W/kg} - \left(6\ \text{W/kg} \times \text{exposed body mass/total body mass}\right). \qquad (9.29)$$

Partial-body SAR distributions in high-pass, birdcage MRI coils operating at 1.5 T (64 MHz) and 3.0 T (128 MHz) are shown in Figures 9.25 and 9.26 for the VH Man and Woman models, respectively [204]. It is interesting to note the similarity of the global pattern of SAR distributions. However, there are some differences for the two field strengths and human models. For example, the peak SAR values occur in the skin (or surface) of the neck and shoulder for the chest coil position, in the skin of arms and the abdomen for the umbilicus coil position, and in the muscles of the knee joint and inner thigh areas for the knee coil position, where the induced circulating RF currents are the highest.

The FDTD computed total and partial-body absorptions and SARs are given in Tables 9.12 and 9.13 for the VH man and VH woman, respectively, for 1 W input power to the 1.5 and 3.0 T birdcage coils centered at the chest, umbilicus, and knees. As expected, the total absorption is higher than partial-body absorption; however, whole-body average SARs are lower than those for partial body locations at the chest, umbilicus, and the knees. Moreover, in general, absorption at 3.0 T is 5%–40% higher than at 1.5 T for the man

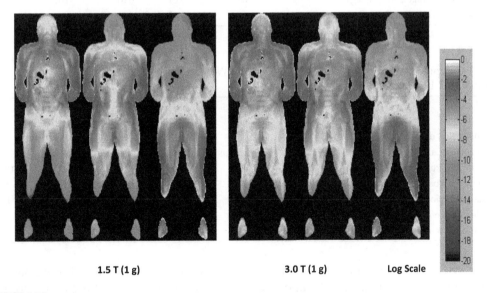

FIGURE 9.25
Partial-body SAR distributions in coronal planes of the VH Man in a birdcage MRI coil: From left to right: partial-body SAR distributions for the chest, umbilicus, and knee coil positions, respectively. Data in the figure are normalized to one watt input power.

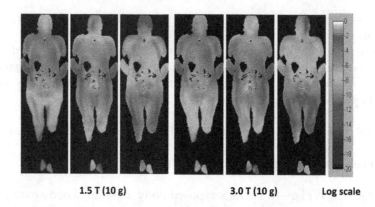

1.5 T (10 g)   3.0 T (10 g)   Log scale

FIGURE 9.26
Partial-body SAR distributions in coronal planes of the VH Woman in a birdcage MRI coil: From left to right: partial-body SAR distributions for the chest, umbilicus, and knee coil positions, respectively. Data in the figure are normalized to one watt input power.

TABLE 9.12

FDTD Computed Absorptions and SARs for the VH Man Model at 1 W Input Power to the 1.5 and 3.0 T Birdcage MRI Coils

Height (m)	1.876					
Mass (kg)	105.64					
Magnetic-flux density (T)	1.5			3.0		
Coil center location	Chest	Umbilicus	Knees	Chest	Umbilicus	Knees
Mass in coil (kg)	52.20	60.43	23.99	52.20	60.43	23.99
Total power absorption (W)	0.91	0.91	0.75	0.98	0.98	0.99
Partial-body power absorption (W)	0.85	0.83	0.56	0.89	0.84	0.82
Whole-body average SAR (W/kg)	0.01	0.01	0.01	0.01	0.01	0.01
Partial-body average SAR (W/kg)	0.02	0.01	0.02	0.02	0.01	0.03

TABLE 9.13

FDTD-Computed Absorptions and SARs for the VH Woman Model at 1 W Input Power to the 1.5 and 3.0 T Birdcage MRI Coils

Height (m)	1.725					
Mass (kg)	82.80					
Magnetic-flux density (T)	1.5			3.0		
Coil center location	Chest	Umbilicus	Knees	Chest	Umbilicus	Knees
Mass in coil (kg)	45.97	50.33	19.80	45.97	50.33	19.80
Total power absorption (W)	0.87	0.97	0.69	1.00	1.00	1.00
Partial-body power absorption (W)	0.82	0.77	0.53	0.91	0.89	0.83
Whole-body average SAR (W/kg)	0.01	0.01	0.01	0.01	0.01	0.01
Partial-body average SAR (W/kg)	0.02	0.02	0.03	0.02	0.02	0.04

model while they vary from 3% to 50% for the woman model for the same input power. It is interesting to note that the total and partial-body absorptions at 1.5 T are higher for the man than the woman model, whereas the situation is reversed at 3.0 T.

The IEC partial-body average SAR limits calculated from the above-mentioned formulas (Equations 9.28 and 9.29) both for 1.5 and 3.0 T coils and for the VH models are

Computational Methods and EM Fields 357

given in Table 9.14. It can be seen that the IEC formulas for partial-body average SAR limits are higher for the Man model than the Woman model because of differences in body mass.

It is noteworthy that the IEC formulas (Equations 9.28 and 9.29) for deriving the partial-body average SAR and their use in specifying the partial-body average SAR limits (see Table 9.14) are based on body mass. They are not related to absorption in specific tissues of the chest, umbilicus, or body extremities. Therefore, it is of interest to compare the IEC partial-body average SAR limits to those provided by FDTD calculations inside anatomical body models.

To illustrate the difference, the partial-body absorbed powers may be computed from multiplying IEC limit (Equation 9.28) by the appropriate mass. Under normal mode operation, the computed partial-body absorbed powers for 1.5 T are 315.65, 327.75, and 196.32 W for the Man model and 255.56, 258.55, and 160.13 W for the Woman model for the chest, umbilicus, and knee positions, respectively. If these numbers are combined with FDTD calculated SARs given in Tables 9.12 and 9.13, they yield the FDTD computed partial-body SAR listed in Table 9.15, which correspond to the powers permitted by the IEC limit for partial-body average SAR. It is noted that the IEC limit values are always higher than the FDTD computations. The IEC limits may be as high as 200% and are about 130% higher, on average, than the FDTD-computed SARs for both anatomical body models inside the MRI coil.

TABLE 9.14

Partial-body Average SAR Limits Calculated from IEC Formulas for 1.5 and 3.0 T Coils for the Visible Man and Visible Woman Models

	Man Model			Woman Model		
Partial-body average SAR	**Chest**	**Umbilicus**	**Knees**	**Chest**	**Umbilicus**	**Knees**
Normal mode operation (W/kg)	6.05	5.43	8.18	5.56	5.14	8.09
First level control (W/kg)	7.05	6.57	8.64	5.67	6.35	8.57

TABLE 9.15

FDTD Partial-body Average SAR Compared with Limits Calculated from IEC Formulas for 1.5 and 3.0 T MRI Coils for the VH Man and Woman Models

Magnetic flux density (T)		1.5			3.0	
Coil center location	**Chest**	**Umbilicus**	**Knees**	**Chest**	**Umbilicus**	**Knees**
Visible Man						
IEC partial-body absorbed power (W)	315.65	327.75	196.32	315.65	327.75	196.32
IEC partial-body average SAR (W/kg)	6.05	5.43	8.18	6.05	5.43	8.18
FDTD partial-body average SAR (W/kg)	5.15	4.46	4.60	5.37	4.52	6.71
IEC/FDTD partial-body average SAR ratio	1.18	1.22	1.78	1.04	1.14	1.21
Visible Woman						
IEC partial-body absorbed power (W)	255.56	258.55	160.13	255.56	258.55	160.13
IEC partial-body average SAR (W/kg)	5.56	5.14	8.09	5.56	5.14	8.09
FDTD partial-body average SAR (W/kg)	4.55	3.96	4.26	5.09	4.55	6.74
IEC/FDTD partial-body SAR ratio	1.33	1.37	2.07	1.09	1.13	1.20

The peak local FDTD calculated SAR values the IEC limits would allow may be calculated from the partial-body or whole-body average SAR using the formula,

$$SAR_{lp} = \left[(SAR_{iec}) / (SAR_{fdtd}) \right] \times \left(SAR_{fdtd1g} \text{ or } SAR_{fdtd10g} \right), \qquad (9.30)$$

where SAR_{lp} is the peak local FDTD calculated SAR values allowed by the IEC, SAR_{iec} is the IEC SAR limit, and SAR_{fdtd} is the FDTD calculated whole-body average SAR at 1 W input power, and SAR_{fdtd1g} and $SAR_{fdtd10g}$ are the FDTD calculated peak SAR for 1 g mass and 10 g mass, respectively, at 1 W input power. The peak SARs normalized to IEC whole-body and partial-body average SAR limits calculated from IEC formulas and FDTD algorithm for 1.5 and 3.0 T coils centered at three body locations of the VH models are given in Tables 9.16 and 9.17.

The IEC local SAR limits for head, trunk, and extremities are 10, 10, and 20 W/kg, respectively, for both normal and first level controlled operation modes. As can be seen from Tables 9.16 and 9.17, the peak local SARs are lower than the FDTD-computed SARs by a large margin in all cases. This implies that the IEC permissible peak local SARs for the chest, umbilicus, and lower extremities could exceed the limit values of 10 and 20 W/kg by an average of three- to sixfold and by as much as tenfold in both male and female patients under the normal operating mode, according to the VH models.

More specifically, the FDTD-calculated average local peak partial-body 1 g and 10 g SARs are 124.94 and 63.57 W/kg, and 133.32 and 64.43 W/kg for the Man and Woman models, respectively, at 1.5 T. Similarly, the FDTD 1 g and 10 g SARs are 117.17 and 65.20 W/kg, and 112.86 and 62.52 W/kg for the Man and Woman models, respectively, at 3.0 T. In addition to the above observation of a factor of three to six times higher than the IEC limits, a clear trend is also seen for the 1 g based local peak SARs, which are twice as high as SAR values based on 10 g of equivalent mass.

TABLE 9.16

Peak SARs Normalized to the IEC Whole-Body and Partial-body Average SAR Limits Calculated from IEC Formulas and FDTD Algorithm for 1.5 and 3.0 T Coils Centered at Three Body Locations of the VH Man Model

	Chest		Umbilicus		Knees	
	SAR_1	SAR_{10}	SAR_1	SAR_{10}	SAR_1	SAR_{10}
Peak local SAR (W/kg)* at 1.5 T						
Values below are normalized to IEC:						
Whole-body 2 W/kg (normal mode operation)	67.55	32.66	141.41	53.32	84.72	67.78
Whole-body 4 W/kg (first level control)	135.30	65.32	282.81	106.63	169.44	135.55
Partial-body SAR (normal mode operation)	107.75	52.02	243.35	91.76	104.87	83.90
Partial-body SAR (first level control)	125.35	60.52	294.69	111.11	110.69	88.56
Peak local SAR (W/kg)[a] at 3.0 T						
Values below are normalized to IEC:						
Whole-body 2 W/kg (normal mode operation)	64.88	36.76	88.93	34.71	130.65	91.25
Whole-body 4 W/kg (first level control)	129.76	73.53	177.86	69.41	261.30	182.50
Partial-body SAR (normal mode operation)	106.99	60.63	160.99	62.82	150.60	105.18
Partial-body SAR (first level control)	124.47	70.53	194.95	76.08	158.96	111.02

[a] SAR_1 and SAR_{10} based on 1 g and 10 g of averaging tissue mass, respectively.

Computational Methods and EM Fields

TABLE 9.17

Peak SARs Normalized to the IEC Whole-body and Partial-body Average SAR Limits Calculated from IEC Formulas and FDTD Algorithm for 1.5 and 3.0 T Coils Centered at three Body Locations of the VH Woman Model

	Peak Local SAR (W/kg)[a] at 1.5 T					
	Chest		Umbilicus		Knees	
	SAR_1	SAR_{10}	SAR_1	SAR_{10}	SAR_1	SAR_{10}
Values below are normalized to IEC:						
Whole-body 2 W/kg (normal mode operation)	47.76	31.47	134.14	37.90	133.94	87.83
Whole-body 4 W/kg (first level control)	95.93	62.95	268.29	75.81	267.87	155.66
Partial-body SAR (normal mode operation)	78.40	51.66	236.53	66.83	169.12	110.90
Partial-body SAR (first level control)	94.06	61.98	292.51	82.65	179.12	117.46
	Peak local SAR (W/kg)[a] at 3.0 T					
Values below are normalized to IEC:						
Whole-body 2 W/kg (normal mode operation)	46.58	31.08	108.61	42.08	111.43	77.98
Whole-body 4 W/kg (first level control)	93.16	62.15	217.22	84.16	222.86	155.96
Partial-body SAR (normal mode operation)	78.46	52.34	194.41	75.32	137.67	96.34
Partial-body SAR (first level control)	94.12	62.80	240.42	93.14	145.82	102.04

[a] SAR_1 and SAR_{10} based on 1 g and 10 g of averaging tissue mass, respectively.

In summary, these results show that in both 1.5 and 3.0 T birdcage MRI coils, the FDTD computed partial-body SARs are higher than values given by the curve-fitting formulas for male and female patients, and the local peak SARs allowed are considerably greater than those specified in the IEC and FDA regulatory limits for both whole-body and partial-body SARs.

9.6 Temperature Elevations Induced in Biological Tissues by EM Power Deposition

9.6.1 Introduction

EM energy impinging on the human body induces currents and fields inside the body. A major biological response from absorption of EM energy in the RF and microwave frequency range is the elevation of tissue temperature. Thus, aside from temperature elevation based biomedical applications, most internationally recognized guidelines for limiting human exposure to EM fields in the RF and microwave range use SAR as the basic dosimetric metric [110,205]. Consequently, the vast majority of studies available in the literature, addressing the topic of human exposure to EM fields, focus their attention on the dosimetric problem of quantifying induced fields and SAR inside the exposed subject. A central premise of these exposure guidelines is to protect exposed subjects against temperature increases exceeding the threshold for induction of adverse thermal effects. Therefore, a large number of investigations have addressed the problem of human exposure to EMFs with a thermal analysis to estimate the temperature increment induced inside the exposed subject.

Another domain in which a thermal analysis can be very useful, or even essential, is that of therapeutic applications where EMFs are deliberately used to cause predefined temperature increases in specific target tissues in the body. Some of the applications include hyperthermia cancer treatment and microwave tissue ablation [206–212]. In such cases, performing a numerical EM and thermal study of the applicator in its intended operating environment, inside the body, can be a valuable aid in designing the applicator, in establishing the clinical protocol (i.e., power to be delivered, time of application, etc.), and for treatment planning purposes.

In the following, an overview of the available analytical formulations to characterize heating induced by EMFs is presented. Some numerical implementations, suitable to study the thermal problem in realistic situations, are summarized with specific examples.

9.6.2 The Bio-Heat Equation

The bio-heat equation (BHE) was originally proposed by Pennes in 1948 to analyze temperature distributions in a resting forearm [213]. Subsequently, it had been modified to study phenomena of heat transport and exchange for the whole body [214,215]. It is an analytical model that describes the temperature distribution $T = T(\mathbf{r},t)$ inside the body. One of the more general formulations of the BHE is given here for temperature rises associated with exposures to EM fields,

$$\nabla \cdot \left(K(\mathbf{r})\nabla T \right) + A(\mathbf{r},T) + Q_v(\mathbf{r}) - RL(\mathbf{r}) - B(\mathbf{r},T)(T - T_B) = C(\mathbf{r})\rho\ (\mathbf{r})\frac{\partial T}{\partial t}\quad [\mathrm{W/m^3}] \quad (9.31)$$

The five terms on the left side of Equation 9.31 represent heat accumulation (or loss) per unit time and per unit volume at a point inside the body. Specifically, the various ways through which heat is transferred, produced, or removed from the tissue are:

- Heat transfer through internal conduction, where K [W/(m °C)] is the tissue thermal conductivity.
- Metabolic heat production [A (W/m³)].
- EM power deposition [Q_v (W/m³)].
- Respiratory heat losses in the lungs [RL (W/m³)].
- Heat exchange due to capillary blood perfusion, which is proportional to blood flow, and is represented by the parameter B [W/(°C m³)], and the difference between blood and tissue temperature ($T_B - T$). Noted that T_B is a function of time [i.e., $T_B = T_B(t)$].

The right side of Equation 9.31 denotes the temperature increase (or decrease) per unit time. The thermal capacitance per unit volume is given by the product between the tissue specific heat, C [J/(kg °C)] and density, ρ (kg/m³).

It should be mentioned that the BHE assumes that heat exchange with blood takes place exclusively via capillary perfusion. In reality, heat exchange also occurs with large blood vessels. This mechanism does not take the form of a distributed exchange throughout the tissue volume, like the $B\ (T - T_B)$ term in the BHE, but instead, the form of a localized exchange at the blood vessel walls. To account for it would require the introduction of an additional term in the BHE [216,217]. Moreover, it would require precise knowledge of the structure of the vasculature inside the biological body, which is not always

Computational Methods and EM Fields

available. However, this mechanism only alters temperature distribution near large blood vessels, and does not significantly affect the overall temperature distribution, especially, the maximum temperature increases elsewhere in an exposed body [218]. Therefore, this mechanism can generally be neglected without significant loss of accuracy, if the principal purpose is to assess safety compliance of a given exposure situation, from the thermal point of view. On the other hand, proper inclusion of large blood vessels may be important when planning hyperthermia or ablation treatments. The presence of a large blood vessel in the target region may cause temperature elevations to remain below the minimum threshold required for an effective treatment.

A first step in using the BHE to compute the temperature increases induced by exposure to EMFs is the evaluation of SAR or local power deposition. In fact, $Q_v = \rho$ SAR is the exogenous heat source responsible for the alteration in temperature profiles inside the exposed subject. Once the Q_v term is determined, the BHE would provide the time evolution of temperature, provided that appropriate initial and boundary conditions are imposed, as discussed later. In this manner, the BHE allows assessment of both the transient response and steady state temperature increases.

An implicit assumption in the above discussion is that the EMF and thermal problems are independent and can be investigated separately or successively. This is equivalent to assuming that EM transients are inconsequential and therefore the SAR distributions are induced instantaneously and can be used as the input for the thermal analysis, and that changes in tissue temperature do not alter the field distribution inside the tissue. Concerning the first assumption, the time constants of the EM and thermal processes are orders of magnitude different, with the EMF reaching its peak value at all parts of the biological body, at most, after a few microseconds, while thermal constants inside living biological tissues are of the order of a few minutes, under usual circumstances. This means that EM transients can indeed be neglected for the thermal analysis. The second assumption, instead, deserves some more attention. In fact, dielectric permittivities of biological tissues are temperature dependent and, therefore, the distribution of EMF could change as heating proceeds and temperature increases. However, this effect may be neglected so long as the temperature elevation is small, that is, on the order of a few degrees Celsius, as is expected for common EMF exposures. If temperature increase is large, and the induced variation in dielectric permittivity is no longer negligible (for example, the heating of food stuff in a microwave oven), the EM and thermal problems must be solved in a coupled manner, iteratively updating the EM solution as heating progresses [219–221].

9.6.2.1 Initial Conditions

The BHE is a partial differential equation in time and space; its solution requires the specification of both initial and boundary conditions. For studies involving RF and microwave induced heating inside the human body, the initial temperature distribution typically is set to the physiological norm, computed as the steady-state solution of Equation 9.31 in the absence of external power deposition ($Q_v = 0$). Thus, the resulting equation is:

$$\nabla \cdot \left(K(\mathbf{r})\nabla T \right) + A_0(\mathbf{r}) - RL(\mathbf{r}) - B_0(\mathbf{r})(T - T_{B0}) = 0 \quad [\mathrm{W/m^3}] \tag{9.32}$$

In this case, thermal parameters do not depend on temperature, and are set to their physiological values, at approximately 37°C. Similarly, the physiological value at rest is used for blood temperature. Note that Equation 9.32 does not contain time derivatives and, therefore, does not require any initial condition to be solved.

9.6.2.2 Boundary Conditions

Boundary conditions are needed to account for the heat exchange between the body surface, namely, the skin, and the external environment, both in the general and steady-state formulations of the BHE as represented by Equations 9.31 and 9.32, respectively. The simplest boundary condition that can be applied is the adiabatic condition, that is, a thermally insulated surface, or the Dirichelet boundary condition, that is, an enforced surface temperature. Adiabatic conditions can be used to model tissue surfaces in close contact with highly insulating materials, such as the catheters used to insert antennas employed in hyperthermia or ablation treatment. In contrast, Dirichelet boundary conditions can be used for surfaces in close contact with a circulating fluid, kept at a constant temperature (forced convection).

Adiabatic and Dirichelet boundary conditions are rather simple, but they are not suitable for representing the general heat exchanges that take place at the skin. A general boundary condition that is obtained by imposing the continuity of the heat flow perpendicular to the surface of the body can be expressed as [222]:

$$-K(\mathbf{r})(\nabla T \cdot \mathbf{n}_0)_S = H(T_S - T_A) + SW(T) \, [W/m^2]$$ (9.33)

where S is the skin surface, and $\mathbf{n}_0$ is the outward unit vector normal to S. The terms on the right side of Equation 9.33 represent the two ways in which heat is exchanged with the environment. In particular, the first term describes heat loss due to convection, and it is proportional to the difference between skin temperature (T_S) and ambient air temperature (T_A) through the convection coefficient H [W/(m²°C)]. The last term represents heat loss due to sweating (SW).

A few words are needed about radiative heat exchange. If one assumes the body surface is surrounded by objects that are all at the same ambient temperature T_A, the expression for heat exchange through radiation from the body surface to the environment, per unit area, is given by [223,224]:

$$Q_r = e\sigma\left(T_S^4 - T_A^4\right) [W/m^2]$$ (9.34)

where e is the surface emissivity, σ is Stefan–Boltzmann's constant, and the temperatures are expressed in degrees Kelvin (K). Under normal conditions, T_S and T_A do not differ significantly from about 300 K, and Equation 9.34 can be approximated as [224]:

$$Q_r = H_r(T_S - T_A) [W/m^2]$$ (9.35)

where H_r is an equivalent convection coefficient. Therefore, the convective term in Equation 9.35 can effectively model both convective and radiative heat exchanges, by using an overall convection coefficient which also takes into account the equivalent convection parameter H_r in Equation 9.35. There are cases, however, in which the surrounding objects are at different temperatures. In such circumstances, the problem becomes very complex and a possible solution, based on the use of an RT method to connect mutually visible surfaces and consider radiant heat transfer between them, has been proposed [225]. However, the simple approach of an equivalent convection is generally sufficient for an accurate analysis of the thermal problem.

It is worthy of mention that the convective boundary condition also can be used to represent an adiabatic condition by simply setting the convective coefficient to zero, or an approximate Dirichelet boundary condition, by using a very high convective coefficient and setting T_A to the imposed surface temperature.

9.6.3 Thermoregulatory Responses

The temperature of the human body is regulated to within a narrow range of about 37°C, in its core. Under normal circumstances, this is accomplished through an exquisite thermoregulatory mechanism involving sweating and vasodilatation. The thermoregulatory mechanism is activated whenever the temperature $T(\mathbf{r})$ in specific parts of the body, where thermal sensors are located, shifts from its basal value $T_0(\mathbf{r})$. In particular, the basal temperature distribution $T_0(\mathbf{r})$, which corresponds to a state of "thermal comfort," is the one obtained in a naked subject when the external air temperature T_A is about 30°C (in a dry environment) [215,226].

Since a part or all of the absorbed EM energy is converted into heat inside the human body, computations of tissue temperature must take into account the thermoregulatory mechanisms in response to the heat input from RF and microwave absorption, starting from a state of thermal comfort [226]. Specifically, the presence of thermoregulatory mechanisms causes some of the terms in Equations 9.31 and 9.33 to vary with body temperature. The first term that shows a dependence on temperature in Equation 9.31 from metabolic heat production, which may be characterized by the following equation [227]:

$$A\left(\mathbf{r}, T(\mathbf{r})\right) = A_0(r)\left(1.1\right)^{(T(\mathbf{r})-T_0(\mathbf{r}))} \tag{9.36}$$

where A_0 is the basal metabolic rate in the tissue. Equation 9.36 shows that metabolic heat production depends only on local tissue temperature. It must be noted that this dependence is not related to thermoregulation, but rather to the fact that metabolic processes are slightly accelerated when the temperature increases.

With regard to the variation of blood flow, there are two different, but essential, phenomena: one for internal tissue perfusion, and the other for peripheral (skin) perfusion. For blood perfusion to the internal tissues, the regulation depends only on local tissue temperature [227,228]. Thus, in a simple model, blood perfusion could be assumed to be at its basal value B_0, until the local temperature reaches 39°C. When the local temperature exceeds 39°C, the blood perfusion starts to increase linearly with temperature in order to enhance the local heat removal process, until the local temperature rises to above a value of about 44°C. At this point, the increasing rate of blood perfusion arrives at a maximum. Accordingly, the internal blood perfusions are modeled by the following expressions:

$$B\left(\mathbf{r}, T(\mathbf{r})\right) = B_0(\mathbf{r}) \quad T(\mathbf{r}) \leq 39°C \tag{9.37}$$

$$B\left(\mathbf{r}, T(\mathbf{r})\right) = B_0(\mathbf{r})\left[1 + S_B\left(T(\mathbf{r}) - 39\right)\right] \quad 39°C < T(\mathbf{r}) < 44°C \tag{9.38}$$

$$B\left(\mathbf{r}, T(\mathbf{r})\right) = B_0(\mathbf{r})(1 + 5S_B) \quad T(\mathbf{r}) \geq 44°C \tag{9.39}$$

The above model of the internal temperature regulation mechanism is rather simple. A more complex temperature control model, instead, would include regulation of blood perfusion in the skin through vasodilatation. In particular, two different signals are used as feedback to regulate vasodilatation: one is the hypothalamic temperature increase $(T_H - T_{H0})$, used as an indicator of the elevation of the body core temperature, and the other is the average skin temperature increase $\overline{\Delta T_S}$, defined as follows:

$$\overline{\Delta T_S} = \frac{\int_S \left(T(r) - T_0(r)\right) dS}{S} \tag{9.40}$$

where S is the skin surface of the body. The two feedback signals are assigned different weights, with a greater importance given to the hypothalamic temperature, and then used, together with local skin temperature, to regulate skin blood flow according to [214,215]:

$$B(\mathbf{r},T(\mathbf{r})) = \left[B_0(\mathbf{r}) + F_{HB}(T_H - T_{H0}) + F_{SB}\overline{\Delta T_S} \right] \cdot 2^{(T(\mathbf{r})-T_0(\mathbf{r}))/6} \tag{9.41}$$

where F_{HB} and F_{SB} are the weights of the hypothalamic and skin temperature signals, respectively.

From the above discussion, it can be noted that blood acts as a heat transfer agent, taking heat away from the inner body parts, whose temperature is higher than that of the blood, and bringing this heat to the body periphery. There, heat is passed to the skin layers, whose temperature is lower than that of the blood, and dissipated through sweating and evaporation. During microwave exposure, the net heat exchange, between blood and the various body tissues, is different from zero, and consequently the blood temperature T_B varies according to the following equation:

$$Q_{BTOT} = C_B \rho_B V_B \frac{\partial T_B}{\partial t} [\text{W}] \tag{9.42}$$

where Q_{BTOT} is the net rate of heat acquisition of the blood from the body tissues, C_B and ρ_B are the blood specific heat and mass density, respectively, and V_B is the total blood volume, assumed equal to about $5\,\text{L}$ [229]. When the thermal equilibrium is reached, the net heat exchange is null, and therefore blood temperature stays at a constant value, slightly higher than the basal one.

The feedback mechanism that regulates sweating (SW in Equation 9.34) is very similar to that regulating peripheral blood flow and can be described as follows [214,215]:

$$SW(\mathbf{r},T(\mathbf{r})) = \left[PI + F_{HS}(T_H - T_{H0}) + F_{SS}\overline{\Delta T_S} \right] 2^{(T(\mathbf{r})-T_0(\mathbf{r}))/10} \tag{9.43}$$

where PI represents "perspiratio insensibilis" (insensible perspiration), that is the basal evaporative heat loss from the skin.

In fact, this model still represents a simplification of the thermoregulatory system of the human body, which is very complex. For example, the skin from different parts of the body does not have the same sweating behavior, as implied by Equation 9.44, and there exist other internal temperature sensors, besides the hypothalamus. Notwithstanding these limitations, and the great variability in thermoregulatory behavior among different subjects, the model can be considered a good starting point to assess thermal responses in a human subject exposed to an EMF. It must also be observed that in most practical situations, induced thermal elevations are very small and thermoregulatory responses may not be invoked, so that basal physiological values for thermal parameters may be assumed for the BHE.

9.6.4 Numerical Methods for Solving Thermal Problems

The combination of the BHE and the thermal boundary condition represent a complicated problem, which can become nonlinear if thermoregulatory mechanisms are considered. Analytical solutions of this problem, neglecting thermoregulation, can only be obtained for simplified body geometries and exposure conditions, which allow an analytical determination of the SAR distribution. For example, an analytical solution in stratified media

Computational Methods and EM Fields 365

may be obtained as an expansion in eigen functions, which are applicable to planar, cylindrical, and spherical multi-layer geometries [230,231]. Also, an analytical solution for the case of a multi-layer slab has been investigated in terms of Green's functions [232]. More complicated solutions, able to take into account thermoregulatory mechanisms, have also been developed, based on a simplified cylindrical segment approximation of the human body [214,215,233,234]. In particular, the thermal behavior of the human body is simulated by means of two systems: a controlling system and a controlled one. The controlled system, modeled by the BHE, determines the temperature distribution inside the body, while the controlling system provides feedback signals able to modify the thermal parameters of the controlled one in order to maintain a constant body core temperature (thermoregulation). The principal limitation of this approach stems from modeling the body as a few homogeneous cylindrical segments, each having a uniform SAR and temperature distribution.

When studying more realistic and detailed geometries, like an anatomically based body model, analytical or cylindrical-segment solutions are no longer feasible, and a numerical approach becomes necessary. One possibility is the development of an FEM solution of the BHE [235,236]. However, the most common approach is to use a FD scheme, which will be discussed in some detail in this section. One of the main reasons for preferring the FD solution, besides its computational efficiency, is that it allows a very simple link with the FDTD method, which is the most popular numerical method for SAR computations. Earlier FD solutions of the BHE—used in conjunction with cubic cell models of the human body—comprised only a few hundred voxels. They used an implicit formulation to avoid the restrictions on the size of the time step. Since these solutions required matrix inversions, they were computationally intensive. As more detailed body models, comprised large number of voxels, became available, new FD solutions were developed. These techniques, based either on explicit or on alternate-direction implicit (ADI) formulations, are discussed in what follows.

9.6.4.1 Explicit FD Formulation

One approach to obtain an FD explicit formulation of the BHE is based on the thermal balance approach [108]. The body under consideration is divided into cubic cells of side δ, and the temperature is evaluated at the center of each cell. Temperatures are computed at equal-time steps, δt. In the following, the expression $T^n(i,j,k)$ represents temperature computed at time $n\delta t$ in the (i,j,k) cell. The FD formulation is derived by imposing the thermal balance to each cell [223], such that

$$Q_{tot}^{n,n+1}(i,j,k) = \Gamma\left(T^{n+1}(i,j,k) - T^n(i,j,k)\right)[\mathrm{J}] \tag{9.44}$$

where $Q_{tot}^{n,n+1}$ is the total heat accumulated (positive) or lost (negative) in the cell during the time interval $n\delta t \div (n+1)\delta t$, $(T^{n+1} - T^n)$ is the variation of the cell temperature in the same time interval, and $\Gamma = C\,\rho\delta^3$ is the thermal capacitance of the cell. The total heat $Q_{tot}^{n,n+1}$ is accumulated (or lost) in the cell through the five mechanisms in the BHE, and, for boundary cells, also through convection to external air and sweating Equation 9.34.

Heat transfer through internal conduction is governed by Fourier's law. For the (i,j,k) cell, the heat $Q_K^{n,n+1}$ entering the cell through conduction from the $(i-1,j,k)$ cell in the time interval, $n\delta t - (n+1)\delta t$, can be derived by exploiting the well-known analogy between heat conduction and electrical current conduction [216,223]. In particular, if K_1 and K_2 are the thermal conductivities of the two cells under examination, heat flows through the series connection of two thermal conductances, equaling $\dfrac{K_1\,\delta^2}{\delta/2}$ and $\dfrac{K_2\,\delta^2}{\delta/2}$, respectively. Therefore, heat flowing from the center of the $(i-1,j,k)$ cell to the center of the (i,j,k) cell, through the boundary face, experiences an overall thermal conductance equal to $\dfrac{2K_1K_2\delta^2}{(K_1+K_2)\delta}$. As a result, we have

$$Q_K^{n,n+1}(i,j,k) = \frac{2K_1K_2}{K_1+K_2}\delta^2 \frac{T^n(i-1,j,k)-T^n(i,j,k)}{\delta}\delta t \tag{9.45}$$

An expression similar to Equation 9.46 holds for heat exchanged with the other neighboring cells.

The contributions of metabolic heat production and EM power deposition are volumetric heat sources, and therefore, the contribution they give to $Q_{tot}^{n,n+1}$ can be immediately derived, and is expressed by Equations 9.46 and 9.47, respectively:

$$Q_A^{n,n+1}(i,j,k) = A(i,j,k)\delta^3\delta t \tag{9.46}$$

$$Q_{Q_v}^{n,n+1}(i,j,k) = Q_v(i,j,k)\delta^3\delta t \tag{9.47}$$

Respiratory losses in the lungs are taken into account by subtracting the volumetric loss RL from the metabolic heat production A in the corresponding cells for the lung.

Finally, the contribution to $Q_{tot}^{n,n+1}$ due to capillary blood perfusion takes the form of a volumetric term and can be represented, similarly to metabolic heat production and exogenous heat deposition, as:

$$Q_B^{n,n+1}(i,j,k) = B(i,j,k)\big(T_B - T^n(i,j,k)\big)\delta^3\delta t \tag{9.48}$$

For boundary cells in contact with air, heat flow through the face is governed by convection rather than conduction. For a generic cell (i,j,k), considering a face in direct contact with air, the heat $Q_H^{n,n+1}$ entering the cell through convection in the time interval, $n\,\delta t \div (n+1)\,\delta t$, is:

$$Q_H^{n,n+1}(i,j,k) = H\big(T_A - T^n(i,j,k)\big)\delta^2\delta t \tag{9.49}$$

Heat losses due to sweating at the skin surface (SW) are converted to a volumetric heat loss term and are directly subtracted from the metabolic heat production term A in the skin cells.

Note that in Equations 9.45, 9.48, and 9.49, the temperature has been referred to the time instant $n\,\delta t$ in order to obtain, at the end, an explicit formulation. Starting from the equations given above, general explicit formulations that hold for each cell are then derived.

9.6.4.2 Stability Criterion

Explicit FD formulations are straightforward to implement and are computationally efficient, but they have a limitation on the maximum time step δt that can be used without incurring numerical instability. The stability criterion for the FD scheme can be obtained through Fourier analysis, which yields the following restriction on δt, derived for internal cells without convective contributions [237]:

$$\delta t \le \frac{1}{6\dfrac{K}{C\rho\delta^2} + \dfrac{B_0}{2C\rho}} \tag{9.50}$$

Computational Methods and EM Fields

Because of the typical values of thermal parameters and convection coefficients for the human body, the stability criterion for the peripheral voxels, where some of the faces exchange heat through convection rather than conduction, is less stringent than that of Equation 9.51. Consequently, Equation 9.51 may be safely assumed as the stability criterion for the overall scheme.

9.6.4.3 ADI Formulation

While the explicit FD formulation of the BHE has been applied to many simulations, it becomes computationally expensive when very small cell sizes are used or when high thermal conductivity materials are present in the domain under study. This stems from the extremely small time steps δt that would be required according to Equation 9.51. In such cases, the ADI formulations can be used [238]. ADI is a general method, developed for numerical solution of parabolic equations. It combines unconditional stability, typical of implicit methods, with the computational efficiency, due to the tri-diagonal nature of the resulting matrices [239–241]. Note that the Fourier heat conduction equation is a typical parabolic equation. While the BHE is no longer parabolic, because of the presence of the term related to blood flow, ADI can still be applied, but it loses its unconditional stability. In any case, for time steps on the order of a few seconds, the scheme has proved to be stable in typical applications. It can yield reductions on the order of ten or more [239] in execution time, over the classical explicit formulation.

The basic idea behind the ADI technique is to extend to the 3-D case the 1-D Crank–Nicolson scheme, which averages the outcome from explicit and the implicit formulation to obtain second-order accuracy both in space and in time variables [223]. In particular, Crank–Nicolson's scheme can be extended to the full 3-D case, by using a sequence of approximate Crank–Nicolson solutions along the three axis, indicated as $T^*(i,j,k)$, $T^{**}(i,j,k)$, and $T^{***}(i,j,k)$, the last one being used as the final estimate for $T^{n+1}(i,j,k)$.

The first approximate solution is obtained using Crank–Nicolson's scheme along the x axis only, while backward differencing is used along y and z:

$$
\begin{aligned}
\frac{K}{\rho C}\frac{1}{2}&\left(\frac{T^*(i-1,j,k)-2T^*(i,j,k)+T^*(i+1,j,k)}{(\delta x)^2}\right.\\
&\left.+\frac{T^n(i-1,j,k)-2T^n(i,j,k)+T^n(i+1,j,k)}{(\delta x)^2}\right)\\
&+\frac{K}{\rho C}\frac{T^n(i,j-1,k)-2T^n(i,j,k)+T^n(i,j+1,k)}{(\delta y)^2}\\
&+\frac{K}{\rho C}\frac{T^n(i,j,k-1)-2T^n(i,j,k)+T^n(i,j,k+1)}{(\delta z)^2}\\
&=\frac{T^*(i,j,k)-T^n(i,j,k)}{\delta t}-\frac{A_0+Q_v+B_0T_B}{\rho C}\\
&+\frac{B_0}{\rho C}\frac{T^*(i,j,k)+T^n(i,j,k)}{2}
\end{aligned}
\tag{9.51}
$$

Extending subsequently Crank–Nicolson's solution along the y axis and the z axis, the following expressions are obtained for the second and third estimates:

$$
\begin{aligned}
&\frac{K}{\rho C}\frac{1}{2}\left(\frac{T^*(i-1,j,k)-2T^*(i,j,k)+T^*(i+1,j,k)}{(\delta x)^2}+\frac{T^n(i-1,j,k)-2T^n(i,j,k)+T^n(i+1,j,k)}{(\delta x)^2}\right)\\
&+\frac{K}{\rho C}\frac{1}{2}\left(\frac{T^{**}(i,j-1,k)-2T^{**}(i,j,k)+T^{**}(i,j+1,k)}{(\delta y)^2}+\frac{T^n(i,j-1,k)-2T^n(i,j,k)+T^n(i,j+1,k)}{(\delta y)^2}\right)\\
&+\frac{K}{\rho C}\frac{T^n(i,j,k-1)-2T^n(i,j,k)+T^n(i,j,k+1)}{(\delta z)^2}\\
&=\frac{T^{**}(i,j,k)-T^n(i,j,k)}{\delta t}-\frac{A_0+Q_v+B_0 T_B}{\rho C}\\
&\quad+\frac{B}{\rho C}\frac{T^{**}(i,j,k)+T^n(i,j,k)}{2}
\end{aligned}
\tag{9.52}
$$

$$
\begin{aligned}
&\frac{K}{\rho C}\frac{1}{2}\left(\frac{T^*(i-1,j,k)-2T^*(i,j,k)+T^*(i+1,j,k)}{(\delta x)^2}+\frac{T^n(i-1,j,k)-2T^n(i,j,k)+T^n(i+1,j,k)}{(\delta x)^2}\right)\\
&+\frac{K}{\rho C}\frac{1}{2}\left(\frac{T^{**}(i,j-1,k)-2T^{**}(i,j,k)+T^{**}(i,j+1,k)}{(\delta y)^2}+\frac{T^n(i,j-1,k)-2T^n(i,j,k)+T^n(i,j+1,k)}{(\delta y)^2}\right)\\
&+\frac{K}{\rho C}\frac{1}{2}\left(\frac{T^{n+1}(i,j,k-1)-2T^{n+1}(i,j,k)+T^{n+1}(i,j,k+1)}{(\delta z)^2}+\frac{T^n(i,j,k-1)-2T^n(i,j,k)+T^n(i,j,k+1)}{(\delta z)^2}\right)\\
&=\frac{T^{n+1}(i,j,k)-T^n(i,j,k)}{\delta t}-\frac{A_0+Q_v+B_0 T_B}{\rho C}\\
&\quad+\frac{B_0}{\rho C}\frac{T^{n+1}(i,j,k)+T^n(i,j,k)}{2}
\end{aligned}
\tag{9.53}
$$

Computational Methods and EM Fields

Starting from the above expressions, it is possible to derive the general ADI formulation which holds for each internal cell. The formulation can also be adapted to boundary cells, where convective heat exchange must be considered, by introducing a fictitious external node.

9.6.5 Temperature Elevations in Subjects Exposed to EMFs

When an EMF impinges on the biological body, a fraction of the incident power is absorbed by the body and is converted into heat in the body tissue. Thus, the absorbed energy can cause temperature increases in various body organs and tissues. If the temperature increase is small, it has little effect and is controlled by the thermoregulatory mechanisms of the body. However, if the temperature increment is large, it can produce irreversible biological damage. For example, a temperature increase of about 4.5°C for more than 30 min would produce neuronal damage [230]. Experiments performed on the rabbit eye indicated that a threshold increase of 3°C–5°C in the lens can induce cataract formation [242–245]. The temperature increase necessary to induce thermal damage to the skin is about 10°C [246,247], while it is 8°C for muscle tissues [248]. Also, experiments performed using laboratory animals have shown various physiological and behavioral effects when the body core temperature rises more than 1°C–2°C [249].

Moreover, most RF protection standards have adopted basic restrictions in order to keep the thermal increments below some agreed upon level. In particular, the value of 4 W/kg averaged over the whole body (SAR_{WB}) had been adopted by exposure guidelines as the threshold for the induction of adverse thermal effects associated with an increase of the body core temperature of about 1°C in animal experiments. Restrictions on local SAR were introduced to limit local temperature increments, since the ratio of the local peak to whole-body averaged SAR can be as high as 20:1 for exposure to a uniform plane wave [248,249]. However, it is important to note that tissue heating during EM exposure not only is strongly influenced by the power dissipated in the local tissue volume, but also by the way in which absorption is distributed in the surrounding area, by the thermal characteristics of the tissue and its neighbors, and finally, by the heat exchange with the external environment. The correlations between local SAR and temperature increases and between SAR distribution and temperature distribution is not straightforward. Indeed, the correlation is influenced both by exposure duration and tissue mass or volume. The following section describes some of the studies and results for both far and near field radiating sources.

9.6.5.1 Temperature Increments in the Human Body Exposed to the Far Field of Radiating RF Sources

In the past, temperature elevations due to EM energy absorption in the human body have been evaluated using several models. The earlier studies were based on simplified cylindrical segments approximating the human body. These studies were limited to modeling the body as few homogeneous cylindrical segments, each one having a uniform SAR and temperature distribution. A subsequent study [228] used a cubic-cell model with tissue inhomogeneity and accounted for the thermoregulatory mechanisms in the BHE. In this case, the BHE was solved using an implicit formulation, which avoided the restriction in the size of the time step. Later, explicit formulations of the BHE have been developed to study thermal responses in anatomically realistic body models [227,250,251]. In these studies, only partial body regions were considered, and thermoregulation mechanisms were neglected.

More recently, the EM and thermal problems have been combined in a detailed (5 mm resolution) anatomical model of the human body [108]. The FDTD method was used to compute the EMF distribution inside the exposed body, while an explicit FD formulation of the BHE, together with a more complete model of the human thermoregulatory system, were developed for calculation of the corresponding temperature increase.

For an incident power density equal to the maximum permissible value in the International Commission on Nonionizing Radiation Protection (ICNIRP) exposure guidelines for the general public [110], Figure 9.27 shows the maximum steady-state temperature increase ΔT_{max} obtained inside the body and in the blood as a function of frequency for a subject wearing shoes, either with or without thermoregulation [108]. It can be seen that the highest ΔT values are obtained at 40 MHz. It is also interesting to note that, when thermoregulation is considered, the increase in blood temperature is practically zero, while the maximum temperature rise in the body can reach 0.72°C. This happens since blood temperature is very close to the body core temperature, which thermoregulation tends to keep as constant, while the maximum temperature increments are usually found in the superficial tissue layers. It is worth noting that at 40 MHz, the maximum steady-state temperature increase (0.72°C in the presence of thermoregulation) is found in the muscle tissues of the ankle. The threshold for the induction of thermal damage in muscle is about 45°C [246] that corresponds to a temperature increase of about 8°C. This temperature differential coincides with the safety factor of 10 promulgated by ICNIRP [110] for occupational exposure in limiting the power density from inducing a thermal effect.

Figure 9.28 Shows the distribution of the maximum steady-state temperature increase for each horizontal layer of the body at (a) 40 MHz and (b) 900 MHz, for an incident power density of 10 W/m². At 40 MHz, the maximum temperature increases are obtained at the level of the ankles, where the maximum local SARs also are located. The result showed that the presence of shoes could influence temperature change. Since shoes are insulators from the thermal point of view, they prevent heat flow from going to the ground through them and promote higher heating within the body. The only exception is in the ankle

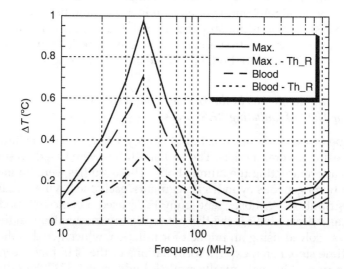

FIGURE 9.27
Maximum steady-state temperature increase (ΔT) in the body and blood of a subject wearing shoes, as a function of frequency, with or without thermoregulation (Th_R) for a P_{inc} equal to the limits set by ICNIRP [110].

Computational Methods and EM Fields

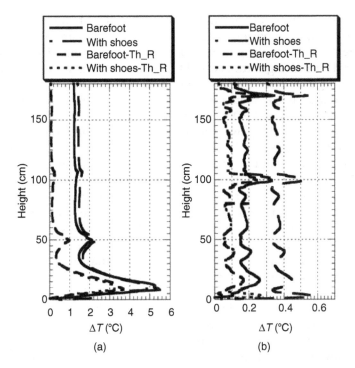

FIGURE 9.28
Layer peak steady-state temperature increase (ΔT) in the absence or presence of thermoregulation (Th_R) for a grounded subject with barefoot or with shoes ($P_{inc} = 10\,W/m^2$). (a) $f = 40\,MHz$; (b) $f = 900\,MHz$.

section, where heating was higher in the barefoot model because of the higher SAR values, at 40 MHz.

Also, the presence of the thermoregulatory mechanisms reduced the temperature increase almost uniformly along the body. Figure 9.28 illustrates clearly the role of blood convection in heat exchanges. In fact, even without active thermoregulation, heat could be spread from the point where its induction is relatively high (e.g., the ankle at 40 MHz) to the rest of the body, by an increase in the temperature of the circulating blood. Therefore, even if power deposition is limited to one body region, temperature elevations may occur throughout the body. This is clearly visible at 40 MHz, where, although power deposition is mainly confined to the ankle region, in the absence of thermoregulation significant temperature elevations (about 1.4°C, $P_{inc} = 10\,W/m^2$—see Figure 9.28a) can occur in the brain. The corresponding elevation in blood temperature elevation is about 1.46°C. It is interesting to note that at 900 MHz, in the absence of active thermoregulation, the brain temperature elevation (0.5°C, $P_{inc} = 10\,W/m^2$—see Figure 9.28b) is higher than blood temperature elevation (0.35°C), as a result of power deposition inside the brain.

9.6.5.2 Temperature Increments in the Head of Cell Phone Users

One consequence of RF power deposition in the human head exposed to the field emitted by a cell phone is temperature increase in the head. In practical situations, in addition to RF power deposition, there are two other causes for temperature increase. The first one is the contact between the phone case and the user's head (ear and cheek, in particular), which blocks the convective heat exchange between the skin layers and the air. It causes the temperature to rise in tissues around the contact zone. Obviously, this heating is not produced by the radiated RF power. The second cause for temperature increase is the heating of the phone itself, due to the power dissipated in the internal circuitry, especially the power amplifier. This heating is transferred to the head tissues via thermal conduction.

Studies on temperature rises in the human head, associated with the field emitted by the cell phone, are usually conducted by using anatomically based head models, a FDTD solution of the EM problem and FD formulations of the BHE [172,175,183,218,251–254]. For example, the dissipation in the power amplifier was simulated by adding a power deposition of 250 mW at 900 MHz and 125 mW at 1800 MHz, uniformly distributed inside the upper part of the phone with 50% efficiency [172]. The heating effects due to SAR, phone contact, and power dissipation in the amplifier were considered separately, and were subsequently added together in order to obtain the temperature elevation. The maximum temperature elevations obtained in the ear and in the brain of a user's head are given in Table 9.18 for 900 and 1800 MHz. The ambient air temperature was assumed to be 24°C and a time interval of 15 min, approximating the duration of a long phone call. Although a steady state would not have been reached, the temperature elevation after 15 min is expected to be close to the steady-state value [175].

The data shown in Table 9.18 reveal some interesting findings. First, the temperature elevation induced inside the brain by SAR alone is less than 0.1°C, especially when the phone was kept in the "cheek" position. This configuration resulted in a marked reduction in power deposition inside the brain. Table 9.18 also shows that the mere contact of the cell phone with the ear and cheek, even in a stand-by mode, in which no RF power is radiated, can cause a temperature elevation in the ear reaching as high as 1.5°C. This is due to the highly insulating properties assumed for the phone's plastic shell. A negligible maximum temperature elevation of about 0.01°C, instead, is obtained in the peripheral brain region. If the contribution from power dissipation in the amplifier is included, the induced temperature elevations were not significantly altered. It must be noted, however, that this result arises from consideration of power dissipation in the power amplifier alone. In the real situation, additional power dissipation is present in the internal circuitry of the

TABLE 9.18

Temperature Elevations Induced in the User's Head After 15 min By a Phone Equipped with a Dual-band Monopole-helix Antenna. Average Radiated Power: 250 mW at 900 MHz and 125 mW at 1800 MHz

Freq. (MHz)	Position	Heating Cause	ΔT_{max} (°C)	ΔT_{max} Brain (°C)
900	Vertical	SAR	0.221	0.061
	"Cheek"	SAR	0.136	0.023[a]
		Contact	1.543	0.012[b]
		Contact + Power Dissipation	1.544	0.012[b]
		Contact + Power Dissipation + SAR	1.581	0.023[a]
1800	Vertical	SAR	0.155	0.036
	"Cheek"	SAR	0.085	0.011[a]
		Contact	1.543	0.012[b]
		Contact + Power Dissipation	1.543	0.012[b]
		Contact + Power Dissipation + SAR	1.549	0.012[b]

[a] ΔT_{max} Brain located in the upper external brain region.
[b] ΔT_{max} Brain located in the lower external brain region.

handset, besides the power amplifier, and hence slightly higher temperature elevations may be expected [253].

The effect of the phone contact on the temperature evolution in the ear region is shown in Figure 9.29. It can be seen that when the phone was put in contact with the ear, the ear temperature experiences a quick decrease. This is because the phone was initially at ambient temperature (24°C), which was lower than the ear temperature. However, soon afterward, the heat supplied by blood and conducted from the neighbouring tissues stopped the decrease. Indeed, the temperature started to elevate, going beyond the initial value, because of the suppressed convective exchange with air.

When all heating sources are considered simultaneously, the results indicated that the maximum temperature elevation in the ear was almost entirely due to the contact effect, with only a very slight contribution due to EM power deposition in the ear region. However, the situation was completely different in the brain region. In fact, the heating effects due to SAR and phone contact tend to heat different parts of the brain. The contact-effect heating occurred in the lower peripheral brain region, and the SAR-induced heating occurred mostly in the upper peripheral brain region. Therefore, these two heating effects are not additive in the brain, and when they are simultaneously present, as opposed to the case when only one is considered, the result is that the portion of the brain affected by heating becomes larger. The peak temperature increase in the brain is therefore governed by the more significant of the two heating causes. At 900 MHz, SAR is more dominant, while at 1800 MHz, due to the lower radiated power; the two heating effects are comparable. Note that the U.S. Federal Communications Commission (FCC) safety rules [158], which restrict the 1-g averaged spatial peak SAR to 1.6 W/kg, are associated with maximum temperature rises in the brain between 0.03°C and 0.09°C. These values are about 50 times lower than the threshold for thermal damage. The ICNIRP safety guideline of a 10-g averaged spatial peak SARs equal to 2 W/kg, results in maximum temperature rises in the brain between 0.1°C and 0.2°C, which is about 25 times lower than the threshold value.

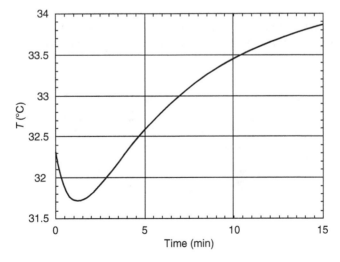

FIGURE 9.29
Time evolution of the temperature at a point on the ear in direct contact with a non-radiating cell phone.

9.7 Correlation between RF Absorption Metrics and Temperature Rise

In recent years, there has been growing concern about the relationship between SAR and tissue temperature elevation, and the appropriateness of various sizes of tissue mass for SAR-induced temperature characterization in anatomically realistic human models [254–259]. It has been suggested that under steady-state exposure conditions, temperature distribution does not correlate well with SAR distribution in voxel based anatomical models of the human body. On the other hand, most of the studies, as described above, were conducted for steady-state scenarios involving exposures of long durations. Thus, they do not address the important issue of shorter duration RF-exposure-induced temperature increases or local "hotspots." Indeed, the time evolution of RF-induced temperature rise in biological tissues has not been appropriately addressed. Moreover, while induced SAR distribution or RF deposition is instantaneous, RF-induced temperature increases or hotspots vary with exposure duration and size of mass of tissue in which RF-induced heating may occur. Both factors—exposure duration and tissue mass—would influence determination of the appropriateness of the size of tissue averaging mass for SAR-induced temperature characterization in voxel based, anatomically realistic human models. This is a most significant issue, especially for RF exposure guidelines based on allowable increase in tissue temperature or proposed to mitigate against tissue temperature rise in RF-exposed human subjects.

This section examines in some detail the correlation between SAR and temperature increase for a human body exposed to both near-field RF sources [258] and far-field plane waves [252,256] as functions of exposure duration, different tissue size, and schemes for averaging metrics, including description of volumetric absorption rate (VAR) [254,255], in addition to SAR as a dosimetry metric.

9.7.1 Near-Field RF Sources

As a practical example of a well-known near-field application, a study was performed by considering a 64-MHz low-pass MRI birdcage coil antenna [260,261]. This antenna has an external shield with a diameter of 78 cm, and a height of 80 cm (Figure 9.30a). The coil antenna is constituted by 16 cylindrical copper legs with a diameter of 2 cm and a height of 65 cm. The legs are uniformly distributed on a cylindrical surface with a diameter of 70 cm

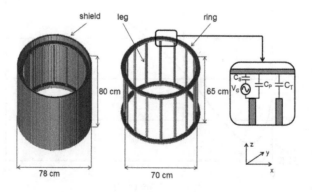

FIGURE 9.30
MRI birdcage coil antenna: (a) Shielded coil; (b) Coil without shield; (c) Capacitive tuning at the leg-ring connection.

Computational Methods and EM Fields

(Figure 9.30b) and are connected to two rings, with a 2×4 cm cross-section, by tuning capacitors (C_T in Figure 9.30c). The capacitances are tuned to achieve the desired resonance frequency. Four 50 Ω generators spaced 90° apart (V_G in Figure 9.30c) provide sinusoidal waveforms with 90° phase shift and are connected between the legs and the upper ring; they are used for exciting the coil antenna at the desired frequency. In addition, there are two tuning capacitors, one in series (C_S) and the other in parallel (C_P) connected to the generator ($C_T = C_S + C_P$) (see Figure 9.30c). This excitation simulates the scheme typically adopted in MRI coil antennas [262], and produces a magnetic field of clockwise circular polarization with respect to the positive z-axis, which is necessary for maximum coupling with nuclear proton spin. A single generator with Gaussian time behavior is used to study the frequency behavior of the reflection coefficient for evaluation of coil resonance frequencies [261].

An anatomical model with 5-mm resolution was adopted from the Virtual Family data set (Duke) with $110 \times 58 \times 360$ cells and 78 different tissues [91]. The values of the permittivity, conductivity, and density of the tissues were taken from the literature [263]. Starting from the Duke model, a partial body model was obtained to focus on the thoracic region of the body. The model was obtained by removing portions of the body far from the coil where the RF power deposition is expected to be negligible and it is shown in the center of Figure 9.24 with its position inside the unshielded coil antenna. The use of the reduced model gives rise to consistent savings of memory occupation and execution time both for EM and thermal simulations, without reducing the accuracy of the computed results [264].

Starting from the FDTD determined power deposition in tissues, the temperature distributions inside the anatomical body model were computed by solving the BHE. The model was divided into 5-mm cubic cells. In addition to evaluation of SAR distributions in W/kg, a different metric for quantifying RF absorption, namely volumetric absorption rate (VAR) in W/m^3 was computed. Absorption-induced temperature rises were then calculated at the center of each cell.

Specifically, SAR was evaluated by adopting the IEEE procedure. This procedure computes average SAR for each cell within the body by building a cubic volume around the cell itself with desired tissue mass; provisions were made such that cubes having one or more faces entirely in air were considered invalid. Only cells with an associated valid averaging volume were assigned the corresponding SAR value. Each cell used to evaluate a valid averaging cube was marked as "used." The invalid but "used" cells were assigned the maximum SAR value among those evaluated in the several cubes in which the cell was used. Finally, a special treatment was required to assign a SAR value to the remaining cells (which are, generally, those close to the external body surface). In summary, The IEEE averaging procedure propagates average SAR values of the inner layers to the boundary layers, where valid averaging cubes cannot be built.

For VAR computations, a simple algorithm was chosen by building around each cell a cube of desired volume regardless of air content in the cube itself, and dividing the total power deposition inside the cube by the cube's volume. This means that for boundary cells, most of the accounted volume will be air with a consequent reduction of computed VAR values. Hence, this procedure tends to smooth out VAR values close to the external body surface.

Thus, SAR and VAR distributions differ both for different exposure metric (mass versus volume-specific absorption) and for different averaging scheme. To assess separately the influence of the two metrics on correlation with temperature increases, their correlation may be evaluated both by considering the entire SAR or VAR distributions computed for each cell within the body, and SAR or VAR distributions limited to cells where only valid SAR-averaging volumes had been built according to IEEE C95.3 procedures. In the second case, boundary cells were excluded and their effect on correlation of different exposure metrics becomes evident. For the results shown below, the mass (or volume) varied from 0.5 g (or cm^3), 1–10 g (or cm^3) in steps of 1 g (or cm^3), and the increments from 10 to 50 g (or cm^3) were in steps of 5 g (cm^3).

Temperature increases as a function of time were computed at several points in a central horizontal section of the anatomical model. Exposure durations ranged from 30 s to 30 min to assess the correlation between SAR or VAR and temperature increase under both initial and steady-state conditions. The input power for the MRI coil antenna was set equal to 40 W.

The correlation was evaluated by performing a regression analysis, based on a least-square linear fit, where temperature increase in each cell was taken as the dependent variable, while the corresponding SAR or VAR value was considered as an independent variable. Scatter plots for temperature increase (ΔT) and averaged SAR or VAR at different exposure times and for various averaging schemes were computed, and correlation coefficients of related fitting lines were used to compare the different metrics. A linear fitting was chosen since the thermal problem is linear and, hence, temperature increases are expected to be proportional to power deposition. The slope of the regression line represents the proportionality coefficient between induced temperature rise and power deposition. The fitting line is forced to pass through the origin, so as to predict zero ΔT, in the absence of power deposition. All cells where temperature increases were not computed (i.e., internal air and blood where only convection takes place) were excluded from this analysis. Different absorption metrics and averaging schemes were compared on the basis of the correlation coefficients for the resulting fitting lines.

An example of SAR, VAR, and ΔT distribution after 30 s of exposure is shown in Figure 9.31 for a central section of the anatomical Duke model. A close correspondence between temperature elevation and SAR can be seen. Figure 9.32 gives a computed scatter plots obtained for temperature increases in the thorax of the Duke anatomical model after 30 s of exposure for SAR averaged over 1 g according to the IEEE 2005 procedure. The figure also shows the fitting line.

Figure 9.33 shows the correlation coefficients of temperature increase for averaging mass (or volume) varying from 0.5 g (cm^3) to 50 g (cm^3) after 30 s of RF exposure. It can be seen

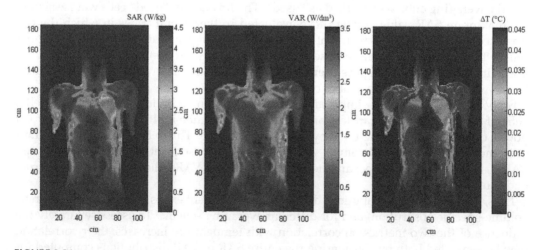

FIGURE 9.31
Two dimensional distributions in a central coronal section of the anatomical Duke model: (a) 1-g averaged SAR, (b) 1-cm^3 averaged VAR, and (c) temperature elevation after 30 s exposure.

Computational Methods and EM Fields

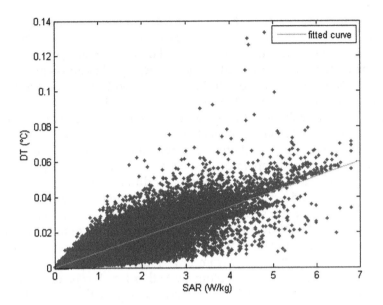

FIGURE 9.32
Scatter plot connecting temperature increase ΔT in the Duke's thorax after 30 s of exposure for SAR_{1g} averaged according to the IEEE 2005 procedure.

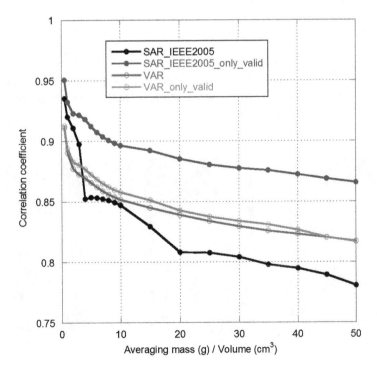

FIGURE 9.33
Correlation coefficients of the linear fitting for different averaging schemes after 30 s of exposure of the anatomical model.

that temperature increase correlates better with SAR for small averaging masses, as compared to VAR, because of the negligible heat transfer effect at the body boundary, especially for mass and volume less than 5 g or 5 cm³. Higher averaging mass and volume can lead to inclusion of different tissues within the averaging cubes and consequently, the correlation worsens. Note that the SARs and VARs evaluated by considering only valid cells provided somewhat different correlation coefficients. They both decreased monotonically with increasing mass or volume, although at different rates. This is the result of inhomogeneity and presence of internal air pockets in the anatomical model, which make SAR and VAR metrics different, especially for inner regions. Moreover, it is interesting to note that the correlation between temperature increase and VAR is only slightly influenced by values calculated at boundary voxels, while greater differences are obtained for SAR.

The scenario under steady-state conditions is represented by the distributions of SAR, VAR, and temperature increase shown in Figure 9.34, following 30 min of RF exposure. In general, compared to SAR, VAR correlates slightly better with temperature distribution. However, as can be seen from Figure 9.35, the correlation coefficients behave similarly for SAR and VAR, in that they both start from low values and improve to a maximum and then leveling out with larger mass or volume, whether for all cells or for only valid cells. In this case, an optimal averaging volume to maximize correlation is 7–8 cm³. For SAR, the correlation with ΔT reaches a maximum between 10 and 15 g followed by an oscillatory behavior for larger mass.

Figure 9.36 presents the maximum correlation coefficients obtained for each metric (SAR or VAR) and the corresponding averaging mass or volume, using the anatomical Duke model for exposure durations ranging from 30 s to 10 min. The correlation coefficients show similar behaviors for SAR and VAR in that they both begin from a lower values and rise to a maximum and then dropping off with increasing exposure time. Results indicate that induced temperature increase correlates better with SAR for shorter exposures (1 min) and smaller averaging mass (0.5 g), but the correlation coefficient remains above 0.9 at 2 min for a 2 g mass. However, the correlation is better with VAR, starting with an exposure time of 90 s. A value of about 1 cm³ appears to be the optimal averaging volume for VAR and for exposures up to 6 min, increasing to 5 cm³ for durations ranging from 7 to 10 min and beyond (i.e., steady state).

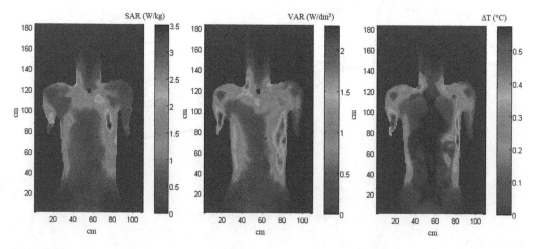

FIGURE 9.34
Increase in a central coronal section of the anatomical Duke model. following 30 min of exposure.

Computational Methods and EM Fields

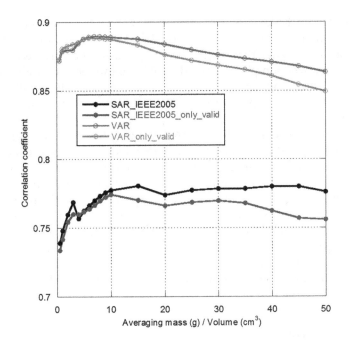

FIGURE 9.35
Correlation coefficients of the linear fitting for different averaging schemes following 30 min of exposure of the anatomical Duke model.

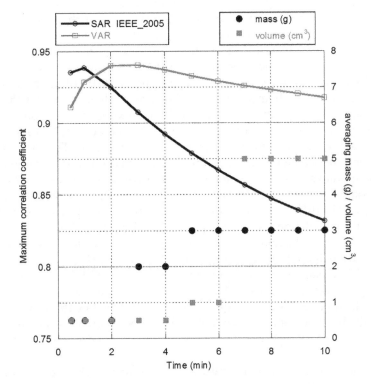

FIGURE 9.36
Maximum correlation coefficient with respect to averaging mass or volume as a function of exposure duration.

380   *Electromagnetic Fields*

These results demonstrate very different phenomena between short exposure and steady-state condition for the human body model. For short exposures, SAR at small averaging masses correlates better than VAR with temperature increase because, in this case, heat diffusion and convection phenomena do not have influence on induced temperature elevation and its distribution. On the contrary, under steady-state conditions, VAR correlates better than SAR with temperature increase due to its smoother behavior close to the body boundaries.

The correlation is better with VAR than SAR, starting from an exposure time of 90 s. It is interesting to note that the correlation between SAR and temperature increase is greatly improved using only valid cells in the short exposure case, where heat convection and conduction effect are yet to begin their influence. However, the correlation slightly worsened for steady state indicating that in this case the complex shape of the human body should be taken into account in the exposure metric. Thus, correlation between SAR and temperature increase is strongly influenced by the different averaging procedure. On the other hand, correlation between VAR and heating is only slightly influenced by inner voxels of the body model. Moreover, the computationally revealed decreasing behavior of the VAR metric close to the boundary appears to better represent the naturally decreasing behavior of temperature close to the body surface.

9.7.2 Far Field Plane Waves

The use of plane waves in the far field is an established approach for investigating EM interaction with dielectric structures, including biological bodies. A plane wave has the advantage of allowing investigation of correlation between SAR, VAR, and temperature increase without such confounding factors as complexities of the source. In this case, a study was chosen to complement observations from the near-field exposure described in the previous section. Specifically, EM simulation was performed by considering a vertically polarized plane wave at the same frequency (64 MHz), impinging on the human body (Duke) model with a spatial resolution of 1 mm. The SAR distributions were computed using the IEEE averaging scheme, while the VAR was evaluated as the volume averaged power deposition. For temperature increase, different exposure durations were included to examine differences in the resulting correlation between power deposition and temperature as a function of duration, including steady-state conditions. The correlation between SAR (or VAR) and induced temperature increase for each cell was determined by performing a regression analysis, where the temperature increase in each cell was taken as the dependent variable, while the corresponding SAR (or VAR) value was considered as the independent one. The different absorption metrics and averaging schemes were compared on the basis of the correlation coefficients of the resulting fitting lines.

As examples, the distributions of SAR averaged over 1 g of mass, VAR averaged over 1 cm^3, and induced temperature increase in the anatomical Duke model after 30 s of exposure to 64 MHz plane waves are presented in Figure 9.37. Likewise, the distributions of SAR averaged over 5 g of mass, VAR averaged over 5 cm^3, and induced temperature increase after 30 min of exposure are given in Figure 9.38. While there are obvious differences among the behavior of all dependent variables between 30 s and 30 min exposures, however, with respect to temperature distribution, the influences of SAR and VAR are very subtle.

The scatter plots of induced temperature increase after 30 s of plane-wave exposure for (a) SAR and (b) VAR given in Figure 9.39 show proportional increases in ΔT for both increasing SAR averaged over 1 g and VAR averaged over 1 cm^3. Thus, a corresponding

Computational Methods and EM Fields 381

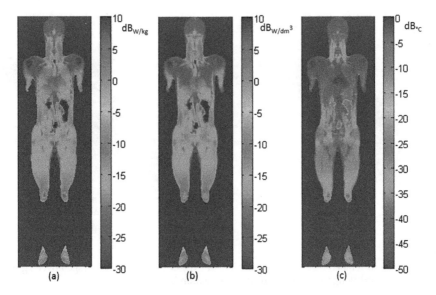

FIGURE 9.37
Distribution of (a) SAR averaged over 1 g of mass; (b) VAR averaged over 1 cm³; and (c) temperature increase in the anatomical Duke model after 30 s of exposure to 64 MHz plane waves.

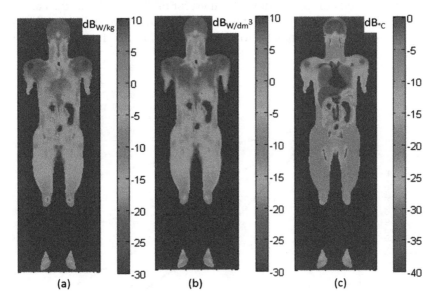

FIGURE 9.38
Distribution of (a) SAR averaged over 5 g of mass; (b) VAR averaged over 5 cm³: and (c) temperature increase in the anatomical Duke model following 30 min of exposure to 64-MHz plane waves.

linear fitting line was derived for SAR and VAR, respectively, and induced temperature increase. A correlation coefficient for both the plane-wave SAR and VAR is 0.984.

Note that in the case of exposure to a near-field MRI source, the correlation coefficients are 0.920 for SAR averaged over 1 g, and 0.890 for VAR averaged over 1 cm³. Thus, plane wave exposures yield a better correlation between the SAR and the temperature increase with respect to the exposure to near-field exposures from this study. Since shorter

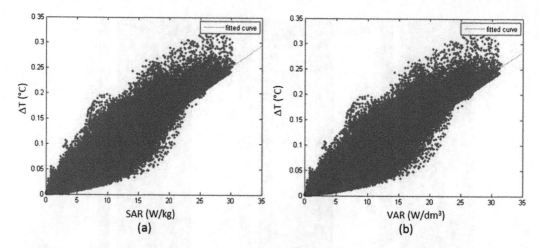

FIGURE 9.39
Scatter plots of induced temperature increase after 30 s of exposure for (a) SAR averaged over 1 g of mass; (b) VAR averaged over 1 cm^3 along the corresponding interpolation lines.

wavelengths are associated with higher frequency RF field, they would also give rise to better correlations.

The maximum correlation coefficients obtained for SAR or VAR and the corresponding averaging mass or volume from the anatomical Duke model are shown in Figure 9.40 for plane-wave RF exposure durations up to 30 min. Note that for short exposures (30 s), the

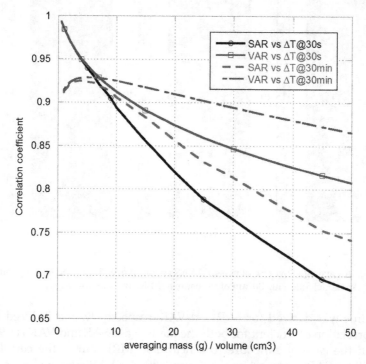

FIGURE 9.40
Correlation coefficients for exposures at 30 s and 30 min, respectively, as a function of the averaging mass (or volume).

Computational Methods and EM Fields

correlation coefficients of ΔT with SAR and VAR are about the same for smaller averaging masses (<5 g) or volumes (<5 cm^3). However at 30 s, the correlation is better with VAR for 5 cm^3 or greater volumes. For the 30-min exposure, the correlation coefficients again display similar behaviors for SAR and VAR in that they both start with slightly lower values and improve to a maximum and then dropping off with increasing mass or volume. For SAR, the correlation with ΔT reaches a maximum for a 3 g mass and then drops off rapidly for 4 g or larger mass. For the 64-MHz plane wave exposure, the most favorable averaging volume to maximize VAR correlation is 4–5 cm^3. For larger volumes, correlation for VAR and ΔT also drops off, but not as rapidly as for SAR.

As mentioned already, most published studies have focused on prolonged or steady-state exposure conditions. In this regard, some of the results discussed here are in general agreement with those reported by McIntosh and Anderson [263] for plane-wave, steady-state exposure (30 min) in the 0.5–6 GHz range. Specifically, McIntosh and Anderson [263] found VAR is better correlated with steady-state temperature increase than SAR. Moreover, they had suggested choosing averaging volume and mass of 10 cm^3 for VAR and 10 g for SAR, respectively. These values are substantially larger than the 3–4 g or 4–5 cm^3 obtained from the current study and discussed above. Therefore, the averaging mass adopted by some of the currently promulgated exposure guidelines may not be appropriate or optimal, as assumed.

9.7.3 A Summary

The discussions in this section clearly show very different phenomena among short and prolonged (including steady state) RF exposures of a human body exposed to near field sources and to far field plane waves. Moreover, these features would vary depending on the metric and size selected for RF energy absorption characterization in biological tissue. Some of the salient features are summarized below.

9.7.3.1 Short RF Exposures

- In *the near-field*, the correlation coefficients with ΔT for SAR and VAR both start at a high level and then monotonically and rapidly decrease with increasing mass or volume.
- SAR for small averaging mass correlates better than VAR with temperature increase and for exposure durations less than 90 s.
- Temperature increase correlates better with SAR for shorter exposures (1 min) and smaller averaging masses (0.5 g), but the correlation coefficient remains above 0.9 at 2 min for a 2 g mass.
- A value of about 1 cm^3 appears to be the optimal averaging volume for VAR and for exposures up to 6 min.
- In *the far-field*, correlation of ΔT with SAR and VAR is about the same for smaller averaging mass (<5 g) or volume (<5 cm^3) for short exposures.

9.7.3.2 Prolonged RF Exposures Including Steady State

- In *the near-field*, the correlation coefficients behave similarly for SAR and VAR; they both start with slightly lower values and improve to a maximum and then leveling out with larger mass or volume, at a comparable pace.

- For SAR, the correlation with ΔT reaches a maximum between 10 and 15 g, followed by a minor oscillatory behavior for larger mass.

- VAR correlates better than SAR with temperature increase.

- A volume of 5–7 cm^3 appears to be the optimal averaging volume for VAR and for exposure durations ranging from 7 to 10 min and beyond (i.e., steady state).

- In *the far-field*, the correlation coefficients display similar behaviors for SAR and VAR. They both start with slightly lower values (but > 0.9) and improve to a maximum and then dropping off with increasing mass or volume, but more rapidly for SAR.

- For SAR, the correlation with ΔT reaches a maximum for a 3 g mass and then drops off rapidly for 4 g or greater mass.

- The correlation for VAR with ΔT is better for 5 cm^3 or larger volumes.

- At 64 MHz, the most favorable averaging volume to maximize VAR correlation is 4–5 cm^3. For larger volume, correlation for VAR and ΔT also drops off, but not as rapidly as for SAR.

9.8 Concluding Remarks

Knowledge of tissue electric and magnetic fields, induced current densities, and SARs is fundamental in studying the biological responses, health effects, and medical applications of EMFs. Complexities of biological tissues and of the incident fields make closed-form analytical solutions impractical, and computer methods are needed to predict the internal fields and their distributions. Great strides are being made in the area of numerical dosimetry using anatomically realistic models of the human body. Among the most valuable of the numerical methods for predicting EMFs and SAR calculations are the impedance method for use at lower frequencies, where quasi-static approximations may be made (<40 MHz for the human body), and the FEM and FDTD methods which may be used at any frequency of interest. For numerical calculations the FDTD method requires a computer memory and computation time that is proportional to N. This is a considerable advantage over the computing methods such as MoM. This chapter described the salient features of these methods and the many bioelectromagnetic exposure conditions for which they have been applied. Because of the limitations on the length of the chapter, only a few of the important recent applications of some of these methods were presented in some detail.

Note that computer-aided numerical methods have matured to a level that they are being increasingly used by researchers in many laboratories for dosimetric calculations for important and meaningful bioelectromagnetic problems. Some of the important developments in the past decade have helped to improve the efficiencies of the various computational codes by techniques such as use of the adaptive or expanding grid rather than the rigid regular grid, elimination of the relatively shielded interior regions of the modeled space at higher frequencies, and use of truncated models of the body at microwave frequencies where there is a lack of coupling between the various regions of the body. Because of accurate modeling of the tissue heterogeneities and shapes, the fine-resolution anatomically realistic models along with numerical computation algorithms have played an important role in emerging technologies with bioelectromagnetic concerns and applications, and will continue to do so in the future.

References

1. Lin, J. C. Computer methods for field intensity predictions. In *CRC Handbook of Biological Effects of Electromagnetic Fields*, C. Polk and E. Postow, eds. CRC Press, Boca Raton, FL, 1986, 273–313.
2. Lin, J. C. and Gandhi, O. P. Computer methods for predicting field intensity. In *Handbook of Biological Effects of Electromagnetic Fields*, C. Polk and E. Postow, eds. CRC Press, Boca Raton, FL, 1996, 337–402.
3. Lin, J. C. and Bernardi, P. Computer methods for predicting field intensity and temperature change in biological systems. In *Handbook of Biological Effects of Electromagnetic Fields, Bioengineering and Biophysical Aspects of Electromagnetic Fields*, F. Barnes and B. Greenebaum, eds. CRC Press, Boca Raton, FL, 2007, 293–380.
4. Lin, J. C. Mechanisms of field coupling into biological systems at ELF and RF frequencies. In *Advances in Electromagnetic Fields in Living Systems*, J. C. Lin, ed. Kluwer/Plenum, New York, vol. 3, 2000, 1–38.
5. Lin, J. C. Coupling of electromagnetic fields into biological systems. In *Electromagnetic Fields in Biological Systems*, J. C. Lin, ed. CRC Taylor/Francis, Boca Raton, FL, 2011, 1–57.
6. Lin, J. C., Bernardi, P., Pisa, S., Cavagnaro, M., and Piuzzi, E. Antennas for medical therapy and diagnostics. In *Modern Antenna Handbook*, C. Balanis, ed. Wiley, Hoboken, NJ, 2008, 1377–1428.
7. Lin, J. C., Bernardi, P., Pisa, S., Cavagnaro, M., and Piuzzi, E. Antennas for biological experiments. In *Modern Antenna Handbook*, C. Balanis, ed. Wiley, Hoboken, NJ, 2008, 1429–1460.
8. Schwan, H. P. and Piersol, G. M. Absorption of electromagnetic energy in body tissues. *American Journal of Physical Medicine & Rehabilitation*, 33, 371, 1954.
9. Schwan, H. P. and Li, K. Hazards due to total body irradiation by radar. *Proceedings of the IRE*, 44, 1572, 1956.
10. Schwan, H. P. and Li, K. The mechanism of absorption of ultrahigh frequency electromagnetic energy in tissue as related to the problem of tolerance dosage. *IRE Transactions on Medical Electronics*, 4, 45, 1956.
11. Johnson, C. C. and Guy, A. W. Nonionizing electromagnetic wave effects in biological materials and systems. *Proceedings of the IEEE*, 60, 692, 1972.
12. Michaelson, S. M. and Lin, J. C. *Biological Effects and Health Implications of Radiofrequency Radiation*. Plenum Press, New York, 1987.
13. Shapiro, A. R., Lutomirski, R. F., and Yura, H. T. Induced fields and heating within a cranial structure irradiated by an electromagnetic plane wave. *IEEE Transactions on Microwave Theory and Techniques*, 19, 187, 1971.
14. Kritikos, H. N. and Schwan, H. P. Hot spot generated in conduction spheres by EM waves and biological implications. *IEEE Transactions on Biomedical Engineering*, 19, 53, 1972.
15. Lin, J. C., Guy, A. W., and Kraft, G. H. Microwave selective brain heating. *Journal of Microwave Power*, 8, 275, 1973.
16. Ho. H. S. and Guy, A. W. Development of dosimetry for RF and microwave radiation. *Health Physics*, 29, 317, 1975.
17. Weil, C. M. Absorption characteristics of multi-layered sphere models exposed to UHF/microwave radiation. *IEEE Transactions on Biomedical Engineering*, 22, 468, 1975.
18. Joines, W. T. and Spiegel, R. J. Resonance absorption of microwaves by the human skull. *IEEE Transactions on Biomedical Engineering*, 21, 46, 1975.
19. Lin, J. C. Interaction of two cross-polarized electromagnetic waves with mammalian cranial structures. *IEEE Transactions on Biomedical Engineering*, 23, 371, 1976
20. Lin, J. C., Guy, A. W., and Johnson, C. C. Power deposition in a spherical model of man exposed to 1–20 MHz electromagnetic fields. *IEEE Transactions on Microwave Theory and Techniques*, 21, 791, 1973; See also corrections *IEEE MTT*, 23, 265, 1975.
21. Kritikos, H. N. and Schwan, H. P. The distribution of heating potential inside lossy spheres. *IEEE Transactions on Biomedical Engineering*, 22, 457, 1975.

22. Johnson, C. C., Durney, C. H., and Massoudi, H. Long-wavelength electromagnetic power absorption in prolate spheroidal models of man and animals. *IEEE Transactions on Microwave Theory and Techniques*, 23, 739, 1975.
23. Durney, C. H., Johnson, C. C., and Massaudi, A. Long wave-length analysis of plane wave irradiation f a prolate spheroidal model of man. *IEEE Transactions on Microwave Theory and Techniques*, 23, 246, 1975.
24. Massoudi, H., Durney, C. H., and Johnson, C. C. Long wavelength electromagnetic power absorption in ellipsoidal models of man and animals. *IEEE Transactions on Microwave Theory and Techniques*, 24, 41, 1977.
25. Guy, A. W., Webb, M. D., and Sorenson, C. C. Determination of power absorption in man exposed to HF electromagnetic fields by thermographic measurements on scale models. *IEEE Transactions on Biomedical Engineering*, 23, 361, 1976.
26. Liversy, D. E. and Chen, K. M. Electromagnetic fields induced inside arbitrary shaped biological bodies. *IEEE Transactions on Microwave Theory and Techniques*, 22, 1273, 1974.
27. Guru, B. S. and Chen, K. M. Experimental and theoretical studies in electromagnetic field induced inside finite biological bodies. *IEEE Transactions on Microwave Theory and Techniques*, 24, 433, 1976.
28. Chen, K. M. and Guru, B. S. Internal EM field and absorbed power density in human torsos induced by 1–500 MHz EM waves. *IEEE Transactions on Microwave Theory and Techniques*, 25, 746, 1977.
29. Hagman, M. J., Gandhi, O. P., and Durney, C. H. Numerical calculation of electromagnetic energy deposition for a realistic model of man. *IEEE Transactions on Microwave Theory and Techniques*, 27, 804, 1979
30. Gandhi, O. P. Electromagnetic absorption in inhomogeneous model of man for realistic exposure conditions. *Bioelectromagnetics*, 3, 81, 1982
31. Armitage, D. W., Leveen, H. H., and Pethig, R. Radio-frequency induced hyperthermia: Computer simulation of specific absorption rate distributions using realistic anatomical models. *Physics in Medicine and Biology*, 28, 31, 1983.
32. Gandhi, O. P., DeFord, J. F., and Kanai, H. Impedance method for calculation of power deposition patterns in magnetically induced hyperthermia. *IEEE Transactions on Biomedical Engineering*, 31, 644, 1984.
33. Gandhi, O. P. and DeFord, J. F. Calculation of EM power deposition for operator exposure to RF induction heaters. *IEEE Transactions on Electromagnetic Compatibility*, 30, 63, 1988.
34. Orcutt, N. and Gandhi, O. P. A 3-D impedance method to calculate power deposition in biological bodies subjected to time-varying magnetic fields. *IEEE Transactions on Biomedical Engineering*, 35, 577, 1988.
35. Orcutt, N. and Gandhi, O. P. Use of the impedance method to calculate 3-D power deposition patterns for hyperthermia with capacitive plate electrodes. *IEEE Transactions on Biomedical Engineering*, 37, 36, 1990
36. Epstein, B. R. and Foster, K. R. Anisotropy in dielectric properties of skeletal muscle. *Medical and Biological Engineering and Computing*, 21, 51, 1983.
37. Zheng, E., Shao, S., and Webster, J. G. Impedance of skeletal muscle from 1 Hz to 1 MHz. *IEEE Transactions on Biomedical Engineering*, 31, 477, 1984.
38. Zhu, X. L. and Gandhi, O. P. Design of RF needle applicators for optimum SAR distributions in irregularly-shaped tumors. *IEEE Transactions on Biomedical Engineering*, 35, 382, 1988.
39. Gandhi, O. P. and Chen, J. Y. Numerical dosimetry at power-line frequencies using anatomically based models. *Bioelectromagnetics*, Supplement 1, 43, 1992.
40. Tofani, S., Ossola, P., d'Amore, G., and Gandhi, O. P. Electric fields and current density distributions induced in an anatomically based model of the human head by magnetic fields from a hair dryer. *Health Physics*, 68, 71, 1995.
41. Harrington, R. F. *Field Computation by Moment Methods*. McGraw-Hill, New York, 1968.
42. Schelkunoff, S. A. Field equivalence theorems. *Communications on Pure and Applied Mathematics*, 4, 43, 1951.

Computational Methods and EM Fields

43. Lin, J. C. and Wu, C. L. Scattering of microwaves by dielectric materials used in laboratory animal restrainers. *IEEE Transactions on Microwave Theory and Techniques*, 24, 219, 1976.

44. Gandhi, O. P., Hagman, M. J., and D'Andrea, J. A. Part-body and multi-body effects on absorption of radio frequency electromagnetic energy by animals and by models of man. *Radio Science*, 14, 155, 1979.

45. Karimullah, K., Chen, K. M., and Nyquist, D. P. Electromagnetic coupling between a thin-wire antenna and a neighboring biological body. *IEEE Transactions on Microwave Theory and Techniques*, 28, 1218, 1980.

46. Chatterjee, I., Hagman, M. J., and Gandhi, O. P. Electromagnetic energy deposition in an inhomogeneous block model for near-field irradiation conditions. *IEEE Transactions on Microwave Theory and Techniques*, 28, 1452, 1980.

47. Wu, T. K. and Tsai, L. L. Electromagnetic fields induced inside arbitrary cylinders of biological tissue. *IEEE Transactions on Microwave Theory and Techniques*, 25, 61, 1977.

48. Wu, T. K. and Tsai, L. L. Scattering from arbitrary-shaped lossy dielectric bodies of revolution. *Radio Sci*, 12, 709. 1977.

49. Poggio, A. J. and Miller, E. K. Integral equation solutions of three-dimensional scatteriny problems. In *Computer Techniques for Electromagnetics*, Mittra, R., ed. Pergamon Press, Elmsford, NY, 1973, 159.

50. Massoudi, H., Durney, C. H., Barber, P. W., and Iskander, M. F. Post resonance EM absorption by man and animals. *Bioelectromagnetics*, 3, 333, 1982.

51. Wu, T. K. Electromagnetic fields and power deposition in body of revolution models of man. *IEEE Transactions on Microwave Theory and Techniques*, 27, 279, 1979.

52. Mautz, J. R. and Harrington, R. F. Radiation and scattering from bodies of revolution. *Applied Scientific Research*, 20, 405, 1969.

53. Harrington, R. F. and Mautz, J. R. Green's functions for surfaces of revolution. *Radio Science*, 7, 603, 1972.

54. Jin, J. *The Finite Element Method in Electromagnetics*. Wiley, New York, 1993.

55. Boyes, W. E., Lynch, D. R., Paulsen, K. D., and Minerbo, G. N. Nodal-based finite element modelling of Maxwell's equations in three dimensions. *IEEE Transactions on Antennas and Propagation*, 40, 642, 1992.

56. Paulsen, K. D., Jia, X., and Sullivan, J. M., jr. Finite element computations of specific absorption rates in anatomically conforming full-body models for hyperthermia treatment analysis. *IEEE Transactions on Biomedical Engineering*, 40, 933, 1993.

57. Yee, K. S. Numerical solutions of initial boundary value problems involving Maxwell's equations in isotropic media. *IEEE Transactions on Antennas and Propagation*, 14, 303, 1966.

58. Taflove, A. and Brodwin, M. E. Computation of the electromagnetic fields and induced temperatures within a model of the microwave-irradiated human eye. *IEEE Transactions on Microwave Theory and Techniques*, 23, 888, 1975.

59. Taflove, A. and Brodwin, M. E. Numerical solution of steady-state EM scattering problems using the time dependent Maxwell's equation. *IEEE Transactions on Microwave Theory and Techniques*, 23, 623, 1975.

60. Taflove, A. Application of the finite-difference time domain method to sinusoidal steady-state electromagnetic-penetration problems. *IEEE Transactions on EM Compatibility*, 22, 191, 1980.

61. Holland, R. THREDE: A free field EMP coupling and scattering code. *IEEE Transactions on Nuclear Science*, 24, 2416, 1977.

62. Kunz, K. S. and Lee, K. M. A three-dimensional finite-difference solution of the external response of an aircraft to a complex transient EM environment: Part 1- The method and its implementation. *IEEE Transactions on Electromagnetic Compatibility*, 20, 328, 1978.

63. Kunz, K. S. and Luebbers, R. J. *The Finite-Difference Time-Domain Method for Electromagnetics*. CRC Press, Inc., Boca Raton, FL, 1993.

64. Taflove, A. *Computational Electrodynamics the Finite-Difference Time-Domain Method*. Artech House, London, 1995.

65. Taflove, A. and Hagness, S. C., eds. *Computational Electrodynamics: The Finite-Difference Time-Domain Method*. Artech House, London, 2000.
66. Spiegel, R. J., Fatmi, M. B. A., Stuchly, S. S., and Stuchly, M. A. Comparison of finite-difference time-domain SAR calculations with measurements. In a heterogeneous model of man. *IEEE Transactions on Biomedical Engineering*, 36, 849, 1989.
67. Chen, J. Y. and Gandhi, O. P. Currents induced in an anatomically based model of a human for exposure to vertically polarized electromagnetic pulses. *IEEE Transactions on Microwave Theory and Techniques*, 39, 31, 1991
68. Sullivan, D. M., Borup, D. T. and Gandhi, O. P. Use of the finite-difference time-domain method in calculating EM absorption in human tissues. *IEEE Transactions on Biomedical Engineering*, 34, 148, 1987.
69. Chen, J. Y. and Gandhi, O. P. Numerical simulation of annular-phased arrays of dipoles for hyperthermia of deep-seated tumors. *IEEE Transactions on Biomedical Engineering*, 39, 209, 1992.
70. Chen, J. Y., Gandhi, O. P., and Conover, D. L. SAR and induced current distributions for operator exposure to RF dielectric sealers. *IEEE Transactions on Electromagnetic Compatibility*, 33, 252, 1991.
71. Luebbers, R., Hunsberger, F. P., Kunz, K. S., Standler, R. B., and Schneider, M. A frequency-dependent finite-difference time-domain formulation for dispersive materials. *IEEE Transactions on Electromagnetic Compatibility*, 32, 222, 1990.
72. Bui, M. D., Stuchly, S. S., and Costache, G. I. Propagation of transients in dispersive dielectric media. *IEEE Transactions on Microwave Theory and Techniques*, 39, 1165, 1991.
73. Sullivan, D. M. A frequency-dependent FDTD method for biological applications. *IEEE Transactions on Microwave Theory and Techniques*, 40, 532, 1992.
74. Luebbers, R. J., Hunsberger, F., and Kunz, K. S. FDTD for Nth order dispersive media. *IEEE Transactions on Antennas and Propagation*, 40, 1297, 1992.
75. Joseph, R. M., Hagness, S. C., and Taflove, A. Direct time integration of Maxwell's equations in linear dispersive media with absorption for scattering and propagation of femtosecond electromagnetic impulses. *Optics Letters*, 16, 1412, 1991.
76. Gandhi, O. P., Gao, B. Q., and Chen, J. Y. A frequency-dependent finite-difference time-domain formulation for induced current calculations in human beings. *Bioelectromagnetics*, 13, 543, 1992.
77. Gandhi, O. P., Gao, B. Q., and Chen, J. Y. A frequency-dependent finite-difference time-domain formulation for general dispersive media. *IEEE Transactions on Microwave Theory and Techniques*, 41, 658, 1993.
78. Furse, C. M., Chen, J. Y., and Gandhi, O. P. A frequency-dependent finite-difference time-domain method for induced current and SAR calculations for a heterogeneous model of the human body. *IEEE Transactions on Electromagnetic Compatibility*, 36, 128, 1994.
79. Gandhi, O. P. and Chen, J. Y. Electromagnetic absorption in the human head for a proposed 6 GHz mobile communication system. *IEEE Transactions on Electromagnetic Compatibility*, 37, 547, 1995.
80. Gandhi, O. P. Some numerical methods for dosimetry: ELF to microwave frequencies. *Radio Science*, 30, 161–177, 1995.
81. Ackerman, M. J. The visible human project. *Proceedings of the IEEE*, 86, 504, 1998.
82. Mason, P. A., Ziriax, J. M., Hurt, W. D., Walters, T. J., Ryan, K. L., Nelson, D. A., Smith, K. I., and D'Andrea, J. A. Recent advancements in dosimetry measurements and modeling. In *Radio Frequency Radiation Dosimetry*, Klauenberg, B. J. and Miklavcic, D., eds. Springer Science+Business Media: Berlin and London, 2000, 141.
83. Available: ftp://starview.brooks.af.mil/EMF/dosimetry_models/.
84. Piuzzi, E., Bernardi, P., Cavagnaro, M., Pisa, S., and Lin, J. C. Analysis of adult and child exposure to uniform plane waves at mobile communication systems frequencies (900 MHz–3 GHz). *IEEE Transactions on Electromagnetics Compatibility*, 53, 38–47, 2011.
85. Centers for Disease Control and Prevention (CDC) Growth Charts. Available: http://www.cdc.gov/growthcharts/.

Computational Methods and EM Fields

86. Leslie, G. and Farkas, M. D. *Anthropometry of the Head and Face*. Elsevier, New York, 1981.

87. Dimbylow, P. Development of the female voxel phantom, Naomi, and its application to calculations of induced current densities and electric fields from applied low frequency magnetic and electric fields. *Physics in Medicine and Biology*, 50, 1047, 2005.

88. Findlay, R. P. and Dimbylow, P. J. FDTD calculations of specific energy absorption rate in a seated voxel model of the human body from 10 MHz to 3 GHz. *Physics in Medicine and Biology*, 51, 2339, 2006.

89. Nagaoka, T., Watanabe, S., Sakurai, K., Kunieda, E. and WatJournal, T. Development of realistic high-resolution whole-body voxel models of Japanese adult male and female of average height and weight and application of models to radio-frequency electromagnetic-field dosimetry. *Physics in Medicine and Biology*, 49, 1–15, 2004.

90. Nagaoka, T. and Watanabe, S. Voxel-based variable posture models of human anatomy. *Proceedings of IEEE*, 97, 2015, 2009.

91. Christ, A., Kainz, W., Hahn, E. G., Honegger, K., Zefferer, M., Neufeld, E., Rascher, W., Janka, R., Bautz, W., Chen, J., Kiefer, B., Schmitt, P., Hollenbach, H-P., Shen, J., Oberle, M., Szczerba, D., Kam, A., Guag, J. W., and Kuster, N. The Virtual Family—development of surface-based anatomical models of two adults and two children for dosimetric simulations. *Physics in Medicine and Biology*, 55, 23, 2010.

92. Li, C., Chen, Z., Yang, L., Lv, B., Liu, J., Varsier, N., Hadjem, A., Wiart, J., Xie, Y., Ma, L., and Wu, T. Generation of infant anatomical models for evaluating the electromagnetic fields exposure. *Bioelectromagnetics*, 36, 10, 2015.

93. Wu, T., Tan, L., Shao, Q., Zhang, C., Zhao, C., Li, Y., Conil, E., Hadjem, A., Wiart, J., Lu, L., Wang, N., Xie, Y., and Zhang, S. Chinese adult anatomical models and the application in evaluation of wideband RF EMF exposure. *Physics in Medicine and Biology*, 56, 2075, 2011.

94. Li, C. and Wu, T. Dosimetry of infant exposure to power-frequency magnetic fields: Variation of 99th percentile induced electric field value by posture and skin-to-skin contact. *Bioelectromagnetics*, 36, 204, 2015.

95. Rush, S., Abildskov, J. A., and McFee, R. Resistivity of body tissues at low frequencies. *Circulation Research*, 12, 40, 1963.

96. Florig, H. K., Hoburg, J. F., and Morgan, M. G. Electric-field exposure from electric blankets. *IEEE Transactions on Power Delivery*, 2, 527, 1987.

97. Hayashi, N., Isaka, K., and Yokoi, Y. Analysis of magnetic-field profiles in electric blanket users. *IEEE Transactions on Power Delivery*, 4, 1897, 1989.

98. Kaune, W. T. and Gillis, M. F. General properties of the interaction between animals and ELF electric fields. *Bioelectromagnetics*, 2, 1, 1981.

99. Guy, A. W., Davidow, S. Yang, G. Y., and Chou, C. K. Determination of electric current distributions in animals and humans exposed to a uniform 60-Hz high-intensity electric field. *Bioelectromagnetics*, 3, 47, 1982.

100. Stratton, J. A. *Electromagnetic Theory*. McGraw-Hill, New York, 1941.

101. Deno, D. W. Currents induced in the human body by high voltage transmission line electric field—Measurement and calculation of distribution and dose. *IEEE Transactions on Power Apparatus and Systems*, 96, 1517, 1977.

102. DiPlacido, J., Shih, C. H., and Ware, B. J. Analysis of the proximity effects in electric field measurements. *IEEE Transactions on Power Apparatus and Systems*, 97, 2167, 1978.

103. Rukspollmuang, S. and Chen, K. M. Heating of spherical vs. realistic models of human and infrahuman heads by electromagnetic waves. *Radio Science*, 14, 51, 1979.

104. Hagman, M. J., Gandhi, O. P., D'Andrea, J. A., and Chatterjee, I. Head resonance: Numerical solutions and experimental results. *IEEE Transactions on Microwave Theory and Techniques*, 27, 809, 1979.

105. Gandhi, O. P., Hunt, E. L., and D'Andrea, J. A. Deposition of EM energy in animals and in models of man with and without grounding and reflector effects. *Radio Science*, 12, 39S, 1977.

106. Deford, J. F., Gandhi, O. P., and Hagman, M. J. Momem-Method solutions and SAR calculations for in homogeneous models of man with large number of cells. *IEEE Transactions on Microwave Theory and Techniques*, 31, 848, 1983.

107. Sullivan, D. M., Gandhi Om, P., and Taflove, A. Use of the finite-difference time-domain method for calculating EM absorption in man models. *IEEE Transactions on Biomedical Engineering*, 35, 179, 1988.

108. Bernardi, P., Cavagnaro, M., Pisa, S., and Piuzzi, E. Specific absorption rate and temperature elevation in a subject exposed in the far-field of radio-frequency sources Operating in the 10–900-MHz range. *IEEE Transactions on Biomedical Engineering*, 50, 295, 2003.

109. Dimbylow P. J. FDTD calculations of the whole-body averaged SAR in an anatomically realistic voxel model of the human body from 1 MHz to 1 GHz. *Physics in Medicine and Biology*, 42, 479, 1997.

110. ICNIRP. Guidelines for limiting exposure to time-varying electric, magnetic, and electromagnetic fields (up to 300 GHz). *Health Physics*, 74, 494, 1998.

111. Dimbylow, P. J. Fine resolution calculations of SAR in the human body for frequencies up to 3 GHz. *Physics in Medicine and Biology*, 47, 2835, 2002.

112. Mason, A. P., Hurt, W. D., Walters, T. J., D'Andrea, J. A., Gajšek, P., Ryan, K. L., Nelson, D. A., Smith, K. I., and Ziriax, J. M. Effects of frequency, permittivity, and voxel size on predicted specific absorption rate values in biological tissue during electromagnetic-field exposure. *IEEE Transactions on Microwave Theory and Techniques*, 48, 2050, 2000.

113. Mazzurana, M., Sandrini, L., Vaccari, A., Malacarne, C., Cristoforetti, L., and Pontalti, R. A semi-automatic method for developing an anthropomorphic numerical model of dielectric anatomy by MRI. *Physics in Medicine and Biology*, 48, 2003.

114. Gajšek, P., Hurt, W. D., Ziriax, J. M., and Mason, A. P. Parametric dependence of SAR on permittivity values in a man model. *IEEE Transactions on Biomedical Engineering*, 48, 1169, 2001.

115. Tinniswood, A. D., Furse, C. M., and Gandhi Om, P. Power deposition in the head and neck of an anatomically based human body model for plane wave exposures. *Physics in Medicine and Biology*, 43, 2361, 1998.

116. Sandrini, L., Vaccari, A., Malacarne, C., Cristoforetti, L., and Pontalti, R. RF dosimetry: a comparison between power absorption of female and male numerical models from 0.1 to 4 GHz. *Physics in Medicine and Biology*, 49, 5185, 2004.

117. Gabriel S., Lau R. W., and Gabriel C. The dielectric properties of biological tissues: III. Parametric models for the dielectric spectrum of tissues. *Physics in Medicine and Biology*, 41, 2271, 1996.

118. Gabriel, C. Compilation of the dielectric properties of body tissues at RF and microwave frequencies. Brooks Air Force, Brooks AFB, TX, Tech. Rep. AL/OE-TR-1996-0037, 1996.

119. Faraone, A., Tay, R. Y.-S., Joyner, K. H., and Balzano, Q. Estimation of the average power density in the vicinity of cellular base-station collinear array antennas. *IEEE Transactions on Vehicular Technology*, 49, 984, 2000.

120. Cicchetti, R. and Faraone, A. Estimation of the peak power density in the vicinity of cellular and radio base station antennas. *IEEE Transactions on Electromagnetic Compatibility*, 46, 275, 2004.

121. Bizzi, M. and Gianola, P. Electromagnetic fields radiated by GSM antennas. *Electronics Letters*, 35, 855, 1999.

122. Altman, Z., Begasse, B., Dale, C., Karwowski, A., Wiart, J., Wong, M. F., and Gattoufi, L. Efficient models for base station antennas for human exposure assessment. *IEEE Transactions on Electromagnetic Compatibility*, 44, 588, 2002.

123. Bernardi, P., Cavagnaro, M., Cristoforetti, L., Malacarne, C., Pisa, S., Piuzzi, E., Pontalti, R., and Vaccari, A. Modelling of BTS antennas: Dependence of the accuracy on FDTD mesh size and implementation criteria. In *Proc. 2nd Int. Workshop on Biological Effects of Electromagnetic Fields, Rhodes, Greece*, Kostarakis, P., ed., 2002, 74.

124. Blanch, S., Romeu, J., and Cardama, A. Near field in the vicinity of wireless base-station antennas: An exposure compliance approach. *IEEE Transactions on Antennas and Propagation*, 50, 685, 2002.

125. Adane, Y., Gati, A., Wong, M.-F., Dale, C., Wiart, J., and Hanna V. F. Optimal modeling of real radio base station antennas for human exposure assessment using spherical-mode decomposition. *IEEE Antennas and Wireless Propagation Letters*, 1, 215, 2002.

Computational Methods and EM Fields

126. Fridén, J. RF exposure compliance boundary analysis of base station antennas using combined spherical–cylindrical near-field transformations. *Electronics Letters*, 39, 1783, 2003.

127. Nicolas, E., Lautru, D., Jacquin, F., Wong, M. F., and Wiart, J. Specific absorption rate assessments based on a selective isotropic measuring system for electromagnetic fields. *IEEE Transactions on Instrumentation and Measurement*, 50, 397, 2001.

128. Lazzi, G. and Gandhi, O. P. A mixed FDTD-integral equation approach for on-site safety assessment in complex electromagnetic environments. *IEEE Transactions on Antennas and Propagation*, 48, 1830, 2000.

129. Gandhi, O. P. and Lam M. S. An on-site dosimetry system for safety assessment of wireless base stations using spatial harmonic components. *IEEE Transactions on Antennas and Propagation*, 51, 840, 2003.

130. Cooper, J., Marx, B., Buhl, J., and Hombach, V. Determination of safety distance limits for a human near a cellular base station antenna, adopting the IEEE standard or ICNIRP guidelines. *Bioelectromagnetics*, 23, 429, 2002.

131. Catarinucci, L., Palazzari, P., and Tarricone, L. Human exposure to the near field of radiobase antennas—A full-wave solution using parallel FDTD. *IEEE Transactions on Microwave Theory and Techniques*, 51, 935, 2003.

132. Bernardi, P., Cavagnaro, M., Pisa, S., and Piuzzi, E. Human exposure in the vicinity of radio base station antennas. In *Proc. EMC Europe 2000 (4th European Symp. Electromagn. Compat.), Brugge, Belgium*, 2000, 187.

133. Meyer, F. J. C., Davidson, D. B., Jakobus, U., and Stuchly M. A. Human exposure assessment in the near field of GSM base-station antennas using a hybrid finite element/method of moments technique. *IEEE Transactions on Biomedical Engineering*, 50, 224, 2003.

134. Bernardi, P., Cavagnaro, M., Pisa, S., and Piuzzi, E. Human exposure to cellular base station antennas in urban environment. *IEEE Transactions on Microwave Theory and Techniques*, 48, 1996, 2000.

135. Martinez-Burdalo M., Nonidez, L., Martin, A., and Villar R. Near-field time-domain physical-optics and FDTD method for safety assessment near a base-station antenna. *Microwave and Optical Technology Letters*, 39, 393, 2003.

136. Bernardi, P., Cavagnaro, M., Cicchetti, R., Pisa, S., Piuzzi, E., and Testa, O. A UTD/FDTD investigation on procedures to assess compliance of cellular base-station antennas with human-exposure limits in a realistic urban environment. *IEEE Transactions on Microwave Theory and Techniques*, 51, 2409, 2003.

137. Lin, J. C. and Bernardi, P. Computer methods for predicting field intensity and temperature change in biological systems. In *Handbook of Biological Effects of Electromagnetic Fields, Bioengineering and Biophysical Aspects of Electromagnetic Fields*, F. Barnes and B. Greenebaum, eds. CRC Press, Boca Raton, FL, 2007, 339–340.

138. Di Benedetto, M. G., Kaiser, T., Molisch, A. F., Oppermann, I., Politano, C., and Porcino, D. *2006 UWB Communication Systems: A Comprehensive Overview*. Hindawi, New York.

139. Lin, J. C. Coupling of electromagnetic fields into biological systems. In *Electromagnetic Fields in Biological Systems*, J. C. Lin, ed. CRC Press/Taylor & Francis Group, Boca Raton, FL, 2012, 40–59.

140. Yang, L. Q. and Giannakis G. B. Ultra-wideband communications. *IEEE Signal Processing Magazine*, 21, 26, 2004.

141. Qiu, R. C., Liu, H. P., and Shen, X. M. Ultra-wideband for multiple access communications. *IEEE Communications Magazine*, 43, 80, 2005.

142. Lin, J. C. Microwave thermoelastic tomography and imaging. In *Advances in Electromagnetic Fields in Living Systems*. Springer, New York, 2005, vol. 4, 41–76.

143. Lin, J. C. Interaction of electromagnetic transient radiation with biological materials. *IEEE Transactions on Electromagnetic Compatibility*, 17, 93, 1975.

144. Lin, J. C., Wu, C. L., and Lam, C. K. Transmission of electromagnetic pulse into the head. *Proceedings of the IEEE*, 63, 1726, 1975.

145. Lin, J. C. Electromagnetic pulse interaction with mammalian cranial structures. *IEEE Transactions on Biomedical Engineering*, 23, 61, 1976.

146. Lin, J. C. and Lam, C. K. Coupling of Gaussian electromagnetic pulse into muscle-bone model of biological structure. *Journal of Microwave Power*, 11, 67, 1976.
147. Lin, J. C. *Microwave Auditory Effects and Applications*. Charles C. Thomas, Springfield, IL, 1978.
148. Lin, J. C. Microwave induced hearing sensation: some preliminary theoretical observations. *Journal of Microwave Power*, 11, 295, 1976.
149. Lin, J. C. On microwave-induced hearing sensation. *IEEE Transactions on Microwave Theory Techniques*, 25, 605, 1977.
150. Lin, J. C. Further studies on the microwave auditory effects. *IEEE Transactions on Microwave Theory Techniques*, 25, 936, 1977.
151. Lin, J. C. Calculations of frequencies and threshold of microwave-induced auditory signals. *Radio Science*, 12/SS-1, 237, 1977.
152. Lin, J. C. The microwave auditory phenomenon. *Proceedings of IEEE*, 68, 67, 1980.
153. Watanabe, Y., Tanaka, T., Taki, M., and Watanabe, S. FDTD analysis of microwave hearing effect. *IEEE MTT*, 48, 2126, 2000.
154. Lin, J. C. and Wang, Z. W. Hearing of microwave pulses by humans and animals: Effects, mechanism, and thresholds. *Health Physics*, 92, 621, 2007.
155. Lin, J. C. and Wang, Z. W. Acoustic pressure waves induced in human heads by RF pulses from high-field MRI scanners. *Health Physics*, 98, 603, 2010.
156. Yitzhak, N. M., Ruppin, R., and Hareuveny, R. Numerical simulation of pressure waves in the cochlea induced by a microwave pulse. *Bioelectromagnetics*, 35, 491, 2014.
157. Gandhi, O. P., Gu, Y. G., Chen, J. Y., and Bassen, H. I. Specific absorption rates and induced current distributions in an anatomically based human model for plane-wave exposures. *Health Physics*, 63, 281, 1992.
158. Evaluating compliance with FCC guidelines for human exposure to radiofrequency electromagnetic fields. FCC, Washington, DC, OET Bulletin 65, August 1997.
159. Human exposure to radio frequency fields from hand-held and body-mounted wireless communication devices—Human models, instrumentation, and procedures—Part 1: Procedure to determine the specific absorption rate (SAR) for hand-held devices used in close proximity to the ear (frequency range of 300 MHz to 3 GHz), IEC Standard, 62209–1, 2005.
160. Toftgard, J., Hornsleth, S. N., and Andersen, J. B. Effects on portable antennas of the presence of a person. *IEEE Transactions on Antennas and Propagation*, 41, 739, 1993.
161. Dimbylow, P. J. and Mann, S. M. SAR calculations in an anatomically realistic model of the head for mobile communication transceivers at 900 MHz and 1.8 GHz. *Physics in Medicine and Biology*, 39, 1537, 1994.
162. Gandhi, O. P., Lazzi, G., and Furse, C. M. Electromagnetic absorption in the human head and neck for mobile telephones at 835 and 1900 MHz. *IEEE Transactions on Microwave Theory and Techniques*, 44, 1884, 1996.
163. Okoniewski, M., and Stuchly, M. A. A study of the handset antenna and human body interaction. *IEEE Transactions on Microwave Theory and Techniques*, 44, 1855, 1996.
164. Hombach, V., Meier, K., Burkhardt, M., Kuhn, E., and Kuster, N. The dependence of EM energy absorption upon human head modeling at 900 MHz. *IEEE Transactions on Microwave Theory and Techniques*, 44, 1865, 1996.
165. Watanabe, S., Taki, M., Nojima, T., and Fujiwara, O. Characteristics of the SAR distributions in a head exposed to electromagnetic fields radiated by a hand-held portable radio. *IEEE Transactions on Microwave Theory and Techniques*, 44, 1874, 1996.
166. Bernardi, P., Cavagnaro, M., and Pisa, S. Evaluation of the SAR distribution in the human head for cellular phones used in a partially closed environment. *IEEE Transactions on Electromagnetic Compatibility*, 38, 357, 1996.
167. Colburn, J. S., and Rahmat-Samii, Y. Human proximity effects on circular polarized handset antennas in personal satellite communications. *IEEE Transactions on Antennas and Propagation*, 46, 813, 1998.
168. Lazzi, G., and Gandhi, O. P. On modeling and personal dosimetry of cellular telephone helical antennas with the FDTD code. *IEEE Transactions on Antennas and Propagation*, 46, 525, 1998.

169. Mangoud, M. A., Abd-Alhameed, R. A., and Excell, P. S. Simulation of human interaction with mobile telephones using hybrid techniques over coupled domains. *IEEE Transactions on Microwave Theory and Techniques*, 48, 2014, 2000.
170. Cerri, G., Russo, P., Schiavoni, A., Tribellini, G., and Bielli, P. A new MoM-FDTD hybrid technique for the analysis of scattering problems. *Electronics Letters*, 34, 438, 1998.
171. Bernardi, P., Cavagnaro, M., Pisa, S., and Piuzzi, E. A graded-mesh FDTD code for the study of human exposure to cellular phones equipped with helical antennas. *The Applied Computational Electromagnetics Society Journal*, 16, 90, 2001.
172. Bernardi, P., Cavagnaro, M., Pisa, S., and Piuzzi, E. Power absorption and temperature elevations induced in the human head by a dual-band monopole-helix antenna phone. *IEEE Transactions on Microwave Theory and Techniques*, 49, 2539, 2001.
173. Jensen, M. A. and Rahmat-Samii, Y. EM interaction of handset antennas and a human in personal communications. *Proceedings of IEEE*, 83, 7, 1995.
174. Rowley, J. T. and Waterhouse, R. B. Performance of shorted patch antennas for mobile communication handsets at 1800 MHz. *IEEE Transactions on Microwave Theory and Techniques*, 47, 815, 1999.
175. Bernardi, P., Cavagnaro, M., Pisa, S., and Piuzzi, E., Specific Absorption rate and temperature increases in the head of a cellular-phone user. *IEEE Transactions on Microwave Theory and Techniques*, 48, 1118, 2000.
176. de Salles, A. A., Fernandez, C. R., and Bonadiman, M. FDTD simulations and measurements on planar antennas for mobile phones. *Proceedings of the SBMO/IEEE MTT-S IMOC*, 1043, 2003.
177. Tinniswood, A. D. Furse, C. M., and Gandhi, O. P. Computations of SAR distributions for two anatomically based models of the human head using CAD files of commercial telephones and the parallelized FDTD code. *IEEE Transactions on Antennas and Propagation*, 46, 829, 1998.
178. Schiavoni, A., Bertotto, P., Richiardi, G., and Bielli, P. SAR generated by commercial cellular phones —Phone modeling, head modeling, and measurements. *IEEE Transactions on Microwave Theory and Techniques*, 48, 2064, 2000.
179. Chavannes, N., Tay, R., Nikoloski, N., and Kuster, N. Suitability of FDTD-based TCAD tools for RF design of mobile phones. *IEEE Antennas and Propagation Magazine*, 45, 52, 2003.
180. Pisa, S., Cavagnaro, M., Lopresto, V., Piuzzi, E., Lovisolo, G. A., and Bernardi, P. A procedure to develop realistic numerical models of cellular phones for an accurate evaluation of SAR distribution in the human head. *IEEE Transactions on Microwave Theory and Techniques*, 53, 2005.
181. Lin, J. C. Cellular mobile telephones and children. *IEEE Antennas and Propagation Magazine*, 44, 142, 2002.
182. Peyman, A., Rezazadeh, A. A., and Gabriel, C. Changes in the dielectric properties of rat tissue as a function of age at microwave frequencies. *Physics in Medicine and Biology*, 46, 1617, 2001.
183. Gandhi, O. M., and Kang, G. Some present problems and a proposed experimental phantom for SAR compliance testing of cellular telephone at 835 and 1900 MHz. *Physics in Medicine and Biology*, 47, 1501, 2002.
184. Schoenborn, F., Burkhardt, M., and Kuster, N., Differences in energy absorption between heads of adults and children in the near field of sources. *Health Physics*, 74, 160, 1998.
185. Guy, A. W., Chou, C. K., and Bit-Babik, G. FDTD derived SAR distributions in various size human head models exposed to simulated cellular telephone handset transmitting 600 mW at 835 MHz. In *24th Bioelectromagnetics Soc. Annu. Meeting*, Quebec, 7, 2002.
186. Wang, J., and Fujiwara, O. Comparison and evaluation of electromagnetic absorption characteristic in realistic human head models of adult and children for 900-MHz mobile telephones. *IEEE Transactions on Microwave Theory and Techniques*, 51, 966, 2003.
187. Hadjem, A., Lautru, D., Dale, C., Wong, M. F., Hanna, V. H., and Wiart, J. Study of specific absorption rate (SAR) induced in two child head models and in adult heads using mobile phones. *IEEE Transactions on Microwave Theory and Techniques*, 53, 4, 2005.
188. Dominguez, H., Raizer, A., and Carpes, Jr., W. P. Electromagnetic fields radiated by cellular phone in close proximity to metallic walls. *IEEE Transactions on Magnetics*, 38, 793, 2002.

189. International Electrotechnical Commission (IEC). International standard, medical electrical equipment Part 2–33: Particular requirements for the basic safety and essential performance of magnetic resonance equipment for medical diagnosis. Geneva: IEC60601-2-33, edition 3.0, 2010.
190. Center for Devices and Radiologic Health (CDRH). Guidance for the submission of pre-market notifications for magnetic resonance diagnostic devices. Rockville: Food and Drug Administration, 1988. http:// www.fda.gov/cdrh/ode/guidance/793.html.
191. Lin, J. C. International guidelines for radio-frequency exposure, especially for the most successful application of electromagnetics in medicine: Magnetic resonance imaging. *IEEE Antennas and Propagation Magazine*, 53-1, 69, 2011.
192. National Electrical Manufacturers Association (NEMA). Characterization of SAR for MRI Systems. Rosslyn, Virginia, USA NEMA Standard MS-8-1993.
193. Collins, C. M. and Smith. M. B. Spatial resolution of numerical models of man and calculated specific absorption rate using the FDTD method: A study at 64 MHz in a magnetic resonance imaging coil. *Journal of Magnetic Resonance Imaging*, 18, 383, 2003.
194. Collin, C. M., Liu, W. Z., Wang, J. H., Gruetter, W., Vaughan, J. T., Ugurbil, K., and Smith. M. B. Temperature and SAR calculations for a human head within volume and surface coils at 64 and 300 MHz. *Journal of Magnetic Resonance Imaging*, 19(5), 650, 2004.
195. Wang, Z. W., Lin, J. C., Mao, W. H., Liu, W., Smith, M. B., and Collins, C. M. SAR and temperature: Calculations and Comparison to Regulatory Limits for MRI. *Journal of Magnetic Resonance Imaging*, 26(2), 437, 2007.
196. Ibrahim, T. S. and Tang, L. Insight into RF power requirements and B_1 field homogeneity for human MRI via rigorous FDTD approach. *Journal of Magnetic Resonance Imaging*, 25(6), 1235, 2007.
197. Wang, Z. W., Lin, J. C., Vaughan, J. T., and Collins, C. M. On Consideration of physiological response in numerical models of temperature during MRI of the human head. *Journal of Magnetic Resonance Imaging*, 28(5), 1303, 2008.
198. Collins, C. M. and Wang, Z. W. Calculation of radiofrequency electromagnetic fields and their effects in MRI of human subjects. *Magnetic Resonance in Medicine*, 65(5), 1470, 2011.
199. Yeo, D. T. B., Wang, Z. W., Loew, W., Vogel, M. W. and Hancu, I. Local specific absorption rate in high-pass birdcage and transverse electromagnetic body coils for multiple human body models in clinical landmark positions at 3T. *Journal of Magnetic Resonance Imaging*, 33(5), 1209, 2011.
200. Wang, Z. W., Penney, C. W., Luebbers, R. J., and Collins, C. M. Poseable male and female numerical body models for field calculations in MRI. In *Proc 16th Annual Meeting ISMRM*, Toronto, Canada, 75, 2008.
201. Gabriel, C. Dielectric properties of biological tissue: Variation with age. *Bioelectromagnetics*, 26(S7), S12, 2005.
202. Gabriel, S., Gabriel, C., and Lau, R. W. The dielectric properties of biological tissues: III. Parametric models for the dielectric spectrum of tissues. *Physics in Medicine and Biology*, 41(11), 2271, 1996.
203. Liu, W., Collins, C. M., and Smith, M. B. "alculations of B1 distribution, specific energy absorption rate, and intrinsic signal-to-noise ratio for a body-size birdcage coil loaded with human subjects at 64 and 128 MHz. *Applied Magnetic Resonance*, 29(1), 5, 2005.
204. Wang, Z. W. and Lin, J. C. Partial-Body SAR calculations in magnetic resonance image (MRI) scanning systems. *IEEE Antennas and Propagation Magazine*, 54(2), 230, 2012.
205. IEEE, Standard for Safety Levels with Respect to Human Exposure to Radio Frequency Electromagnetic Fields, 3 kHz to 300 GHz, IEEE Standard C95.1, 2005.
206. Beckman, K. J., Lin, J. C.,Wang, Y., Illes, R. W., Papp, M. A., and Hariman, R. J. Production of reversible and irreversible atrio-ventricular block by microwave energy. The 60th Scientific Sessions, American Heart Association, Anaheim, CA, 1987; also in *Circulation*, 76, 1612, 1987.
207. Lin, J. C., Beckman, K. J., Hariman, R. J., Bharati, S., Lev, M., and Wang, Y. J., Microwave ablation of the atrioventricular junction in open heart dogs. *Bioelectromagnetics*, 16, 97, 1995.
208. Lin, J. C., Hariman, R. J., Wang, Y. G. and Wang, Y. J. Microwave catheter ablation of the atrioventricular junction in closed-chest dogs. *Medical & Biological Engineering & Computing*, 34, 295, 1996.

Computational Methods and EM Fields

209. Lin, J. C. Catheter microwave ablation therapy for cardiac arrhythmias. *Bioelectromagnetics*, 20(S4), 120, 1999.
210. Huang, S. K. S. and Wilber, D. J. eds. *Radiofrequency Catheter Ablation of Cardiac Arrhythmias: Basic Concepts and Clinical Applications*, 2nd ed. Futura, Armonk, NY, 2000.
211. Lin, J. C. Biophysics of radiofrequency ablation. In *Radiofrequency Catheter Ablation of Cardiac Arrhythmias: Basic Concepts and Clinical Applications*, S. K. S. Huang and D. J. Wilber, eds. 2nd ed. Futura, Armonk, NY, 2000, 13–24.
212. Lin, J. C. Hyperthermia therapy. In *Encyclopedia of Electrical and Electronics Engineering*, J. G. Webster, ed. Wiley, New York, 1999, vol. 9, 450–460.
213. Pennes, H. H. Analysis of tissue and arterial blood temperatures in resting forearm. *Journal of Applied Physiology*, 1, 93, 1948.
214. Stolwijk, J. A. J. and Hardy, J. D. Control of body temperature. In *Handbook of Physiology - Reaction to Environmental Agents*, D. H. K. Lee, ed. American Physiological Society, Rockville, MD, 1977, 45.
215. Spiegel, R. J. A review of numerical models for predicting the energy deposition and resultant thermal responses of humans exposed to electromagnetic fields. *IEEE Transactions on Microwave Theory and Techniques*, 32, 730, 1984.
216. Mooibroek, J. and Lagendijk, J. J. W. A fast and simple algorithm for the calculation of convective heat transfer by large vessels in three-dimensional inhomogeneous tissues. *IEEE Transactions on Biomedical Engineering*, 38, 490, 1991.
217. Kolios, M. C., Sherar, M. D., and Hunt, J. W. Large blood vessel cooling in heated tissues: a numerical study. *Physics in Medicine and Biology*, 40, 477, 1995.
218. Van Leeuwen, G. M. J., Lagendijk, J. J. W., Van Leersum, B. J. A. M., Zwamborn, A. P. M., Hornsleth, S. N., and Kotte, A. N. T. J. Calculation of change in brain temperatures due to exposure to a mobile phone. *Physics in Medicine and Biology*, 44, 2367, 1999.
219. Ma, L., Paul, D.-L., Pothecary, N., Railton, C., Bows, J., Barratt, L., Mullin, J., and Simons, D. Experimental validation of a combined electromagnetic and thermal FDTD model of a microwave heating process. *IEEE Transactions on Microwave Theory and Techniques*, 43, 2565, 1995.
220. Torres, F. and Jecko, B. Complete FDTD analysis of microwave heating process in frequency-dependent and temperature-dependent media. *IEEE Transactions on Microwave Theory and Techniques*, 45, 108, 1997.
221. Lu, C.-C., Li, H.-Z., and Gao, D. Combined electromagnetic and heat-conduction analysis of rapid rewarming of cryopreserved tissues. *IEEE Transactions on Microwave Theory and Techniques*, 48, 2185, 2000.
222. Gordon, R. G., Roemer, R. B., and Horvath, S. M. A mathematical model of the human temperature regulatory system – Transient cold exposure response. *IEEE Transactions on Biomedical Engineering*, 23, 434, 1976.
223. Ozisik, N. *Heat Transfer: A Basic Approach*. New York: Mc Graw Hill, 1985.
224. Gagge, A. P. and Nishi, Y. Heat exchange between human skin surface and thermal environment. In *Handbook of Physiology—Reaction to Environmental Agents*, D. H. K. Lee, ed. American Physiological Society, Rockville, MD, 1977, 69.
225. Haala, J. and Wiesbeck, W. Modeling microwave and hybrid heating processes including heat radiation effects. *IEEE Transactions on Microwave Theory and Techniques*, 50, 1346, 2002.
226. Adair, E. R. Thermal physiology of radiofrequency radiation (RFR) interactions in animals and humans. In Klauenberg, B. J., Grandolfo M. and Erwin D. J., eds. *Radiofrequency Radiation Standards*. Plenum Press, New York, 1995, 245.
227. Hoque, M. and Gandhi, O. P. Temperature distributions in the human leg for VLF-VHF exposures at the ANSI recommended safety levels. *IEEE Transactions on Biomedical Engineering*, 35, 442, 1988.
228. Chatterjee, I. and Gandhi, O. P. An inhomogeneous thermal block model of man for the electromagnetic environment. *IEEE Transactions on Biomedical Engineering*, 30, 707, 1983.
229. Guyton, A. C. *Textbook of Medical Physiology*. W.B. Saunders Company, 1991.

230. Bardati, F., Gerosa, G., and Lampariello, P. Temperature distribution in simulated living tissues irradiated electromagnetically. *Alta Freqência*, XLIX, 61, 1980.

231. Durkee, J. W., Antich, P. P., and Lee C. E. Exact solutions to the multiregion time-dependent bioheat equation. I: Solution development. *Physics in Medicine and Biology*, 35, 847, 1990.

232. Vyas, R. and Rustgi, M. L. Green's function solution to the tissue bioheat equation. *Medical Physics*, 19, 1319, 1992.

233. Way, W. I., Kritikos, H., and Schwan, H. Thermoregulatory physiological responses in the human body exposed to microwave radiation. *Bioelectromagnetics*, 2, 341, 1981.

234. Charny, C. K., Hagmann, M. J., and Levin, R. L. A whole body thermal model of man during hyperthermia. *IEEE Transactions on Biomedical Engineering*, 34, 375, 1987.

235. Scott J. A. A finite element model of heat transport in the human eye. *Physics in Medicine and Biology*, 33, 227, 1988.

236. Labonté, S., Blais, A., Legault, S. R., Ali, H. O., and Roy, L. Monopole antennas for microwave catheter ablation. *IEEE Transactions on Microwave Theory and Techniques*, 44, 1832, 1996.

237. Wang, J. and Fujiwara, O. FDTD computation of temperature rise in the human head for portable telephones. *IEEE Transactions on Microwave Theory and Techniques*, 47, 1528, 1999.

238. Pisa, S., Cavagnaro, M., Piuzzi, E., Bernardi, P., and Lin, J. C. Power density and temperature distributions produced by interstitial arrays of sleeved-slot antennas for hyperthermic cancer therapy. *IEEE Transactions on Microwave Theory and Techniques*, 51, 2418, 2003.

239. Peaceman, D. W. and Rachford, H. The numerical solution of parabolic and elliptic differential equtions. *Journal of the Society for Industrial and Applied Mathematics*, 3, 28, 1955.

240. Douglas, J. On the numerical integration of $u_{xx} + u_{yy} = u_t$ by implicit methods. *Journal of the Society for Industrial and Applied Mathematics*, 3, 42, 1955.

241. Douglas, J. Alternating direction methods for three space variables. *Numerische Mathematik*, 4, 41, 1962.

242. Emery, A. F., Kramar, P., Guy, A. W., and Lin, J. C. Microwave induced temperature rises in rabbit eyes in cataract research. *Journal of Heat Transfer*, 97(1), 123, 1975.

243. Guy, A. W., Lin, J. C., Kramar, P. O., and Emery, A. F. Effect of 2450 MHz radiation on the rabbit eye. *IEEE Transactions on Microwave Theory and Techniques*, 23, 492, 1975.

244. Appleton, B., Hirsch, S. E. and Brown, P. V. K. Investigation of single-exposure microwave ocular effects at 3000 MHz. *Annals of the New York Academy of Sciences*, 247, 125, 1975.

245. Sliney, D. H., and Stuck, B. E. Microwave exposure limits for the eye: applying infrared laser threshold data. In *Radiofrequency Radiation Standards*. Plenum Press, New York, 1994, 79.

246. Hardy, J. D., Wolff, H. G., and Goodell, H. *Pain Sensations and Reactions*. Williams and Wilkins, Baltimore, MD, 1952.

247. Foster, K. R., and Erdreich, L. S. Thermal models for microwave hazards and their role in standards development, *Bioelectromagnetics*, 20, 52, 1999.

248. Riu, P. J. and Foster, K. R. Heating of tissue by near-field exposure to a dipole: a model analysis. *IEEE Transactions on Biomedical Engineering*, 46, 911, 1999.

249. Lin, J. C., Guy, A. W., and Caldwell, L. R. Thermographic and behavioral studies of rats in the near field of 918 MHz radiations. *IEEE Transactions on Microwave Theory and Techniques*, 25, 833, 1977.

250. Cherry, P. C. and Iskander, M. F. Calculations of heating patterns of an array of microwave interstitial antennas. *IEEE Transactions on Biomedical Engineering*, 40, 771, 1993.

251. Bernardi, P., Cavagnaro, M., Pisa, S., and Piuzzi, E. SAR distribution and temperature increase in an anatomical model of the human eye exposed to the field radiated by the user antenna in a wireless LAN. *IEEE Transactions on Microwave Theory and Techniques*, 46, 2074, 1998.

252. Wainwright, P. Thermal effects of radiation from cellular telephones. *Physics in Medicine and Biology*, 45, 2363, 2000.

253. Gandhi, O. M., Li, Q. X., and Kang, G. Temperature rise for the human head for cellular telephones and for peak SARs prescribed in safety guidelines. *IEEE Transactions on Microwave Theory and Techniques*, 49, 1607, 2001.

254. McIntosh, R. L. and Anderson, V. SAR versus VAR, and the size and shape that provide the most appropriate RF exposure metric in the range of 0.5–6 GHz. *Bioelectromagnetics*, 32, 312, 2011.

Computational Methods and EM Fields

255. McIntosh, R. L. and Anderson, V. SAR versus Sinc: What is the appropriate RF exposure metric in the range 1–10 GHz? Part II: Using complex human body models. *Bioelectromagnetics*, 31, 467, 2010.
256. Cavagnaro, M., Pisa, S., Piuzzi, E., and Lin, J. C. Correlation between electromagnetic power absorption and induced temperature elevation in the human body for plane wave exposure. In *BioEM-2014 Conference*, Cape Town, South Africa, 2014.
257. Pisa, S., Cavagnaro, M., Piuzzi, E., and Lin, J C. Influence of tissue mass and exposure duration on correlation between radio frequency energy absorption and induced temperature elevation. *URSI General Assembly and Symposium*, Beijing, China, 2014.
258. Pisa, S., Cavarnaro, M., and Lin, J. C. The influence of averaging schemes and exposure duration on the correlation between temperature elevation and rf power absorption metrics in MRI scans. *IEEE Microwave Magazine*, 17(7), 14, 2016.
259. Murbach, M., Neufeld, E., Capstick, M., Kainz, W., Brunner, D. O., Samaras, T., Pruessmann, K. P., and Kuster, N. Thermal tissue damage model analyzed for different whole-body SAR and scan durations for standard MR body coils. *Magnetic Resonance in Medicine*, 431, 421–431, 2014.
260. Jin, J. *Electromagnetic Analysis and Design in Magnetic Resonance Imaging*. CRC Press, Boca Raton, FL, 1999.
261. Lin, J. C., Bernardi, P., Pisa, S., Cavagnaro, M., and Piuzzi, E. Antennas for medical therapy and diagnostics. In *Modern Antenna Handbook*, C. Balanis, ed. Wiley, 2008, 1377–1428.
262. Vaughan, J. T., Adriany, G., Snyder, G. J., Tian, J., Thiel, T., Bolinger, L., Liu, H., DelaBarre, L., and Ugurbil, K. Efficient high frequency body coil for high-field MRI. *Magnetic Resonance in Medicine*, 52, 851, 2004.
263. Andreuccetti, D., Fossi, R., and Petrucci, C. An Internet resource for the calculation of the dielectric properties of body tissues in the frequency range 10 Hz–100 GHz. Available http://niremf.ifac.cnr.it/tissprop/IFAC-CNR, Florence (Italy). Based on data published by C. Gabriel et al., 1997.
264. Pisa, S., Bernardi, P., Cavagnaro, M., and Piuzzi, E. Power absorption and temperature elevation produced by magnetic resonance apparatus in the thorax of patients with implanted pacemakers. *IEEE Transactions on Electromagnetic Compatibility*, 52, 32, 2010.

10

Experimental Dosimetry

Rodolfo Bruzon and Hakki Gurhan
University of Colorado Boulder

CONTENTS

10.1 Introduction 400
10.2 Experimental Dosimetry of Static and ELF Electromagnetic Fields.......401
    10.2.1 EF Measurement 401
        10.2.1.1 Electrostatic Field Meters...401
        10.2.1.2 ELF EF Meters 402
    10.2.2 Magnetic Field Measurement..403
        10.2.2.1 Induction Coil Magnetometer.......................................403
        10.2.2.2 Fluxgate Magnetometer 404
        10.2.2.3 Hall Effect Magnetometer..405
        10.2.2.4 SQUID Magnetometer...406
10.3 RF Experimental Dosimetry 408
    10.3.1 RF Fields..408
        10.3.1.1 EFs, Magnetic Fields, and Power Density 408
        10.3.1.2 Plane waves 409
        10.3.1.3 Field Zones (Near Field and Far Field)........................409
        10.3.1.4 Guided Waves 410
        10.3.1.5 Polarization..411
    10.3.2 Dielectric Properties of Biological Tissue 411
        10.3.2.1 Permittivity, Conductivity, and Permeability 411
        10.3.2.2 Dielectrophoresis 412
    10.3.3 RF Measurement Instrumentation 413
        10.3.3.1 Power Meters..413
        10.3.3.2 Spectrum Analyzers 421
        10.3.3.3 Network Analyzers..422
    10.3.4 RF Measurements 423
        10.3.4.1 EF Measurements...423
        10.3.4.2 Magnetic Field Measurements 424
10.4 RF Dosimetry...425
    10.4.1 SAR 425
    10.4.2 SAR Measurements 426
        10.4.2.1 Measuring SAR with EF Probes....................................426
        10.4.2.2 Differential Power Technique...426
        10.4.2.3 Calorimetric Techniques 426

10.5 RF *in vitro* Exposure Systems	428
10.5.1 TEM Cell	428
10.5.2 Rectangular Waveguide	429
10.5.3 Radial Waveguide	430
10.5.4 Horn Antenna	430
Acknowledgments	430
References	431

10.1 Introduction

The first part of this chapter focuses on sensors that are commonly used in measurements of static and low-frequency electric and magnetic fields. The second part is dedicated to radio frequency (RF) experimental dosimetry.

Electric and Magnetic Fields are vector quantities characterized by both strength and direction. Electric and Magnetic sensors measure these quantities in various ways. The units of measure for an electric field (EF) in the International System of Units (SI) are Newton per coulomb (N/C) or volts per meter (V/m). The strength of a magnetic field is measured in units of ampere turns per meter and the magnetic flux density is measured in Tesla in the SI; the units are in Oersted and Gauss, respectively, in the CGS System. One Tesla is equal to 10^4 Gauss.

Electric and Magnetic field sensors can be divided into vector component and scalar magnitudes types. Vector meters measure separately the three vector components of an electric and magnetic field. Total field or scalar meters measure the magnitude of the vector electric and magnetic field. Three orthogonal sensors are required to measure the components of the electric and magnetic field in all three dimensions [1].

In the laboratory, the intensity and homogeneity of the electric and magnetic field are usually controlled. The common procedure to determine the homogeneity of an electric and magnetic field is to measure directly the electric and magnetic field strength or its absolute value as a function of the space coordinates. In general, a high-sensitivity meter is sensitive to electric and/or magnetic field but also to electrical and/or magnetic interferences. The optimal meter is one that meets the requirements of a specific application.

According to Maxwell's equations any time-varying source will generate electric and magnetic fields. However, at low frequency, the electric and magnetic field are very weakly coupled and are treated independently. In the same way, the measurement methods for the electric and magnetic field will be presented separately here.

RF is a term that is often used to describe the oscillation rate of electromagnetic radiation spectrum, where electric and magnetic fields are inextricably coupled. RF extends over a wide range of frequencies, from 3 kilohertz (3 kHz) to 300 gigahertz (300 GHz) [2]. RF waves are mainly used in telecommunication services such as cellular communication, TV broadcasting, amateur radio, and satellite communications. There are other uses of RF energy including radar, industrial RF processing systems for rapid heating and drying of materials and microwave ovens. Microwave ovens use RF emitters, typically magnetrons to heat food, as power outputs of 600 to 1200 watts are available at low costs in the frequency band near 2.7 GHz. Industrial heaters and sealers create RF radiation which quickly heats the materials. And radars are widely used by traffic enforcement and air traffic control centers. Since the use of these services has been increased exponentially over the past decades, background levels of RF radiation have also increased.

Experimental Dosimetry 401

Radio waves belong to the category of non-ionizing radiation, meaning that there is not enough energy in a single photon to ionize a typical ion or molecule. Non-ionizing radiation has enough energy to move atoms in a molecule around or cause them to vibrate. RF radiation has higher energy than extremely low-frequency (ELF) radiation in a single photon, but it has lower energy in a single photon than some other kinds of non-ionizing radiation, like visible light and infrared [3].

In order to estimate a potential health risk to general public and possible occupational hazards, ELF and RF fields should be quantified by measurements. Sections 10.3 and beyond will focus on the issue of RF field measurements and absorbed RF energy measurements.

10.2 Experimental Dosimetry of Static and ELF Electromagnetic Fields

10.2.1 EF Measurement

An EF strength meter consists of two parts, the probe or field sensor, and the detector. The probe produces an electrical signal proportional to the EF which is then processed by the detector circuit. EF measurements are extremely easily be distorted by the presence of nearby objects. Conducting objects have a significant effect on EFs. Conducting bodies placed within an EF would concentrate the EF around the conducting body. The human body is a conducting object that also distorts the EF. Holding the instrument too close to a conducting body to measure the EF will result in an erroneous reading. In general, proximity effects are a function of distance between the observer and measurement location, measurement height above ground and the electric potential of the observer.

10.2.1.1 Electrostatic Field Meters

The range of sensitivity of electrostatic field meters is from 10 V/m to 2000 kV/m. The upper limit of field meter measurement is usually dictated by the breakdown of air, which is around 20 kV/cm [4]. Fields mills (also called generating voltmeters) determine EF strength by measuring modulated, capacitively induced charges or currents on metal electrodes. In shutter type meter (Figure 10.1), the sensing electrode is periodically exposed to and shielded from the EF by a grounded, rotating shutter [5]. The charge q_s induced on the sensing electrode and the current i_s between the sensing electrodes and grounds are both proportional to the EF strength E normal to the electrode:

$$q_s(t) = \varepsilon_0 E a_s(t) \text{ and } i_s(t) = \varepsilon_0 E \frac{\mathrm{d}a_s(t)}{\mathrm{d}t} \tag{10.1}$$

where ε_0 is the permittivity of free space and $a_s(t)$ is the effective exposed area of the sensing electrode at time t. Thus, the field strength can be determined by measuring the induced charge or current (or voltage across the impedance Z).

Shutter-type field mills are operated at the ground or at a ground plane, but a cylindrical field mill can be used to measure EF at points removed from a ground plane. A cylindrical field mill consists of two half-cylinder sensing electrodes. Charges induced on the two sensing electrodes are varied periodically by rotating the sensing electrodes about the cylinder axis at a constant angular frequency ω_c [5]. The charge q_c induced on a half cylinder of length L and the current i_c between the half cylinders are given by

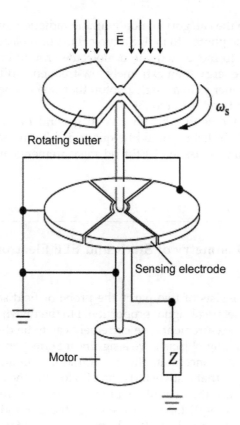

FIGURE 10.1
Shutter-type field mills for measurement of the strength and polarity an electrostatic field [5].

$$q_c = 4\varepsilon_0 r_c LE \sin\omega_c t \text{ and } i_c = 4\varepsilon_0 r_c LE \cos\omega_c t \quad (10.2)$$

where r_c is the cylinder radius. Thus, the EF strength can be determined from a measurement of the induced charge or current.

Another type of EF meter uses a vibrating plate to generate an AC signal that is proportional to the electric field strength. EF meters utilizing an AC carrier type system are most common is high quality EF monitoring systems. This AC signal is produced by modulating a capacitance pickup in an EF and the amplitude of the AC signal created is proportional to the modulation amplitude for any given EF. These instruments are extremely reliable and require little power and its speed of response is typically around 0.5 s [4].

10.2.1.2 ELF EF Meters

In contrast to the magnetic sensors there are fewer sensor types for low-frequency EFs showing sufficient sensitivity. Three types of EF meters have been used to characterize ELF EF: free body meters, ground reference meters and electro-optic meters. In free body meters, the magnitude of the alternating EF is determined by measuring the induced current oscillating between two halves of an electrically isolated conductive body which makes up the probe or sensor. The free-body meter is suitable for survey-type measurements because it is portable, allows measurements above the ground plane, and does not require a ground reference [6].

Experimental Dosimetry 403

Commercial field meters are usually rectangular in shape, and typical dimensions are on the order of 10 cm. The charge Q on half of the field meter is proportional to the incident EF E along the meter axis:

$$Q = A\varepsilon_0 E \qquad (10.3)$$

where ε_0 is the permittivity of free space and A is a constant proportional to the surface area.

For electrostatic fields, the components are real scalars that are independent of time. For steady state, time harmonic fields, the components are complex phasors with repetitions dependent on $e^{j\omega t}$, where ω is the angular frequency and t is the time, are suppressed [5]. For the spherical geometry, $A = 3\pi a^2$, where a is the sphere's radius. Since the current I between the two halves is equal to the time derivative of the charge, for time harmonic fields, it can be written as

$$I = j\omega A\varepsilon_0 E \qquad (10.4)$$

This allows E can be determined from the measured current.

Ground referenced meters are normally used with the probe or sensor located on a grounded surfaces. Ground reference meters determine the magnitude of the field by measuring the induced current ground. The currents induced into the probes of free body and ground references meters are proportional to the time derivative of the EF; for this reason, the waveform of the current no longer reflects that of the EF when harmonics are present in the field. To avoid these measurement errors, a stage of integration is often incorporated into the signal processing circuitry to recover the waveform of the field [6].

The underlying physics for performing measurements with electro-optic meters differs from that of free body meters described above, but both types of meters are used in a similar fashion. Electro-optic meters are typically based on Pockel's effect, in which a crystal changes length and dielectric constant in an EF, changing the interference fringes of a light beam. Further discussions of the various types of EF meters and their principles of operation are found in reference [7].

While the IEEE standard recommends the use of free body meters for characterizing power line fields [8], an International Electrotechnical Commission (IEC) standard describes the use of electro-optic type field meters which utilize the Pockel's effect to determine the EF strength as well as free body and ground reference-type field meters [9].

10.2.2 Magnetic Field Measurement

There are many technologies to sense magnetic fields, most of them based on the intimate connection between magnetic and electric phenomena. Each technique has unique properties that make it more suitable for particular applications. The main characteristics of the most common magnetometers are shown in Table 10.1.

10.2.2.1 Induction Coil Magnetometer

The principle behind the search-coil magnetometer is Faraday's law of induction. This law states that if the magnetic flux through a coiled conductor changes, a voltage proportional to the rate of change of the flux (ϕ) is generated between the leads:

$$V(t) = -\mathrm{d}\phi/\mathrm{d}t \qquad (10.5)$$

TABLE 10.1

Magnetometers Characteristics

Instrument	Range (mT)	Resolution (nT)	Bandwidth (Hz)	Comment
Induction coil	10^{-10} to 10^6	Variable	10^{-1} to 10^6	Cannot measure static fields
Fluxgate	10^{-4} to 0.5	0.1	dc to 2×10^3	General purpose magnetometer
Hall effect	0.1 to 3×10^4	100	dc to 10^8	General purpose and good performance for fields above 1T
SQUID	10^{-9} to 0.1	10^{-4}	dc to 5	Highest sensitivity magnetometer

Source: Adapted from Macintyre, Steven. 1999. "Magnetic Field Measurement." *The Measurement, Instrumentation and Sensors Handbook on CD-ROM.* doi:10.1201/9780415876179.ch48.

The flux through the coil will change if the coil is in a magnetic field that varies with time. For example, if the coil is rotated in a uniform static field or if the coil is moved through a non-uniform field or placed in a time-varying field, a voltage will be generated. Since magnetic induction B is flux density then a loop with cross-sectional area A (NA if the coil has N turns) will have a terminal voltage

$$V(t) = -\mathrm{d}(\boldsymbol{B} \cdot \boldsymbol{A})/\mathrm{d}t \qquad (10.6)$$

for spatially uniform magnetic induction fields. Equation 10.2 states that a temporal change in B or the mechanical orientation of A relative to B will produce a terminal voltage.

An important advantage of induction magnetometers is that they are completely passive sensors for time-changing fields: they do not require any internal energy source to convert magnetic field into electrical signal. In that case, the only power consumption associated with a search coil is that needed for signal processing [10]. To study in-depth the topic and to see the part of signal conditioning for the different magnetometers presented, see [11 and 18].

10.2.2.2 Fluxgate Magnetometer

The fluxgate magnetometer is a versatile instrument that has the ability to measure the vector components of magnetic fields from DC to several kHz. The major advantage of fluxgate magnetometers over search coils is their ability to precisely measure static magnetic field generated by direct-currents. Fluxgate magnetometers have low noise levels and relatively large dynamic ranges and thus are often the best selection for measurements if resolution in the nT range is required.

The fluxgate is a transducer that converts a magnetic field into an electric voltage. This device involves two coils, a primary and a secondary, wrapped around a common high permeability ferromagnetic core. An alternating current through one coil magnetizes the core to saturation and induces a pulsing current in the other coil (Figure 10.2). The magnetic induction of this core changes in presence of an external magnetic field [12]. As the core permeability and magnetic field alternates from a low value to high value, it produces a voltage pulse at the signal winding output that has amplitude proportional to the magnitude of the external magnetic field and a phase indicating the direction of the field. According to Faraday's law, a changing flux will produce a voltage at the terminals of the

Experimental Dosimetry

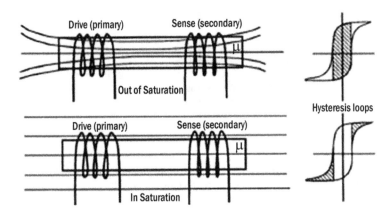

FIGURE 10.2
Operating principle of fluxgate magnetometer. Output signal becomes modulated by driving the core into and out of saturation. The shaded regions in hysteresis loops indicate the regions of operation [19].

signal winding that is proportional to the rate of change flux. For DC and low-frequency magnetic fields, the signal winding voltage is:

$$V(t) = nA \frac{d(\mu_0 \mu_e H)}{dt} = nA\mu_0 H \quad (10.7)$$

where H is the component of the magnetic field being measured; n is the number of turns on the signal windings; A is the cross-sectional area of the signal winding and $\mu_e(t)$ is the effective relative permeability of the core.

The most common type of fluxgate magnetometer uses the second harmonic. The voltage output from the sense coil consists of even-numbered harmonics of the excitation frequency. For readout, the second harmonic is extracted and rectified. The voltage associated with this harmonic is proportional to the external magnetic field [13–14]. The frequency of the signal is twice the excitation frequency since the saturation to saturation transition occurs twice each excitation period. A detailed explanation, recent achievements in the technology and design of fluxgate sensors can be seen in [15, 16].

10.2.2.3 Hall Effect Magnetometer

The Hall Effect device is the most familiar and widely used sensor for measuring strong magnetic fields. The zero offset and $1/f$ noise of the Hall voltage amplifier limit the performance of a Hall Effect gaussmeter for low field strength measurements. When a conductor is placed in a magnetic field perpendicular to the direction of the electron flow, they will be deflected from a straight path. As a consequence, one plane of the conductor will become negatively charged and the opposite side will become positively charged. The voltage between these planes is called the Hall Voltage [17]. These sensors produce a voltage proportional to the applied magnetic field and also sense the polarity.

The Hall Effect is a consequence of the Lorentz force law, which states that a moving charge q, when acted upon by a magnetic induction field B, will experience a force F that is at right angles to the field vector and the velocity vector v of the charge as expressed by the following equation:

$$F = -q(E + v \times B) \quad (10.8)$$

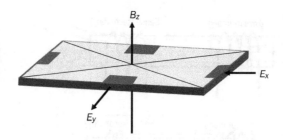

FIGURE 10.3
Simplified scheme of Hall Effect sensor. A magnetic field B_z applied normal to the surface of the sensor, which conducts a current along the x-direction, will generate a voltage along the y-direction which is known as the Hall Voltage.

The Hall Effect device consists of a flat, thin rectangular conductor or semiconductor with two pairs of electrodes at right angles to one another (Figure 10.3).

An EF E_x is applied along x. When a magnetic field B_z is applied perpendicular to the surface of the device, the free charge, which is flowing along the x-axis as result of E_x, will be deflected toward the y or Hall Voltage axis. This will cause a buildup of the charge along the y-axis that will create an EF which produces a force opposing the motion of the charge. This EF is described by $E_y = v_x B_z$, where v_x is the average drift velocity of the electrons (or majority carriers). In a conductor that contains n free charges per unit volume having an average drift velocity of v_x, the current density $J_x = qnv_x$ and $E_y = J_x B_z / qn = R_H J_x B_z$ where R_H is called the Hall coefficient. The Hall Effect is very small in metallic conductors, but a semiconductor gives a much larger effect. The faster the electrons are moving, the stronger the force they experience and the greater the Hall Voltage produced at equilibrium. A semiconductor is treated in terms of the mobility μ of the majority carrier (electron or hole) and conductivity σ. In this case, $E_y = \mu E_x B_z$ and $E_x = J_x / \sigma$. Therefore $E_y = (\mu/\sigma) J_x B_z$ and $R_H = \mu/\sigma$. The value of R_H varies substantially from one material to another and is both temperature and field magnitude dependent.

Semiconductor materials, such as Indium Arsenide (InAs) exhibit lower temperature dependence of the Hall Voltage compared to Silicon (Si) and Indium Antimonide (InSb) and the working range of InAs is also superior. InAs, because of its combined low temperature coefficient of sensitivity (<0.1%/°C), low resistance, and relatively good sensitivity, is the material favored by commercial manufacturers of Hall Effect devices [18].

10.2.2.4 SQUID Magnetometer

The superconducting quantum interference device (SQUID) magnetometers are the most sensitive of all magnetic field measuring instruments. These sensors operate at temperatures near absolute zero and require special thermal control systems (cooling with liquid helium at 4.2 K or liquid nitrogen at 77 K). SQUID is based on the interactions of the electric currents and magnetic fields observed when certain materials are cooled below a superconducting transition temperature. At this temperature, the materials become superconductors and they lose all resistance to the flow of electricity.

The SQUID measures the magnitude of the superconductor critical current through a Josephson junction, which consists of two superconductors separated by a thin non-conducting barrier through which electrons can tunnel in accord with quantum phenomena. The current in a superconductor is carried by so-called Cooper pairs

Experimental Dosimetry

(pairs of electrons with opposite momentum and spin). If two superconductors are weakly connected, Cooper pairs can exchange between them. The Josephson current is affected by the presence of a magnetic field so it is a very sensitive indicator of the flux density [17].

In Figure 10.4, the general structure of a Josephson junction and the voltage-current (V–I) relationship is shown. Two superconductors (niobium) are separated by a thin insulating layer (aluminum oxide). When the temperature of the junction is reduced to below −269°C, a superconductor current will flow in the junction with 0 V across the junction. The magnitude of this current, called the critical current I_c is a periodic function of the magnetic flux present in the junction [11].

A simple SQUID system consists of room temperature electronics and a low-temperature probe containing the SQUID sensor, configured with an integrated input coil to measure changes in current. Connecting the input coil to a detection coil allows measurement of magnetic fields [20]. A simplified circuit used to measure the voltage across the SQUID loop is shown in Figure 10.5. The coil on the left side applies both a dc and a 100 kHz flux to the SQUID loop; the dc flux cancels the flux being measured and the 100 kHz is used

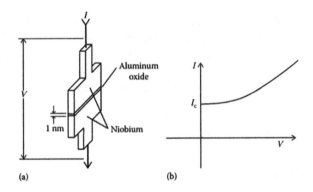

FIGURE 10.4
(a) The Josephson junction of a superconductor such as niobium separated by a thin insulating layer. (b) The voltage (V) versus current (I) curve shows that a superconducting current flows through the junction with zero volts across the junction.

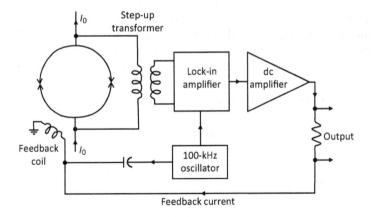

FIGURE 10.5
Simplified circuit used to measure the voltage across the SQUID loop. The output voltage is proportional to the feedback current which keeps the total quasi-static flux in the loop, thus minimizing the 100-kHz component into the lock-in amplifier [21].

408   *Electromagnetic Fields*

to facilitate a narrowband, lock-in type of measurement. The output is proportional to the feedback current and, hence, to the amount of flux required to cancel the measured flux [21].

Biomedical research is one of the more important applications of SQUID magnetometers. The highest sensitivity exhibit SQUID sensors, with noises of about 5 fT/Hz they enable to detect fT magnetic field (in typical application pT). Therefore, the SQUID magnetometers are commonly used to analyze of magnetic field resulting from brain activity (magnetoencephalography). In the specialized literature, we can find several papers and handbooks interesting that discuss different aspects of the magnetometers [22–23].

10.3 RF Experimental Dosimetry

10.3.1 RF Fields

An RF field has both an EF and a magnetic field component, and in the near field the intensity of the RF environment at a given location needs to be specified in terms of units specific for each component [24]. The majority of the time, the term electromagnetic field or RF field can be used to signify the existence of electromagnetic or RF energy. Radio waves and microwaves are a form of electromagnetic energy. Electric and magnetic energy are moving together through space at the speed of light. The terms electromagnetic field and electromagnetic energy also apply to DC and low frequencies, even though coupling between the electric and magnetic fields is weak.

10.3.1.1 EFs, Magnetic Fields, and Power Density

In the introductory chapter, EFs and magnetic fields are discussed in detail. Briefly, an EF is a vector-force field used to represent the forces between electric charges. If the distribution of electric charges changes with time, then EF will also change. A magnetic field is proportional to the electric currents and spin polarization in magnetic materials. If the current path or the permanent magnet moves or the current magnitude changes with time, the magnetic field will also change with time. A time-varying EF creates a magnetic field and a time-varying magnetic field creates an EF [25].

In case of the isotropic radiator at a point O which is fed with a power of P watts, the power flows outwards from the origin and must flow through the spherical surface, S, of radius, r. [Figure 10.6]

Then, we can define the power density, P_d at the point Q as:

$$P_d = \frac{P}{4\pi r^2} \tag{10.9}$$

Poynting's theorem defines the relationship between the power density to the E-field and H-field vectors as defined below:

$$P_d = \vec{E} \times \vec{H} \tag{10.10}$$

Where E (EF strength) is in volts per meter (V/m), H (magnetic field strength) is in amperes per meter (A/m) and P_d (power density) is in watts per square meter (W/m²). This

Experimental Dosimetry

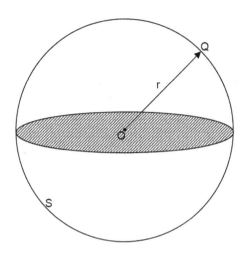

FIGURE 10.6
Isotropic radiator.

indicates the amount of radiated power passing through each square meter of a surface perpendicular to the direction away from the source. The magnitude of the power density (peak power density) in free space is thus:

$$|P_d| = |E||H| = \frac{E^2}{120\pi} \quad (10.11)$$

since ratio of E to H is the intrinsic impedance of the medium which is 120π in free space.

$$\eta = E/H \quad (10.12)$$

If the source is sinusoidal, then the average power density is half of the peak power density.

10.3.1.2 Plane waves

A wave in which the wave fronts are planar is called plane waves. E-field, H-field, and the direction of propagation (k) are all mutually perpendicular. This becomes increasingly the case, the farther the point of observation is from a point or other radiating source [Figure 10.7].

10.3.1.3 Field Zones (Near Field and Far Field)

Electromagnetic fields close enough to a source that fields often may not be approximated by a plane wave are called near fields. The field is often more non-propagating in nature and is also called as fringing field, reactive field or induction field. In the near-field region, E-field and H-field are not necessarily perpendicular, and it is s not easy to characterize the fields. Therefore, both the E-fields and H-fields must be measured separately at distances less than about $\lambda/2\pi$ from a field source, where λ is the wavelength. If objects are placed near a source, this may have a strong effect on the nature of the near fields. For instance, placing a probe near a source to measure the field may change the nature of field remarkably. This needs to be considered as an important factor in measurement accuracy for measurements made very near a source [26].

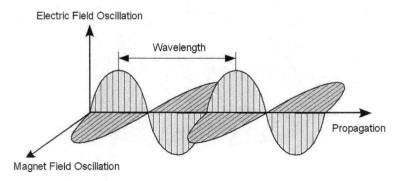

FIGURE 10.7
Electromagnetic radiation.

Electromagnetic fields far enough away from the source producing them that the fields are approximately plane wave in nature are called far fields. The mathematical expression to determine the boundary between the near-field and far-field region is:

$$r = \frac{2L^2}{\lambda} \quad (10.13)$$

Where r is the distance from the source, L is the aperture of the source antenna and λ is the wavelength of the fields.

This region is also called the free-space region, and the fields have a predominantly plane wave character. EF strength and magnetic field strength in plane waves are distributed very uniformly. And both the electric and magnetic fields are perpendicular to the direction that an electromagnetic wave is propagating. For that reason, making measurements in the far field and calculations for far-field energy absorption are much easier than for near-field energy absorption [27].

10.3.1.4 Guided Waves

At higher frequencies transmission along a guiding structure is best represented in terms of wave propagation. In the MHz range two conductor lines are widely used. At microwave frequencies and above, power losses in two conductor lines become excessive. Therefore, in GHz region waveguides are usually used as guiding structures.

10.3.1.4.1 Standing Waves

When a transmission line is terminated in its characteristic impedance as an open circuit or short circuit, incident waves and reflected waves would be equal in magnitude and their combination forms a pattern called a standing wave. If the load impedance is not zero (a perfect short circuit) or infinite (a perfect open circuit) and is not equal to the characteristic impedance, the magnitude of reflected wave is not equal to the incident wave. Thus, a similar pattern to standing waves forms with maxima and minima.

Standing wave ratio (SWR) is the ratio of maximum field strength to minimum field strength along the direction of propagation of two waves traveling in opposite directions on a transmission line [28]. Sometimes, the term VSWR is used to explicitly denote the voltage ratio.

Experimental Dosimetry

$$S = E_{max} / E_{min} \tag{10.14}$$

Where S is the standing wave ratio, E_{max} is the maximum value of the magnitude of the EF intensity anywhere along the line and E_{min} is the minimum value of the magnitude of the EF intensity anywhere along the line. SWR is a measure of reflection.

$$S = (1 + \rho)/(1 - \rho) \tag{10.15}$$

Where ρ is the ratio of the reflected wave's magnitude to the incident wave's magnitude and it's called as reflection coefficient.

10.3.1.4.2 Waveguides

A waveguide is often a hollow conducting structure which is capable of guiding electromagnetic waves from one place to another. Most commonly used waveguides are rectangular or circular, and they usually consist of a hollow metallic tube. Electromagnetic fields propagating in waveguides are called modes which is the sum of a series of characteristic field patterns. Waveguides are able to transport a number of different propagation modes. The stimulus frequency must be greater than the critical frequency of the relevant mode for a mode to propagate. When the stimulus frequency increases, the number of the modes capable of propagation also increases.

10.3.1.5 Polarization

Orientations of the incident E field and H field vectors with respect to the absorbing object is called polarization and have a very strong effect on the strength of fields inside the object [29]. The incident-field vector E, H, or K (vector in the direction of propagation) defines polarization for objects those have circular symmetry about the long axis (like human body). The polarization is called E-polarization if E is parallel to the long axis, H-polarization if H is parallel to the long axis, and K-polarization if k is parallel to the long axis. These three polarizations are illustrated in terms of a prolate spheroidal model in Figure 10.8. A prolate spheroid is a surface of revolution obtained by rotating an ellipse about its major axis.

10.3.2 Dielectric Properties of Biological Tissue

10.3.2.1 Permittivity, Conductivity, and Permeability

The dielectric properties of a biological tissue are the result of the property of the material that reflects how the material affects the incident waves at the molecular and cellular level as explained in Chapter 4 in this volume. Dielectric properties are experimentally determined by measuring complex relative permittivity, $\hat{\varepsilon}$ and presented by the formula below as a function of frequency:

$$\hat{\varepsilon} = \varepsilon' - j\varepsilon'' \tag{10.16}$$

Where ε' is the relative permittivity of the material and ε'' is the out of phase loss factor which is also expressed as:

$$\varepsilon'' = \sigma / \varepsilon_0 \omega \tag{10.17}$$

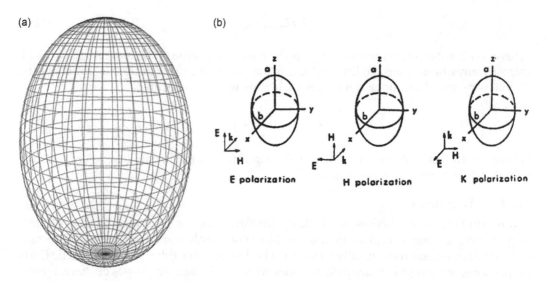

FIGURE 10.8
(a) A prolate spheroid. (b) Polarization of an incident field with respect to the absorbing object.

where σ is the conductivity of the material, ε_0 is the permittivity of the free space and ω is the frequency of the field.

As we see from the equation above, permittivity of a biological tissue is a function of frequency and in general permittivity decreases with frequency. This means that the charges in the tissue are lacking in their response to the applied fields in higher frequencies. Biological tissues have a very high dielectric constants compared to homogeneous liquids, and generally soft tissues show continuous decrease in permittivity when frequency increases.

Permittivity is a measure of how easily charge displacement occurs in a material. If an applied E-field give rise to many induced dipoles per unit volume or a high net alignment of permanent dipoles per unit volume, that means the charge displacement give rise to polarization and higher permittivity. Materials which are affected by the polarization of bound charges and orientation of permanent dipoles are called dielectrics. Conductivity is a measure of how much drift of conduction charges occur for a given applied E-field. A large drift give rise to ionic conductivity in a material. Materials which are affected by drift of conduction charges (both electronic and ionic) are called conductors.

At higher field strength there are experimental observations which predict non-linear molecular and cellular polarization. Field strengths of the order of 10^6 V/m may initiate polarization mechanisms which affect the cellular function. These higher fields may cause the dielectric breakdown within the membrane and leads to cell destruction [30].

The magnetic permeability of biological tissues is very close to that of free-space, and magnetic losses are negligible. That means most biological tissues are essentially nonmagnetic.

10.3.2.2 Dielectrophoresis

Dielectrophoresis is the motion of particles caused by electrical polarization effects in inhomogeneous (non-uniform) EFs. The induced motion is thus determined by the dielectric properties of the particle. Pethig (1986) demonstrated the possibility of manipulating single cells, or of separating more than 10^3 cells per second [31]. It is discussed further in Chapter 5 in this volume.

Experimental Dosimetry

10.3.3 RF Measurement Instrumentation

10.3.3.1 Power Meters

10.3.3.1.1 Diode Detectors

The diode or multi-diode power sensor is often the preferred option for modern power meter applications. These sensors employ one or more diodes to rectify the RF signal and produce an equivalent DC signal in order to determine the EF and the power level entering the load. Diode based RF power sensors have two major advantages. First, they are able to measure signals down to very low levels of power, as low as −165 dBm, and this is much lower than is possible when using heat-based RF power sensors. Second, they are able to respond faster than heat-based types.

A diode detector's DC output voltage is proportional to power at low signal levels and proportional to the peak RF voltage at higher levels. Below about −20 dBm (30 mV peak carrier voltage), diodes behave as non-linear resistors since the RF input is not high enough to cause the diodes to fully conduct in the forward direction [Figure 10.9].

The RF detector curve will usually have three regions; square law, linear, and compression [Figure 10.10]. The top 20 dB of the detector range is called as "linear range," output circuitry and measurement algorithms are adjusted to compensate for the change to the linear mode of operation. However, in the linear range the power in the harmonics has a much greater effect.

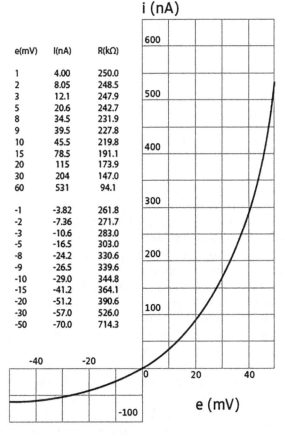

FIGURE 10.9
I–V curve showing "non-linear resistor" characteristic [33].

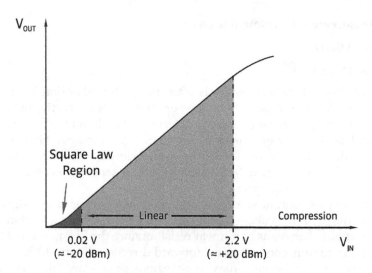

FIGURE 10.10
Square-law, linear, and compression region of a detector circuit [33].

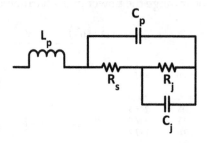

FIGURE 10.11
Schottky diode equivalent circuit: where R_j and C_j are junction resistance and capacitance, L_p and C_p are package parasitics consist of an inductance and capacitive impedance, R_s is the series resistance.

The region below that linear range is called the square-law region due to the fact that the output voltage would be a function of the square of the EF. In this low power range, the output voltage would be linearly related to the square of the input voltage of the RF signal, and thus be linearly proportional to the detected power. In this region, diode detectors operate almost like the thermistor sensors, but with much faster speeds and much wider dynamic range [32].

A Schottky diode is also known as hot-carrier diode. It consumes less power than the P–N junction diode and it is widely used for RF applications as a detector. It is a metal semiconductor diode and the switching speed is often limited by the recombination time for the carriers in the semiconductor. In a Schottky diode, the voltage drop normally ranges between 0.15 and 0.45 volts while in a PN junction semiconductor diode, the voltage drop is between 0.6 to 1.7 volts. This lower voltage drop and faster recombination lifetimes provide higher switching speed and better system efficiency. In a Schottky diode, a semiconductor–metal junction is formed between a semiconductor and a metal, which creates a Schottky barrier. A Schottky diode with equivalent circuit is shown in Figure 10.11.

Until recently, more diode sensors use a two or more of embedded diode elements. Some of them are padded with larger attenuation to allow them to be in the square-law region while operating at higher powers. In order to extend the useful range of the power sensor,

Experimental Dosimetry

complex algorithms are used in the power meter instrumentation. These algorithms can detect when the power from one sensor exceeds the square-law region, and let power meter to take its readings from one of the attenuated diodes. Some commercially available power sensors are listed in Table 10.2.

10.3.3.1.2 RF Thermocouples

Thermocouples are commonly used for measuring low RF power levels. RF thermocouple power sensors possess a square-law detection characteristic. The input RF power is proportional to the DC output voltage from the thermocouple sensor [33]. A thermocouple is created by joining two dissimilar metal wires together. A small voltage is produced in response to a temperature difference between the hot and cold junctions which is typically just a few tens of microvolts per °C. The principle for thermocouple operation is as follows:

When one end of a conductor is heated, the electrons at the hot end are more thermally energized than the electrons at the cooler end. These thermally energized electrons begin to diffuse toward the cooler end. Even though charge neutrality is maintained, this redistribution of electrons creates a negative charge at the cool end and an equal positive charge at the hot end. Therefore, heating one end of a conductive material to a temperature higher than the opposite end creates an electrostatic voltage due to the redistribution of thermally energized electrons throughout the entire material. This is the basic principle of thermocouples and it is called the Seebeck effect [34].

When one side of two connected copper wires is hotter than the other, the electrons diffuse from the hot side to the cold side. Since the electrons diffuse uniformly, a voltmeter placed between two sides does not detect voltage difference. This happens because the other wire of the same metal produces an identical Seebeck voltage. As a result, a net voltage of 0 V is measured at the measurement points.

If one side of copper wire is replaced by iron with the same temperature difference, the difference in transport properties between copper and iron will cause a voltage difference between both junctions. In other words, the free electrons at the warmer side of copper have different speed than the free electrons at the warmer side of the iron. Then the electrons flow from the warmer side to the colder side and this creates potential difference between both junctions [Figure 10.12].

The energy available from a single thermocouple is very small. Therefore, arrays of thermocouples are used to construct thermoelectric devices capable for measuring small amounts of power and small temperature changes. More sensitive devices can be made by connecting thermocouples in series to increase the size of the voltage difference and in parallel to increase the current capacity. Such an array of thermocouples is called a thermopile. A diagram illustrating the thermopile principle is shown in Figure 10.13.

No voltage is produced at the measurement junction; instead, a voltage is developed along each wire as the temperature changes [35]. This is one of the most misunderstood issues regarding the thermocouples. When there is a temperature difference between the ends of the wires current flow can take place. Since two differing metals have different Seebeck coefficients, voltage difference is observed at the receiving end and as a result that produces a voltage difference at the meter point [Figure 10.14].

Different metals, metal alloys, and semiconductor materials are used to make thermocouples. The materials listed in Table 10.3 form the basis for the commonly available thermocouples. Their thermoelectric sensitivities (Seebeck coefficients) can vary significantly in magnitude and can have a positive or negative value. For example, if the two selected materials are the iron and the constantan which have Seebeck coefficients of

TABLE 10.2

Some Commercially Available Power Sensors

Supplier	Power Sensor* Power Meter	Frequency Range	Dynamic Range	VSWR	Remark
Power sensors in matched load configuration and related power meter					
Hewlett-Packard	HP8478B	10 MHz–18 GHz	—	1.1–1.75	Thermistor
Rohde & Schwarz	NRV-Z52	dc–26.5 GHz	1 µW–100 mW	1.11–1.22	Thermocouple, up to 30 W available
Marconi	6913/6914S	10 MHz–26.5/46 GHz	1 µW–100 mW	1.1–1.4/3.6	Thermocouple, up to 3 W available
Boonton	51100(9E)	10 MHz–18 GHz	10–100 µW	1.18–1.28	Thermocouple
Hewlett-Packard	HP8485A	50 MHz–26.5 GHz	1 µW–100 mW	1.10–1.25	Thermocouple
	HP8487A	50 MHz–50 GHz	1 µW–100 mW	1.10–1.50	Thermocouple
	HPR/Q/W8486A	26.5–40/33–50/75–110 GHz	1 µW–100 mW	1.4/1.5/1.08	Rectangular waveguide, thermocouple
Rohde & Schwarz	NRV-Z6	50 MHz–26.5 GHz	1 nW–20 mW	1.2–1.4	Diode
Marconi	6923/6924S	10 MHz–26.5/46 GHz	0.1 nW/0.1–10 µW	1.12–1.5/3.6	Diode
Hewlett-Packard	HP8487D	50 MHz–50 GHz	0.1 nW–10 µW	1.15–1.89	Diode
Rohde & Schwarz	*NRVS/D	dc–26.5 GHz	0.4 nW–30 W	—	One/two channel
Boonton	*4230A	10 kHz–100 GHz	0.1 nW–25 W	—	—
Marconi	*6960B	30 kHz–46 GHz	0.1 nW–30 W	—	—
	*6970	30 kHz–46 GHz	0.1 nW–30 W	Hand portable	
Hewlett-Packard *HP437B	100 kHz–110 GHz	0.07 nW–25 W	—	—	

(Continued)

TABLE 10.2 (*Continued*)

Some Commercially Available Power Sensors

| Supplier | Power Sensor* | | | | |
	Power Meter	Frequency Range	Dynamic Range	VSWR	Remark
Power analyzer					
Hewlett-Packard	HP84812/13/14A	500 MHz–18/26.5/40 GHz	0.6 μW–100 mW	1.25–1.60	Resolution 100 ps
	*HP8990A	500 MHz–40 GHz	0.5 pW–100 mW	—	Rise/fall time 5 ns
Peak power sensors and related power meter					
Rohde & Schwarz	NRV-Z31/33	0.03–6 GHz	1 μW–20 mW/1 mW–20 W	1.05–1.33	With NRVS
Hewlett-Packard	HP84812/3/4A	500 MHz–18/26.5/40 GHz	1 pW–100 mW	1.25/1.35/1.50	—
Boonton	56340	500 MHz–40 GHz	—	1.25–2.00	Dual diode risetime<15 ns
	*HP8990A	500 MHz–40 GHz	—	—	—
Boonton	4500A	1 MHz–40 GHz	0.1 μW–100 mW	—	—
Feedthrough power sensor and related power meter					
Rohde & Schwarz	NAS-Z7	1.71–1.99 GHz	0.01–30 W	<1.15	a_D > 26 dB, GSM, DCS1800/1900
	*NAS	0.001–1.99 GHz	10 mW–1200 W	—	—

Source: Adapted from Webster, John G., and Halit Eren. 2014. Measurement, Instrumentation, and Sensors Handbook, Second Edition: Electromagnetic, Optical, Radiation, Chemical, and Biomedical Measurement.

* Designates item is power sensor.

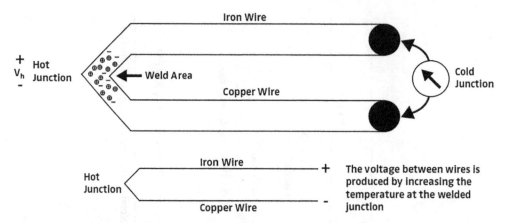

FIGURE 10.12
Diagram illustrating a thermocouple [33].

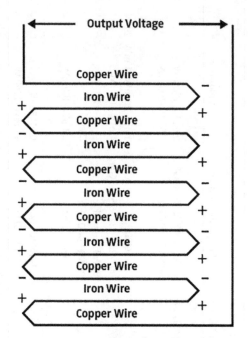

FIGURE 10.13
Diagram illustrating a thermopile [33].

approximately +19 μV/°C and −35 μV/°C, respectively, then the difference between these two coefficients results in a thermocouple sensitivity about +54 μV/°C at 0°C.

Classification of thermocouple types is associated with their useable temperature range, sensitivity and accuracy. The commonly used materials are chromium, copper, nickel, iron, platinum, and rhenium. Commonly known thermocouples are K-type, J-type, E-type, and T-type. K-type thermocouple is made of chromel and alumel, J-type thermocouple is made of iron and constantan, E-type thermocouple is made of chromel and constantan, T-type thermocouple is made of copper and constantan [36].

Experimental Dosimetry 419

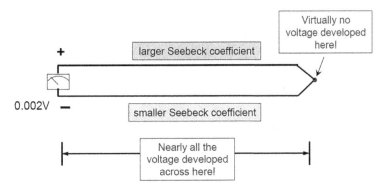

FIGURE 10.14
Thermocouple having different Seebeck coefficients [34].

TABLE 10.3

The Seebeck Coefficients (Thermoelectric Sensitivities) of Some Common Materials at 0°C (32°F)

Material	Seebeck Coeff.[a]	Material	Seebeck Coeff.[a]	Material	Seebeck Coeff.[a]
Aluminum	3.5	Gold	6.5	Rhodium	6.0
Antimony	47	Iron	19	Selenium	900
Bismuth	−72	Lead	4.0	Silicon	440
Cadmium	7.5	Mercury	0.60	Silver	6.5
Carbon	3.0	Nichrome	25	Sodium	−2.0
Constantan	−35	Nickel	−15	Tantalum	4.5
Copper	6.5	Platinum	0	Tellurium	500
Germanium	300	Potassium	−9.0	Tungsten	7.5

[a] Units are μV/°C

Thermal responses of several different types of thermocouples are shown in the chart below [Figure 10.15]. The useful temperature range of the copper-constantan "type T" thermocouple is limited as compared to the other thermocouples. Different types of thermocouples have different sensitivities and linearity ($\Delta V/\Delta T$). Thermocouples having a more limited temperature range are inclined to have better linearity characteristics [37]. Some higher temperature thermocouples are not intended for measuring temperatures below 0°F(−18°C) because of poor linearity.

Figure 10.15 Thermal responses of several different types of thermocouples (E-type: Chromel–Constantan, J-type: Iron–Constantan, T-type: Copper–Constantan, K-type: Chromel–Alumel, C-type: Tungsten 5% Rhenium–Tungsten 26% Rhenium, R-type: Platinum 13% Rhodium–Pure Platinum, S-type: Platinum 10% Rhodium–Pure Platinum).

Due to their small size and thus small thermal mass, thermocouples have much faster response time (several to tens of milliseconds range) and larger dynamic range than either thermistors or calorimeters. They also exhibit a higher level of sensitivity than thermistor RF power sensors and for that reason they can be used for detecting power levels down to several microwatts.

On the other hand, their relatively low sensitivity (usually 50 μV/°C (28 μV/°F)) limits their usefulness when the RF power level is less than several microwatts. The thermocouple represents a low impedance source, as the thermal noise voltage is proportional to the resistance.

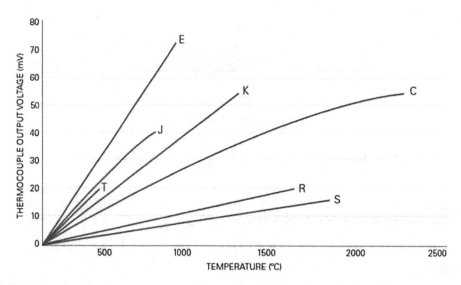

FIGURE 10.15
Thermal responses of several different types of thermocouples (E-type: Chromel–Constantan, J-type: Iron–Constantan, T-type: Copper–Constantan, K-type: Chromel–Alumel, C-type: Tungsten 5% Rhenium–Tungsten 26% Rhenium, R-type: Platinum 13% Rhodium–Pure Platinum, S-type: Platinum 10% Rhodium–Pure Platinum) [36].

Long cable lengths may require a shield and grounding to bring noise down to an acceptable level. The longer the cable, the more susceptible it is to radiated noise. This problem can also be improved by better signal filtering, and analog-to-digital conversion but it cannot be eliminated. Thermocouple meters generally average 100 points for each measurement, which will increase the signal-to-noise ratio (SNR) by approximately 10 because the noise goes down proportionally to the square root of the number of averaged samples.

Like other sensors, thermocouples also require calibration with a precision source. Since they are typically DC blocked, this precision source must be a low frequency AC source.

10.3.3.1.3 Calorimeters

Calorimeters are often considered the most accurate and traceable of power measurement systems over a wide range of frequency and power levels. The calorimeter includes a liquid cooled RF load that absorbs the RF energy. This load is kept in a heat exchanger, and a closely coupled thermopile is used to sense the change in temperature by producing a DC voltage directly proportional to the applied RF power. A heat exchanger removes the heat picked up by the fluid and runs it off to ambient air or another liquid. The cooled fluid is then recirculated into the load in a closed loop.

Since the fundamental measurement is temperature, a calorimeter can provide highly accurate RF power measurements traceable to NIST. Even though these systems are highly stable and can handle very large power, they are slow to respond and heavy [40].

10.3.3.1.4 RF Thermistors and Bolometers

An RF bolometer is a system where the RF measuring element is a thermally sensitive object that produces an electrical signal dependent on temperature change. The most common systems currently use a thermistor, a thermally sensitive resistor, in a DC bridge system. The DC bridge is electrically balanced, and when an RF signal is applied to the thermistor element, the element heats up. As a result, dissipated power in the thermistor tends to lower the resistance and reduces bias to maintain the balance of the bridge.

Experimental Dosimetry

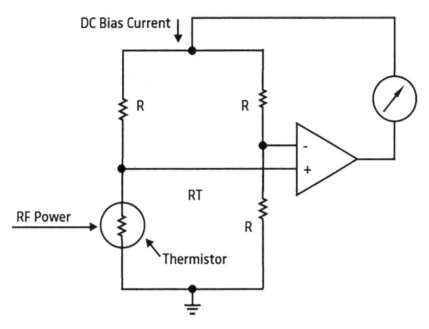

FIGURE 10.16
Thermistor sensor diagram [33].

The decrease in bias is related to the power absorbed by the thermistor. The total power dissipated by the thermistor is the sum of the power due to the DC bias and the incoming RF power. Thermistor's dissipation due to the DC bias can be measured by multiplying bridge current by bridge voltage and dividing it by four since the three other resistors have negligible temperature coefficient of resistance. And the power dissipated due to RF heating can be measured by subtracting this value (DC only power) from its total (DC + RF) power. Thermistors have linearity but they have a relatively small dynamic range (typical 10 µW–10 mW). Since the thermistor is equally sensitive to RF or DC power, using a precision DC source is helpful to produce a known power. By doing this, the balancing circuit can be calibrated relative to the DC power absorbed.

The circuit diagram of a thermistor sensor is shown in Figure 10.16.

10.3.3.2 Spectrum Analyzers

A spectrum analyzer is a specialized type of receiver, which displays the amplitude, power or a noise density of a signal on the y-axis versus the frequency of the signal on the x-axis. The frequency scale is in most cases linear; the vertical axes can be either linear or logarithmic. Thus, it could be considered a frequency-sensitive power meter; but still a spectrum analyzer (SA) cannot be classified as a true power meter, because it is intended to measure the power that falls within the resolution bandwidth filter while RF power meters typically measure the total power.

A spectrum analyzer breaks down a signal into its various frequency components and shows the strength of each component. A pure sine wave will only show a single peak while waveforms other than sine waves will show numerous peaks that correspond to the different frequency components that make up the waveform. There might be a large peak at the base frequency, followed by a series of other peaks at higher frequencies with lower amplitudes. Some commercially available spectrum analyzers are listed in Table 10.4.

TABLE 10.4

Some Commercially Available Spectrum Analyzers

Company/Model	Frequency Range	Min. Res. Bandw.	Amplitude Accuracy	Remarks
Anritsu				
MS2602A	100 Hz–8.5 GHz	—	1.1 dB	—
Avantek				
3365	100 Hz–8 GHz	10 Hz	—	Portable, tracking
3371	100 Hz–26.5 GHz	10 Hz	—	Portable, tracking
R3272	9 kHz–26.5 GHz	300 Hz	1 dB	External mixer 325 GHz
Hewlett-Packard				
HP4196A	2 Hz–1.8 GHz	1 Hz	1 dB	—
HP8590L	9 kHz–1.8 GHz	1 kHz	1.7 dB	—
HP8560E	30 Hz–2.9 GHz	1 Hz	1.85 dB	Portable
HP8596E	91 kHz–12.8 GHz	30 Hz	2.7 dB	—
HP8593E	9 kHz–22 GHz	30 Hz	2.7 dB	—
HP8564E	9 kHz–40 GHz	1 Hz	3 dB	—
HP8565E	9 kHz–50 GHz	1 Hz	3 dB	—
Marconi				
2370	30 Hz–1.25 GHz	5 Hz	5 Hz	With frequency extender
2383	30 Hz–4.2 GHz	3 Hz	1 dB	Tracking
Rohde & Schwarz				
FSEA30	20 Hz–3.5 GHz	1 Hz	1 dB	—
FSEB30	20 Hz–7 GHz	1 Hz	1 dB	—
FSEM30	20 Hz–26.5 GHz	1 Hz	1 dB	External mixer 110 GHz
Tektronix				
2714	9 kHz–1.8 GHz	300 Hz	2 dB	AM/FM demodulation 50 Ω/75 Ω
2784	100 Hz–40 GHz	3 Hz	1.5 dB	Counter 1.2 THz, external mixer 325 GHz

Source: Adapted from Webster, John G., and Halit Eren. 2014. Measurement, Instrumentation, and Sensors Handbook, Second Edition: Electromagnetic, Optical, Radiation, Chemical, and Biomedical Measurement.

Spectrum analyzers cover a broad range of frequencies and they give a quick analysis of the spectral power distribution of a signal. Also spectrum analyzers have a large dynamic range, a resolution bandwidth of a few hertz, and a feasible frequency resolution. A key attribute of a spectrum analyzer is its displayed average noise level (DANL). DANL also called as the sensitivity of the spectrum analyzer. In general, sensitivity ranges from –135 dBm to –165 dBm. Optimum sensitivity can be achieved by using the narrowest resolution bandwidth possible, sufficient averaging, a minimum RF-input attenuation, and/or a preamplifier.

10.3.3.3 Network Analyzers

The network analyzer with a probe system is first calibrated so that the reflection coefficient measurements are referenced to the probe's aperture plane, then the network analyzer is used for measuring the scattering parameters (*S*-parameters) while the exposure

TABLE 10.5

Some Commercially Available Network Analyzers

Company	Frequency Minimum	Maximum (GHz)	Method	Cal. Methods
Hewlett-Packard HP 8510	45 MHz	110	Heterodyne	SOLT, TLR, LRL, LRM, TRM
Wiltron	45 MHz	110	Heterodyne	SOLT, TLR, LRL, LRM, TRM
Rhode & Schwarz	10 Hz	4	Heterodyne	SOLT, TLR, LTL, LRM, TRM
AB Millimeterique	2 GHz	800	Heterodyne	TLR, LRL, proprietary

Source: Adapted from Webster, John G., and Halit Eren. 2014. Measurement, Instrumentation, and Sensors Handbook, Second Edition: Electromagnetic, Optical, Radiation, Chemical, and Biomedical Measurement.

chamber was either empty or loaded with a sample. S-parameters describe the electrical behavior of linear electrical networks. The output signal of the network analyzer includes values for the reflection coefficient (S_{11}) and the insertion loss (S_{21}). S_{11} is used to determine the Voltage Standing Wave Ratio (VSWR) and a value of zero means a perfect match (no loss). S_{21} represents forward gain between the input signal and the output signal.

A network analyzer that only measures the amplitude properties is called Scalar Network Analyzer. On the other hand, Vector Network Analyzers (VNA's) can measure phase as well as the amplitude response. Therefore, VNA's are very useful to characterize the exposure chambers in vitro studies. Some commercially available network analyzers are listed in Table 10.5.

10.3.4 RF Measurements

10.3.4.1 EF Measurements

EF measuring devices consist of a dipole antenna and a detector. Dipole antenna is preferred to be electrically and physically small in order to make measurements in high frequencies. The dipole can consists of a two pieces of wire or two short strips. And the detector diode produces a signal capable of being read by a meter [Figure 10.17].

The detector may be either a diode or a thermal sensor. Both of them are square law detectors which provide DC output proportional to the square of E field. The diode rectifies the generated RF voltage so that the monitoring device can store the value. Most commonly used thermal sensor is a thermocouple. Particularly, at higher frequencies and for higher fields thermocouples are preferred.

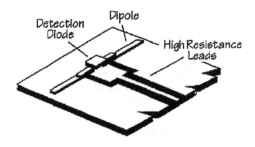

FIGURE 10.17
Dipole sensor [38].

Since the voltage difference between the dipole terminals is proportional to the E field parallel to the axis of the dipole, it is possible to obtain the strength of the E field by monitoring the voltage across the dipole terminals.

In order to transmit the voltage or current between the detector and the monitoring electronics, leads are being used. However, leads are very sensitive to the presence of E field. Therefore electromagnetic interference may occur. It is possible to reduce this interference by using high resistance leads and high impedance amplifiers in the monitoring device. Low-pass filters can be placed between the detector and the leads if further reduction of interference is desired. Also placing the leads perpendicular to the direction of the incident E field reduces the interference.

The dipole is sensitive only to the E field parallel to the axis of the dipole and the detector does not sense the E field perpendicular to the axis of the dipole. In practice, probes are often geometrically constructed into a structure of three orthogonal elements, one to sense the E-field in each direction. The summation of the DC outputs of all three sensor elements will give us the magnitude of the E-field.

10.3.4.2 Magnetic Field Measurements

H-Field measuring devices consist of two components, the pickup and the detector. The detector could be either a diode or a thermocouple [Figure 10.18]. For the H-field, the pickup is an electrically and physically small loop antenna. This small loop antenna is sensitive only to the H-field component perpendicular to the plane of the loop. A time-varying H-field produces a voltage in the loop which is proportional to the loop's area and the frequency of the H-field's time variation. Therefore, the loop should be large enough to be sensitive to weak fields at low frequencies. There is a trade-off here since the H-field probe should be small enough to minimize the perturbation of the field being measured.

Loop antennas may be sensitive to E-field if the loop is terminated by an electrical load. In this case, coupling of the electrical field component parallel to the plane of the loop occurs. This effect of E-field coupling can be minimized by the probe calibration.

H-field and E-field antennas are usually remote from the detector in order to minimize the perturbation of the measured field and electromagnetic interference, because leads can also cause unwanted pickup of fields in measurements. To overcome this problem, the

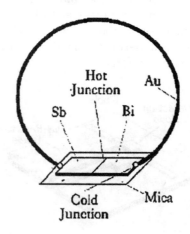

FIGURE 10.18
Thermocouple loop probe [38].

Experimental Dosimetry 425

conductive connection between the probe and the associated monitoring device can be replaced by fiber optic leads [38].

10.4 RF Dosimetry

RF dosimetry is the quantification of the magnitude and distribution of absorbed electromagnetic energy in biological objects which are exposed to RF fields. Absorbed energy is directly related to the EM fields inside the object. Depending on the size and shape of the object, its electrical properties, its polarization, and the frequency of the incident fields, the internal and incident EM fields can be quite different. In RF, the dosimetric quantity commonly used is known as Specific Absorption Rate (SAR).

10.4.1 SAR

The transfer of the energy from electric and magnetic fields to any object is defined in terms of the SAR. Although SAR is directly associated with heat absorption, it is also associated with local E and H intensity, so concept is useful in dosimetry associated with non-thermal as well as thermal mechanisms producing bioelectromagnetic effects. SAR is the time derivative (rate) of the incremental energy (dW) absorbed by (dissipated in) an incremental mass (dm) contained in a volume element (dV) of a given density (ρ).

$$\mathrm{SAR} = \frac{\mathrm{d}}{\mathrm{d}t}\left(\frac{\mathrm{d}W}{\mathrm{d}m}\right) = \frac{\mathrm{d}}{\mathrm{d}t}\left(\frac{\mathrm{d}W}{\rho\mathrm{d}V}\right) \tag{10.18}$$

SAR is expressed in the units of watts per kilogram (W/kg) and SAR is related to the EF at a point by:

$$\mathrm{SAR} = \frac{\sigma|E|^2}{\rho} \tag{10.19}$$

Where σ is the conductivity of the object (S/m), ρ is the mass density of the tissue (kg/m^3) and E is the rms EF strength (V/m). Therefore, if three of the quantities in Eqn (10.19) are known inside the object, the fourth also can be found easily at that point.

SAR is also related to the increase in temperature at a point by:

$$\mathrm{SAR} = \frac{c\Delta T}{\Delta t} \tag{10.20}$$

Where ΔT is the change in the temperature (°C), ΔT is the duration of the exposure (seconds), and c is the specific heat capacity (J/kg °C). The rapid conversion of the energy in the applied field to random motions of the ions and molecules means that in most cases the SAR is equivalent to a heat source that leads to a temperature rise which in turn can change chemical reaction rates. The local SAR represents the magnitude of the SAR in a small portion of an exposed biological object. The average (whole-body) SAR is the magnitude of the spatially averaged SAR throughout an exposed biological object [39].

The SAR is a function of the incident fields, the frequency, the geometry, and the properties of the absorber. It should be noted that not all RF incident on an object is absorbed since some is reflected. The peak SAR occurs for resonances at about 80 MHz for a standing man and at about 600 MHz for the rat for E polarization which means that the resonant frequency is related to the length of the body.

The SAR is generally higher for E-polarization, lowest for H-polarization and intermediate for K-polarization. According to a rule of thumb, the SAR is higher when the incident E-field is more parallel to the body than perpendicular to it and when the cross-section of the body perpendicular to the incident H-field is comparatively larger. However, for H polarization, the incident E-field is perpendicular to the body and the cross-section of the body perpendicular to the incident H-field is comparatively smaller. Both conditions lead to a lower average SAR.

10.4.2 SAR Measurements

Sometimes non-uniform exposures occur or incident power density cannot be measured. In such cases SAR is a way to measure RF energy absorption and that makes SAR very useful in dosimetry. There are several techniques to measure SAR in biological systems:

10.4.2.1 Measuring SAR with EF Probes

By using EF Probes in a tissue which is exposed to RF, we can measure SAR if dielectric properties of the tissue are known. This method is useful when measuring the SAR at specific point in the tissue. The average field strength can be measured directly with an implantable probe containing one or more diodes mounted on a dielectric substrate and attached with high resistive leads to a voltage measurement instrument.

10.4.2.2 Differential Power Technique

This method allows us to calculate absorbed power inside the radiation chamber by subtracting transmitted and reflected power from incident (forward) power. In glass and dielectric waveguides scattering losses also need to take into account due to end face roughness, surface roughness, and sidewall roughness. Differential power technique method is limited to closed exposure systems such as Transverse Electromagnetic Mode (TEM) Cells and hollow waveguides. In this method, power meters are connected to the exposure systems by directional couplers to measure incident, reflected and transmitted power. When live animals are exposed to RF fields inside the system, the values of those three measurements alter as animals move since absorption is a function of the animal's orientation relative to field polarization. The advantage of this method is that it provides real-time measurements of absorbed power. However this technique has a couple of disadvantages. First, when multiple animals are exposed to RF fields at the same time, the SAR result would give as average dose rate for the group instead of a value of individual animal. Thus, there may be substantial variability between animals and hot spots may not be observed. It's optimum to expose animals individually. Second, it may be impossible to measure the power absorption if the RF energy absorption rate is very low. The reason for that is the measurement error in the power meter exceeds the computed power difference.

10.4.2.3 Calorimetric Techniques

If we assume that all the RF energy absorbed by a biological target is converted to heat, then the calorimetric method measures the heat added to that biological target. In the

Experimental Dosimetry

initial stage, an animal cadaver is exposed to radiation with a short exposure at high power. By doing this, heat loss errors due to conduction and convection during the exposure are reduced. After that, thermalized energy added to the cadaver can be measured with calorimeter.

There are two well-known calorimetric techniques which are very helpful to measure average SAR in animal phantoms and cadavers. During the experiments, it has been assumed that there are no notable differences between the dielectric properties of the cadaver and the live animal. This may not always be the case, as discussed in Chapter 4.

10.4.2.3.1 Twin-Well Calorimetry

Twin-well calorimeters are instruments which measure average SAR very accurately. It consists of two-thin walled aluminum wells, each of which will accommodate a cadaver. Both wells are thermally insulated from each other and from the outside. In this technique, pairs of cadavers of identical in age and mass are used. In such a system, calorimetry errors are cancelled. Both of the cadavers are placed in a well of the calorimeter in equilibrium, a differential curve representing the residual differential body heat is produced as equilibrium is restored. A reliable exponential decay toward thermal equilibrium can be produced. The twin-well calorimeter measures the addition of heat introduced by the exposure. When a known amount of heat is added to one of the cadavers, superimposed on the decay portion of the initial differential curve, the added curved area can be calculated. Irradiations for dosimetry are made by removing both cadavers from calorimeter to their holders and exposing one of them and then promptly returning both cadavers to the calorimeter to measure the heat added to the exposed cadaver. The temperature difference between the wells is measured by a thermopile circuit and output of which is suitably amplified. The SAR is calculated from the measured caloric increase, cadaver mass, and the exposure time. The structure of twin well calorimeter is shown in Figure 10.19.

An improvement of the method reduced the measurement time and increased the accuracy by using the microprocessor system which controls the calorimeter. The microprocessor program controls the rate at which heat is applied to the unexposed cadaver. That way, equilibrium is established in as short a period of time using the twin-well calorimeter as a "thermal" balance [40].

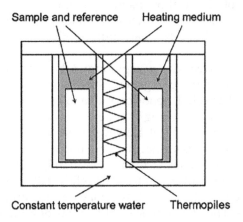

FIGURE 10.19
Structure of twin-well calorimeter [41].

10.4.2.3.2 Dewar-Flask Calorimeter

The Dewar-flask method of calorimetry is a relatively simple, straightforward way of determining the whole-body average SARs of animal cadavers [42]. This method uses the difference between the average temperature of the cadaver before and after being exposed to RF radiation. Irradiated cadaver is immersed in a Dewar-flask containing a medium at a known temperature. Water is usually used as a heat transfer medium. And then, the equilibrium temperature of the mixture is measured. Generally, in order to estimate the pre-exposed whole-body temperature of the exposed cadaver, calorimetry is conducted on a sham cadaver of similar weight. The whole-body temperature of the sham is then assumed to be the initial whole-body temperature of the irradiated cadaver. Finally, the whole-body temperature is determined from the theory of mixtures and the knowledge of the average specific heat capacity of the animal. The SAR in (W/kg) is determined by:

$$\text{SAR} = C_s \left[T_e \left(\text{exposed} \right) - T_e \left(\text{control} \right) \right] / \text{ exposure time in seconds} \qquad (10.21)$$

Where C_s is the specific heat of the cadaver and T_e is the rationalized temperature of the cadaver upon insertion in the calorimeter.

The method itself is simple by design, but it requires a long time to measure equilibrium temperature. The immersion of the cadaver can be done only once and two cadavers are needed for each SAR determination. Moreover, the average specific heat capacity of the cadaver must be known since the body's composition is complex and this capacity cannot be accurately determined.

10.5 RF *in vitro* Exposure Systems

10.5.1 TEM Cell

The TEM cells provide exposure conditions closest to free- space propagation of plane waves; it was introduced by Crawford in 1974 [43]. Both ends of a rectangular section of transmission line are tapered in order to adapt to round coaxial connectors. Its flat conductor ensures a TEM mode of propagation inside, up to the frequency at where higher order wave modes are excited. These higher order wave modes limit the usable bandwidth. The main advantages of a TEM cell are the quasi-uniform EF (*E*-field) inside and its versatility [44].

The coupling efficiency between the waveguide and the test object is frequently small, so that the high power may be required to get the desired exposure levels. The field homogeneity volume inside the TEM cell depends on the ratio between the cell's dimensions and the operating frequency band. Designing a proper experiment requires knowing the internal field distribution inside the TEM cell. However, measuring the field strength inside the cell can be tiresome and imprecise, since the field probe should be isotropic and electrically isolated, non-perturbing, and easy to insert even in rather inaccessible corners [45].

Desta et al. [46] exposed L929 murine fibroblast cells at 835 MHz to determine the effect of RF-radiation energy emitted by wireless phones on ornithine decarboxylase (ODC) activity in cultured cells. The exposure system consists of a model CC110 Crawford cell (height 47.8 cm, depth 22.9 cm, width 15.2 cm) and a sham-exposure chamber with similar dimensions. Forward power into the Crawford cell and reflected power from the Crawford

Experimental Dosimetry 429

cell are measured by HP 432A and HP432B power meters. After 8 hours of exposure to an average SAR from 1 W/kg up to 15 W/kg, no statistically significant difference in ODC activity was found between RF-radiation exposed and sham-exposed cells at non-thermal SARs.

Sarimov et al. [47] studied Human Lymphocytes by exposing them at different frequencies in the range of 895–915 MHz for 30 minutes and 1 hour. Lymphocytes are obtained from seven healthy people. Exposure was performed in TEM cell. Input, reflected and output powers are measured by using a power meter, Hewlett-Packard 435A and a coaxial directional coupler, Narda 3001–20. Then, based on these measurements, SAR is calculated. Results indicated changes in chromatin conformation and individual sensitivity of human lymphocytes to MW exposure.

Nikolovski et al. [48] reevaluated the TEM cell system developed by Litovitz et al. [49] and utilized by Penafiel et al. [50] for the exposure of cells in T-25 flasks at 835 MHz. The system, consisting of two Crawford TEM cells for simultaneous RF and sham exposure of four T-25 flasks per TEM cell, was modified to enable blinded exposures, forced cooling and repeatable positioning of the flasks. The overall average SAR within the medium of 6.0 W/kg at 1 W input power obtained as compared to the previous study reporting an average SAR within the medium of 2.5 W/kg at an input power of 0.96 W. The temperature increase of 0.13°C/(W/kg) reduced to 0.045°C/(W/kg) by applying active air flow cooling.

10.5.2 Rectangular Waveguide

Similar to the TEM Cell, the rectangular waveguide is quite a versatile structure. This exposure system consumes considerable less power. A rectangular waveguide supports TM and TE modes but not TEM modes and operates over a limited range of frequencies. Different configurations are also considered to determine the optimum orientation and positioning of the cell cultures inside the rectangular waveguide. For instance, system performance may be achieved when the rectangular waveguide is terminated by a matched load and EF is parallel to the sample. Also, rectangular waveguides are standardized in a variety of sizes and designations such as WG waveguide and WR waveguide to enable waveguides from different manufacturers to be used together [51].

Bismoto et al. [52] designed a thermostatted waveguide exposure system by using a rectangular cavity made of a waveguide (110 mm × 55 mm × 500 mm) and exposed 3 mL of myoglobin solution to 1.95 GHz microwave radiation for 2.5 hours at 30°C. The presence of the RF field did not cause any change in this spectral region, independently from the protein concentration that was variable in the range 1–20 µM.

Zeni et al. [53] exposed unstimulated lymphocyte cultures for 2 hours at 900 MHz. The exposures have been carried out in an exposure chamber which was made of a rectangular waveguide (124 × 248 × 500 mm) under strictly controlled conditions of temperature and dosimetry. The results indicated that 900 MHz RF fields failed to induce DNA damage in human peripheral blood leukocytes following acute exposure (2 h) at both 0.3 and 1 W/kg SAR values.

Gerber et al. [54] used WR 340 brass waveguide to expose T-25 flask, which contains the cell suspension at 2.45 GHz. The SAR for the system was between 9 and 11 W/kg and was monitored by the measurement of absorbed power in the culture medium. The temperature rise due to the RF (~0.3°C) is compensated by lowering the circulator temperature in the cell culture by same amount, so that it remained around 37°C. Dosimetry evaluation showed high SAR values such as 10 W/kg can be used without producing a temperature rise with the temperature-controlled waveguide.

Prisco et al. [55] designed exposure systems based on a simple WG structure. Four 8 ml samples and two 15 ml samples are exposed at 900 MHz. A temperature increase of 0.2°C ± 0.1°C is measured only in the 8 ml samples following a 1 h exposure with 1 W/kg SAR.

10.5.3 Radial Waveguide

A radial transmission line can overcome limitations in both TEM cells and rectangular waveguide since it can simultaneously expose large numbers of sample. Another advantage of these systems is the circular uniformity of the exposure.

The electromagnetic design of an example of this structure is discussed, and an extensively bench-tested realization is described in [56]. Referred to 1 W of net forward power, the following SAR data were obtained: at 835.62 MHz, 16.0 ± 2.5 mW/kg (mean ± SD) with range (11–22); at 2450 MHz, 245 ± 50 mW/kg with range (130–323).

Hansen et al. [57] was exposed a number of 120 hamsters with mobile communication signals at 383 and 900 MHz. The variation of the dissipated energy within the animals could be reduced to less than 30% though the objects were not restrained. Whole-body SARs of 80 mW/kg were applied. An extreme degree of uniformity together with a high-power efficiency due to the confinement of the radiation is obtained.

10.5.4 Horn Antenna

A horn antenna is widely used at microwave frequencies above 300 MHz. Horn antennas provide high gain, low VSWR and relatively wide bandwidth. Since these exposure systems allow many samples to be exposed simultaneously, they are useful for making large experiments. These are the principal systems currently used for frequencies over 2.45 GHz [58]. However, these systems have low efficiency due to the low-power incident densities and poor homogeneity.

Vijayalaxmi et al. [59] also used two horn antennas operating at 2.45 and 8.2 GHz to expose T25 flasks in an incubator inside an anechoic room. Exposures were conducted at 1.75 m from the opening of the antenna at a frequency of 2.45 GHz and 1.46 m at 8.2 GHz. Numerical dosimetry confirmed low efficiencies (0.1 and 0.34 (W/kg)/W at 2.45 and 8.2 GHz, respectively). SAR homogeneities were given in terms of a dose distribution function.

Peinnequin et al. [60] studied apoptosis by exposing Jurkat cells at 2.45 GHz by using a custom-made horn antenna (19 cm × 23 cm) in a horizontal direction. This device produces a homogeneous 5 mW/cm^2 field in cell incubator. These exposure conditions weakly increase cell culture media temperature by 0.1 ± 0.05°C. SAR is evaluated calorimetrically and it was 4 W/kg. Placing control plates in the left part of the incubator (near a microwave-absorbing screen) decreased microwave exposition to less than 0.1 mW/cm^2. Jurkat cell sensitivity to Fas-induced apoptosis was slightly increased under these irradiation conditions.

Acknowledgments

We thank Professors Frank Barnes and Ben Greenebaum for comments and suggestions on the manuscript.

References

1. Edelstein, A. 2007. "Advances in Magnetometry." Journal of Physics: Condensed Matter 19 (16): 165217. doi:10.1088/0953-8984/19/16/165217.
2. Markov, M. S. "Dosimetry of Magnetic Fields in the Radiofrequency Range." In Radio Frequency Radiation Dosimetry and its Relationship to the Biological Effects of Electromagnetic Fields, pp. 239–245. Springer Netherlands, 2000.
3. Durney, C. H., H. Massoudi, and M. F. Iskander. *Radiofrequency Radiation Dosimetry Handbook.* Salt Lake City: Dept Of Electrical Engineering, Utah Univ, 1986.
4. Vosteen, W. E. "A review of current electrostatic measurement techniques and their limitations." Paper presented at Electrical Overstress Exposition, San Jose, CA, 24–26 April, 1984.
5. Hill, D. A. and K. Motohisa. "Electric-Field Strength." In *Measurement, Instrumentation, and Sensors Handbook: Electromagnetic, Optical, Radiation, Chemical, and Biomedical Measurement,* edited by J. G. Webster and H. Eren, 1–12. Boca Raton: CRC Press, 2014.
6. Misakian, M. "Extremely Low Frequency Electric and Magnetic Field Measurement Methods." In Gaseous Dielectrics VIII, edited by L. G. Christophorou and J. K. Olthoff, 451–457. Boston, MA: Springer, 1998.
7. IEEE Std 1308–1994, *IEEE Recommended Practice for Instrumentation: Specifications for Magnetic Flux Density and Electric Field Strength Meters-10Hz to 3 kHz,* The Institute of Electrical and Electronics Engineers, Inc., New York (1994).
8. IEC Publication 833. Measurement of Power. Frequency Electric Fields, (International Electrotechnical. Commission, Geneva, Switzerland, 1987).
9. Misakian, M. "ELF Electric and Magnetic Field Measurement Methods." In *IEEE International Symposium on Electromagnetic Compatibility,* 150–155. Dallas, TX: IEEE, 1993. doi:10.1109/ISEMC.1993.473761.
10. Kunihisa, T. "Induction Coil Magnetometers." In High Sensitivity Magnetometers: Smart Sensors, Measurement and Instrumentation, edited by A. Grosz, M. J. Haji-Sheikh and S. C. Mukhopadhyay, 1–39. Switzerland: Springer International Publishing, 2017.
11. Fagaly, R. L. and A. S. Macintyre. "Magnetic Field Measurement." In *Measurement, Instrumentation, and Sensors Handbook: Electromagnetic, Optical, Radiation, Chemical, and Biomedical Measurement,* edited by J. G. Webster and H. Eren, 1–32. Boca Raton: CRC Press, 2014.
12. Ripka, P. 1992. "Review of Fluxgate Sensors." Sensors and Actuators: A. Physical. doi:10.1016/0924–4247(92)80159-Z.
13. Janicke, J. M. The Magnetic Measurement Handbook. New Jersey: Magnetic Research Press, 1994.
14. Caruso, M. J. and T. Bratland. 1998. "A New Perspective on Magnetic Field Sensing." *Sensors and Actuators: A. Physical* 15: 34–47. doi:10.1023/B:EDPR.0000034021.12899.11.
15. Primdahl, F. 1979. "The Fluxgate Magnetometer." Journal of Physics E: Scientific Instruments 12 (4): 241–53. doi:10.1088/0022-3735/12/4/001.
16. Ripka, P. 2003. "Advances in Fluxgate Sensors." Sensors and Actuators, A: Physical 106: 8–14. doi:10.1016/S0924-4247(03)00094-3.
17. Popovich, R. S. *Hall Effect Devices,* Second Edition. London: Taylor & Francis, 2003. doi:org/10.1201/NOE0750308557.
18. Macintyre, S. "Magnetic Field Measurement." In The Measurement, Instrumentation and Sensors Handbook on CD-ROM, 1999. doi:10.1201/9780415876179.ch48.
19. Lenz, J., and S. Edelstein. 2006. "Magnetic Sensors and Their Applications." *IEEE Sensors Journal* 6 (3): 631–649. doi:10.1109/JSEN.2006.874493.
20. Fagaly, R. L. "Principles and Technology of SQUIDs." In *Measurement, Instrumentation, and Sensors Handbook: Electromagnetic, Optical, Radiation, Chemical, and Biomedical Measurement,* edited by J. G. Webster and H. Eren, 1–15. Boca Raton: CRC Press, 2014.
21. Van Duzer, T. and C. W. Turner. *Principles of Superconductive Devices and Circuits.* New York: Prentice Hall, 1999.

22. Korepanov, V., R. Berkman, L. Rakhlin, Y. Klymovych, A. Prystai, A. Marussenkov, and M. Afanassenko. 2001. "Advanced Field Magnetometers Comparative Study." Measurement: Journal of the International Measurement Confederation 29 (2): 137–146. doi:10.1016/S0263-2241(00)00034–8.
23. Tumanski, S. 2011. Handbook of Magnetic Measurements. *Nature* 96. doi:10.1038/096087b0.
24. www.fcc.gov/engineering-technology/electromagnetic-compatibility-division/radio-frequency-safety/faq/rf-safety.
25. Webster, J. G., and H. Eren, eds. *Measurement, Instrumentation, and Sensors Handbook, Second Edition: Electromagnetic, Optical, Radiation, Chemical, and Biomedical Measurement.* CRC press, 2014.
26. Hooker, G. 1995. "A Practical Guide to the Determination of Human Exposure to Radiofrequency Fields." *Occupational and environmental medicine* 52 (7): 496.
27. Gajšek, P. "Radiofrequency Measurements and Sources." In *Radio Frequency Radiation Dosimetry and Its Relationship to the Biological Effects of Electromagnetic Fields,* 309–319. Springer Netherlands, 2000.
28. *IEEE Std C95.3-2002 (Revision of IEEE Std C95.3-1991): IEEE Recommended Practice for Measurements and Computations of Radio Frequency Electromagnetic Fields with Respect to Human Exposure to such Fields,100 kHz–300 GHz.* S.l.: IEEE, 2002.
29. Hurt, W. D. "Absorption Characteristics and Measurement Concepts." In Radio Frequency Radiation Dosimetry and Its Relationship to the Biological Effects of Electromagnetic Fields, 39–52. Springer Netherlands, 2000.
30. Gabriel, C., S. Gabriel, and E. Corthout. 1996. "The Dielectric Properties of Biological Tissues: I. Literature Survey." *Physics in Medicine and Biology* 41 (11): 2231.
31. Pethig, R. 1996. "Dielectrophoresis: Using Inhomogeneous AC Electrical Fields to Separate and Manipulate cells." *Critical Reviews in Biotechnology* 16(4): 331–348.
32. Dunsmore, J. P. *Handbook of Microwave Component Measurements: With Advanced VNA Techniques.* John Wiley & Sons, 2012.
33. www.boonton.com/~/media/Boonton/Reference%20Guides/WTG_RefGuide_F1128_sm_web.ashx.
34. www.ti.com/lit/ml/slyp161/slyp161.pdf.
35. http://www.ni.com/white-paper/53184/en/.
36. www.efunda.com/designstandards/sensors/thermocouples/thmcple_theory.cfm.
37. Morris, A. S. 2001. "Measurement and Instrumentation Principles." Measurement Science and Technology 12(10): Oxford: Butterworth Heineman, 475 pp.
38. Cecelja, F. 1998. "Experimental Dosimetry for High Frequencies." *Measurement and Control* 31 (6): 179–184.
39. Chou, C. K., H. Bässen, J. Osepchuk, G. Balzano, R. Petersen, M. Meitz, R. Cleveland, J. Lin, and L. Heynick. "Radio Frequency Electromagnetic Exposure." *Journal of Bioelectromagnetics* 17 (1996): 195–208.
40. Elder, J. A. and D. F. Cahill, eds. *Biological Effects of Radiofrequency Radiation.* Health Effects Research Laboratory, Office of Research and Development, US Environmental Protection Agency, 1984.
41. Akiyama, T., K. Wake, T. Arima, S. Watanabe, and T. Uno. Whole-body averaged SAR measurements for small phantom by calorimetric method. In 2012 *International Symposium on Antennas and Propagation (ISAP)*, 692–695. IEEE, 2012.
42. Padilla, Jimmy M., and R. R. Bixby. Using Dewar-flask calorimetry and rectal temperatures to determine the specific absorption rates of small rodents. No. USAFSAM-TP-86-3. SCHOOL OF AEROSPACE MEDICINE BROOKS AFB TX, 1986.
43. Crawford, M. L. 1974. "Generation of Standard EM Fields Using TEM Transmission Cells." *IEEE transactions on Electromagnetic Compatibility* 4: 189–195.
44. Iftode, C. and S. Miclaus. 2012. "Design and Validation of a TEM Cell Used for Radiofrequency Dosimetric Studies." *Progress In Electromagnetics Research* 132: 369–388.
45. Guy, A. W., C. K. Chou, and J. A. McDougall. 1999. "A Quarter Century of In Vitro Research: A New Look at Exposure Methods." *Bioelectromagnetics* 20 (8): 522–522.

Experimental Dosimetry

46. Desta, A. B., R. D. Owen, and L.W. Cress. 2003. "Non-thermal Exposure to Radiofrequency Energy from Digital Wireless Phones Does Not Affect Ornithine Decarboxylase Activity in L929 Cells." *Radiation Research* 160 (4): 488–491.

47. Sarimov, R., L. O. G. Malmgren, E. Marková, B. R. R. Persson, and I. Y. Belyaev. 2004. "Nonthermal GSM Microwaves Affect Chromatin Conformation in Human Lymphocytes Similar to Heat Shock." *IEEE Transactions on Plasma Science* 32 (4): 1600–1608.

48. Nikoloski, N., J. Fröhlich, T. Samaras, J. Schuderer, and N. Kuster. 2005. "Reevaluation and Improved Design of the TEM Cell In Vitro Exposure Unit for Replication Studies." *Bioelectromagnetics* 26 (3): 215–224.

49. Litovitz, T. A., D. Krause, M. Penafiel, E. C. Elson, and J. M. Mullins. 1993. "The Role of Coherence Time in the Effect of Microwaves on Ornithine Decarboxylase Activity." *Bioelectromagnetics* 14 (5): 395–403.

50. Penafiel, L. M., T. Litovitz, D. Krause, A. Desta, and J. Michael Mullins. 1997. "Role of Modulation on the Effect of Microwaves on Ornithine Decarboxylase Activity in L929 Cells." *Bioelectromagnetics* 18 (2): 132–141.

51. Ramo, S., J. R. Whinnery, and T. Van Duzer. *Fields and Waves in Communication Electronics.* John Wiley & Sons, 2008.

52. Bismuto, E., F. Mancinelli, G. d'Ambrosio, and R. Massa. 2003. "Are the Conformational Dynamics and the Ligand Binding Properties of Myoglobin Affected by Exposure to Microwave Radiation?" *European Biophysics Journal* 32 (7): 628–634.

53. Zeni, O., M. Romano, A. Perrotta, M. B. Lioi, R. Barbieri, G. d'Ambrosio, R. Massa, and M. R. Scarfi. 2005. "Evaluation of Genotoxic Effects in Human Peripheral Blood Leukocytes Following an Acute In Vitro Exposure to 900 MHz Radiofrequency Fields." *Bioelectromagnetics* 26 (4): 258–265.

54. Gerber, H. L., A. Bassi, M. H. Khalid, C. Q. Zhou, S. M. Wang, and C. C. Tseng. 2006. "Analytical and Experimental Dosimetry of a Cell Culture in T-25 Flask Housed in a Thermally Controlled Waveguide." *IEEE Transactions on Plasma Science* 34 (4): 1449–1454.

55. De Prisco, G., G. d'Ambrosio, M. L. Calabrese, R. Massa, and J. Juutilainen. 2008. "SAR and Efficiency Evaluation of a 900 MHz Waveguide Chamber for Cell Exposure." *Bioelectromagnetics* 29 (6): 429–438.

56. Moros, E. G., W. L. Straube, and W. F. Pickard. 1999. "The Radial Transmission Line as a Broad-Band Shielded Exposure System for Microwave Irradiation of Large Numbers of Culture Flasks." *Bioelectromagnetics* 20 (2): 65–80.

57. Hansen, V. W., A. K. Bitz, and J. R. Streckert. 1999. "RF Exposure of Biological Systems in Radial Waveguides." *IEEE Transactions on Electromagnetic Compatibility* 41 (4): 487–493.

58. Paffi, A., F. Apollonio, G. A. Lovisolo, C. Marino, R. Pinto, M. Repacholi, and M. Liberti. 2010. "Considerations for Developing an RF Exposure System: A Review for In Vitro Biological Experiments." *IEEE Transactions on Microwave Theory and Techniques* 58 (10): 2702–2714.

59. Vijayalaxmi. 2006. "Cytogenetic Studies in Human Blood Lymphocytes Exposed in Vitro to 2.45 GHz Or 8.2 GHz Radiofrequency Radiation." *Radiation Research* 166 (3): 532–538.

60. Peinnequin, A., A. Piriou, J. Mathieu, V. Dabouis, C. Sebbah, R. Malabiau, and J. C. Debouzy. 2000. "Non-thermal Effects of Continuous 2.45 GHz Microwaves on Fas-Induced Apoptosis in Human Jurkat T-Cell Line." *Bioelectrochemistry* 51 (2): 157–161.

11

Overcoming the Irreproducibility Barrier: Considerations to Improve the Quality of Experimental Practice When Investigating the Effects of Low-Level Electric and Magnetic Fields on In Vitro Biological Systems

Lucas Portelli
Kirsus Institute, Zürich

CONTENTS

11.1 Introduction 435
11.2 Some Additional Spatio-temporal Considerations of *In Vitro*
 Bioelectromagnetic Experimentation 437
    11.2.1 Culture Container Architecture Considerations 438
    11.2.2 Electric and Magnetic Field Dosimetry Considerations 439
    11.2.3 Culture Medium Dynamic Factors 444
    11.2.4 Cell Cultures Dynamic Factors 444
    11.2.5 Additional Dynamic Factors 447
11.3 Concepts on Monitoring and Controlling Dynamic and Complex
 Bioelectromagnetics Systems 448
11.4 Uncertainty, Variation, Validation, and Quality Assurance 449
11.5 Experimental Design, Implementation, and Reporting Considerations 452
    11.5.1 The Sensitivity Approach to Causality 453
    11.5.2 The Human Factor 453
11.6 Conclusions 454
Acknowledgments 455
References 455

11.1 Introduction

Reports of biological effects of low-level electric and magnetic effects have been generated for the last ~50 years with emphasis on one or more of the multiple branches of the sciences involved in bioelectromagnetics. For some of these observations, reproducibility has been elusive, to the point of affecting consensus of the scientific community, policy, funding, and further research in this discipline. To explain, and ultimately transcend this occurrence, one may refer to the present-day replication crisis in biological and medical sciences alone, where it is proposed that a large portion of contemporary studies is irreproducible [Begley and Ellis, 2012; Freedman and Inglese, 2014]. The reason behind these observationns are numerous and may be linked back to fundamental errors in experimental design in general [Colquhoun, 2014; Halsey et al., 2015; Ioannidis, 2005; Loiselle and Ramchandra, 2015]. While suggestions and recommendations to amend those fundamental errors exist, they have been primarily aimed and limited at helping remedy those general sources of experimental variability and irreproducibility from the traditional biological experimentation point of view [Foster and Skufca, 2016].

Bioelectromagnetics is a branch of science which attempts to study complex phenomena by harmonizing diverse tools and research cultures from Physics, Chemistry, Biology, and several engineering disciplines at unison. Therefore, one can argue that practical bioelectromagnetics experimentation may involve additional factors and complications than those found in "traditional" disciplines (which in fact, it does) [Paffi et al., 2015a, b]. However, while such extra factors and complications entail further possibility for error, they also offer the possibility for improvement. This has been the view of many dedicated bioelectromagnetics researchers over the years who have produced a wealth of resources containing advancements of many aspects of experimental design, performance, and reporting [Bassen et al., 1992; Bassett et al., 1974; Kaune, 1995; Kuster and Schönborn, 2000; Markov, 2017; Misakian et al., 1993c; Negovetic et al., 2005; Simkó et al., 2016; Valberg, 1995; Vijayalaxmi, 2016]. Such references show many of the traditional and more specific pitfalls and solutions endemic to bioelectromagnetics research. However, regardless of this available wealth of specific and general information on the subject, experimental variability seems to still be very prominent [Lin, 2014a, b]. Perhaps, as a result of this, an increasing number of researchers are coming into the realization that experimental replication and testing of mechanistic ideas is unavoidably dependent on the quality of the experimental performance and reporting [Hiscock et al., 2017].

In essence, this chapter assumes that the root of experimental variability and irreproducibility may rely on the notions that:

- Cellular systems are perhaps the most complex machines we are aware of, and as such, we do not yet have a sufficient understanding of many of its structures, interconnections, or functions. The relevant operation timeframes and spatial details of these systems span for several orders of magnitude (μm to cm and μs to days) with nonlinear and feedback (feed forward) loop architectures which as a result exhibit great potential for amplification, with recursive, memory, delay, and resonance traits [Barnes and Kandala, 2018; Gomez-Cabrero and Tegnér, 2017; Kwok, 2010; Lazebnik, 2004].

- Bioelectromagnetics experimental design, validation, performance, and reporting are based on some (presumably adequate) degree of spatio-temporal approximations of the actual physical phenomenon and system under study (reductionist approach) [Ahn et al., 2006] for which scientific justification is many times unclear, unjustified, or based on technical limitations.

- The mechanism (or most likely mechanisms) by which low-level electric and magnetic fields affect cellular systems is not yet established [Barnes, 2017; Barnes and Greenebaum, 2015, 2016, 2017; Binhi and Prato 2017a, b, 2018; Hiscock et al., 2017; Kattnig, 2017; Krylov and Larkin, 2017].

- Cellular systems respond to changes in their internal and immediate external environment only (the *microenvironment*) [Barthes et al., 2014].

Overcoming the Irreproducibility Barrier

- Bioelectromagnetics experiments have been shown to have contradictory outcomes and the existing cohort of data is not of sufficient quality to rule out the existence of biological effects [Greenebaum, 2017; Portelli, 2017; Portelli et al., 2017a; Simkó et al., 2016].

These notions result in the several (not necessarily uncorrelated) realizations:

- The current degree of spatio-temporal resolution of physical, chemical, and biological factors adopted to generate the models which used for designing, simulating, validating, performing, interpreting, and reporting contemporary experimental bioelectromagnetics research may not be sufficient to accurately reproduce the relevant cellular functions and environmental factors from the cells perspective [Portelli et al., 2017a]. For example, our basic understanding of the factors defining macrodosimetric electric and magnetic (and other environmental parameters) exposure may not be sufficient to assess microdosimetric exposure at the cellular level [Hart and Palisano, 2017].
- Our incomplete understanding of the mechanism of interaction of these fields with biological systems (should it exist), and our incomplete (or approximated) understanding of the biological system itself, obscures the relationship between macrodosimetric exposure and actual biologically relevant dose, substantially complicating the relative significance of experimental results [Hansson Mild and Mattsson, 2017].
- The extreme complexity, uncertainty, and variability associated with bioelectromagnetics experimentation as a whole is prone to undermine the evidence of causality, which can only be asserted via sensitivity and uncertainty analysis of competing factors (but which is seldom performed satisfactorily) [Miller, 2017; Vaughan and Weaver, 2005].

By considering these premises, one can at least partially visualize how the current uncertain state of the art, although discouraging, is not surprising. With this in mind, the author makes an attempt at listing some additional details which can be useful for the focused bioelectromagnetics researcher when attempting to break the irreproducibility barrier. As such, the goal of this chapter is not to start with known fundamentals of bioelectromagnetics practical experimentation, for which material can be found in the works cited throughout this chapter. Instead it aims to compile, complement, and emphasize some additional concepts and factors which may be influential in generating and perpetuating the current experimental irreproducibility and variability in our field and which must be kept in mind to finally transcend it. Although this chapter has been focused in *in vitro* and low-level Extremely Low Frequency exposures, its conclusions and recommendations may extend to exposures on other ranges of the electromagnetic spectrum accordingly.

11.2 Some Additional Spatio-temporal Considerations of *In Vitro* Bioelectromagnetic Experimentation

All biological processes depend on environmental conditions with different degrees of sensitivity. Therefore, isolation of such systems from their surrounding environment (minimizing input-output unknowns to-and-from the system being studied) is fundamental in order to enable its characterization and further scientific scrutiny. Once the system under study is decoupled from the environment, a cohort of such parameters (including some specific stimulus) is re-introduced in a controlled, predictable, and monitored manner. pH, temperature, protein concentration, mechanical forces (flow, vibration, pressure), and some forms of electric and magnetic fields have been shown to be substantially influential to biological systems under this approach [Horswill et al., 2007].

Many experiments on cell biology, microbiology, and molecular biology are almost always performed inside or with the aid of standard laboratory incubation systems which serve to create controlled physical environments that partially emulate natural or special conditions in a repeatable manner. It is important to acknowledge that such factors are only important in reference to the environment that is inside the cell or in immediate proximity to the cellular surface (i.e., within the cellular microenvironment). Within these minute spatial domains, physical, chemical, and biological factors form structures, substantial gradients, and time-dependent processes and transients, which can signal cells in a multitude of ways [Keenan and Folch, 2008]. Such complex and minute details in the cellular microenvironment are essential to the kinetics of cell growth, development, and function and therefore on clinical outcomes [Barthes et al., 2014].

It is expected, that once under sufficiently controlled environmental conditions, groups of cellular and microbiological cultures can be grown and maintained with reasonably predictable outcomes. However, within these artificial microenvironments, the observation of effects is only possible when the biological reaction is sufficiently large to overcome the noise resulting from the inherent fluctuations and inhomogeneities imposed by the exposure system itself. In this regard, there are several considerations which may be important to consider. Some of them are described below.

11.2.1 Culture Container Architecture Considerations

A fundamental part of the cellular microenvironment under the control of the researcher is the culture container (e.g., Petri dish, flasks). In full organisms, cells are usually in a state of collaboration ruled by complex positive and negative control loops within specific structures in which microenvironmental parameters are generated and regulated. However, this is in great part silenced in the case of unorganized cells *in vitro* as culture containers' microenvironments are, in principle, considerably simpler that those observed *in vivo*. Here these parameters are less complex as they contain less and smaller influences of competing molecular change [Vaughan and Weaver, 2005]. Therefore, in principle, microenvironments in culture spaces generated for *in vitro* experimentation can be controlled within tighter boundaries and therefore present fewer obstacles in the event of replication of such conditions (in great part a result of artificial design).

However, naturally, the notion of replication depends on the rigorousness of the accuracy and precision under which such replication is deemed successful. In this sense, microenvironmental details may not be well described by typical macroenvironmental observations, measurements, or approximations form the sense that the biological response to the omitted details is bounded within reasonable (and known) limits. Although the use of such containers is so widespread and standardized, small differences in their surface micro- and nanotopographies are normal, and cell viability and behavior can vary significantly as a function of the material properties to which cells adhere. For example, several authors have pointed out that cultures behave differently between glass and polystyrene containers, so much to the point of irreproducible results [Blackman, 2017; Marinkovic et al., 2016].

Overcoming the Irreproducibility Barrier 439

One study systematically characterized the features of the culture surfaces on polystyrene culture containers (e.g., roughness and wetness), showing substantial differences between commercial manufacturers. Most importantly, this study showed differences in doubling time ranging from 5% to 80% for of human mesenchymal cells, solely as a function of manufacturer (and hence, as a function of the culture surface materials and/or features) [Zeiger et al., 2013]. Differences of similar order were observed depending on the surface treating method [Hosoya et al., 2017], additional surface coatings and additives, some of which are routinely added to polystyrene containers with the goal of enhancing cell adhesion and differentiation, while only to very specific cell lines [Marinkovic et al., 2016]. Many of the forms of 3D cultures are more desirable to test some drug efficacies since they allow the generation of more physiologically relevant (but not less complex) microenvironments. However, differences of the same order are reported for systematic studies comparing conventional 2D cultures with multiple 3D modalities [Breslin and O'Driscoll, 2016; Luca et al., 2013].

A commonly applied (and simple) strategy to mitigate such effects is to consistently use the same culture architecture, method and container manufacturer throughout experiments (following protocol). However, such approach only transfers the responsibility to the manufacturer and their quality assurance capabilities, rather than the researcher himself. Therefore, this approach, while comfortable and practical, should be used with caution. Ideally, the researcher should introduce a quality system which allows him to reasonably test the sensitivity of his cellular model to such variables periodically. This procedure, and its results, along with the culture container specifications should be well described in the experimental report, and upon replication, the researcher must be aware of such possible sources of variability.

11.2.2 Electric and Magnetic Field Dosimetry Considerations

With the exception of experimentation with static magnetic fields, induced electric fields will always appear in the wet culture container, with their magnitude, frequency, and spatial orientation depending on the specific factors involved. One must realize that, unlike the magnetic field, the induced electric field will present substantial distortions at the cellular level when compared with the applied or induced electric field calculated or measured from a macrodosimetric perspective. This becomes evident when analyzing known solutions for the Laplace equation describing the electric field resulting from the presence of a spherical structure with distinct electrical properties to the enveloping medium upon the application of a homogeneous electric field. Such configuration generates localized gradients along the two poles perpendicular to the applied field. This notion by itself makes most of the *in vitro* exposures performed in single-cell systems essentially non-homogeneous in nature when looked from the cell's perspective [Takuma and Techaumnat, 2010]. In general, the induced electric field is not always oriented along circles in a plane perpendicular to the magnetic field direction (i.e., circumferential). Even in a spatially nearly uniform magnetic field, the radially directed electric field may deviate substantially from direct proportionality with frequency [Polk, 1990]. An additional complication is that cell membranes are not smooth. They contain protruding microscopic structures (e.g., the glycocalyx in eukaryotic cells) which are electrically charged and therefore can transduce electrical signals to mechanical torques into the cytoskeleton (perhaps as an extension of the mechanism for detecting fluid shears). Heterogeneity in the induced electric field in the cell vicinity can have effects in cellular systems via interaction with these fields depending on their specific spatial distribution [Hart and Palisano, 2017].

A factor of potential importance is that cells exist as individual units in culture only under certain conditions (i.e., low seeding concentration, no aggregation, etc.). Given sufficient quorum, cells tend to aggregate and often form more complex structures which start to resemble their natural state. The simplest cases entail the formation of layers and clusters [Tremel et al., 2009]. More complex cases entail the formation of multiple morphologies of intricate designs with distinguishable different features in all three dimensions (see Figure 11.1). Such morphologies depend on multiple factors other than the type of biological organism such as culture container architecture (e.g. 2D, 3D, under flow, etc.), surface coating, extracellular stimulation, cellular quorum, etc. While these increasingly complex structures resemble more to the cellular natural state in terms of microenvironmental conditions (and also in terms of microdosimetric electric and magnetic field exposures), these microenvironments are not necessarily simpler, easier to replicate or less variable than in the cases where cells are isolated.

Several studies have explored the exposure differentials introduced by more detailed structures at the cellular, subcellular and multicellular scale in comparison with traditional

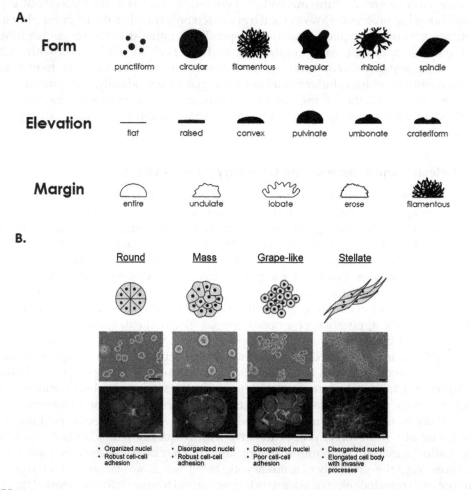

FIGURE 11.1
(A) Bacterial colony morphology diversity example. From: https://commons.wikimedia.org/wiki/File:Colony_morphology.svg. (B) Structure of 3D cultures formed by a panel of 25 breast cancer cell lines. From: [Kenny et al., 2007].

models. For example, numerical simulations have shown that the complexity of current flow near cell clusters can introduce significant induced electric field differentials in the vicinity of cell surfaces (c.a. ±50% for spherical cells). Differentials of the same order result from the introduction of dissimilar cellular shapes (spheres versus rods) [Hart, 1996; Hassan et al., 2003; Stuchly and Xi, 1994] and significantly dissimilar exposures are prescribed to cells in stacks or clusters [Hart, 2011; Wang et al., 1993]. Furthermore, the possibility of electrical coupling between cells, e.g., due to gap junctions, can considerably increase the induced electric field inside of cellular clusters, depending on multiple details such as the specific type of culture and the degree of aggregation [Fitzsimmons et al., 1994; Hart, 1996; Stuchly and Xi, 1994]. With regard of such numerical simulations, decreasing the complexity in non-symmetrical models as these (e.g., from 3D to its 2D geometrical equivalent) may show additional differentials in the induced electric fields distributions [Tarao et al., 1998].

It is important to realize that the results cited correspond to distortions resulting from imposing homogeneous electric fields to isolated cell models in conductive and homogeneous medium. In contrast, the electric field in practical exposure situations in bioelectromagnetics research is inherently inhomogeneous due to the presence of other cells in the vicinity and due to the size and shape of the culture container, medium composition and field generation systems (and their relative positioning in space). For example, when the imposed magnetic field is homogeneous and perpendicular to the culture plane for the case of adherent cultures (typically adhered to the bottom of the cell container), the induced electric field vortex will be located at the center of the culture surface and its magnitude will grow linearly as a function of the radius making electric field exposure variable for cultures (except for the case of annular culture containers where the gradient is significantly minimized [Liburdy, 1992]. As consequence, the number of cells, the magnitude and the direction of the electric fields to which cultures are exposed depends on the location of the cells within the culture container, where about 50% of the cells are exposed to electric fields that range from 0% to 70% of the maximum induced electric field on a round culture container (Petri dish). On the other hand, when the imposed magnetic field is homogeneous and parallel to the culture plane, the induced electric field vortex will be located on a line parallel to the culture surface and separated from it by about half of the height of the culture liquid. In this case, the electric field maximum magnitude is significantly diminished from the previous case, but most of the cells on the culture plane are exposed to reasonably homogeneous fields in comparison with the previous case [Bassen et al., 1992]. More homogeneous (or inhomogeneous) exposures can be achieved via customized culture containers or specially designed coil systems (e.g., annular ring culture wells [Liburdy, 1992], gradient coils [Makinistian, 2016], etc.). At this level, the introduction of small (but real) structural differentials in numerical models show that dosimetric estimations can be substantially different from the analytical solution and related approximations at certain frequencies. A simple example is the effect of the shape of the culture medium when inside a culture container, i.e., the meniscus, formed because of the surface tension of such liquid on contact with a gaseous medium [Schuderer and Kuster, 2003].

In addition, the presence of unwanted artifacts or extra components in the electric or magnetic fields in the culture environment can complicate resultant exposures if not properly controlled. For example, several systematic surveys have shown that the inherent static and time-varying background magnetic fields inside and around the typical biological laboratory environment and equipment, which may greatly differ from natural levels, can span over several orders of magnitude and exist in diverse spatial distributions. These fields have been shown to come as a result of power distribution and usage from point-sources (e.g., motors, heaters, relays, permanent magnets) as well as wide-sources (e.g., powerlines, building structure) [Gresits et al., 2015; Hansson Mild et al., 2003; Hansson Mild et al., 2009; Makinistian and Belyaev, 2018; Moriyama et al., 2005; Portelli et al., 2013]. These signals have been shown to have rich harmonic content including additional frequencies to the "nominal" frequencies that are normally considered during experimental design, validation, execution, and reporting. For example, several surveys have shown transients with components ranging from ~3 kHz to 10 MHz (intermediate frequencies) near powered equipment and an integral part of at least some of the experimental exposures studied [Aerts et al., 2017; Herrala et al., 2017; Portelli, 2012; Roivainen et al., 2014]. Equipment required for such measurements requires non-trivial effort as they pose additional complications due to the time-frequency diversity found in such fields [Knockaert et al., 2017; Setiawan et al., 2017a; Setiawan and Leferink, 2017b]. For this reason, their mitigation as well as complete characterization in bioelectromagnetic experimental reports is often lacking. In addition, the presence of those transients has been shown to interact in various ways with measurement devices resulting in substantial variabilities in their uncertainties [Leferink et al., 2016]. Additionally, sharp and localized gradients may exist within the bioelectromagnetics laboratory, instrumentation, and exposure systems in different ways. For example, very localized gradients can exist in the vicinity of sharp conductive materials (e.g., wires, edges) when these are immersed in an imposed electric or magnetic field [Lekner, 2013]. For example, numerical modeling has shown the appearance of large spatial gradients (>200%) in standard culture space locations which were generated from the interaction of an homogeneous imposed magnetic field and the microscope's objective and other parts [Chatterjee et al., 2001]. Interestingly, slight (1°) objective/coil misalignment have revealed distortion of the imposed homogeneous magnetic field of up to 193% several millimeters away from the focal plane, which in turn generated distortions in the induced electric field of up to 136% in homogeneous culture medium [Publicover et al., 1999]. Therefore, microscope objectives and similar instrumentation which have metallic components (springs, screws, studs, etc.) should be considered when evaluating the resultant electric and magnetic fields at the cellular level.

Another way in which unwanted spatio-temporal artifacts can be introduced is with the presence of partially magnetized (or saturated) ferromagnetic materials. These can exist in magnetically relevant coatings (e.g., nickel-chrome based) which may be part of traditional laboratory instrumentation (e.g., microscopes, etc.) and also part of magnetic shields which may be part of the exposure system in use. Many shielding architectures of the culture volume have been proposed over the years for bioelectromagnetics research and are treated in detail elsewhere [Misakian et al., 1993c; Portelli, 2012]. A caveat is that such materials can sustain sharp gradients in small spaces (μm range) for long times (which is the basis for magnetic recording technology [Speliotis and Morrison, 1966]) and introduce higher frequencies due to nonlinearities introduced by localized saturation and hysteresis [Celozzi et al., 2008]. In addition, such gradients can be generated by proximity to active currents in woven patterns such as Peliter thermal actuators and other semiconductors used for specialized culture applications [Portelli et al., 2017b]. Artifacts can be generated even by the existence of unwanted frequency components in the signal generation or amplification stages of the bioelectromagnetics exposure system if not properly isolated from the power distribution network and parasitic currents. To avoid these cases, sufficient decoupling on the design stage is fundamental.

In the same way, unwanted (and many times unaccounted) static and time-varying electric fields can be present in the culture environment fields inside and around the bioelectromagnetics laboratory environment and equipment due to accumulation of charge and

Overcoming the Irreproducibility Barrier 443

time-varying potentials. For example, electric fields can be generated by the potential drop of electrically powered equipment (e.g., motors, heating resistors, etc.) and even by the coils of the bioelectromagnetics exposure system when not properly shielded [Caputa and Stuchly, 1996]. In the latter case, these fields have been shown to be as high as 300 V/m in the culture space [Schuderer et al., 2004]. Sharp and localized electric field gradients are also possible in the vicinity of sharp conductors (e.g., wires, edges) when immersed in such artifacts [Lekner, 2013].

An important detail is that such extra sources of electric and magnetic fields are not necessarily in phase (especially currents on ground systems) and are generated in different points in space. As a result, this leads to the possibility of resultant fields in culture which are elliptically polarized. While this may be especially true near electrically powered equipment, like inside a typical biological laboratory, it is perhaps true for most of the fields found in human environments, rendering the linearly polarized fields as a special case only [Ainsbury et al., 2005; Deno, 1976; Kaune, 1995; Methner and Bowman, 2000]. In contrast, most bioelectromagnetics research design, performance, validation, and reporting assumes that the fields involved are linearly polarized with only a few exceptions [Burch et al., 2000].

Elliptically polarized fields can result in complex and inhomogeneous exposures on conductive medium (such as biological systems and wet culture containers) since the induced currents are highly dependent on the phase difference of the imposed fields [Matsumoto et al., 2000]. Because of this, investigating the effects of polarized fields *in vitro* requires extra considerations for which the reader is encouraged to refer to the references listed. Simplified calculations exist for aqueous medium, showing that when applying a homogeneous but circularly polarized magnetic field, the induced electric field vector will rotate with constant magnitude (never vanishing). In contrast, the induced electric field vector resulting from an homogeneous and linearly polarized field will only oscillate along a fixed direction (passing through zero) [Misakian, 1991; Misakian, 1997].

Measurement of polarized fields requires extra considerations. Single axis field meters may be used to measure the maximum magnetic field by orienting the probe until a maximum reading is indicated (in case measurements are performed only on one axis). In the case measurements are performed in three axes (either with a well-positioned one-axis field meter (orthogonal positioning within ~5° [Portelli et al., 2013]) or with three-axis meters), the resultant magnetic field (Root-mean-square (RMS)) is given by the sum of the squares of each orthogonal RMS field component. The maximum magnetic field is less than (circularly or elliptically polarized) or at most equal (linearly polarized) to the resultant magnetic field and the difference between the two quantities will depend on the degree of polarization. Such underestimation can be compensated by techniques which allow for the measurement of the angle between pairs of signals (some of them needing less than one complete cycle) [Micheletti, 1991]. In case accurate angular measurements are not possible, circularly polarized fields (worst case) will correspond to a resultant measurement which is larger than the maximum field by a factor of $\sqrt{2}$ [Misakian et al., 1993a]. While this is valid for band-limited signals, it can be extended to wider bands with additional effort.

From this section, one can see how the traditional practice of electric and magnetic field exposure assessment based on macrodosimetric approximations (homogeneous medium conditions) may disregard microscopic features capable of introducing substantial variations when examined from the cellular spatio-temporal point-of-view. Such cases can result in important differentials between applied fields and actual exposures at the microscopic level (and potentially doses, provided that such fields have biological relevance).

444   *Electromagnetic Fields*

More importantly, the reported exposures in past and current experimental literature as well as most current experimental design are based on macrodosimetric perspectives only. This can result, for example, in reported exposures which can be apparently identical from a macrodosimetric perspective while radically different from the microdosimetric perspective (for example, by having different levels of cellular aggregation, a factor that rarely reported with a substantial degree of certainty). Under these conditions, such apparently identical exposures could not be reliably grouped or compared, and in the case that the fields tested are biologically relevant, it could certainly lead to conflicting results. Therefore, improving traditional models to increasingly include the microenvironment details, as well as standardized methods to quantify, interpret, and report exposures from a microscopic perspective may help reproducing experimental conditions within tighter levels of accuracy and may also help to reach more reasonable levels of experimental reproducibility in bioelectromagnetics.

11.2.3 Culture Medium Dynamic Factors

Most experimental reports that deal with *in vitro* systems, typically describe the culture medium as homogeneous with predetermined (and invariable) electrical (and biochemical) properties. These quantities are reported based on direct measurements or on simple estimations (which sometimes are qualitative rather than quantitative). However, for a significant fraction of bioelectromagnetics experiments, there is the possibility that substantial changes can be introduced in its physical, chemical, biochemical and electrical properties [Freshney, 2010; Hahlbrock, 1975]. Such changes can come as a direct cause of the dynamic nature of cellular metabolism and environmental influences which depend on multiple factors of the experimental design and methodology (e.g., evaporation/condensation, chemical reactions with the environment (e.g., CO_2, light), cellular concentration, etc. [Grzelak et al., 2001]). In view of this possibility, the bioelectromagnetics researcher must be aware of the relative implications of such dynamic factors of the size of the biological effects studied.

11.2.4 Cell Cultures Dynamic Factors

Cell morphology (size and shape) is irregular and dynamic (see Figure 11.2). Cells regularly change shape and size as part of the necessary myriad of functions performed; and the degree to which these changes occur depends many factors, including the life cycle of the cell and cues from the neighboring microenvironment. These changes might happen in fractions of a second to hours and morphological differentials might range from infinitesimal to several cellular diameters depending on the specific cell in question. Because of this, the resulting exposure from a microscopic perspective can be highly variable on the same cell over the course of an experiment (See Section 11.2.2).

In addition to the individual cell morphology changes, cellular units divide and usually re-accommodate over the culture space introducing more variability in microdosimetric exposures [Weiss, 1945, 1961; Weiss and Garber, 1952]. During the course of an experiment, cell number differentials may range from a few percent in several days (e.g., neurons), to orders of magnitude in some hours (e.g., bacteria) and the cell division rate usually obeys environmental cues like cellular quorum usually being maximal during the "logarithmic growth" phase and more stagnant in other phases. Depending on the cellular system in question, some of them aggregate in a non-homogeneous way and form structures of diverse morphologies [Kirisits et al., 2005] while some of them remain solitary (e.g., blood

Overcoming the Irreproducibility Barrier 445

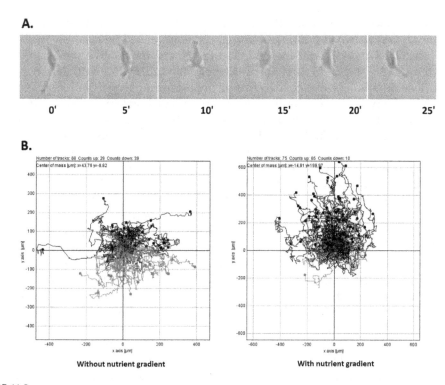

FIGURE 11.2
(A) Single HT1080 (human fibrosarcoma) cell observed over a period of 20 minutes (5 minutes intervals) showing morphological changes in all the observable surfaces. (B) Locomotion history of HT1080 cells over a period of several hours with and without nutrient gradients.

cells, amoebas) (See Figure 11.1). Locomotion velocities are varied and ranging from a few μm/hour (e.g., human connective tissue cells) to several hundreds of μm/second in some bacteria [Skoge et al., 2016]. These speeds (or any of the cellular behavior and function) are not constant, but depend on microenvironmental cues, such as pH, temperature, etc., which have optimal and sub-optimal combinations [Aly et al., 2008; Hobi et al., 2014]. There are secondary behaviors which may be also of interest. For example, the position of a cell within a group of cells (distance from the "wavefront" in 2-D migration) acts as a limiting factor to the velocity of cells, adding more complexity to the concept of cellular quorum [Tremel et al., 2009]. These facts together can result in substantially different (variable) and dynamic cellular microenvironmental spatial configurations over a period of time, unavoidably resulting in dynamic rather than static microenvironmental conditions and exposures (i.e., electric and magnetic fields, pH, biochemical concentrations, etc.).

Several factors need to be considered to minimize potential experimental variations in such inherently dynamic systems. For example, since relatively small differences can be amplified and compounded by biological processes over time; one such factor is to accurately control the initial conditions, such as cell numbers at the beginning of the experiment. In this regard, the ability to control such condition depends on the quality of the cytological methods and devices utilized. However, the quality of cell counts has been shown to be sensitive to various cell and medium physical properties (cell morphology (size and shape), electrical conductivity, light absorbance, etc.), operator (user), cell pre-processing methods (detachment (in the case of adherent cultures), dilution, and resuspension), concentration, and other details specific to the methods and devices used. Some comparisons between multiple manual, semi-automated, and automated methods have reported inter-device, inter-method, and inter-operator relative precision variabilities as low as in the single digits [Cadena-Herrera et al., 2015; Prathalingam et al., 2006]. However, it is perhaps safe to state that relative precisions ranging from 10% to 20% can be achieved with the typical methods available in common laboratory practice and relatively good care to exceptional care to detail [Camus et al., 2011; Ongena et al., 2010], while equal to larger variations are commonplace when more relaxed methodologies (standard to most laboratories) are employed. Several theoretical as well as practical methods have been proposed to improve these values for specific cases [Petrunkina et al., 2010]. In the case of automatic or semi-automatic counters, for example, calibration values are typically warranted which are specific to cell lines/types, concentration ranges, and medium utilized.

It must be kept in mind that most (if not all) such calibration and verification procedures do not provide direct means to improve (or measure) the accuracy of the methods and devices. Instead only relative comparisons based on applying the different methods to a sample used as reference (precision) which real or true number of cells (or particles) is not exactly known but also estimated indirectly. Such concepts are different. While accuracy quantifies the difference between a measurement and the true absolute value, precision quantifies the variability range of a measurement [Cork et al., 1983; Orear, 1958]. Put in simple and practical terms, for example: consider a batch of 100 cells (true number of cells) that is counted several times utilizing a certain device and method (resulting in estimations: 101, 99, 112, 87, 89, 92, and 95 cells). Then, a relative measure of the accuracy of the device and method utilized for such quantization can be calculated to be 3.6% (i.e., (|mean of the measurements − true number of cells|)/true number of cells) while a relative measure for the precision can be calculated to be ±7.9% (i.e., ±std. dev. (measurements)/true number of cells). The variations observed in the counts presented in this example are commonplace and stem from multiple sources which are specific to the devices and methods themselves. One fundamental complication is that the true number of cells (i.e., the number 100 in the example above) is not known in a practical situation. Instead, the best estimation of this number is the mean of the measurements performed. This fact only allows for the estimations of precision and accuracy to be relative for the devices and methods utilized, instead of absolute. The resulting limitation when utilizing standard counting devices and methods is that the possible comparisons are only relative, while the biological systems operate and respond to the absolute numbers.

As a partial solution to this problem, fields like hematology have explored the generation of quality standards involving the use of reference solutions in which the number of cells (or particles) is indirectly standardized via references and inter-comparison methods [Briggs et al., 2014; England et al., 1994]. However, how far away this is from the real true value in a practical case is not clear. In other words, in a typical biological experiment, the "known" number of cells is not completely known − but it only can be said that the number of cells in such experiment can be repeated within certain known range (if the same device and method are used in experimental replications). Therefore, being the case that absolute cell number calibrations are typically not possible, the cytometry methods must be described in detail in the experimental report in a way that such procedure can be repeated reliably.

Biochemical processes are another dynamic aspect of cellular systems which may be of importance. In recognition of the potential impact of this factor, additional effort is sometimes introduced in traditional biological experimentation to improve the size of the biological responses to some introduced stimulus. Many microbiological experiments,

Overcoming the Irreproducibility Barrier 447

for example, are performed in which the cell cycle has been synchronized via external (bio)chemical agents (or deprivation of such) [Futcher et al., 1999]. Besides cell cycle, there are many known sustained autonomous oscillatory biochemical processes [Brasen et al., 2012; Ehrengruber et al., 1996; Novák and Tyson, 2008; Petty, 2006; Rapp, 1979; Stark et al., 2007] with periods ranging from fractions of a second to days [Maroto and Monk, 2008]. Oscillations in intracellular and extracellular ion concentrations (e.g., CA^{+2}) [Falcke and Malchow, 2003], insulin production [Bergsten, 2002], and electrical potentials [Wachtel, 1985; Koshiya and Smith, 1999] are widely documented and studied examples. With this in mind, one may find certain support for the notion that, just as their (bio)chemical counterparts, electric and magnetic field exposures (and potentially the resulting true doses at the cellular level) are, in principle, also dynamic as the elicited biological responses would depend on the cellular biochemical status at that particular moment of exposure. Therefore, the bioelectromagnetics researcher must be aware of such inherent variations while at the same time trying to minimize the artifacts they can introduce.

11.2.5 Additional Dynamic Factors

Of the physical parameters composing the experimental exposure environment, temperature may be the most widely controlled in biological experimentation and perhaps the most universally influential. Previous measurement campaigns have shown not only static, but also oscillatory and transient differentials between and within culture containers ranging from fractions to several degrees and from several minutes to hours. The duration and magnitude of such differences depended on the container's size and shape as well as other multiple factors (type of incubator, relative positioning, forced flow effects, etc.) affecting the heat exchange rates between the environment and the culture medium. Additionally, such factors were also dependent on the type of perturbation (e.g., door opening, insertion, withdrawal, relocation) and the amount of medium [Portelli, 2017].

Static, transient or oscillatory thermal signals may be able to significantly interact with biological systems since chemical reaction rates are governed by forms of the Arrhenius equation, where the temperature dependency is exponential [Dewey, 2009]. Additionally, simple derivations from the Nernst equation (dealing with the fundamental balance of ion concentrations at the cell membrane) show direct dependence not on only the magnitude of the thermal differential, but in its rate-of-change ($\Delta T/\Delta t$) [Barnes, 1984]. Several lines of evidence show that small and transitory thermal differentials and signals can have biological relevance [Portelli, 2017, 2018; Portelli et al., 2017b]. As a result, transient and inhomogeneous thermal microenvironments in standard culture containers can potentially introduce undesired experimental variations. For example, small thermal differentials within (or outside) the culture containers may create local concentrations of nutrients and growth factors by changing the fluid dynamics within the dish [Paffi et al., 2015b]. Such can be the case of exposures under microscopes (where energy due to light irradiance is localized) or due to thermal transients and inhomogeneities introduced by the exposure system or handling protocols [Portelli, 2017]. In addition, such transients and differentials are different from those experienced *in vivo* where larger thermal constants and blood flow reduce the amplitude and frequency of possible perturbations.

The reader can imagine that transients or inhomogeneities in other microenvironmental factors such as forces (pressure [Akasaka and Matsuki, 2015; Johnson and Flagler, 1950; Marquis et al., 2012], vibration/sound [Muehsam and Ventura, 2014], shear stress [Martinez et al., 2016]), etc. also carry the possibility of resulting in substantial biological effects.

11.3 Concepts on Monitoring and Controlling Dynamic and Complex Bioelectromagnetics Systems

There are several microenvironmental variables which are (potentially) biologically relevant and therefore must be well characterized to be replicated within reasonable bounds. Therefore, it is easy to imagine that a fundamental technical recommendation for sensors is that they have the widest spatio-temporal capabilities (i.e., small, fast, accurate, and precise) to be able to be used *in situ* to perform real-time measurements in such microenvironments. In practice, however, some considerations must be kept in mind to minimize unavoidable variabilities, uncertainties, and substantial experimental design complications.

One such consideration is that practical measurements can only provide values which correlate to the true value of the target parameter only for certain conditions. Such conditions usually involve certain spatio-temporal limits within which special considerations must be taken. For example, electric and magnetic field artifacts in proximity with the experimental exposures (i.e., steep gradients, additional harmonics) may be hard to detect or characterize depending on the spatio-temporal limits of the designated sensing systems [Chatterjee et al., 2001; Misakian, 1993a; Publicover et al., 1999; Speliotis and Morrison, 1966]. In turn, such possible artifacts should be studied *a priori* via numerical simulation and calculations which at least provide bounds to spatio-temporal characteristics. In this way, proper actions can be taken from the design stage of the exposure system and meaningful validations can be performed within the abilities (uncertainties) of the instruments on hand. Additionally, sensors also introduce spatio-temporal distortions to the parameter measured and potentially to several others. For example, consider the case of a thermocouple in a Petri dish. This thermocouple, can introduce substantial changes (inhomogeneities) to the thermal time constant of the dish, potential biological (and chemical) contamination in the cultures and even elliptical polarizations can appear as a result of linearly polarized fields interacting with its conductive material [Lekner, 2013]. Therefore, all such potential issues must be thoroughly characterized to fully assess the relevance (and practicality) of the measurements performed.

In many cases, measurements *in situ* are not possible due to spatial constraints. In such cases, alternatives need to be implemented to estimate (directly or indirectly) these parameters within reasonable bounds. Numerical modeling is one alternative for estimation of bounds within which the system will perform as long as such models are subject to validation. In the case of monitoring, one alternative is to perform measurements in identical and parallel conditions. For example, if an experiment is to be performed in a six-well plate, a group of sensors can be placed permanently in one of the wells, while cell cultures are in the others during the duration of the experiment. The requirement for this experimental design relies on the researcher having done a calibration with identical groups of sensors in all six-well plates under controlled conditions that mimic those to be found during the experiment itself (i.e., same incubator, same exposure system, same handling, same medium volume, etc.). In this way, the measurements performed during the experiment (with the remaining group of sensors) will be bound by the uncertainty previously determined [Portelli et al., 2017b].

Another consideration is that biological systems have the ability to respond to short transients as well as to more long-lasting environmental differentials that take place during cellular culture, exposure, and handling (for all physical parameters involved). Therefore, monitoring and control need to be performed continuously and with enough resolution in both frequency- and time-domains. However, traditionally, close control and monitoring

Overcoming the Irreproducibility Barrier 449

of environmental parameters is limited to only the time-periods in which the experimental electric and magnetic fields exposures are performed. In many cases, such exposures comprise only a small fraction of the time in which the biological system exists in the timeframe of the duration of the experiment. For example, a typical experimental electric and magnetic field exposure could be comprised of exposing some cell culture for one hour a day, 5 days a week for 2 weeks, corresponding to only 10 hours out of a total of 336 hours, or only about 3% of the total time in which the cell exists in the culture microenvironment. In such case, the environmental parameters are recorded and controlled only for 3% of the total time, while omitting this data for the times in which the biological system is under "normal" incubation conditions. Environmental parameters during these "normal" periods can be much more variable than during exposures and therefore, the biological relevance of such stimuli greater than the electric and magnetic field exposures [Portelli, 2017]. Therefore, it is recommended that the "normal" incubation conditions also be thoroughly described, validated, monitored, and controlled. Additionally, to accurately record and monitor possible transients and long-standing differentials which may be biologically relevant, the bioelectromagnetics researcher may implement time-frequency recordings. Such type of solutions is being explored in the regulatory arena as an alternative to frequency-only electromagnetic compatibility limits [Knockaert et al., 2017; Setiawan and Leferink, 2017b; Setiawan et al., 2017a]. Additionally, these measurements may be combined using techniques which include additional spatial information [Bowman and Methner, 2000; Methner and Bowman, 2000].

In view of these unavoidable facts, a useful notion for the bioelectromagnetics researcher is that the best control for a parameter is to not have to control it (the same can be said about measurements). In other words, experimental systems and methods designs which minimize the environmental and experimental variations within a known range must be favored. This will not only minimize the need for technological complications, but also minimize the distortions and artifacts introduced by measurement equipment and even interaction with the samples. Finally, the considerations presented in this section may be extended to other environmental factors not explicitly mentioned without loss of generality and can help when designing the exposure system and experimental method to minimize unavoidable variabilities and uncertainties.

11.4 Uncertainty, Variation, Validation, and Quality Assurance

In order to understand the fundamental limits to which experimental conditions can be replicated, one needs to start with an analysis of uncertainty and variation of the experimental factors involved. Uncertainty and variation are different concepts. Briefly, uncertainty describes the probability distribution around a nominal value and is associated with the calibration and validation of the device in question [BIPM, 2008; Negovetic et al., 2005]. In other words, uncertainty characterizes the range of values within which the true value is asserted to lie (with some level of confidence). In the case of sensor measurements, the uncertainty budget can be interpreted as the combination of the precision and accuracy (bias, or distance from the true value) of that device and method.

On the other hand, variation refers to the variations from the measured mean but as a function of changes during exposure. Examples of exposures which have temporal and spatial variation arise in measurements near electrically powered equipment (when its function requires intermittence), habitational environments (due to human dynamics), experimental exposure of animals (due to movement around their cage), and similar situations [Misakian et al., 1993b; Negovetic et al., 2005; Portelli et al., 2013]. As another example, consider thermal measurements performed in a bioelectromagnetics exposure system. The sensor itself, may present a combined uncertainty (considering the sensor absolute and relative errors, method and additional factors needed to ascertain a temperature measurement) of 1°C over the range of interest (e.g. Gaussian distribution, $k = 2$) [BIPM, 2008]. However, during the whole course of the experiment, the temperature of the sample is expected to vary as much as ±3°C in time and have a homogeneity of ±30% within the culture container designated volume.

In practice, the use of a numerical model that describes the physical parameters involved (simulation) can be useful, but it can only be considered relevant once confirmed via real and trustworthy measurements (i.e., validated). In short, validation refers to a set of procedures which assure that the device and methods (or numerical simulations) in question are functioning within reasonable bounds, when analyzed, tested, or compared against known and trustworthy references. Another instance of system validation in bioelectromagnetics practice may be comprised, for example, of performing measurements of the magnetic field generated by a Helmholtz coil exposure system at a number of places defined in space with a calibrated reference sensor. To declare such validation as successful, the resulting magnitudes must fall within acertain range (determined by the combined uncertainty budget of the system) of the numerical simulation or analytical solution (if applicable), confirming that such field generation system is functioning appropriately. It is important to notice that the definition of such ranges (as well as the measurements performed as part of an effective validation procedure) must be performed under the same conditions under which the exposure system will be functioning. As a simple example, one may imagine that if an exposure system is comprised of a Helmholtz coil inside of a biological incubator, the measurements would have to be performed with the incubator operating under the same conditions as it would be during an experiment (e.g., fully functioning, door closed, etc.).

Ultimately, the uncertainty budget of the specific sensor and measurement method will delineate the restrictions (and quality) within which the validation is acceptable, by listing all variables that can affect its accuracy and precision. It is important to consider that such uncertainty budget will be valid as long as the conditions of the measurement to be performed are within those there stipulated. For instance, in the case of the measurement of electric and magnetic fields, the bioelectromagnetics researcher must be careful to fully characterize the sensors with sources which are similar to the sources that need to be validated in the experimental system. The reason is that the relative size, shape, and position of both the source and the sensor may have substantial impact in the measurement uncertainty [Misakian and Fenimore, 1996, 1997; Portelli, 2012]. For induction-coil-based sensors, for example, substantial uncertainty (>14% (1-axial) > 19% (3-axial)) is expected close or around (<3 diameters) small magnetic field dipoles (depending on relative orientation) [Misakian, 1993a, 1994]. Because of the dependence on these factors, measurement error may be much greater than the uncertainty declared by the commercial manufacturer when the sources measured differ from those used for factory calibration [Sieni and Bertocco, 2006]. Additionally, due to these facts, one can realize that validation of electric and magnetic field inhomogeneities has hard physical limits. As a result, the presence of sharp gradients in bioelectromagnetics experiments (e.g., <10 mm [Chatterjee et al., 2001; Publicover et al., 1999]) can sometimes only be asserted reliably only via numerical simulation. Since the same is true when testing

Overcoming the Irreproducibility Barrier

palliative measures for such gradients, it is recommended to avoid their appearance (to practice preventive design) whenever possible.

Complete validation may be an extensive procedure for the day-to-day operation of bioelectromagnetics experiments. However, some level of confirmation that the generated microenvironmental parameters are within the accepted ranges is important, as there are multiple possibilities for variation. One such reason is the simple wear and tear of the equipment from normal use. This source of variation may be significant since bioelectromagnetic experimental setups tend to be handcrafted *ad hoc* systems. That is, created as a solution which results of a specific set of requirements dictated by a specific set of experimental goals (non-generalizable or intended to be adapted to other purposes) and performed at relatively small scale (sometimes even only one copy). It is common for these systems to be discarded or dismantled after the series of experiments are performed. Therefore, they are mostly designed and built in artisanal ways, making them experimental in nature. Furthermore, manufacturing and testing under strong Quality Assurance systems which are commonplace in larger endeavors like industrial devices with significantly larger markets and volumes (mass-produced biomedical devices, auto industry, etc.) is in such cases, prohibitive. Because of this, these systems' software and hardware are subject to possible errors and uncertainties which make failures, malfunctions, or imperfections in their design and operation not uncommon. Furthermore, due to the typical multidisciplinarity of the field, these devices may be designed, built, and calibrated in one location (and by one set of scientists (typically engineers)) and then transported and installed in another location to be operated by another set of scientists. Such transportation, reassembly and differences in operation make the system prone to be damaged or modified in substantial ways. Because of this, it is recommended that the bioelectromagnetics researcher implement procedures, methods, and systems with which quick validation procedures (i.e., confirmation, verification) can be performed periodically, *in situ*, and by the operator. This should also be the case for all other aspects of the experiment such as biochemical assays and other instrumentation.

Quality assurance procedures and methods should also extend to aspects of the experiment other than the exposure system (e.g., biochemical assays, handling, incubation, etc.). The reason resides in the notion that exposure systems and methods are integral. In other words, the techniques, assays, manipulation, testing, and exposures together with the sequence and timing in which these are performed should be treated as an inseparable "tool." If such is the case that, for example, one of the assays which form part certain original "tool" is to be applied in a different part of the experimental sequence, then the resulting "tool" will be different. In order for this new "tool" to be reliable, it must be subjected to rigorous testing and validation. Therefore, the bioelectromagnetics researcher must install Quality Assurance methods and policies which maintain a level of control over the allowed variation ranges in the technical, physical, chemical, and biological experimental parameters. The reason lies in that due to the interconnectedness of these integral systems, small modifications to any of the involved parameters (e.g., change of culture container size, change of medium volume, change in seeding concentration, etc.) may result in substantial changes in other parameters (e.g., changing the thermal time-constant of the culture container and incubation system, the air-flow within the culture volume, the direction, orientation and magnitude of the induced electric fields, etc.) which may have substantial biological relevance. Therefore, it is recommended to perform a full-requalification of the entire exposure system and method upon any small modification to any of the experimental parameters to determine the extent of the effects caused on the environmental conditions at the cellular level.

11.5 Experimental Design, Implementation, and Reporting Considerations

Adequate bioelectromagnetics experimental design starts with sufficiently through literature research. Systematic reviews and meta-analyses can be helpful to draw conclusions from the existing wealth of information [Mattsson and Simkó, 2014; Golbach et al., 2016]. Additionally, it may be helpful to implement a rating system which assigns a score according to the quality of each experimental exposure described [Uman, 2011]. Such classification, for example, should range from light requirements for pilot experiments to much stricter ones for established effects. In this way, such classification can reflect the reality of bioelectromagnetics literature with some clarity and aid directing further research efforts effectively [Cuppen, 2016]. In the case of technical considerations, the bioelectromagnetics researcher must be particularly careful in avoiding traditional sources of potential experimental failure, making special emphasis in the biological methods and the microenvironmental perspective. In this regard, many problems and solutions have been identified and exist in the literature cited in this book. Some of these potential problems are not intentional or widely known but are commonplace. For example, misidentified cell lines (publishing studies about one type of cell when rather the experiments were performed on another) is a recurring problem in biomedical science to this day affecting large portions of the published and ongoing research activities [Halffman and Horbach, 2017; Horbach and Halffman, 2017]. Additionally, it is imperative to design the experiment from a study replication perspective in which the microenvironmental factors are thoroughly considered [Portelli, 2017]. Therefore, the experimental exposure system and methods should be treated as a unit in which sequence and timing of the exposures, assays, and manipulation are properly designed, executed, and thoroughly documented. For this, extra documentation can be provided in the form of supplemental photographic material (even video) to the written and visual descriptions found in a standard scientific publication, when appropriate. Static and time-varying microenvironmental conditions must be fully described within reasonable bounds.

Sometimes, the variability of the initial conditions between experiments (or samples) cannot be further minimized. In such cases, a commonly utilized technique is to use same biological sample as both the "exposed" and "control" sample. That is, to do the exposures at discrete intervals in time (exposed time-period) and compare the outcomes with the intervals in which no exposure (control time-period) is taking place (provided that all other physico-chemical environmental variables lay within a reasonable range) [Meiboom and Gill, 1958]. However, it is arguable that if, for example, cytological methods are not sufficiently accurate, the initial conditions in the samples can be different enough that different responses from identical experiments could still be expected. In order to minimize such possibility, the examination of the data can be done in an experiment-by-experiment basis in contrast to aggregation of the results, as long as those results are sufficiently meaningful. Along the same lines, an adequate experimental design to minimize cytometry variations would include such cytological devices and methods in the experimental protocol with extensive experimental description in the resulting report. In some cases, this might be necessary if all means to reduce the uncertainty of such methods have been exhausted without reaching the desired levels. Additionally, a standardized validation solution can be utilized which will ensure the correct functioning of the devices and methods (from experiment to experiment) and will provide for a means to replicate such tests in further experimental replication attempts.

11.5.1 The Sensitivity Approach to Causality

In combination with the uncertainty in all experimental parameters including measurement systems and methods, one must consider that biological systems are very complex (i.e., nonlinear with great potential for amplification, time-dependent, sensitive to initial conditions, memory (recurrence, feedback, delay), oscillatory, and greatly interconnected). As a result, some authors have made it obvious that, in the presence of such systems, causality is not clear [Miller, 2017]. This is perhaps especially true when talking of small signals (i.e. low-level electric and magnetic fields) with the concept that the resulting biological effects could also be small. Therefore, in view of these premises, experimental efforts to study the bioeffects of low-level electric and magnetic fields need to be designed in a way in which the relative sensitivity of such systems can be observed over ranges of experimental variables (e.g., field, temperature, cell concentration, etc.) [Marino et al., 2008; Sobieszczanski-Sobieski, 1990; Weaver et al., 1999]. In such way, a measure of the weight of each of the experimental variables in the context of the biological system and exposure can be observed. The careful researcher must always be vigilant of factors that could introduce variations that are not mentioned here, and perform sensitivity analyses in order to quantify their potential biological relevance. In some cases, these parameters will be intertwined in ways in which it may be difficult to draw conclusions about their relative effect size (should there be any). This is the case, for example, of the induced electric fields due to a vertically-imposed imposed magnetic field on a wet culture container like a Petri dish. Here, the electric and magnetic fields to which individual cells are exposed will not be the same for homogeneous imposed magnetic fields generated with coil configurations typically used in bioelectromagnetics research (e.g., Helmholtz coils). Similarly, complex combinations of electric and magnetic fields can appear in more infrequent culture techniques [Edmondson et al., 2014; El-Ali et al., 2006] depending on the spatial configuration of the system. Nevertheless, regardless of the experiment in question, the elucidation of the source of the observed effects, starting with the separation of the electric and magnetic field effects (e.g., using an annular Petri dish [Liburdy, 1992]) almost inevitably calls for clever experimental designs, unconventional techniques and unusual amounts of effort.

11.5.2 The Human Factor

With the considerations summarized in this chapter, it is clear that there are several instances in which a "human factor" is involved in multiple aspects of bioelectromagnetics experimentation, many times introducing uncertainties that can substantially degrade detrimental effects to the experimental quality. One such case, is the introduction of random errors ranging from differentials in traditional laboratory techniques (e.g., pipetting, handling, transportation, etc.) to the measurement or reporting of exposure electric and magnetic field exposure conditions [Portelli et al., 2017a]. Many instances of such case can be avoided by appealing to cell culture automation (i.e., robots, assembly lines, etc.) [Daniszewski et al., 2017]. However, it must be kept in mind that such systems may entail extra considerations like the introduction of substantial electric and magnetic field artifacts [Gresits et al., 2015; Hansson Mild et al., 2003; Hansson Mild et al., 2009; Makinistian and Belyaev, 2018; Moriyama et al., 2005; Portelli et al., 2013]. Along the same lines, data automation is also to be considered. Automatic data handling involves several possibilities, (i.e., automated experimental blinding, randomized signal generation, e.g., randomized generation of sham/exposures), monitoring, and logging, etc, which can be advantageous.

Poor project management and lack of quality assurance can lead to issues intertwined with the innate multidisciplinarity found in bioelectromagnetics which the careful bioelectromagnetics researcher should be aware of. For example, a common occurrence is that a core bioelectromagnetics team lacks expertise in one or more of the aspects involving an experimental endeavor, resulting in the hiring (outsourcing) of such service elsewhere. While this responsibility delegation, in principle, may be appealing and at the same time appear to an external observer as an adequate solution, it can often generate problems. A common example is that of the biology-oriented core group leading a bioelectromagnetics experimentation endeavor, while hiring the generation of an exposure system from an external partner as a service. In practice, this approach often results in experimental reports that lack fundamental information about important details of the exposure parameters which may only depend on the operator (e.g., not reporting the Petri dish size utilized) resulting in poor quality publications with potentially irreproducible exposures and results [Portelli et al., 2017a; Simko et al., 2016]. In such cases, it is clearly not enough to refer to a secondary (or complementary) publication which describes the exposure system in detail, but it is necessary to have much closer collaboration with the external partner (than may be possible) or to have that level of expertise in-house instead, in order to produce a scientific report with the minimal level of quality necessary. In fact, substantial participation from all experts involved in the bioelectromagnetics experiment is fundamental in all stages of the work (from planning to publication) in order to take advantage of such expertise collective and avoid futility. Furthermore, it is strongly recommended that one or more the members of the core team to have an acceptable level of familiarity with the fundamentals (and details) of the bioelectromagnetics discipline itself. Although at first glance, the multidisciplinary combination of the knowledge and presence brought by all members of the core team should suffice, this is sometimes not the case, as there are multiple particularities which only appear at the crossroads of all disciplines but are not normally covered by any of them in detail. Many of these unique details to bioelectromagnetics can be found in this book and in the reference material. In fact, the amount of details involved can be such that it is enough to warrant the emergence of bioelectromagnetics as a distinct branch of science and consequently the bioelectromagnetics researcher as a standalone complete professional who is an expert in such particularities. Therefore, efforts must also be made at the educational level so that the problems rooted in the multidisciplinary nature of bioelectromagnetics are transcended.

11.6 Conclusions

This chapter puts forward the notion that traditional practice of electric and magnetic field exposure effects assessment is based on spatio-temporal models built on approximations of physical, chemical, and biological experimental aspects which may obscure details with the potential to introduce substantial experimental variations. Such premise not only can explain the current uncertain state of affairs in bioelectromagnetics experimentation but also offers a view into solutions that may allow finally transcending the irreproducibility barrier.

Therefore, a reasonable first step into further experimentation should be to generate bioelectromagnetics experiments, systems, and methods which are designed, calibrated, validated, operated, monitored from a perspective that considers the cellular spatio-temporal point-of-view with sufficient depth of detail. Also, the necessity for uncertainty and

Overcoming the Irreproducibility Barrier 455

variability determination, validation, quality assurance, and sensitivity analysis as a means to assess causality needs to be understood and applied.

Like in any other discipline, improving the expected outcome implies seeing the details where others have failed. Moving forward, perhaps we must only recognize one simple but righteous universal truth: things will be as simple as they are instead of as simple as we need them to be.

Acknowledgments

This work was only funded by my own personal resources and based on experience and discussions which were acquired thanks to the interaction with multiple scientists and friends over the years. To all of them, thank you. Additionally, thanks to Profs. Ben Greenebaum for providing good reference material for his own chapters and Prof. Frank Barnes for useful discussions and collaborations over the years.

References

Aerts S, Calderon C, Valič B, Maslanyj M, Addison D, Mee T, Goiceanu C, Verloock L, Van den Bossche M, Gajšek P, Vermeulen R. 2017. Measurements of intermediate-frequency electric and magnetic fields in households. *Environmental Research* 154:160–170.

Ahn AC, Tewari M, Poon CS, Phillips RS. 2006. The limits of reductionism in medicine: could systems biology offer an alternative? *PLoS Medicine* 3(6):e208.

Ainsbury EA, Conein E, Henshaw DL. 2005. An investigation into the vector ellipticity of extremely low frequency magnetic fields from appliances in UK homes. *Physics in Medicine and Biology* 50(13):3197.

Akasaka K, Matsuki H. 2015. *High Pressure Bioscience*. Springer, New York, NY.

Aly AA, Cheema MI, Tambawala M, Laterza R, Zhou E, Rathnabharathi K, Barnes FS. 2008. Effects of 900-MHz radio frequencies on the chemotaxis of human neutrophils in vitro. *IEEE Transactions on Biomedical Engineering* 55(2):795–797.

Barnes FS. 1984. Cell membrane temperature rate sensitivity predicted from the Nernst equation. *Bioelectromagnetics* 5(1):113–115.

Barnes FS. 2017. External Electric and Magnetic Fields as a Signaling Mechanism for Biological Systems. In Markov, M. ed. *Dosimetry in Bioelectromagnetics*. CRC Press, Boca Raton, FL.

Barnes FS, Greenebaum B. 2015. The effects of weak magnetic fields on radical pairs. *Bioelectromagnetics* 36(1):45–54.

Barnes F, Greenebaum B. 2016. Some effects of weak magnetic fields on biological systems: RF fields can change radical concentrations and cancer cell growth rates. *IEEE Power Electronics Magazine* 3(1):60–68.

Barnes F, Greenebaum B. 2017. Comments on Vladimir Binhi and Frank Prato's A physical mechanism of magnetoreception: Extension and analysis. *Bioelectromagnetics* 38(4):322–323.

Barnes FS, Kandala S. 2018. Effects of time delays on biological feedback systems and electromagnetic field exposures. *Bioelectromagnetics* 39: 249–252.

Barthes J, Özçelik H, Hindié M, Ndreu-Halili A, Hasan A, Vrana NE. 2014. *Cell Microenvironment Engineering and Monitoring for Tissue Engineering and Regenerative Medicine: The Recent Advances.* BioMed research international.

Bassen H, Litovitz T, Penafiel M, Meister R. 1992. ELF in vitro exposure systems for inducing uniform electric and magnetic fields in cell culture media. *Bioelectromagnetics* 13:183–198.

Bassett CA, Pawluk RJ, Pilla AA. 1974. Acceleration of fracture repair by electromagnetic fields. A surgically noninvasive method. *Annals of the New York Academy of Sciences* 238:242–262.

Begley CG, Ellis LM. 2012. Drug development: Raise standards for preclinical cancer research. *Nature* 483(7391):531–533.

Bergsten P. 2002. Role of oscillations in membrane potential. cytoplasmic Ca^{2+} and metabolism for plasma insulin oscillations. *Diabetes* 51(1):S171–S176.

Binhi VN, Prato FS. 2017a. A physical mechanism of magnetoreception: Extension and analysis. *Bioelectromagnetics* 38(1):41–52.

Binhi VN, Prato FS. 2017b. Biological effects of the hypomagnetic field: An analytical review of experiments and theories. *PloS one* 12(6):e0179340.

Binhi VN, Prato FS. 2018. Nonspecific biological effects of weak magnetic fields depend on molecular rotations. arXiv preprint arXiv:1802.02903.

BIPM, IEC, IFCC, ISO, IUPAC, IUPAP, OIML. 2008. Evaluation of measurement data—Guide to the expression of uncertainty in measurement. Joint Committee for Guides in Metrology, JCGM 100: 2008.

Blackman C. 2017. Potential Causes for Nonreplication of EMF BioEffect Results, and What to Do about It. In Markov, M. ed. *Dosimetry in Bioelectromagnetics.* CRC Press, Boca Raton, FL.

Bowman JD, Methner MM. 2000. Hazard surveillance for industrial magnetic fields: II. Field characteristics from waveform measurements. *Annals of Occupational Hygiene* 44(8):615–633.

Brasen JC, Barington T, Olsen LF. 2012. On the mechanism of oscillations in neutrophils. *Biophysical Chemistry* 148(1):82–92.

Breslin S, O'Driscoll L. 2016. The relevance of using 3D cell cultures, in addition to 2D monolayer cultures, when evaluating breast cancer drug sensitivity and resistance. *Oncotarget* 7(29):45745–45756.

Briggs C, Culp N, Davis B, d'Onofrio G, Zini G, Machin SJ. 2014. ICSH guidelines for the evaluation of blood cell analysers including those used for differential leucocyte and reticulocyte counting. *International Journal of Laboratory Hematology* 36(6):613–627.

Burch JB, Reif JS, Noonan CW, Yost MG. 2000. Melatonin metabolite levels in workers exposed to 60-Hz magnetic fields: Work in substations and with 3-phase conductors. *Journal of Occupational and Environmental Medicine* 42(2):136–142.

Cadena-Herrera D, Esparza-De Lara JE, Ramírez-Ibañez ND, López-Morales CA, Pérez NO, Flores-Ortiz LF, Medina-Rivero E. 2015. Validation of three viable-cell counting methods: manual, semi-automated, and automated. *Biotechnology Reports* 7:9–16.

Camus A, Camugli S, Lévêque C, Schmitt E, Staub C. 2011. Is photometry an accurate and reliable method to assess boar semen concentration? *Theriogenology* 75(3):577–583.

Caputa K, Stuchly MA. 1996. Computer controlled system for producing uniform magnetic fields and its application in biomedical research. *IEEE Transactions on Instrumentation and Measurement* 45(3):701–709.

Celozzi S, Lovat G, Araneo R. 2008. *Electromagnetic Shielding.* John Wiley & Sons, Hoboken, NJ.

Chatterjee I, Hassan N, Craviso GL, Publicover NG. 2001. Numerical computation of distortions in magnetic fields and induced currents in physiological solutions produced by microscope objectives. *Bioelectromagnetics* 22:463–469.

Colquhoun D. 2014. An investigation of the false discovery rate and the misinterpretation of p-values. *Royal Society Open Science* 1(3):140216.

Cork RC, Vaughan RW, Humphrey LS. 1983. Precision and accuracy of intraoperative temperature monitoring. *Anesthesia and Analgesia* 62(2):211–214.

Cuppen, J. 2016. Personal Communication.

Daniszewski M, Crombie DE, Henderson R, Liang HH, Wong RC, Hewitt AW, Pébay A. 2017. Automated Cell Culture Systems and Their Applications to Human Pluripotent Stem Cell Studies. SLAS TECHNOLOGY: Translating Life Sciences Innovation:2472630317712220.

Deno DW. 1976. Transmission line fields. *IEEE Transactions on Power Apparatus and Systems* 95(5):1600–1611.

Dewey WC. 2009. Arrhenius relationships from the molecule and cell to the clinic. *International Journal of Hyperthermia* 25(1):3–20.

Edmondson R, Broglie JJ, Adcock AF, Yang L. 2014. Three-dimensional cell culture systems and their applications in drug discovery and cell-based biosensors. *Assay and Drug Development Technologies* 12(4):207–218.

Ehrengruber MU, Deranleau DA, Coates TD. 1996. Shape oscillations of human neutrophil leukocytes: characterization and relationship to cell motility. *The Journal of Experimental Biology* 199(4): 741–747.

El-Ali J, Sorger PK, Jensen KF. 2006. Cells on chips. *Nature* 442(7101):403–411.

England JM, Rowan RM, Assendelft OV, Bull BS, Coulter WH, Fujimoto K, Groner W, Jones AR, Koepke JA, Lewis SM, Shinton NK. 1994. Guidelines for the evaluation of blood cell analysers including those used for differential leucocyte and reticulocyte counting and cell marker applications. *International Journal of Laboratory Hematology* 16(2):157–174.

Falcke M, Malchow D, eds. 2003. *Understanding Calcium Dynamics: Experiments and Theory*. Springer Science & Business Media, New York.

Fitzsimmons RJ, Ryaby JT, Magee FP, Baylink DJ. 1994. Combined magnetic fields increased net calcium flux in bone cells. *Calcified Tissue International* 55: 376–380.

Foster KR, Skufca J. 2016. The problem of false discovery: Many scientific results can't be replicated, leading to serious questions about what's true and false in the world of research. *IEEE Pulse* 7(2):37–40.

Freedman LP, Inglese J. 2014. The increasing urgency for standards in basic biologic research. *Cancer Research* 74(15):4024–4029.

Freshney R. 2010. *The Culture of Animal Cells: A Manual of Basic Technique and Specialized Applications*. Wiley-Blackwell, New York, NY.

Futcher B. 1999. Cell cycle synchronization. *Methods in Cell Science* 21(2):79–86.

Golbach LA, Portelli LA, Savelkoul HF, Terwel SR, Kuster N, de Vries RB, Verburg-van Kemenade BL. 2016. Calcium homeostasis and low-frequency magnetic and electric field exposure: A systematic review and meta-analysis of in vitro studies. *Environment International* 92:695–706.

Gomez-Cabrero D, Tegnér J. 2017. Iterative systems biology for medicine–Time for advancing from network signature to mechanistic equations. *Current Opinion in Systems Biology* 3:111–118.

Greenebaum, B. 2017. Necessary Characteristics of Quality Bioelectromagnetic Experimental Research. In Markov, M. ed. *Dosimetry in Bioelectromagnetics*. CRC Press, Boca Raton, FL.

Gresits I, Necz PP, Jánossy G, Thuróczy G. 2015. Extremely low frequency (ELF) stray magnetic fields of laboratory equipment: A possible co-exposure conducting experiments on cell cultures. *Electromagnetic Biology and Medicine* 34:244–250.

Grzelak A, Rychlik B, Bartosz G. 2001. Light-dependent generation of reactive oxygen species in cell culture media. *Free Radical Biology & Medicine* 30:1418–1425.

Hahlbrock K. 1975. Further studies on the relationship between the rates of nitrate uptake, growth and conductivity changes in the medium of plant cell suspension cultures. *Planta* 124:311.

Halffman W, Horbach SPJM. 2017. The ghosts of HeLa: How cell line misidentification contaminates the scientific literature. *PloS one* 12(10):e0186281.

Halsey LG, Curran-Everett D, Vowler SL, Drummond GB. 2015. The fickle P value generates irreproducible results. *Nature Methods* 12:179–185.

Hansson Mild K, Wilén J, Mattsson MO, Simkó M. 2009. Background ELF magnetic fields in incubators: A factor of importance in cell culture work. *Cell Biology International* 33(7):755–757.

Hansson Mild K, Mattsson MO, Hardell L. 2003. Magnetic fields in incubators a risk factor in IVF/ICSI fertilization? *Electromagnetic Biology and Medicine* 22(1):51–53.

Hansson Mild K, Mattson MO. 2017. Dose and Exposure in Bioelectromagnetics. In Markov, M. ed. *Dosimetry in Bioelectromagnetics*. CRC Press, Boca Raton, FL.

Hart FX. 1996. Cell culture dosimetry for low-frequency magnetic fields. *Bioelectromagnetics* 17:48–57.

Hart FX. 2011. Investigation systems to study the biological effects of weak physiological electric fields. In Pullar, C. ed. *The Physiology of Bioelectricity in Development, Tissue Regeneration, and Cancer*. CRC Press, Boca Raton, FL.

Hart FX, Palisano JR. 2017. Glycocalyx bending by an electric field increases cell motility. *Bioelectromagnetics* 38(6):482–493.

Hassan N, Chatterjee I, Publicover NG, Craviso GL. 2003. Numerical study of induced current perturbations in the vicinity of excitable cells exposed to extremely low frequency magnetic fields. *Physics in Medicine and Biology* 48:3277–3293.

Herrala M, Kumari K, Blomme A, Khan MW, Koivisto H, Naarala J, Roivainen P, Tanila H, Viluksela M, Juutilainen J. 2017. Assessment of health risks of intermediate frequency magnetic fields. In EMBEC & NBC 2017:719–722. Springer, Singapore.

Hiscock HG, Mouritsen H, Manolopoulos DE, Hore PJ. 2017. Disruption of magnetic compass orientation in migratory birds by radiofrequency electromagnetic fields. *Biophysical Journal* 113(7):1475–1484.

Hobi N, Siber G, Bouzas V, Ravasio A, Pérez-Gil J, Haller T. 2014. Physiological variables affecting surface film formation by native lamellar body-like pulmonary surfactant particles. *Biochimica et Biophysica Acta (BBA)-Biomembranes* 1838(7):1842–1850.

Horbach SP, Halffman W. 2017. The ghosts of HeLa: How cell line misidentification contaminates the scientific literature. *PloS one* 12(10):e0186281.

Horswill AR, Stoodley P, Stewart PS, Parsek MR. 2007. The effect of the chemical, biological, and physical environment on quorum sensing in structured microbial communities. *Analytical and Bioanalytical Chemistry* 387(2):371–380.

Hosoya K, Takahashi K, Oya K, Iwamori S. 2017. Simultaneous process of surface modification and sterilization for polystyrene dish. *Vacuum* 148:69–77.

Ioannidis JP. 2005. Why most published research findings are false. *PLoS medicine* 2(8):e124.

Johnson FH, Flagler EA. 1950. Hydrostatic pressure reversal of narcosis in tadpoles. *Science* 112:91–92.

Kattnig DR. 2017. Radical-pair based magnetoreception amplified by radical scavenging: Resilience to spin relaxation. *The Journal of Physical Chemistry B.* 121(44):10215–10227.

Kaune WT. 1995. Comment on "designing EMF experiments: What is required to characterize 'exposure'?". *Bioelectromagnetics* 16(6):402–404.

Keenan TM, Folch A. 2008. Biomolecular gradients in cell culture systems. *Lab on a Chip* 8(1):34–57.

Kenny PA, Lee GY, Myers CA, Neve RM, Semeiks JR, Spellman PT, Lorenz K, Lee EH, Barcellos-Hoff MH, Petersen OW, Gray JW. 2007. The morphologies of breast cancer cell lines in three-dimensional assays correlate with their profiles of gene expression. *Molecular Oncology* 1(1):84–96.

Kirisits MJ, Prost L, Starkey M, Parsek MR. 2005. Characterization of colony morphology variants isolated from pseudomonas aeruginosa biofilms. *Applied and Environmental Microbiology* 71(8):4809–4821.

Knockaert J, Vanseveren B, Desmet J. 2017. Discussion on Preconditions for reproducible measurements on power conversion harmonics between 2 and 150 kHz. In 24th International Conference on Electricity Distribution. CIRED.

Koshiya N, Smith JC. 1999. Neuronal pacemaker for breathing visualized in vitro. *Nature* 400(6742):360–363.

Krylov VV, Larkin M. 2017. Biological effects related to geomagnetic activity and possible mechanisms. *Bioelectromagnetics* 38(7):497–510.

Kuster N, Schönborn F. 2000. Recommended minimal requirements and development guidelines for exposure setups of bio-experiments addressing the health risk concern of wireless communications. *Bioelectromagnetics* 21:508–514.

Kwok R. 2010. Five hard truths for synthetic biology. *Nature News* 463(7279):288–290.

Lazebnik Y. 2004. Can a biologist fix a radio?—or, what I learned while studying apoptosis. *Biochemistry (Moscow)* 69(12):1403–1406.

Leferink F, Keyer C, Melentjev A. 2016. Static energy meter errors caused by conducted electromagnetic interference. *IEEE Electromagnetic Compatibility Magazine* 5(4):49–55.

Lekner J. 2013. Conducting cylinders in an external electric field: Polarizability and field enhancement. *Journal of Electrostatics* 71(6):1104–1110.

Liburdy RP. 1992. Biological interactions of cellular systems with time-varying magnetic fields. *Annals of the New York Academy of Sciences* 649(1):74–95.

Lin JC. 2014a. Reassessing laboratory results of low-frequency electromagnetic field exposure of cells in culture. *IEEE Antennas and Propagation Magazine* 56(1):227–229.

Lin JC. 2014b. Reexamining biological studies of effect of low-frequency electromagnetic field exposure on cells in culture. *IEEE Microwave Magazine* 15(4):26–55.

Loiselle D, Ramchandra R. 2015. A counterview of 'An investigation of the false discovery rate and the misinterpretation of p-values' by Colquhoun (2014). *Open Science* 2(8):150217.

Luca AC, Mersch S, Deenen R, Schmidt S, Messner I, Schafer KL, Baldus SE, Huckenbeck W, Piekorz RP, Knoefel WT, Krieg A, Stoecklein NH. 2013. Impact of the 3D microenvironment on phenotype, gene expression, and EGFR inhibition of colorectal cancer cell lines. *PloS One* 8:e59689.

Makinistian L. 2016. A novel system of coils for magnetobiology research. *Review of Scientific Instruments*, 87(11):114304.

Makinistian L, Belyaev I. 2018. Magnetic field inhomogeneities due to CO_2 incubator shelves: A source of experimental confounding and variability? *Open Science* 5(2):172095.

Marinkovic M, Block TJ, Rakian R, Li Q, Wang E, Reilly MA, Dean DD, Chen XD. 2016. One size does not fit all: Developing a cell-specific niche for in vitro study of cell behavior. *Matrix Biology* 52:426–441.

Marino S, Hogue IB, Ray CJ, Kirschner DE. 2008. A methodology for performing global uncertainty and sensitivity analysis in systems biology. *Journal of Theoretical Biology* 254(1):178–196.

Marquis RE, Macdonald AG, Hall AC, Pickles DM, Kendig JJ, Grossman Y, Heinemann SH, Hogan PM, Besch SR, Sebert P, Rostain JC. 2012. *Effects of High Pressure on Biological Systems* (Vol. 17). Springer Science & Business Media, New York, NY.

Markov M. 2017. *Dosimetry in Bioelectromagnetics*. CRC Press, Boca Raton, FL.

Maroto M, Monk N, eds. 2008. *Cellular Oscillatory Mechanisms*. Springer Science & Business Media, New York, NY.

Martinez LJ, Pinedo CR, Gutierrez JO, Cadavid H. 2016. Growth rates of dynamic dermal model exposed to laminar flow and magnetic fields. *Research on Biomedical Engineering* 32(1):55–62.

Matsumoto T, Hayashi N, Isaka K. 2000. Quantification of coupling between two-dimensional low-frequency magnetic fields and a spherical model of biological substance. *Electronics and Communications in Japan (Part II: Electronics)* 83(4):50–60.

Mattsson MO, Simkó M. 2014. Grouping of experimental conditions as an approach to evaluate effects of extremely low-frequency magnetic fields on oxidative response in in vitro studies. *Frontiers in Public Health* 2:132–132.

Meiboom S, Gill D. 1958. Modified spin-echo method for measuring nuclear relaxation times. *Review of Scientific Instruments* 29(8):688–691.

Methner MM, Bowman JD. 2000. Hazard surveillance for industrial magnetic fields: I. Walkthrough survey of ambient fields and sources. *The Annals of Occupational Hygiene* 44(8):603–614.

Micheletti R. 1991. Phase angle measurement between two sinusoidal signals. *IEEE Transactions on Instrumentation and Measurement* 40(1):40–42.

Miller W. 2017. The Conundrum of Dosimetry: Its Applications to Pharmacology and Biophysics Are Distinct. In Markov, M. ed. *Dosimetry in Bioelectromagnetics*. CRC Press, Boca Raton, FL.

Misakian M. 1991. In vitro exposure parameters with linearly and circularly polarized ELF magnetic fields. *Bioelectromagnetics* 12(6):377–381.

Misakian M. 1993a. Coil probe dimension and uncertainties during measurements of nonuniform ELF magnetic fields. *Journal of Research of the National Institute of Standards and Technology* 98(3):287.

Misakian M. 1994. Three-axis coil probe dimensions and uncertainties during measurement of magnetic fields from appliances. *Journal of Research of the National Institute of Standards and Technology* 99:247–247.

Misakian M. 1997. Vertical circularly polarized ELF magnetic fields and induced electric fields in culture media. *Bioelectromagnetics* 18(7):524–526.

Misakian M, Bell GK, Bracken TD, Fink LH, Holte KC, Hudson JE, Johnson GB, McDermott TJ, Mukherji RC, Olsen RG, Rauch GB, Sebo SA, Silva JM, Wong PS. 1993b. A protocol for spot measurements of residential power frequency magnetic fields. *IEEE Transactions on Power Delivery* 8(3):1386–1395.

Misakian M, Fenimore C. 1996. Distributions of measurement error for three-axis magnetic field meters during measurements near appliances. *IEEE Transactions on Instrumentation and Measurement* 45(1):244–249.

Misakian M, Fenimore C. 1997. Distributions of measurement errors for single-axis magnetic field meters during measurements near appliances. *Bioelectromagnetics* 18(3):273–276.

Misakian M, Sheppard AR, Krause D, Frazier ME, Miller DL. 1993c. Biological, physical, and electrical parameters for in vitro studies with ELF magnetic and electric fields: A primer. *Bioelectromagnetics* 14(2):1–73.

Moriyama K, Sato H, Tanaka K, Nakashima Y, Yoshitomi K. 2005. Extremely low frequency magnetic fields originating from equipment used for assisted reproduction, umbilical cord and peripheral blood stem cell transplantation, transfusion, and hemodialysis. *Bioelectromagnetics* 26(1):69–73.

Muehsam D, Ventura, C. 2014. Life rhythm as a symphony of oscillatory patterns: electromagnetic energy and sound vibration modulates gene expression for biological signaling and healing. *Global Advances in Health and Medicine* 3(2):40–55.

Negovetic S, Samaras T, Kuster N. 2005. *EMF Health Risk Research: Lessons Learned and Recommendations for the Future*. Monte Verita, Switzerland.

Novák B, Tyson JJ. 2008. Design principles of biochemical oscillators. *Nature Reviews Molecular Cell Biology* 9(12):981–991.

Ongena K, Das C, Smith JL, Gil S, Johnston G. 2010. Determining cell number during cell culture using the scepter cell counter. *Journal of Visualized Experiments: JoVE* 2010(45).

Orear J. 1958. Notes on statistics for physicists. No. UCRL-8417. SCAN-9709037.

Paffi A, Apollonio F, Liberti M, Sheppard A, Bit-Babik G, Balzano, Q. 2015a. Culture medium geometry: The dominant factor affecting in vitro RF exposure dosimetry. *International Journal of Antennas and Propagation*. 2015, Article ID 438962, 10 pages

Paffi A, Liberti M, Apollonio F, Sheppard A, Balzano Q. 2015b. In vitro exposure: Linear and non-linear thermodynamic events in Petri dishes. *Bioelectromagnetics* 36: 527–537.

Petrunkina AM, Harrison RAP. 2010. Systematic misestimation of cell subpopulations by flow cytometry: A mathematical analysis. *Theriogenology* 73(7):839–847.

Petty HR. 2006. Spatiotemporal chemical dynamics in living cells: From information trafficking to cell physiology. *Biosystems* 83(2):217–224.

Polk C. 1990. Electric fields and surface charges induced by ELF magnetic fields. *Bioelectromagnetics* 11(2):189–201.

Portelli LA. 2012. Device for controlling the electric, magnetic and electromagnetic fields in biological incubators. PhD dissertation, University of Colorado.

Portelli LA. 2017. Uncertainty Sources Associated with Low-Frequency Electric and Magnetic Field Experiments on Cell Cultures. In Markov, M. ed. *Dosimetry in Bioelectromagnetics*. CRC Press, Boca Raton, FL.

Portelli LA. 2018. Low-level Thermal Signals: An Understudied Aspect of Radio-Frequency Field Exposures with Potential Implications on Public Health. In Markov, M. ed. *Mobile Communications and Public Health*. CRC Press, Boca Raton, FL.

Portelli LA, Falldorf K, Thuróczy G, Cuppen J. 2017a. Retrospective estimation of the electric and magnetic field exposure conditions in in vitro experimental reports reveal considerable potential for uncertainty. *Bioelectromagnetics* 39(3):231–243

Portelli LA, Kausik A, Barnes FS. 2017c. Effects of small and rapid temperature oscillations on adherent cell cultures: Exposure system, experimental method and a pilot study on human cancer cells. In EMBEC & NBC 2017:707–710 Springer, Singapore.

Portelli LA, Schomay TE, Barnes FS. 2013. Inhomogeneous background magnetic field in biological incubators is a potential confounder for experimental variability and reproducibility. *Bioelectromagnetics* 34(5):337–348.

Prathalingam NS, Holt WW, Revell SG, Jones S, Watson PF. 2006. The precision and accuracy of six different methods to determine sperm concentration. *Journal of Andrology* 27(2):257–262.

Publicover NG, Marsh CG, Vincze CA, Craviso GL, Chatterjee I. 1999. Effects of microscope objectives on magnetic field exposures. *Bioelectromagnetics* 20:387–395.

Rapp PE. 1979. An atlas of cellular oscillators. *Journal of Experimental Biology* 81(1):281–306.

Roivainen P, Eskelinen T, Jokela K, Juutilainen, J. 2014. Occupational exposure to intermediate frequency and extremely low frequency magnetic fields among personnel working near electronic article surveillance systems. *Bioelectromagnetics* 35(4):245–250.

Schuderer J, Kuster N. 2003. Effect of the meniscus at the solid/liquid interface on the SAR distribution in Petri dishes and flasks. *Bioelectromagnetics* 24:103–108.

Schuderer J, Oesch W, Felber N, Spät D, Kuster N. 2004. In vitro exposure apparatus for ELF magnetic fields. *Bioelectromagnetics* 25:582–591.

Setiawan I, Keyer C, Leferink F. 2017a. Smarter concepts for future EMI standards. In Electromagnetic Compatibility (APEMC), IEEE Asia-Pacific International Symposium:47–49.

Setiawan I, Leferink F. 2017b. Time-Frequency Diversity Measurements in Power Systems. 32nd URSI GASS, Montreal, Canada.

Sieni E, Bertocco M. 2006. Nonuniform low frequency magnetic field measurements. In Instrumentation and Measurement Technology Conference, Proceedings of the IEEE:2194–2199.

Simkó M, Remondini D, Zeni O, Scarfi MR. 2016. Quality matters: Systematic analysis of endpoints related to "cellular life" in vitro data of radiofrequency electromagnetic field exposure. *International Journal of Environmental Research and Public Health* 13(7):701.

Skoge M, Wong E, Hamza B, Bae A, Martel J, Kataria R, Keizer-Gunnink I, Kortholt A, Van Haastert PJ, Charras G, Janetopoulos C. 2016. A worldwide competition to compare the speed and chemotactic accuracy of neutrophil-like cells. *PloS one* 11(6):e0154491.

Sobieszczanski-Sobieski J. 1990. Sensitivity of complex, internally coupled systems. *AIAA journal* 28(1):153–160.

Speliotis DE, Morrison JR. 1966. A theoretical analysis of saturation magnetic recording. *IBM Journal of Research and Development* 10(3):233–243.

Stark J, Chan C, George AJ. 2007. Oscillations in the immune system. *Immunological Reviews* 216(1):213–231.

Stuchly MA, Xi W. 1994. Modelling induced currents in biological cells exposed to low-frequency magnetic fields. *Physics in Medicine and Biology* 39:1319–1330.

Takuma T, Techaumnat B. 2010. Analytical Calculation Methods. In *Electric Fields in Composite Dielectrics and their Applications*:127–156. Springer, Netherlands.

Tarao H, Hayashi N, Isaka K. 1998. Characterization of electric fields induced by ELF magnetic fields in biological model of eccentric double-layered sphere, *IEEJ Transactions on Fundamentals and Materials* 118(5):475–482.

Tremel A, Cai A, Tirtaatmadja N, Hughes BD, Stevens GW, Landman KA, O'Connor AJ. 2009. Cell migration and proliferation during monolayer formation and wound healing. *Chemical Engineering Science* 64(2):247–253.

Uman LS. 2011. Systematic reviews and meta-analyses. *Journal of the Canadian Academy of Child and Adolescent Psychiatry*, 20(1):57.

Valberg PA. 1995. Designing EMF experiments: What is required to characterize "exposure"? *Bioelectromagnetics* 16(6):396–401.

Vaughan TE, Weaver JC. 2005. Molecular change signal-to-noise criteria for interpreting experiments involving exposure of biological systems to weakly interacting electromagnetic fields. *Bioelectromagnetics* 26(4):305–322.

Vijayalaxmi. 2016. Biological and health effects of radiofrequency fields: Good study design and quality publications." *Mutation Research-Genetic Toxicology and Environmental Mutagenesis* 810:6–12.

Wachtel H. 1985. Synchronization of Neural Firing Patterns By Relatively Weak ELF Fields. In *Biological Effects and Dosimetry of Static and ELF Electromagnetic Fields*:313–328. Springer, New York, NY.

Wang W, Litovitz TA, Penafiel LM, Meister R. 1993. Determination of the induced ELF electric field distribution in a two-layer in vitro system simulating biological cells in nutrient solution. *Bioelectromagnetics* 14:29–39.

Weaver JC, Vaughan TE, Martin GT. 1999. Biological effects due to weak electric and magnetic fields: The temperature variation threshold. *Biophysical Journal* 76(6):3026–3030.

Weiss P, Garber B. 1952. Shape and movement of mesenchyme cells as functions of the physical structure of the medium contributions to a quantitative morphology. *Proceedings of the National Academy of Sciences* 38(3):264–280.

Weiss P. 1961. Guiding principles in cell locomotion and cell aggregation. *Experimental Cell Research* 8:260–281.

Weiss P. 1945. Experiments on cell and axon orientation in vitro: The role of colloidal exudates in tissue organization. *Journal of Experimental Zoology Part A: Ecological Genetics and Physiology* 100(3):353–386.

Zeiger AS, Hinton B, Van Vliet KJ. 2013. Why the dish makes a difference: quantitative comparison of polystyrene culture surfaces. *Acta Biomaterialia* 9(7):7354–7361.

12

Radio Frequency Exposure Standards

K. R. Foster
University of Pennsylvania

C.-K. Chou
C.-K. Chou Consulting

R. C. Petersen[*]
R. C. Petersen Associates, LLC

CONTENTS

12.1   Introduction 464
12.2   Overview: Science-Based Exposure Standards 466
       12.2.1   IEEE Standards 467
       12.2.2   ICNIRP (1998) Guideline 469
12.3   Dosimetric Considerations 470
       12.3.1   Primary Quantities 471
       12.3.2   Derived Dosimetric Quantities 472
12.4   More Detailed Review of IEEE C95.1-2005 and ICNIRP (1998, 2010) 472
       12.4.1   Shared Features 472
       12.4.2   Development of Limits 474
       12.4.3   Perspective 479
       12.4.4   National Limits 483
       12.4.5   Other "Thermal" Standards 488
       12.4.6   Other Suggested Limits: The BioInitiative Report 489
12.5   Approaches to Critical Reviews of the Literature 491
12.6   Two Sets of Distinctions 494
12.7   Current Health Issues 495
       12.7.1   Electromagnetic "Hypersensitivity" 495
       12.7.2   Cancer 496
12.8   Precautionary Principle 497
       12.8.1   EC Commentary 498
       12.8.2   Precaution-Based Exposure Limits 501
       12.8.3   Other Precautionary Measures 501
12.9   Future Challenges with RF Standards/Guidelines 503
12.10 Conclusion 506
References 506

---

[*] Deceased.

12.1 Introduction

There is no doubt that radiofrequency (RF) energy is hazardous to humans at some level of exposure and that limits to exposure are needed for workers and ordinary citizens. Harm from exposure to RF energy may occur directly, through direct action on the body, or indirectly by interaction of RF energy with other objects or systems in the environment (for example, by causing interference to an implanted medical device that results in harm to the patient).

In the following discussion, RF refers to the part of the electromagnetic spectrum from 3 kHz–300 GHz, and EMF refers generically to electromagnetic fields without specifying the frequency. Following conventional definitions,[*] harm refers to physical injury or damage to an individual's health, a hazard is a potential source of harm, and risk is the chance or probability that a person will be harmed or experience an adverse health effect if exposed to a hazard. The frequency range of chief concern is 0.1 MHz–300 GHz (a subset of the RF band), which is the range where tissue heating is considered to be the dominant hazard mechanism but the limits at lower frequencies will be briefly discussed as well.

In its *Framework for Developing Health-based EMF Standards*[†] (WHO, 2006), the EMF Project of the World Health Organization (WHO) describes "science-based exposure limits that will protect the health of the population from EMF exposure." While the Framework does not explicitly define "science-based," it describes a standards-setting process that begins with a critical review of the relevant scientific literature, establishing exposure limits to avoid established hazards, and extending to "considerations regarding the overall practicability of the standard, compliance procedures and the use of precautionary measures" (Table 12.1). The process relies on a careful review of the scientific data by qualified experts, but also allows for stakeholder participation in setting exposure limits.

This chapter will focus on two science-based exposure limits as related to several national and regional/local exposure limits, but toward the end will also discuss precautionary-based limits adopted in some jurisdictions. The main emphasis is on the Institute of Electrical and Electronics Engineers (IEEE) Standard C95.1-2005, for which two of the three present authors (C.-K. Chou and R. Petersen) have played significant leadership roles. Some of the present material has been adapted from previous writings by these authors (Chou and Petersen, 2008; Chou, 2015; Petersen, 2009). For a recent review of RF exposure limits from a different (non-IEEE) perspective, see Wood (2017).

This chapter describes the major scientific rationales of the limits but does not attempt to summarize them in full detail. (The limits[‡] are highly complex and detailed, and readers who wish to apply any of the exposure limits referred to in this chapter should consult with the original documents as well as any accompanying explanatory information).

For perspective, three kinds of standards have been developed to ensure safe use of electromagnetic energy over the RF spectrum: exposure standards, assessment standards, and electromagnetic compatibility standards for medical devices. These can be voluntary (as with the IEEE standards) or mandatory (implemented in government regulations).

---

[*] www.ccohs.ca/oshanswers/hsprograms/hazard_risk.html.

[†] World Health Organization (WHO). Framework for developing health-based EMF standards, WHO Geneva: 2006. (www.who.int/peh-emf/standards/EMF_standards_framework%5b1%5d.pdf?ua=1).

[‡] Some limits are described by their developers as standards, others as guidelines. For some legal purposes these terms may have different meanings, and for other purposes they might be equivalent. An attempt will be made in this chapter to respect the terminology used by the groups responsible for development of the different sets of limits.

Radio Frequency Exposure Standards

TABLE 12.1

Idealized Process of Developing Science-Based Exposure Limits (Adapted from WHO (2006))

Procedure	Considerations
Select scientific database	Types of studies
	Criteria for inclusion
Perform risk assessment	Hierarchy of studies
	Criteria for evaluation
	Weight-of-evidence
Determine threshold levels	Interpretation of threshold
	Biological effects
	Interaction mechanisms
Select safety factors	Multiple tiers/different populations
	Level of scientific uncertainty
Set exposure limits	Basic restrictions
	Reference levels
	Frequency extrapolation
Ensure overall practicability	Explanatory supporting document
	Compliance measures
	Monitoring system

- *Exposure standards* are "basic standards of personal protection that generally refer to maximum levels to which whole or partial body exposure is permitted from any number of EMF emitting devices." (*Framework*). Examples are IEEE C95.1-2005 (IEEE, 2005) and ICNIRP (1998). These two limits, which were developed independently, together with limits by the U.S. Federal Communications Commission (FCC, 1996) form the basis of most national standards throughout the world apart from those in Russia, China, and some Eastern European countries. Other standards are influential within specific domains, for example, the Threshold Limit Values® of the American Conference of Governmental Industrial Hygienists (ACGIH) are widely influential for occupational health and safety in the USA, and CENELEC—ENV 50166-2 is widely used in the European Union (EU).

- *Assessment standards* "describe how compliance with exposure or emission standards may be ensured" (*Framework*). Examples of standards for assessing compliance of RF exposure sources with exposure standards include IEEE 1528-2013 (IEEE International Committee on Electromagnetic Safety (ICES) TC34), and IEC 62209-1-2016 (International Electrotechnical Commission TC106), which specify protocols and test procedures for determining compliance of a mobile phone handset placed against the head, and IEEE ICES C95.3-2002 and IEC 62232:2017 for determining RF exposure from cellular base stations or other transmitters distant from the body. The overall goal of these standards is to provide unambiguous procedures for assessing compliance with the exposure standards that yield repeatable results. Other standards establish procedures for certifying compliance of specific products such as microwave ovens with product safety standards.

- *EMI (electromagnetic interference) standards* "set various specifications for electrical devices and are generally based on engineering considerations, e.g., to minimize electromagnetic interference with other equipment and/or to optimize the efficiency of the device." (*Framework*). Examples in this category are compatibility standards such as developed by the American National Standards Institute (ANSI), International Organization for Standardization (ISO), Consumer Electronics Association (CEA) and other groups. Other standards ensure a minimum level of electromagnetic immunity for medical devices to prevent harm to patients using them. For example, the Association for the Advancement of Medical Instrumentation (AAMI) is a U.S.-based professional organization with an extensive standards program that establishes electromagnetic immunity standards for many kinds of medical equipment.

Standards are only part of the mechanisms used by technologically advanced countries to ensure safe use of the electromagnetic energy. Invariably, standards exist in the context of administrative rules and legal precedents that shape their meaning and application. In addition, health agencies may issue advisories regarding the safe use of RF technologies including some that fall under the rubric "precaution."

12.2 Overview: Science-Based Exposure Standards

Table 12.1 provides an idealized outline of the development of science-based exposure standards, from the WHO *Framework*. The process begins with a "comprehensive and critical scientific review undertaken by a panel of recognized experts." The review includes "an evaluation of the scientific literature, determination of threshold levels, choice of safety factors for different populations at risk, and derivation of exposure limits." It continues with an evaluation of the "overall practicability of the standard, compliance procedures and the use of precautionary measures."

The following discussion focuses on two major science-based limits, IEEE C95.1-2005 (IEEE, 2005) with an amendment in 2010 to specify ceilings for contact currents (IEEE, 2010), and ICNIRP (1998). The frequency range covered by IEEE C95.1-2005 is 3 kHz–300 GHz while ICNIRP (1998) covers the range "up to 300 GHz," including frequencies approaching but not including static fields. A third set of guidelines, ICNIRP (2010) applies to electric and magnetic fields, nominally within the frequency range 1 Hz–100 kHz (but the document extends these limits up to 10 MHz). ICNIRP (2010) revises ICNIRP (1998) guidelines for electric and magnetic fields up to 10 MHz. The present discussion is chiefly concerned with guidelines at frequencies above the range in which neuro-stimulatory effects (e.g., electric shock) are the limiting hazards, e.g., >100 kHz.

While the IEEE and ICNIRP limits differ in some respects, they are quite similar in both their overall approach and in the limits themselves, and the two sets of guidelines can be considered as paradigm cases of a family of science-based limits that have been adopted, sometimes with modification, by most countries throughout the world. Both IEEE and ICNIRP guidelines are subject to periodic revision. ICNIRP reaffirmed its 1998 RF guidelines in 2009 (ICNIRP, 2009). At present writing, both IEEE C95.1-2005 and ICNIRP (1998) guidelines are undergoing major revision, with approval anticipated late in 2018. This chapter refers to the versions that are currently in force as of this writing (early 2018).

Both sets of limits are explicitly designed to protect against established adverse effects of exposure to RF fields. Thus, the documentation for IEEE C95.1-2005 states "The purpose of this standard is to provide exposure limits to protect against established adverse effects to human health induced by exposure to RF electric, magnetic and electromagnetic

Radio Frequency Exposure Standards

fields over the frequency range of 3 kHz to 300 GHz," while ICNIRP (1998) states its goal as to "establish guidelines for limiting EMF exposure that will provide protection against known adverse health effects." Both sets of limits incorporate safety margins to address the uncertainties in establishing thresholds for hazards. However, neither group explicitly invoked the Precautionary Principle (PP) or other social factors in establishing limits.

12.2.1 IEEE Standards

The IEEE C95.1 standard (current versions are IEEE C95.1-2005 with an amendment in 2010) was developed by the IEEE International Committee on Electromagnetic Safety (ICES), which operates as one of many standards setting groups within the IEEE Standards Association (IEEE-SA) (Figure 12.1) and is subject to its procedures. ICES develops several standards related to EMF safety, including exposure standards for the frequency range 0–3 kHz and 3 kHz–300 GHz, standards for RF safety programs, measurements, warning signs (among others) (Table 12.2). ICES Technical Committee 95 (TC95) oversees the work of several subcommittees that set RF exposure limits. In total, ICES has about 150 members

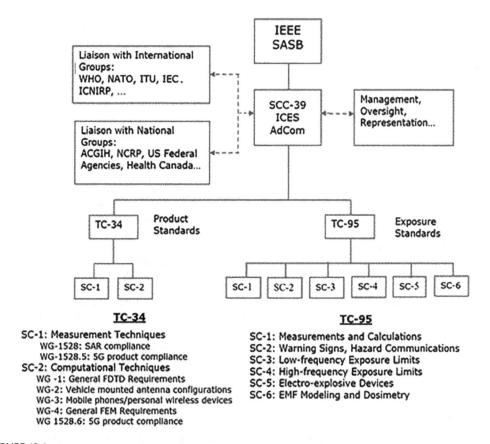

FIGURE 12.1
Organizational structure of International Committee on Electromagnetic Safety (ICES). This committee operated under the Standards Board of IEEE Standards Association (IEEE SASB). It has two Technical Committees (TC-34 and TC-95) for, respectively, product and exposure/safety standards. Each Technical Committee in turn has several subcommittees which in turn have working groups for different subtasks. (www.ices-emfsafety.org/committees/adcom/)

TABLE 12.2

IEEE International Committee on Electromagnetic Safety (ICES) Family of Standards

Technical Committee	Subcommittees	Standards	Titles
TC95	SC1 (techniques, procedures, instrumentation, and computation)	C95.3-2002	Recommended practice for measurements and computations of RF EMFs with respect to human exposure to such fields, 100 kHz to 300 GHz (reaffirmed 2008)
		C95.3.1-2010	Recommended practice for measurements and computation of electric, magnetic, and EMFs with respect to human exposure to such fields, 0 Hz–100 kHz
		1460-1996	IEEE guide for the measurement of quasi-static magnetic and electric fields (reaffirmed 2002, 2008, incorporated into C95.3.1-2010)
		PC95.3-201X	Draft recommended practice for measurements and computations of electric, magnetic, and electro-magnetic fields with respect to human exposure to such fields, 0 Hz to 300 GHz
TC95	SC2 (terminology, units of measurement and hazard communication)	C95.2-1999	IEEE standard for RF energy and current flow symbols (reaffirmed 2005)
		C95.7-2014	Recommended practice for RF safety programs – 3 kHz to 300 GHz
TC95	SC3 (safety levels with respect to human exposure, 0–3 kHz)	C95.6-2002	IEEE standard for safety levels with respect to human exposure to EMFs, 0 to 3 kHz (reaffirmed 2007)
TC95	SC4 (safety levels with respect to human exposure, 3 kHz–300 GHz)	C95.1-2005	IEEE standard for safety levels with respect to human exposure to RF EMFs, 3 kHz to 300 GHz
		C95.1a-2010	Amendment 1: specifies ceiling limits for induced and contact current, clarifies distinctions between localized exposure and spatial peak power density
TC95	SC3/4	C95.1-2345-2014	IEEE standard for military workplaces – force health protection regarding personnel exposure to electric, magnetic, and EMFs, 0 Hz to 300 GHz
		PC95.1-201X	Draft standard for safety levels with respect to human exposure to electric, magnetic, and EMFs, 0 Hz to 300 GHz (revision—incorporates C95.1-2005 and C95.6–2002)
TC95	SC5 (safety levels with respect to electro-explosive devices)	C95.4-2002	IEEE recommended practice for determining safe distances from RF transmitting antennas when using electric blasting caps during explosive operations (reaffirmed 2008)
TC34	SC1 (SAR evaluation - measurement techniques)	1528-2013	Recommended practice for determining the peak spatial-average SAR in the human head from wireless communications devices: measurement techniques (similar to IEC 62209-1)
TC34	SC2 (SAR evaluation computational techniques)	IEC/IEEE 62704-1:2017	Determining the peak spatial-average SAR in the human body from wireless communications devices, 30 MHz to 6 GHz - Part 1: General requirements for using the finite difference time domain (FDTD) method for SAR calculations
		IEC/IEEE 62704-2:2017	Determining the peak spatial-average SAR in the human body from wireless communications devices, 30 MHz to 6 GHz - Part 2: Specific requirements for FDTD modeling of exposure from vehicle mounted antennas
		IEC/IEEE 62704-3:2017	Determining the peak spatial-average SAR in the human body from wireless communications devices, 30 MHz to 6 GHz - Part 3: Specific requirements for using the FDTD method for SAR calculations of mobile phones

Radio Frequency Exposure Standards

TABLE 12.3

Evolution of IEEE C95.x Safety Standards

Year	Standard	Major Innovation
1960		USASI C95 Radiation Hazards Project and Committee chartered
1966	USAS C95.1-1966 (10 MHz to 100 GHz)	Based on simple thermal model
		Frequency independent limit (100 W/m²)
1974	ANSI C95.1-1974	Limits for E^2 and H^2
1982	ANSI C95.1-1982	Incorporates dosimetry (SAR)
1991	IEEE C95.1-1991	Introduction of two tiers
	IEEE C95.1-1997	Reaffirmation of C95.1-1997
2002	IEEE C95.6-2002	(0–3 kHz)
2006	IEEE C95.1-2005	Extends to lower frequencies (3 kHz–300 GHz)
2010	IEEE C95.1a-2010	Amendment of C95.1-2005 – specifies ceiling limits for induced and contact current
2014	IEEE C95.1-2345-2014 (0–300 GHz)	(NATO/IEEE agreement)
2014	IEEE C95.7-2014	IEEE recommended practice for RF safety programs, 3 kHz to 300 GHz
2015		NATO adopted C95.1-2345-2014

from government, academia, industry, and the public in 29 countries (although the number of active participants in the process at any point in time may vary).

The history of IEEE RF safety limits has been described in detail elsewhere (Osepchuk and Petersen, 2003; Petersen, 1998). In brief, the current IEEE C95.1-2005 standard has its origin in the Tri-Service research program on possible health hazards of RF energy that was established in the early 1950s by the U.S. Defense Department. This Program funded research projects on biological effects of RF energy at ten U.S. Universities and hosted a series of research meetings on the topic (Michaelson, 1971). In 1953, Herman P. Schwan from the University of Pennsylvania and one of the grantees of the Program, proposed an exposure limit of 100 W/m² based on his calculations of heating of the body by RF energy (Schwan, 1992). This proposal eventually led to the development of the first RF exposure standard (USAS C95.1-1966). This standard was initially developed under the auspices of the United States of America Standards Institute (USASI) (now the ANSI); eventually sponsorship changed to the IEEE-SA, where it is now developed by ICES. The standard has subsequently undergone five revisions with the most recent full release being approved in 2005 and amended in 2010 (Table 12.3). At present writing (early 2018), the standard is undergoing another of its periodic revisions and updating (as required by IEEE-SA rules), and is expected to be approved in 2018. Consequently, the present IEEE C95.1-2005 represents the result of more than a half century of continuous standards development work. While it was initially begun under sponsorship of an American organization, the continued development of this standard is now an international effort under the IEEE Standards Association.

12.2.2 ICNIRP (1998) Guideline

ICNIRP (1998) guideline is developed by the International Commission on Nonionizing Radiation Protection (ICNIRP), a non-governmental nonprofit organization registered in Germany. ICNIRP[*] traces its history to a meeting at WHO in 1969 on RF safety (Repacholi,

---

[*] www.icnirp.org.

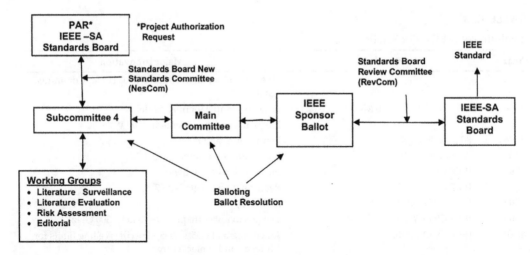

FIGURE 12.2
Process of developing IEEE RF exposure standards. From Petersen (2009).

2017). This led to a series of meetings and workshops on the topic in the early 1970s and formation of ICNIRP in 1992. ICNIRP is presently recognized as a collaborating non-governmental organization by the WHO and the International Labour Organization (ILO), which gives it wide international influence.

ICNIRP's mandate is to "establish exposure guidelines for nonionizing radiation ranging from static electric and magnetic fields through the infrared." In addition, it publishes numerous reviews, statements, workshop proceedings, and other materials on health- and safety-related to nonionizing EMFs ranging from DC fields through the infrared.

ICES and ICNIRP differ considerably in membership and procedures. ICES[*] operates under the rules of the IEEE-SA, which provides for an open consensus process, with regularized procedures, multiple rounds of balloting, open publication of its meeting records on the Internet, and other methods to ensure transparency (Figure 12.2). ICES attempts to be inclusive, by encouraging broad participation by stakeholders (including employees of industry and members of the public), and uses a formalized process to provide transparency and balance.

By contrast, ICNIRP is much smaller and far less organizationally complex than ICES. It consists of a 14-member Commission and with an additional 25 experts participating in Scientific Expert Groups (SEGs). Most of these experts are employed by government agencies and academia from around the world (but predominantly from Europe) but it has no representatives from industry. Despite these differences, both groups have developed quite similar standards/guidelines.

12.3 Dosimetric Considerations

In assessing an individual's exposure to RF fields, it is useful to distinguish between *exposure* (fields measured outside the body) and *dose* (induced fields within the body). Apart from some surface effects that occur outside the skin surface, one can assume that

---

[*] www.ices-emfsafety.org/.

Radio Frequency Exposure Standards

hazardous effects of RF exposure are related to field strengths at specific locations within the body. A recent, elementary introduction to RF exposure limits, chiefly from a European perspective and emphasizing exposure assessment is by Staebler (2017).

12.3.1 Primary Quantities

- *External field strength,* electric field E (measured in volts/meter, V/m); magnetic field H (amperes/m, A/m), or magnetic flux density B (in tesla, T). In the bioeffects literature, the magnetic-flux density is often stated in units of gauss (10^{-4} T). For RF exposure assessment, external field strength is typically more useful at the lower end of the applicable range of the limits, where exposures are in the near field of sources and the electric and magnetic fields are essentially independent. Such fields are not properly termed radiation (they do not propagate through space).
- *Incident power density,* S, in watts/meter square, W/m² (principally useful in far fields of radiators where the exposure consists of EMFs propagating through space, i.e., electromagnetic radiation).

Relevant measures of dose are:

- *Current density within the body* J_i (in A/m²), principally useful at low frequencies. A related measure is internal field strength E_i (V/m) (or *in situ* electric field), which is related to the current density by Ohms Law:

$$J_i = \sigma E_i \tag{1}$$

Where J_i and E_i are the current density and electric field inside the body (A/m² and V/m) and σ (S/m) is the conductivity of tissue at the measurement point. In 1998, ICNIRP defined its basic restriction at lower RFs in terms of current density, but in 2010 changed its basic restriction to internal electric field following IEEE C95.6-2002 (as well as changing the limits below 10 MHz).

- *Contact current* J (in A), which is passed into the body through contact with an external charged object.
- *Specific absorption rate,* SAR (in W/kg), which is a measure of the rate of energy deposition in the body. SAR as a dosimetric quantity was proposed to replace "absorbed power density" by C. C. Johnson (one of the pioneers in RF bioeffects research in the U.S.) and D. Justesen and was formally defined by the National Council on Radiation Protection and Measurements in 1981 (Johnson, 1975; Justesen, 1975; NCRP, 1981). It is now the standard measure of dose rate for RF bioeffects studies. The SAR is related to the RMS electric field strength E in tissue by:

$$SAR = \frac{\sigma E^2}{\rho} \tag{2}$$

where ρ is the mass density of tissue (kg/m³). For a tutorial on measurement of SAR, see the review by Chou et al. (1996) and other chapters of this volume.

The SAR can be defined at single points in space (as the incremental power deposition based on the electric field strength at that point (Eq. 2)), as a quantity averaged over a defined mass and shape of tissue (for example, 10-gram average SAR in a cube), or as an average value over the entire body (whole-body averaged SAR or simply whole-body SAR).

12.3.2 Derived Dosimetric Quantities

The biological effects of RF exposure are typically (but not exclusively) correlated with RF-induced increases in tissue temperature. Over the past decade, numerous computer modeling studies have been conducted using detailed image-based models of the whole body or head that estimated SAR and subsequent temperature increases in the body (for a review, see Foster et al., 2018).

Quantities that are useful to characterize the thermal response of tissue to RF energy include

- *Local tissue temperature T or increase in temperature* ΔT above baseline (pre-exposure) level.
- *Heating factor H*, defined as the ratio of the peak steady-state increase in tissue temperature (ΔT) to the peak spatial-average SAR at any location in the body (denoted by psSAR).

$$H = \frac{\Delta T_{max}}{psSAR} \; (°C \, kg/W) \tag{3}$$

H depends on the size and shape of the volume or mass of tissue over which the SAR is averaged, and on local heat transfer rates near the averaging mass (Foster et al., 2017).

- *Thermal dose* CEM43, which is defined as the number of minutes that tissue must be held at 43°C to sustain the same thermal damage that would be produced by holding it at a tissue temperature T_c for time Δt. CEM43 is obtained from the temperature – time relation:

$$CEM43 = \Delta t R^{43-T_c} \tag{4}$$

where Δt is the time of exposure at tissue temperature T_c. For time-varying temperatures, Eq. 4 would be replaced by an integral over time. The base R in Eq. 4 is taken to be 0.25 for $T < 43°C$ and 0.5 for $T > 43°C$. For an extensive review of thermal damage thresholds see Yarmolenko et al. (2011).

12.4   More Detailed Review of IEEE C95.1-2005 and ICNIRP (1998, 2010)

Both sets of limits are highly complex and technical. The following discussion reviews their major similarities and differences.

12.4.1   Shared Features

Both IEEE C95.1-2005 and ICNIRP (1998, 2010) incorporate two sets of distinctions: two tiers (which broadly correspond to limits for the public and occupational exposures, although

Radio Frequency Exposure Standards 473

the definitions differ somewhat between the two limits). A second set of distinctions is between basic restrictions and reference levels (limits for induced fields or absorbed power within in the body and field strength or power density measured outside the body). These distinctions are described using different terminology between the two limits.

- *Two tiers*: In ICNIRP the two tiers correspond to limits for the general public and occupational exposures. IEEE C95.1-2005 defines a different, but essentially equivalent pair of tiers: "action levels" (for the general public or areas lacking an RF safety program) and "controlled environments" which are generally workplaces where an RF safety program has been implemented. In the next revision, IEEE C95.1 will use the terminology "persons in unrestricted environments" for the lower tier and "persons permitted in restricted environments" for the upper tier. To simplify discussion below, the two tiers in both limits will be referred to as upper and lower tier.

- *Basic restrictions and reference levels*: IEEE and ICNIRP both provide two classes of guidance: basic restrictions in terms of quantities that are directly relevant to health effects (exposures within the body), and maximum permissible exposure (MPE) levels or reference levels that are measurable outside the body. Reference levels are secondary limits that are defined in terms of quantities that can be directly measured in operational settings using standard instrumentation, and are designed to ensure that compliance with the reference levels will ensure compliance with the basic restrictions as well.

The basic restrictions are principally set on the basis of biological/biophysical considerations to limit the dose. The reference levels limit the exposure in terms of quantities that are measurable with conventional RF safety equipment. They were developed from engineering modeling studies that determined the fields induced within the body in the presence of an external field. These calculations were done assuming "worst case" exposure conditions (with the body oriented in the field to absorb the most energy), and will overestimate the internal fields under typical exposure conditions. Consequently, the reference levels provide an additional measure of conservatism beyond those in the basic restrictions. In the future revision, IEEE C95.1 will have new definitions for the basic restrictions as "dosimetric reference limits" (DRLs) and MPE as "exposure reference levels" (ERLs).

In additional, both IEEE C95.1-2005 and ICNIRP (1998) specify limits for whole-body and local exposures. Limits for whole-body exposures are expressed in terms of whole-body SAR (total watts absorbed by the body divided by body mass). Limits for local exposures are expressed in terms of the peak value of SAR averaged over 10 g of tissue (10 g psSAR) within the body. These averaging masses are specified as 10 g of "contiguous tissue" (ICNIRP) or 10 g of tissue "in the shape of a cube" (IEEE). Additionally, both sets of limits specify averaging times (6 or 30 minutes) and averaging areas (areas of body surface over which local exposures are to be averaged).

Adding to the complexity, IEEE C95.1-2005 and ICNIRP limits are defined in different terms in different frequency ranges. For IEEE C95.1-2005:

- 3 kHz to 5 MHz: The IEEE standard considers the maximum *in situ* electric field as the controlling criterion. The limits vary in different regions of the body.

- 100 kHz to 3 GHz: The standard considers the SAR in the body as the controlling criterion. The basic restrictions are given in terms of whole-body average SAR (for whole-body exposure) or peak 10 g average SAR (10 g psSAR), with MPE expressed in terms of the external power density or field strength incident on the body.

- 3 GHz to 300 GHz: The standard defines power density incident on the body as the controlling criterion, and both the basic restriction and MPE are defined in terms of this quantity.

- 3 GHz to 6 GHz: Both absorbed power (SAR) and incident power density on the body are allowed for demonstration of compliance.

  ICNIRP (1998) has similar definitions, but maintains defining the basic restriction in terms of SAR up to 10 GHz. Its more recent edition (ICNIRP, 2010) applies between 1 Hz–100 kHz, including limits up to 10 MHz.

12.4.2 Development of Limits

The process of developing the IEEE and ICNIRP limits can be understood in terms of the stages of standards development described in the *Framework*. These will be briefly reviewed below, first for IEEE C95.1-2005, then more briefly for ICNIRP.

Figure 12.2 gives an overview of the process of establishing the IEEE RF exposure standard. The process begins when ICES submits a "Project Authorization Request" (PAR) to the IEEE Standards Association Standards Board. After the PAR is approved, several working groups within ICES carry out the process of drafting the standard. These working groups maintain an ongoing surveillance of the scientific literature to identify relevant papers as they appear, critically review the literature, draft the limits and its documentation. After several rounds of balloting within Subcommittee (SC) 4, TC95 and IEEE-SA, and resolution of any dissenting opinions, the draft standard is approved as an IEEE Standard by the IEEE Standards Board.

The ICES standard was developed through a series of stages that are conceptually similar to those described by the WHO *Framework*:

a. *Evaluation of the scientific literature*

   IEEE C95.1-2005 was developed after an elaborate literature surveillance and review. ICES maintains an online database of literature* which as of February 2018 includes 3676 references to relevant papers. The literature review used to develop IEEE C95.1-2005 was summarized in a collection of twelve narrative reviews published in a supplementary issue in 2003 in the journal Bioelectromagnetics by individual members of IEEE ICES TC95/SC4. The standard itself, a 250-page document, also provides a detailed rationale for the standard with 1143 references.

   ICNIRP carried out a similar extensive review. Its 1998 RF guidelines were released in a 28 page journal article (ICNIRP, 1998); followed with a 378 page narrative literature review that reaffirmed its 1998 guidelines (ICNIRP, 2009).

b. *Determination of limiting hazards and threshold levels*

   At frequencies below about 100 kHz, the limiting hazard (i.e., that occurring at the lowest exposure level) in considered by both IEEE C95.1-2005 and ICNIRP (1998) to be electrostimulation of tissue, either from electric fields that are induced within the body by exposure to external fields, or from contact currents that result when a person touches a charged conductive object. Depending on the current level, these effects can range from minor sensory phenomena (e.g., phosphenes,

---

* http://ieee-emf.com/database.cfm.

Radio Frequency Exposure Standards

which are visual stimuli from low-level electrical currents in the retina that are induced by exposure of the head to time-varying magnetic fields) to electric shock, burns, and death from cardiac fibrillation. IEEE C95.1-2005 provided a brief description of the thresholds for electrical stimulation, and referred to more extended discussion in the companion standard (IEEE C95.6-2002) (IEEE, 2002) for frequencies below 3 kHz.

As a function of frequency, the thresholds for nerve excitation generally show a broad minimum around power distribution frequencies (50–60 Hz) and increase at higher frequencies. Eventually, about above 0.1 MHz, they exceed the thresholds for noticeable heating and thermal effects become the limiting phenomena. The potential thermal hazards considered by both group to represent limiting hazards are:

Whole-body exposure. Both sets of limits were designed on the understanding that the most reliable and sensitive indicator of potential harm is behavioral disruption. This effect has been observed in several species (mice, rats, and monkeys) after extended (minutes or more) whole-body exposures exceeding about 4 W/kg at several frequencies. "Behavioral disruption" occurs when an exposed animal ceases to carry out an assigned task (e.g., for rats, pushing a lever for food reward) and switches to another behavior (in rats, spreading saliva on the tail, which is a behavioral mechanism for thermoregulation in that species). These responses are often (but not always) accompanied by an increase in core body temperature of about 1°C (IEEE C95.1-2005, p. 36). Behavioral disruption is not an adverse effect in itself, but it is a behavioral response to a significant and possibly excessive thermal burden on the animal.

Local exposure. Both committees (ICES and ICNIRP) designed the limits for local exposure to limit local heating of tissue, which might be excessive even though the total thermal load on the body might be small. Table 12.4 (from IEEE C95.1-2005) summarizes "critical temperature levels" in various species, organs, or tissues that were used to develop the standard. In IEEE C95.1-2005 the limiting effect for setting local exposure limits was considered to be cataract formation in rabbits, which has been experimentally produced by RF exposures at local SARs above 150 W/kg for 30 minutes or more, sufficient to raise lens temperature above 41°C (Table 12.4).

Contact currents. IEEE C95.1-2005 defines contact current as a "current induced in a biological medium via a contacting electrode or other source of current." A typical accident scenario occurs when a grounded individual touches or grasps a charged conductor, allowing RF current to enter the body. Depending on the frequency and current density in the body, this can result in electrical shock and nerve stimulation (low frequencies) and/or burns. Below about 0.1 MHz shocks are the dominant adverse effect, while at higher frequencies the limiting hazards are thermal in nature. Under some conditions, both electrical shock and thermal damage to tissue can occur. The threshold for hazard depends on the electrical potential of the surface, the area of skin that is in contact with the conductor, and the electrical resistance in the current path to ground.

IEEE C95.1-2005 defined two sets of limits for contact currents, one for the frequency range 3 kHz–100 kHz (to protect against shocks) and the second for 100 kHz–3 GHz (against burns). The standard defined two sets of limits, for "touching" and "grasping" contact with assumed contact areas of 1 and 15 cm^2, respectively. Additional provisions protect against spark discharges which can occur when a worker touches a surface at high electrical potential and potentially cause startle reactions leading to a workplace accident.

    c. *Choice of safety factors for different populations at risk.*

TABLE 12.4

Thermal Effects (Adapted from C95.1-2005, Table C.3, p. 98)

Endpoint	Species/Organ/Tissue	Threshold (°C)	Exposure Duration	Reference
Heat stroke	Human (core temperature)	>42°C ≥ 40.5°C		Bynum et al. (1978)
	Human (brain temperature)		Minutes or more	Cabanac (1983)
CNS deterioration	Human (CNS)	42–43°C		Bynum et al. (1978)
Skin necrosis	Human	43°C	10–12 h	Dewhirst et al. (2003)
Fetal abnormalities	Rat (whole body)	2–2.5°C increase	Tens of minutes up to 1 h	Edwards et al. (2003)
Behavioral disruption	Rat (whole-body); monkey (whole-body)	1°C increase	40–60 min	de Lorge (1983, 1984); d'Andrea et al. (1977)
Cataract	Rabbit (eye)	>41°C	>30 min	Kramár et al. (1987); Guy et al. (1975); Carpenter et al. (1960)
Convulsions	Mouse	T_{re} = 44°C		Wright (1976)
Increase in permeability blood brain barrier	Rat	>40°C brain temperature	4 h	Merritt et al. (1978); Finnie et al. (2001, 2002); Sharma and Hoopes (2003)

IEEE C95.1-2005 defines "safety factor" as:

> a multiplier (≤ 1) or a divisor (≥ 1) used to derive maximum permissible exposure values, which provides for the protection of individuals, and uncertainties concerning threshold effects due to pathological conditions or drug treatment, uncertainties in reaction thresholds, and uncertainties in induction models.

The following is a brief review of "safety factors" as considered in IEEE C95.1-2005 with additional comments to describe more recent considerations. As used below, "safety factor" is taken to be the ratio of the threshold exposure for hazard to the MPE (ICNIRP uses an equivalent term, reduction factor).

Safety factors for whole-body exposures (>100 kHz). Historically, most attention in developing RF exposure limits has focused on whole-body exposure, which perhaps is a consequence of the fact that most animal experiments involved whole-body exposure. The hazard threshold, from behavioral disruption experiments in several species of animals, corresponds to a whole-body exposure of about 4 W/kg and increases in core body temperature of about 1°C. IEEE C95.1-2005 (as well as ICNIRP (1998)) set basic restrictions of 0.4 and 0.08 W/kg for whole-body exposures for the upper and lower tiers. This implies safety factors of 10 or 50, respectively, for upper and lower tier exposures based on the animal data.

For humans, the actual safety factors are likely to be somewhat higher, for two reasons:

a. Humans have more efficient thermoregulatory systems than animals and under ordinary environmental conditions can tolerate heat loads considerably higher than 4 W/kg, depending on work load. The basal metabolic rate of humans is

Radio Frequency Exposure Standards

equivalent to a power production of about 1 W per kg of body mass. The presumed threshold for hazard of 4 W/kg whole-body exposure is comparable to the rate of heat generated in humans during moderate exercise at a rate of 4 mets, typical of the exercise level during a brisk walk. The exposure limits (0.08 and 0.4 W/kg whole-body exposure) correspond to the rate of heat generation in the body during very slight exercise.

Also:

b. The computer models used to derive reference levels assume "worst case" exposure scenarios, for example, positioning the body in the incident RF field so as to absorb the most energy. In real-world exposure scenarios, one can expect that the exposed individual will not be positioned so as to absorb the maximum fraction of incident energy, and will move about in the field. Consequently, the actual safety factors for whole-body exposure under real-world exposure conditions will most likely be above the factors of 10 and 50 assumed in designing the standard.

However, the safety factors with respect to local exposures to parts of the body may be different, and cases can be found where whole body exposure of an individual at reference levels might lead to local exposures to parts of the body that exceed the basic restrictions. For example, Dimbylow (2002) calculated that exposure of a grounded individual to vertically oriented electric fields at 50 MHz may induce SARs in the leg that exceed the ICNIRP basic restrictions. Ensuring compliance with both ICNIRP basic restrictions (whole body and local SAR) would require invoking additional limits on currents through the limb.

Safety factors for low-frequency exposures (<100 kHz). Safety factors for exposures of the body to electric or magnetic fields below 0.1 MHz are less well established. At these frequencies, reference levels in IEEE C95.6-2002, C95.1-2005 and ICNIRP (1998, 2010) were set through a combination of computer modeling to estimate induced currents in the body, and biophysical models to estimate thresholds for electrostimulation of body tissues. The rationale for these choices is described at length in the standards documents and their references.

Few direct experimental data exist to directly establish thresholds for hazardous electrical stimulation effects in the frequency range covered by the RF exposure limits. At frequencies for which electrical stimulation is a concern (<0.1 MHz), the body is very poorly coupled to external fields. In the absence of direct contact with a charged conductor, impractically strong fields measured outside the body would be required to induce sufficient currents within the body to excite tissue. In some medical treatments using pulsed magnetic fields, stimulation of excitable tissue may be a concern (if it is not in fact the desired result of treatment). For example, in transcutaneous magnetic stimulation (TMS), brief (millisecond) pulses of very strong magnetic fields (Tesla range) are applied to the brain with the intent of stimulating brain tissue. Potential adverse effects of TMS as applied clinically are usually mild. However, at very high levels of stimulation, TMS waveforms can induce seizures in animals and presumably could do the same in humans (Wasserman, 1996). As another example, gradient magnetic field pulses in MRI imaging can induce peripheral nerve stimulation due to induced electric currents in the body, which limits the imaging parameters that can be used safely. IEEE safety limits do not apply to medical procedures in any event.

Consequently, the safety factors against tissue stimulation are somewhat uncertain, with little direct experimental support apart from particular medical procedures, and must be estimated through modeling studies. Apart from very specialized circumstances, chiefly medical mishaps, few if any injuries are reported from exposures to electric or magnetic fields below 0.1 MHz that do not involve contact with charged conductors and it appears that the standards are sufficiently protective. Apart from close approach to high powered broadcast antennas, there are few if any situations in ordinary occupational or nonoccupational settings where RF field levels in environments accessible to humans can approach the reference levels in any event.

Safety factors for local exposures. Both limits define basic restrictions for local exposure to RF fields below 3–6 GHz (IEEE C95.1-2005) or 10 GHz (ICNIRP, 1998) in terms of 10 g psSAR (10 and 2 W/kg for upper and lower tiers respectively in both sets of limits). These limits were set from experiments showing that the threshold for producing cataracts in rabbits corresponds to a local SAR of 100–140 W/kg in the eye for more than 30 minutes, which is sufficient to raise the temperature of the lens to >41°C (Table 12.4).

As a practical matter, thermal pain avoidance would probably force most individuals to remove themselves from exposure before cataracts or other thermal injury to the eye occurred, given the high sensitivity of the cornea and eyelid to thermal stimuli. For example, Oizumi et al. (2013) calculated that in humans exposed to 2.45 GHz plane waves, "the skin temperature around the eye reached the pain threshold of 43°C before the lens temperature reaches its threshold [for thermal damage] of 41°C."

Since the publication of IEEE C95.1-2005, numerous modeling studies have appeared, that used detailed image-based models of the head and body together with thermal analysis to estimate heating factors and the increases in tissue temperature (for a review, see Foster et al., 2018).

These studies indicate that above about 0.1 GHz, RF exposures at the upper tier limit of 10 W/kg for 10 g psSAR will lead to a maximum temperature increase of 2°C–3°C in a person in ordinary room environments, with steady state temperature increases developing after several minutes. Above about 1 GHz, both the local SAR and peak temperature increases are located very close to the body surface and this may be the case in many exposure situations at lower frequencies as well. In ordinary room environments, skin temperature is about 33°C–34°C and the threshold for thermal pain is about 43°C–44°C. This implies a safety factor of 3–5 for the upper tier limit, relative to the threshold for cutaneous thermal pain under ordinary environmental conditions.

Thresholds for thermal injury to tissue are similar to those for thermal pain; the difference is that tissue must be maintained at a hazardous temperature for some time before thermal injury occurs. As described in two recent reviews on thermal injury, both resulting from IEEE and ICNIRP sponsored workshops (Foster and Morrissey, 2011; Sienkiewicz et al., 2016), the thresholds for thermal injury are described in terms of the thermal dose CEM43, rather than in terms of a fixed temperature threshold. The thermal dose contains an exponential time-temperature relation (Eq. 4), which implies that thermal damage can occur if tissue is exposed to at temperatures somewhat below the threshold for thermal pain for sufficiently long times. However, in most situations, pain avoidance would an effective protective mechanism against RF burns for individuals with normal ability to sense thermal pain.

The usefulness of CEM43 for setting exposure limits is reduced by limitations in the literature on thermal damage to tissue, with few studies providing sufficiently detailed thermal dosimetry to allow precise estimates of CEM43 at the threshold for observable thermal damage (Yarmolenko et al., 2011). In addition, most thermal injury studies applied relatively large thermal doses that would produce severe thermal damage, and data are lacking for thresholds for minimal tissue damage from small thermal doses which would be relevant for setting RF exposure limits.

Radio Frequency Exposure Standards 479

The central nervous system is exceptionally sensitive to thermal damage, with damage thresholds for the brain reported to be about 0.1 min CEM43 (Yarmolenko et al., 2011). This is consistent with physiological data indicating that the blood brain barrier and other damage occurs in animals with thresholds for detectable effects at brain temperatures of 39°C–40°C (Wang et al. 2014). Kodera et al. (2018) estimated that exposures to the head from dipole antennas radiating at 1, 3, or 10 GHz at occupational local exposure limits for the head (10 W/kg averaged over 10 g of tissue) will increase the temperature of localized regions of the brain by up to about 1°C. The temperature increases would be in peripheral areas of the brain (only) where the local brain temperature is a degree or so below core brain temperature due to thermal interactions of the head and the environment. These RF-induced temperature increases are anticipated to be well below thresholds for thermal injury to the brain.

However, the thresholds for minimal brain injury from mild heating to localized regions of the brain of the sort predicted by Kodera et al. are not precisely established, and the thermal calculations are not experimentally validated. Consequently, it is difficult to estimate precisely the safety factors for such exposures. As a practical matter, the predicted increases in brain temperature are steady state values, which would require ten minutes or more of constant exposure to be achieved. Normal movements of the exposure source relative to the head over such times will average exposures and reduce the peak temperature increase. Moreover, the calculated temperature elevations are comparable to those that occur naturally due to environmental and exertional effects as well as in the range of diurnal variations in brain temperature.

Safety factors for contact currents. Both IEEE C95.1-2005 and ICNIRP limits on contact currents are designed to protect against both shocks and burns. However, they are based on very limited data in the frequency range covered by IEEE C95.1-2005 and ICNIRP (1998), chiefly on two human studies; for a review, see Tell and Tell (2018). Important variables include skin impedance, current distribution across the area of conductor in contact with the body, frequency, and pressure with which the conductor is held against the skin. These variables, which are insufficiently explored by experimental studies, make it impossible to assess safety factors for limits on contact current with any precision given the many potential scenarios involving contact current exposure.

As a result of these complexities, the "safety factors" inherent in both the IEEE and ICNIRP limits are uncertain in many respects. ICNIRP (1998) states:

> there is insufficient information on the biological and health effects of EMF exposure of human populations and experimental animals to provide a rigorous basis for establishing safety factors over the whole frequency range and for all frequency modulations.

That said, the apparent absence of reported injuries from exposures compliant with ICNIRP (1998) and IEEE C95.1-2005 limits indicates that they are protective against the hazards for which they were designed.

12.4.3 Perspective

Despite their independent development, the two limits (IEEE C95.1-2005 and ICNIRP (1998, 2010)) are quite similar even though they differ in some details. Table 12.3 compares reference levels of the two limits, while Table 12.5 compares basic restrictions while Table 12.6 presents a more detailed comparison.

The most conspicuous differences between IEEE C95.1-2005 and ICNIRP (1998, 2010) are in the lower end of the frequency range (<1 MHz) where the ICNIRP and IEEE limits

TABLE 12.5

Basic Restrictions in ICNIRP (1998), IEEE C95.1-2005, and FCC (1997) limits compared*

Standard or Guideline	ICNIRP (1998) 100 kHz–10 GHz (BR same as reference levels above 10 GHz)	IEEE C95.1-2005 100 kHz–3 GHz (BR same as reference levels above 3 GHz) W/kg	FCC (1997) 300 kHz–6 GHz (for portable devices, used within 20 cm of body) W/kg
SAR Limit for Local Exposure (W/kg)	General public: 2 (head, trunk), 4 (limbs)	Action Level (equivalent to general public): 2 (unspecified part of body) 4 (extremities and pinnae)	General public: 1.6 (unspecified body part) 4 (hands, wrists, feet, ankles)
	Occupational: 10 (head and trunk), 20 (limbs)	Persons in Controlled Environment (equivalent to occupational): 10 (unspecified part of body) 20 (extremities and pinnae)	Occupational: 8 (unspecified body part) 20 (hands, wrists, feet, ankles)
Averaging Mass (g)	Peak SAR averaged over any 10 g of contiguous tissue	Peak SAR averaged over any 10 g of tissue in shape of cube	Peak SAR averaged over any 1 g of tissue in shape of cube
SAR limit for whole body exposure (W/kg)	General public: 0.08	Action Level (equivalent to general public): 0.08	General public: 0.08
	Occupational: 0.4	Persons in Controlled Environment (equivalent to occupational): 0.4	Occupational: 0.4
	Averaged over whole body	Averaged over whole body	Averaged over whole body

* Simplified from ICNIRP (1998), IEEE C95.1-2005, and FCC (1997). Readers should consult with original documents for numerous technical details in table footnotes in original documents.

TABLE 12.6

Comparison of ICNIRP and IEEE Limits

Parameter	ICNIRP (1998) Guideline	IEEE C95.1-2005 Standard	ICNIRP 201x Guideline(Draft as of Current Writing)	IEEE C95.1-201x Standard (Draft as of Current Writing)
Frequency range covered	1Hz–300 GHz	3 kHz–300 GHz	100 kHz–300 GHz	0 Hz–300 GHz
Tiers	Two (occupational, general public)	Two (persons in controlled environment (upper); action level (lower tier))	Two (occupational, general public)	Two (persons in restricted environment (upper tier)); persons in unrestricted environment (lower tier))
Exposure/ Dose distinction?	Yes. Dose: Basic restriction (SAR)	Yes Dose: Basic restriction (SAR)	Yes. Dose: Basic restriction	Yes Dose: dosimetric reference limit (DRL), epithelial power density
	Exposure: Reference level (incident power density)	Exposure: Maximum permissible exposure (MPE) (incident power density)	Exposure: reference level (incident power density)	Exposure: exposure reference level (incident power density)

(Continued)

Radio Frequency Exposure Standards

TABLE 12.6 (*Continued*)

Comparison of ICNIRP and IEEE Limits

Parameter	ICNIRP (1998) Guideline	IEEE C95.1-2005 Standard	ICNIRP 201x Guideline(Draft as of Current Writing)	IEEE C95.1-201x Standard (Draft as of Current Writing)
Most significant biological endpoint	Behavioral disruption (associated with ~1°C temperature rise)	Behavioral disruption (associated with ~1°C temperature rise)	Behavioral disruption (associated with ~1°C temperature rise)	Behavioral disruption (associated with ~1°C temperature rise)
Limiting whole-body-averaged SAR (applicable frequency range)	0.4 W/kg (occupational) 0.08 W/kg (general public) 100 kHz–10 GHz	Controlled environment: 0.4 W/kg Action level: 0.08 W/kg 100 kHz–3 GHz	Occupational: 0.4 W/kg) General public: 0.08 W/kg 100 kHz–6 GHz	Persons in restricted environment: 0.4 W/kg Persons in unrestricted environment: 0.08 W/kg 100 kHz–6 GHz
Averaging time (f > 100 kHz)	6 min (f ≤ 10 GHz) decreasing to 10 s at 300 GHz (upper and lower tiers)	6 min (f ≤ 3 GHz) then decreasing to 10 s at 300 GHz (different frequency dependence in upper and lower tiers)	30 min for whole body exposure, 6 min for local exposure	30 min for whole-body exposure and 6 min for local exposure
Limiting localized SAR and applicable frequency range	Occupational: 10 W/kg averaged over 10 g contiguous tissue General public: 2 W/kg averaged over 10 g contiguous tissue 100 kHz–10 GHz	Controlled environment:10 W/kg averaged over 10 g cubic tissue Action level: 2 W/kg averaged over 10 g cubic tissue 100 kHz–3 GHz	Occupational: 10 W/kg averaged over 10 g cubic tissue General public: 2 W/kg averaged over 10 g cubic tissue 100 kHz–6 GHz	Persons in restricted environment: 10 W/kg averaged over 10 g cubic tissue Persons in unrestricted environment: 2 W/kg averaged over 10 g cubic tissue 100 kHz–6 GHz
Specific limits for high peak, low average power pulses	Yes, based on evoked auditory response ("microwave hearing")	Yes, based on the stun-effect	Yes, based on fluence for exposures < 6 min	Yes, based on fluence for mm-wave pulses
Provision for RF safety program	Not specifically	Yes, IEEE C95.7–2014. The BRs and MPEs of the lower tier (action level) are linked to an RF safety program to mitigate against exposures that could exceed the BRs and MPEs of the upper tier	Not specifically	Yes, IEEE C95.7–2014. The DRLs and ERLs of the lower tier are linked to an RF safety program to mitigate against exposures that could exceed the DRLs and ERLs of the upper tier.

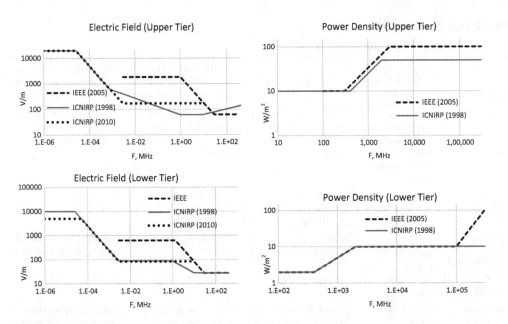

FIGURE 12.3
Comparison of C95.1-2005, ICNIRP (1998) and ICNIRP (2010) exposure limits (MPEs/reference levels). The frequency ranges covered are 3 kHz–300 GHz (IEEE C95.1-2005), "up to" 300 GHz (but excluding static fields) (ICNIRP, 1998) and 1 Hz–10 MHz (ICNIRP, 2010).

differ by a factor of 50 (Figure 12.3). This is chiefly due to different estimates of thresholds for electrical excitation of tissue by the two groups (Reilly, 2005). The real-world consequence of these differences is limited given the few opportunities for human exposure to fields at levels exceeding either set of limits (apart from some medical treatments). The major reported forms of RF injury involve burns and shock, and result from contact currents as opposed to exposure to fields in air. WHO and the standards setting groups themselves have attempted to "harmonize" (bring into agreement) voluntary (ICNIRP and IEEE) and national limits to create a consistent set of international limits. The ICNIRP and IEEE limits are presently quite similar, but wide variations in national limits still remain.

RF injuries in the real world. IEEE C95.1-2005 summarized "various considerations relevant to RF safety." In order of decreasing likelihood of producing injury in real-world exposure these are:

- RF shocks and burns (from contact currents when an individual comes in contact with a conductor that is charged to high voltage at RF frequencies)
- Localized RF heating effects (for example, from too-close approach to high-powered RF equipment)
- Surface heating effects (e.g., from millimeter wave sources, where the energy is absorbed close to the skin surface)
- Whole-body heating effects (e.g., from far-field exposure to an RF transmitter)
- Microwave hearing effects (referring to auditory sensations elicited when the head is exposed to pulsed RF energy of high peak power but low duty cycle, which IEEE C95.1-2005 does not consider to be an adverse effect)

Radio Frequency Exposure Standards 483

RF shocks and burns represent a real occupational hazard to workers in settings where high-powered RF equipment is present. Most reported RF injuries result from contact with circuits or antennas that are charged to high RF voltage, and they can be life threatening. The incidence of such accidents is not well established since many apparently are not reported. One website* for radio operators has a discussion by several RF technicians about "my first RF burn" from touching activated antennas. Hocking and Westerman (1999) gave a harrowing account of "radiofrequency electrocution" in a worker from touching an activated circuit in TV broadcasting equipment operating at 196 MHz. Workers can receive serious RF burns from contact with an ungrounded construction crane erected in the vicinity of an AM radio tower due to induced RF currents in the crane, necessitating special precautions in construction work near the towers (Ustuner, 2012). RF burns to patients are recognized (if rare) complications of medical treatments involving RF ablation, electrosurgery, diathermy, or other medical procedure using RF energy.

One factor that limits the incidence of serious injury from RF energy is the painful nature of RF burns. Given the opportunity, an exposed individual will withdraw from RF exposure before injury occurs. Pain avoidance generally protects individuals from inadvertent burns from other causes as well. For example, a cook can reach into an oven to turn over a steak under the broiler, exposing his/her hand to levels of infrared energy that far exceed any plausible exposure limit; thermal pain forces the cook to withdraw from the oven before sustaining a burn. By contrast, many injuries (sometimes lethal) have occurred when a cook or bystander inadvertently tips a pot of boiling liquids onto his/her body. Preventing such injuries is a matter of safe work (cooking) practices and not regulating the temperature of the water. Similarly, protecting workers against injury from RF exposure in the workplace requires a combination of safe work practices together with RF exposure limits.

12.4.4 National Limits

Few countries have the resources or expertise to undertake the large efforts needed to develop their own science-based limits. Around the world, most countries have adopted ICNIRP (1998) limits (sometimes with "precautionary" modifications). Others have adopted limits that are broadly consistent with the IEEE-ICNIRP family of limits, or entirely different limits (Dhungel et al., 2014). For a comprehensive (but somewhat dated) review of national limits see Stam (2011); see also an online summary by GSMA (an organization of companies producing GSM wireless devices)[†] and a more limited table of limits at a WHO website.[‡]

The information below is believed to be accurate as of the present writing but the regulations frequently change. In addition, national limits are invariably accompanied by rules for their application, which may include special provisions for "sensitive" locations such as schools and hospitals, and the limits may vary with technology (e.g., different limits for mobile phone base station versus broadcast transmitters). The following comments are, at best, a very partial review of a complex and frequently changing set of regulations in place across the world.

---

[*] www.eham.net/articles/34231.

[†] www.gsma.com/publicpolicy/consumer-affairs/emf-and-health/emf-policy.

[‡] http://apps.who.int/gho/data/node.main.EMF?lang=en.

For local body exposures (e.g., from mobile phone handsets), the GSMA website indicates that 150 countries or territories have adopted ICNIRP limits while 19 countries (e.g., Bolivia, Canada, India, Iran, Iraq, S. Korea) have adopted the U.S. (FCC) limits (which in turn were derived from an earlier version of the IEEE standard (C95.1-1991), which in turn were adopted by ANSI as ANSI/IEEE C95.1-1992 (IEEE, 1992). Only two sets of limits (FCC, 1996; ICNIRP, 1998) appear to be in use for mobile phone handsets, perhaps reflecting the fact that major manufacturers test handsets for compliance with only these two limits and it would be impractical for countries to impose their own, different, SAR limits given the international market for mobile phones.

For far-field exposures such as from wireless base station antennas, the situation is more complicated. According to GSMA, as of 2016, 125 countries and territories have adopted ICNIRP (1998), 11 follow FCC limits of 1996 or IEEE C95.1-1991, and 36 have adopted "other" limits. A very partial tabulation of country-specific limits is at the WHO website.[*]

European Union. Most EU nations have adopted the ICNIRP (1998) limits, following recommendations of the Council of the European Union in 1999 (European Union, 1999) (for the general public) and 2013 (European Union 2013) (for occupational exposures). However, the Treaty on European Union allows individual jurisdictions to adopt stricter limits and a minority of EU countries has done so at the national level. In addition, various cities and regions have adopted their own limits that are different from the national limits of their countries. Adding to the complexity, some EU nations that were formerly part of the Warsaw Pact during Soviet times still maintain older, and much lower, limits of the former Soviet Union, sometimes in modified form, while others have moved towards the ICNIRP limits. The diversity of limits across Europe reflects, in part, the fact that local jurisdictions can regulate RF exposures from transmitting facilities (and revise them to respond to local political concerns) and in part from history (e.g., being a former part of the Soviet Union and or one of its Warsaw Pact allies and consequently inheriting a regulatory framework influenced by that of the Soviet Union).

This has led to a complex patchwork of RF exposure limits in effect across the EU. For example, at the national level, Greece has adopted national limits that are 70% of ICNIRP limits, or 60% of ICNIRP limits within specified distances of schools, hospitals, and other "sensitive" locations. Italy has adopted limits of 20% of ICNIRP at 1 GHz (1 W/m² for the general public) but has adopted much lower limits in homes, schools, playgrounds, and places where people may stay for longer than 4 hours, with an "attention value" of 0.1 W/m² as averaged over any 24-hour period.

As another example, France has adopted ICNIRP limits at the national level, but Paris has adopted much more restrictive exposure limits for RF fields emitted by cellular base stations (as opposed to other sources of RF signals). According to a March 2017 news report, the city has reached an agreement with cellular providers to accept a limit of 5 V/m at cellular frequencies in indoor areas (1–2% of ICNIRP limits depending on frequency if measured in terms of incident power density) (Le Hir, 2017). Belgium has allowed its various regions to set their own exposure limits in lieu of setting a national limit. Wallonia, a region in southern Belgium, has adopted what is probably the lowest limit in Europe, 3 V/m "per antenna" over an unspecified frequency range, in areas accessible to the public (0.5% of the ICNIRP limit at 900 MHz). The limits are reduced to 0.6 V/m in schools, day care centers, and hospitals (0.02% of ICNIRP guidelines expressed in terms of incident power density). These restrictions apply to cellular base station antennas, and not

---

[*] http://apps.who.int/gho/data/node.main.EMFLIMITSPUBLICRADIOFREQUENCY?lang=en.

Radio Frequency Exposure Standards 485

to broadcast transmitters, many of which operate at far higher power levels than cellular base stations.

Among Eastern European countries, Poland, Belarus, Georgia, Ukraine, Lithuania (among others) have adopted much lower limits than ICNIRP (in some cases the same as and in other cases higher than the old Soviet limits). By contrast, Bulgaria, Hungary, and Romania have adopted ICNIRP limits, and Slovenia has adopted ICNIRP limits while adding an additional reduction factor of 10 for "sensitive" areas such as schools and hospitals.

U.S. In the USA, the current FCC guidelines (approved in 1996) were derived from earlier limits proposed in a 1986 report of the National Council on Radiation Protection and Measurements (NCRP)[*] together with the 1992 edition of the IEEE limits (ANSI/ IEEE C95.1-1992). The FCC limits for whole-body exposure are similar to ICNIRP and IEEE. However, the peak spatial SAR limits for "portable" devices (including mobile phones) are lower than IEEE C95.1-2005 and ICNIRP (1998) (1.6 versus 2 W/kg for the public) and specify a smaller averaging mass of tissue (1 versus 10 g averaging mass). Consequently, the current FCC limits on RF exposures from cellular handsets and other transmitters used against the body are somewhat more conservative than current IEEE and ICNIRP limits.

Canada. Limits in Canada (Health Canada Safety Code 6) (Health Canada, 2015) are chiefly based on ICNIRP (1998) with a modest further reduction in reference levels at some frequencies due to dosimetric studies that show that the safety factor of 50 for whole-body exposure is not maintained for children exposed under certain conditions (Dimbylow 2002). For example, the whole-body SAR in a model of a 5-year-old child standing in a 60 MHz field can exceed basic restrictions of both ICNIRP and pre-2015 Safety Code 6 by about 5%. For its part, Toronto has adopted RF limits for cellular base stations that are 1% of the national limits in effect when the city ordinance was adopted (an earlier edition of Canadian Safety Code 6).

India. In 2008, India had formerly adopted ICNIRP limits for RF exposure, for both local and far-field exposure. In 2012, India revised its RF exposure limits for cellular base stations (not other transmitting facilities) to 1/10 of ICNIRP (1998) and its local exposure limits (for mobile phones) from the ICNIRP limits (2 W/kg for 10 g psSAR) to the lower U.S. limits (1.6 W/kg for 1 g psSAR).[†]

Russian Federation. Exposure limits in effect in Russia have historically been far lower than those in the West, and the current limits have not changed significantly since Soviet times. The following discussion is largely based on a 2012 review by Repacholi et al. (2012). For more recent reviews, see Grigoriev (2017) and Bukhtiyarov et al. (2015). Older reviews of the Soviet/Russian/Eastern European standards are also available (McRee, 1979; Gajšek et al., 2002).

The present Russian exposure limits for far-field exposures to RF energy from communications base stations (Sanitary Norms and Regulations, SanPiN 2.1.8/2.2.4.1190-03) are 0.25 W/m² for occupational exposures and 0.1 W/m² for general public exposures. However, the laws are complex. Different (higher) limits apply, for example, for workers in "production environments" than for other occupational exposures, and the limits also vary with source of exposure (e.g., different limits for RF exposure from cellular base stations than from broadcast transmitters) (Tables 12.7).

---

[*] NCRP Report 86, Biological Exposure Criteria for Radiofrequency Electromagnetic Fields, NCRP, Bethesda MD 1986.
[†] www.dot.gov.in/journey-emf.

TABLE 12.7

RF Exposure Limits of Russian Federation for Occupational and General Public Exposure (Adapted from Repacholi et al. (2012))

1996 Public. Russian State Sanitary and Epidemiological Surveillance Committee	300 MHz–300 GHz, 2 W/m²/h, with an upper limit of 0.25 W/m² for an 8 h day, from RF equipment	SanPiN 2.2.4/2.1.8.055-96. Physical environmental factors. Electromagnetic factors of the RF range [Russian Standard, 1996]
2003 Public and occupational mobile phone users and base stations	Basic limits for public and workers from telecom equipment (300 MHz–2.4 GHz). 0.1 W/m² for public from base stations; 0.25 W/m² for workers on base stations for ≥8 h shifts or 10 W/m² for ≤0.2 h/day. Mobile phone head exposure ≤1 W/m² determined by phone emitting ≤0.03 W/m² at 37 cm from phone. Recommends limiting mobile phone call time as much as possible and limiting possibility of use by children age <18 years, pregnant women and pacemaker wearers	SanPiN 2.1.8/2.24.1190-03. Hygienic requirements for the siting and operation of land mobile radio communication equipment. Moscow: Russian Federation

Detailed scientific justifications for the Russian limits, comparable to the critical reviews that IEEE, ICNIRP, and various Western health agencies have compiled, are not readily accessible to Western readers and may not exist. As described by Repacholi et al. (2012), the Russian limits are based on the concept that

> people should not have to compensate for any effects produced by RF exposure, even though they are not shown to be adverse to health (pathological). ... Exposure limits are then set that do not cause any possible biological consequence among the population (regardless of age or gender) that could be detected by modern methods during the RF exposure period or long after it has finished.

In addition, Russian limits vary with the duration of exposure in a way that is quite different from Western limits. IEEE and ICNIRP limits, and national limits that derive from these, specify averaging times of 6 or 30 minutes to take into account the thermal inertia of the body (i.e., heating effects). By contrast, the Russian limits are set at levels far below those capable of producing significant heating of the body, and restrict cumulative exposure over a working day.

These differences reflect long-held views of experts in the Soviet Union/Russian Federation that RF energy is biologically active, even at very low exposure levels (compared to Western exposure limits). The Soviet/Russian medical literature has many papers on health and biological effects of RF energy going back to the 1960s or before, many of which report biological effects or medical problems at very low levels of exposure (for reviews in English, see Repacholi et al. (2012) and Pakhomov et al. (2000)). In addition, the medical literature in the former Soviet Union contains many reports, going back for more than half a century, on use of millimeter waves (<200 W/m²) to treat a variety of problems with many claims of therapeutic benefit. Millimeter wave therapy is still practiced in Russia; Betskii et al. (2000) cites 92 papers on mm-wave therapy and with extensive (and to the present writers quite speculative) discussion about its mechanisms of action.

To a Western reader, much of this literature is difficult to evaluate, in part because of very brief descriptions of methodology and in part because of apparent absence of currently accepted measures for quality control such as blinding and use of concurrent sham

Radio Frequency Exposure Standards 487

controls. More broadly, this work clearly reflects a different understanding of public health research than in Western medicine. For example, Bukhtiyarov et al. (2015) listed effects of occupational exposures to EMFs of unspecified characteristics:

> Asthenic syndrome (initial phase of disease) – patient complaints: headache, high fatigability, irritability, occasional heart pains. Autonomic changes vagotonic type usually (hypotension, bradycardia, etc.).
>
> Asthenovegetative syndrome (neurocirculatory dystonia hypertensive type in moderate and expressed stages of disease) – besides deepening of asthenic manifestations there are vegetative disorders connected with vegetative nervous system sympathetic part tone prevalence by way of vascular instability with hypertensive and vasoconstrictive reactions.
>
> Hypothalamic syndrome, with paroxysmal states in form of sympatho-adrenal crisis. In time of crisis there are the possibility of paroxysmal ciliary arrhythmia and ventricular premature beats. Hyperexcitability, emotional instability. Signs of early atherosclerosis, coronary heart disease (ischemia), essential hypertension.

Needless to say, none of these conditions is recognized by Western health agencies as occupational health effects of EMF exposure (of whatever sort). To the extent that the scientific evidence for such reported problems can be evaluated by the present authors, it appears to be based largely on observational reports of nonspecific symptoms in small number of workers, as opposed to controlled and blinded studies with adequate exposure assessment. (Chapter 6 in BMA discusses mm and THz waves and their effects in more detail.)

Despite the obvious benefits of harmonization of standards, it has been difficult to reconcile Russian with Western limits. For their part, Western health agencies would be loath to drastically revise their present RF exposure limits based on health claims that are not supported by their own extensive reviews of the scientific literature. The inclusion criteria for Western health-agency reviews, for example, adequate exposure assessment, would undoubtedly exclude much of the Russian literature, particularly from the Soviet era. On the other hand, some Russian scientists who are prominent in the Russian EMF community continue to assert that exposure to RF energy at levels far below Western limits is harmful to health (e.g., Grigoriev, 2017). As a practical matter, some former Warsaw Pact countries that have now joined the EU (e.g., the Czech Republic, Latvia, and Slovakia) have adopted exposure limits similar to those of most of the rest of the EU, while others retain older and lower limits of the former Soviet Union.

The exposure limits in effect around the world have many complications and the numerical limits provide only part of the story. The limits vary by whom they apply to, and under what circumstances. For example, Russian occupational limits vary with different occupational groups and for different sources of RF exposure. This is perhaps necessary for practical reasons: it would be difficult to craft low exposure limits for cellular base stations and apply them as well to high-powered RF sources including broadcast transmitters that may operate in the same environments, or RF industrial heaters and medical devices that may expose many people to relatively high levels of RF energy, albeit in specialized environments.

Also, in Russia, China, and a number of other countries, different exposure limits apply to military versus civilian settings. For example, IEEE standard C95.1-2345-2014 "IEEE Standard for Military Workplaces—Force Health Protection Regarding Personnel Exposure to Electric, Magnetic, and Electromagnetic Fields, 0 Hz to 300 GHz" was adopted in 2015 by NATO as a replacement for NATO STANAG 2345 (Edition 3). This IEEE standard defines

488   *Electromagnetic Fields*

a third tier, Zone 2, with exposure limits above the higher tier in C95.1-2005 for military personnel with specialized RF training in mitigating high-intensity exposures.

Clearly, the limits in IEEE C95.1-2005 and ICNIRP (1998) together with national limits are not "bright lines" that separate safe from unsafe exposures. They are, rather, more akin to speed limits on a highway that are intended to avoid unsafe practices, but also reflect practical considerations, including the desire to allow use of the RF spectrum. These practical considerations clearly vary depending on circumstances of exposure. Moreover, they incorporate large (if somewhat uncertain) safety factors against thresholds for demonstrable injury.

12.4.5 Other "Thermal" Standards

Other standards/guidelines also address thermal hazards, but incorporate different tradeoffs between practicality and safety. In some cases, their safety factors against thermal hazards are considerably lower than those of IEEE C95.1-2005 and ICNIRP (1998).

For example, product safety standards (IEC 60601-1:2015 for medical electronic equipment, IEC-60950 for information technology equipment including laptops) limit the temperature of the cases of consumer-facing devices (so-called touch temperature). The limits are low enough that an individual who picks up a hot device will have time to put it down before sustaining a burn, but long-term contact of the device with the body can and (in rare cases has) led to serious injury. One case report describes a full thickness burn to the thigh of a 43-year-old man who, after imbibing 100 g of alcohol, fell asleep while watching videos on his laptop computer (Tsang et al., 2011). Less serious thermal injury to the skin (erythema *ab igne*) has been reported in young people from playing computer games using their laptop computers (Arnold and Itin, 2010).

As another example, plumbing codes* limit the temperature of hot water that is delivered at showers and baths, generally to 49°C. That would give a consumer sufficient time to remove a child who had been accidentally placed in an excessively warm bath before scald injury is sustained. They do not protect an individual from harm from excessively long immersion in warm (but not thermally painful) water; one death has been reported of an elderly diabetic individual who apparently became unconscious and remained in a warm bath for 3 hours which raised his core body temperature to 41°C (Kim et al., 2006). Limitations on domestic hot water temperatures reflect a tradeoff between the need to inhibit growth of *Legionella* bacteria in hot water tanks (which requires holding water at temperatures above 50°C) while accommodating consumer demand for hot water for household chores and hot showers, and also preventing scald injuries. While both sets of limits (touch temperature for electronics, water tap temperatures in plumbing codes) are effective in preventing most injuries, they do not provide perfect safety, and would not prevent injuries from long-term exposures at temperatures below those causing thermal pain.

As a final example, ICNIRP limits for far infrared energy for the skin (ICNIRP, 2006) are chiefly designed to protect against burns from brief exposures to intense laser pulses that cause injury before the victim can withdraw from exposure. For longer duration exposures, the limits rely on pain avoidance to induce the individual to withdraw from exposure. "No formalized limit is provided for longer exposure durations [>10 sec] because of the strong dependence upon ambient thermal environmental conditions" the ICNIRP guideline states. For such exposures, the guidelines defer to occupational heat

---

* For a lengthy discussion see www.phcppros.com/articles/1828-hot-water-system-temperatures-and-the-code.

Radio Frequency Exposure Standards 489

stress limits. This approach contrasts with that of ICNIRP limits for RF exposure, which apply to the frequency range just below that covered by the far infrared limits and which protect against-long term exposures (i.e., steady-state temperature increases) with no consideration of ambient thermal environmental conditions or activity level of an individual.

12.4.6 Other Suggested Limits: The BioInitiative Report

A variety of groups have recommended exposure limits of their own. Some of these have played a role in public controversies about the safety of RF energy although they may lack legal standing or other official status.

The BioInitiative Report, published by a self-selected group of (at present) 28 scientists and other individuals[*] is undoubtedly the most widely known such report (Blackman et al., 2012). The report originally appeared in 2007, but was revised and expanded in 2012 with additional material added more recently; all of this material is incorporated in a single online document. The Report presently consists of 28 sections (some available in both 2007 and 2012 versions that are included in the same document) that are authored by individuals or small numbers of coauthors. These sections review topics related to EMF (both power frequency and RF fields) and health. The overall conclusions of the Report, written by the two co-editors and not presented as a consensus statement of the entire group of authors, are dire: "the body of evidence at hand suggests that bioeffects and health impacts can and do occur at exquisitely low exposure levels: levels that can be thousands of times below public safety limits."

The 2007 edition recommends an "interim precautionary limit" for RF fields of 1 mW/m^2 (outdoors) and "an even lower exposure level inside buildings, perhaps as low as [0.1 mW/m^2]. The later (2012) recommendations call for a "cumulative outdoor limit" of 0.3 nW/cm^2, which is three orders of magnitude below the report's 2007 recommendation.

These recommendations are quite different from IEEE, ICNIRP, and national limits derived from them. The BioInitiative Report does not frame the limits as excluding demonstrably hazardous exposures, nor does it indicate exposure levels that the authors consider to be safe. The whole premise of the Report is that EMF exposure is potentially hazardous at arbitrarily low exposure levels, both at powerline frequencies and over unspecified parts of the RF frequency range, even though clear evidence of hazards may be lacking.

Moreover, the BioInitiative recommendations are not fleshed out in sufficient detail to be generally applied in the many different exposure scenarios that might occur in occupational and nonoccupational settings. IEEE and ICNIRP limits are complicated by the need to account for occupational versus general public exposure, the frequency-dependence of thresholds for hazards, and local-body versus whole-body exposure and other issues that are not considered in the BioInitiative Report.

Rather, the "precautionary recommendations" of the BioInitiative Report are aimed at limiting everyday exposures of citizens to RF fields from now-commonplace technologies (such as mobile phones, cellular base stations, Wi-Fi, wireless-enabled utility meters and, in a different frequency range, fields from electrical distribution systems) that have become politically contentious in many places (and which the authors of the Report consider harmful). However, exposures at far higher levels than these produce are commonly encountered in modern society, particularly in occupational settings near high-powered RF sources, and in some medical settings. The 2007 recommendations, if applied across

---

[*] www.bioinitiative.org/.

the board to any RF exposure to any individual in any environment, would preclude many industrial, broadcasting, and medical applications of RF energy, many of which provide important benefits to safety or health. The 2012 recommendations, consistently applied, would probably preclude any use of the RF spectrum that results in transmission of RF energy at any practically useful level into habitable spaces.

The BioInitiative Report has been widely criticized by health agencies in several countries. In its devastating review of the original version the Health Council of the Netherlands (2008) concluded:

> In view of the way the BioInitiative report was compiled, the selective use of scientific data and the other shortcomings mentioned above, the Committee concludes that the BioInitiative report is not an objective and balanced reflection of the current state of scientific knowledge. Therefore, the report does not provide any grounds for revising the current views as to the risks of exposure to electromagnetic fields.

To illustrate some problems that "selective use of scientific data" can cause in health risk assessments, the Report includes a table listing 66 reported biological effects of RF exposure, at SAR levels ranging from 0.064 mW/kg to 2 W/kg. Nearly all of these reported effects occurred at exposure levels below (and most cases, very far below) IEEE C95.1-2005 and ICNIRP (1998) limits. This table underlies the Report's conclusion (2012 edition) that "the body of evidence at hand suggests that bioeffects and health impacts can and do occur at exquisitely low exposure levels: levels that can be thousands of times below public safety limits."

The lowest reported effect in that table in terms of SAR (with an estimated SAR in the head of 0.064 mW/kg) refers to a 2003 study by Zwamborn et al. That table describes the Zwamborn study as showing that "well-being and cognitive function [are] affected in humans exposed to GSM-UMTS cell phone frequencies." The BioInitiative Report does not qualify this statement, or describe contradictory findings by other investigators.

Zwamborn et al. measured cognitive function and (by questionnaire) the feelings of well-being in 36 individuals exposed to simulated cellular telephone signals, half of whom had previously reported subjective complaints from cellular base stations. The overall goal of the study was to determine whether these "sensitive" individuals would experience such effects when exposed to RF fields under well-controlled conditions in a double-blinded study. Although the Zwamborn study appeared to be carefully done, it was only published in an institute report and not in a peer reviewed journal, and would consequently have failed to meet the inclusion criteria for most health agency reviews.

The Zwamborn report concluded

> From the 30 cognitive function tests [in 48 subjects tested], we found that eight cognitive function tests are statistically significant.

The report went on:

> It is noted that the dimension of the changes observed in the Well Being [using a particular survey test] for UMTS-like exposure, though statistically significant, is relatively small...
>
> An important scientific issue is the fact that relations that are found must be reproducible. Since this research is the first one to find a statistically significant relation on Well Being ... reproduction of our research by a research group independent of TNO [the organization in which the study had been done] is necessary.

Three years later, Regel et al. (2006) reported a follow-up study using a similar experimental design as the Zwamborn study with a much larger number of subjects and up to

Radio Frequency Exposure Standards

ten times higher exposure levels, and could not confirm the original findings. Regel et al. concluded that "the reported effects [by Zwamborn et al.] on brain functioning were marginal and may have occurred by chance." Another follow-up study by Eltiti et al. (2007) involving 175 "electrically sensitive" individuals was also negative apart from a small apparent effect that the investigators subsequently traced to a methodological issue (the order of presentation of stimuli in the experimental procedure).

A subsequent meta-analysis of health effects of RF EMFs from mobile phone base stations (Röösli et al., 2010) cited the Zwamborn study but excluded it from the analysis as not meeting the inclusion criteria for the review. The authors concluded: "our review does not indicate an association between any health outcome and radiofrequency electromagnetic field exposure from MPBSs [mobile phone base stations] at levels typically encountered in people's everyday environment."

Whether Zwamborn's original "statistically significant" findings were false positive results, due to some nonrandom error or unrecognized bias, or might have reflected a real but small effect is impossible to know. In any event, the effects as originally reported appear to be too small to have any significance to the subject and were not found in subsequent studies involving much higher exposure levels. None of these complexities are described in the BioInitiative Report and the Zwamborn study has been given little or no weight in health agency reviews.

12.5 Approaches to Critical Reviews of the Literature

The identified hazards of exposure to RF energy that underlie both IEEE C95.1-2005 and ICNIRP (1998) result from short-term (acute) exposures and would be obvious to an affected individual – burns and shocks. This view is generally supported by health-agency reviews in many different countries that have consistently found no convincing evidence of health hazards from RF exposure below recommended limits. (Many of these can be accessed at the ICES website.)[*] These conclusions have not changed over the years, in the face of a rapidly increasing body of literature on RF bioeffects.

In reviewing scientific evidence related to potential health hazards, health agencies, and standards-setting organizations typically conduct critical reviews (as opposed to simply collecting lists of reported effects). This entails assessing the quality of individual studies, searching for consistencies in findings across different studies, assessing the relevance of biological effects to human health.

The need for critical reviews of the diverse and often inconsistent literature in this field has long been recognized by the EMF standards setting community. This entails the need for expert judgment given the diverse and uneven nature of the literature. For example, NCRP Report 86 (NCRP, 1986) remarked:

> [It is] necessary to make difficult decisions in arriving at these conclusions [about potential RF hazards]. Because the biological data base is drawn from reports varying in quality from poor to excellent, one must be aware that the data forming the basis of this [report] also vary in quality. Thus, value judgments had to be made concerning the data base discussed.

---

[*] www.ices-emfsafety.org/expert-reviews/.

492   *Electromagnetic Fields*

IEEE C95.1-2005 describes in more detail:

> Many novel experimental studies have been published in the peer reviewed scientific literature, and while of interest, cannot be applied to setting standards for allowable human exposure to RF energy. A number of these studies suffer from poor design, inappropriate or no controls, inadequate dosimetry, physical artifacts, defective measurements, or improper statistical analysis. Other studies suffer from erroneous conclusions and lack of scientific detail. Many published studies failed to replicate or support initially reported effects of RF exposure. The results of other published studies, of high-quality design or exceptional importance, although not independently replicated in the published literature, were seriously considered as part of the risk assessment because supporting evidence was available in that literature... Painstaking review by experts of the papers in the scientific database was the only dependable means of sorting the meaningful data from the mediocre or unusable data. These reviews, performed as part of the process for establishing this standard, were careful to differentiate between evidence for a biological effect and that for an adverse human health effect...

As time went on, strategies for reviewing health and environmental effects literature have evolved and become more formalized. Early-adopted strategies have included establishing criteria for choosing studies for review (e.g., for RF bioeffects studies, appropriate dosimetry, publication in a peer-reviewed journal, and appropriate controls including sham controls concurrent with exposed groups).

More recently, health agencies have stressed the need for a "weight of evidence" review. Thus, as the WHO explained in its Environmental Health Criteria review of health effects of extremely low frequency (ELF) fields (WHO, 2007):

> All studies, with either positive or negative effects, need to be evaluated and judged on their own merit, and then all together in a weight of evidence approach. It is important to determine how much a set of evidence changes the probability that exposure causes an outcome. Generally, studies must be replicated or be in agreement with similar studies. The evidence for an effect is further strengthened if the results from different types of studies (epidemiology and laboratory) point to the same conclusion.

As Ågerstrand and Beronius (2016) explained:

> In general terms, WoE [weight of evidence] evaluation and SR [systematic reviews] are processes of summarizing, synthesizing and interpreting a body of evidence to draw conclusions, e.g., regarding the relationship between a chemical exposure and adverse health effect. As such, these processes differ from the traditional method for risk assessment by promoting the use and integration of information from all available evidence instead of focusing on a single key study.

A systematic review (SR) is a further refinement that is characterized by Ågerstrand and Beronius (2016):

> ...a clearly stated objective with pre-defined eligibility criteria for studies; an explicit, reproducible methodology; a systematic search that attempts to identify all studies that would meet the eligibility criteria; an assessment of the validity of the findings of the included studies; and a systematic presentation, and synthesis of the characteristics and findings of the included studies... The main point is that both concepts [WoE and SR] provide an alternative to the traditional praxis of identifying a key study and instead promote the use of entire bodies of evidence to reach conclusions regarding health and environmental hazards and risks.

The rise of evidence-based medicine has led to widespread use of SRs and meta-analyses (a related methodology that combines results from multiple studies using specialized statistical analysis) to assess the effectiveness of diagnostic and treatment methods, exemplified, for example, in the extensive series of Cochrane reviews on topics in clinical medicine. More recently, there has been an increased emphasis on use of SRs for assessment of environmental health risks. In addition, protocols for conducting SRs have become formalized in guidelines such as the PRISMA statement (Moher et al., 2009), EQUATOR (Simera et al., 2010), and CONSORT (Schulz et al., 2010) for clinical trials. The PRISMA paper, in particular, has been cited more than 6000 times as of 2017, according to the Web of Science.

A full SR of the entire RF bioeffects literature done to the very high standards of these latest checklists would be an overwhelming task, because of the size of the literature and the many research questions that have been raised. However, high-quality narrative reviews of the RF bioeffects literature have been published by health agencies that attempt to be both critical and comprehensive (at least in their coverage of recent literature); a few SRs and meta-analyses have appeared on more specific topics related to health and safety.

As examples of the latter, two extensive reviews of possible genotoxic effects of RF energy have appeared in recent years. While genotoxicity is not an adverse health effect in itself, it may be a marker for carcinogenicity of an agent and thus is of great interest for risk assessment.

The first, by Veschaeve et al. (2010), was a comprehensive review (but not a formal SR using PRISMA or other criteria) of more than 180 *in vitro* and *in vivo* studies related to possible genotoxicity of RF fields covering a very wide range of biological endpoints and exposure levels, conducted as part of ICNIRP's comprehensive literature review. The authors cited a number of "positive" studies (i.e., reported genetic damage from RF exposure) together with many negative studies. They concluded:

> ..no entirely consistent picture emerges. Many of the positive studies may well be due to thermal exposures, but a few studies suggest that biological effects can be seen at low levels of exposure. Overall, however, the evidence for low-level genotoxic effects is very weak.

The second review, by Vijayalaxmi and Prihoda (2012), was a meta-analysis of 88 *in vitro* studies on human cell lines published between 1990 and 2011. The exposure levels varied widely, from 0.0004 to 5 W/kg. The investigators concluded that (1) while many of the studies reported "statistically significant" effects from exposure, the effect sizes were generally small and comparable to background variability, and (2) there was evidence of publication bias (selective publication of positive versus negative studies). Overall, "there was no consistent pattern in all RF exposure characteristics on all genotoxicity endpoints," the authors concluded, and overall the studies did not support possible carcinogenic effects of RF energy in humans. Smaller studies covered in the review tended to report larger effects, which is a well-known statistical artifact of null hypothesis significance testing using the criterion of $p < 0.05$ to define a "statistically significant" effect (which is the usual approach used in bioeffects studies) (Colquhoun, 2014). Both reviews acknowledge that numerous "statistically significant" effects had been reported over a very wide range of exposures in a variety of experimental preparations, but discounted their significance because of the lack of consistency in the findings.

Critics of groups that develop RF safety standards and guidelines (including ICES and ICNIRP) and health agencies sometimes allege that these groups have ignored reports of biological effects from RF exposure at low levels (i.e., below thresholds for currently accepted limits) in formulating their recommendations. But the situation is different: experts, including those working with ICNIRP and ICES, have devoted considerable time to analyzing such studies but have not (so far) found persuasive evidence of a real health effect given the totality of evidence. In view of the immense literature that presently exists on RF bioeffects and the cumulative nature of scientific knowledge, very strong new evidence would most likely be required to cause health agencies to drastically change their opinions on possible health effects of RF energy (even as they continue to acknowledge the need for further research on the topic.)

12.6 Two Sets of Distinctions

In reviewing this literature, two fundamental sets of distinctions have been made by standards setting organizations: biological effect versus health effect and "established" versus "not established" or "possible" effects.

"Biological effects" versus "health hazards". This distinction relates to the relevance of scientific reports to possible human health risks. IEEE C95.1-2005 considers biological effects as "alterations of the structure, metabolism, or functions of a whole organism, its organs, tissues, and cells. Biological effects can occur without harming health and can be beneficial." The standard defines "adverse health effect" as "a biological effect characterized by a harmful change in health."

ICNIRP (1998) has a similar definition: "An adverse health effect causes detectable impairment of the health of the exposed individual or of his or her off-spring; a biological effect, on the other hand, may or may not result in an adverse health effect."

Established versus "possible" effect. This distinction relates to the strength of evidence for the existence of an effect. IEEE C95.1-2005 defines an "established effect" as "when consistent findings of that effect have been published in the peer-reviewed scientific literature, with evidence of the effect being demonstrated by independent laboratories, and where there is consensus in the scientific community that the effect occurs for the specified exposure conditions."

ICNIRP (1998) states that its guidelines are based on established effects. In a 2002 report that describes its evaluation process, (ICNIRP, 2002)[*] ICNIRP states that "any single observation or study may indicate the possibility of a health risk related to a specific exposure. However, risk assessment requires information from studies that meet [a lengthy statement of] quality criteria as listed in the Appendix" of that report.

More succinctly, then-ICNIRP chair Paolo Vecchia (2005) in a conference paper defined an "established effect" as:

> An effect is considered established when it is consistently indicated by different studies meeting adequate requirements of:
>
> - Scientific quality
> - Replicability
> - Coherence with other research

It is useful to consider terms such as "possible" and "established" in a Bayesian sense, referring to the strength of belief in a scientific conclusion, which may range from near certainty (if the evidence is very strong) to mere suspicion. At one end of this spectrum, multiple lines of evidence from well-done studies with similar conclusions can lead to high confidence that an effect (or health hazard) exists. At the other end

---

[*] International Commission on Non-Ionizing Radiation Protection. "General approach to protection against non-ionizing radiation." Health Physics 82, no. 4 (2002): 540–548.

Radio Frequency Exposure Standards

of the spectrum, a single poor-quality study can raise suspicions even though it falls far short of proof. Proving the *absence* of an effect or health hazard corresponds, in a Bayesian sense, to showing that the posterior probability for the effect (hazard) is zero, which cannot be done with any finite amount of evidence if the prior probability for the effect is nonzero (i.e., if some evidence had previously raised suspicions about the existence of an effect or health hazard). The best that one can do is to collect a large amount of high-quality data and, if it is sufficiently negative, conclude that the effect is very unlikely to exist. (An alternative argument, showing that a claimed effect violates a physical law and is therefore impossible, is difficult to make compellingly with biological phenomena.)

This use of "possible" is consistent with that of the International Agency for Research on Cancer (IARC), whose carcinogen classifications reflect, essentially, various levels of suspicion that an agent or exposure causes cancer. IARC defines "carcinogenic" as where there is "convincing evidence that the agent causes cancer." A "possible carcinogen" is one having "limited evidence of carcinogenicity in humans and less than sufficient evidence of carcinogenicity in experimental animals." IARC has evaluated more than one thousand agents and exposures, and to date has judged only one of them to be "probably not carcinogenic."

Characterizing a hazard as "established" or "possible" relates to just one component of risk assessment, hazard identification, using the now-standard definitions of the famous National Research Council (NRC) 1983 report that is widely known as the "Red Book" (NRC, 1983). Identifying a potential hazard is not enough. To set effective exposure limits or other effective management strategy, one needs more information, including the dose-response relation. Risk assessment is distinct from risk management:

> Risk assessment is the use of the factual base to define the health effects of exposure of individuals or populations to hazardous materials and situations. Risk management is the process of weighing policy alternatives and selecting the most appropriate regulatory action, integrating the results of risk assessment with engineering data and with social, economic, and political concerns to reach a decision. (NRC, 1983)

While the IEEE standards for RF safety, taken as a group, incorporate some elements of risk management (e.g., providing for RF safety programs and describing warning signs), the exposure limits themselves are designed without reference to social, economic, and political concerns and avoid policy recommendations; the same can be said about the ICNIRP guidelines.

12.7 Current Health Issues

Currently, two health issues in particular are subjects of controversy, and have often resulted in calls to revise RF exposure limits:

12.7.1 Electromagnetic "Hypersensitivity"

Many people report nonspecific symptoms (headaches, anxiety, and sleep problems) that they consider to be caused by exposure to EMF from various technologies including fluorescent light bulbs, power lines, and RF fields from Wi-Fi, cellular base stations, or cellular phone handsets. Some of those people are so badly affected that they cannot function normally in modern society, and a fraction of them have taken (literally) to living in caves or in trailers in forests (Foster, 2017). While there is no doubt that these individuals have serious problems, no consistent evidence has emerged so far from properly blinded and controlled studies that demonstrate a link between actual exposure to EMF and the symptoms that Electromagnetic Hypersensitivity (EHS) individuals report. EHS individuals in such studies typically report symptoms when they believe that they are exposed to EMF, as opposed to actually being exposed. Both health agency reviews (e.g. Danker-Hopfe et al., 2016) and systematic scientific reviews by individual scientists (e.g., Rubin et al., 2010) support this conclusion. WHO in its Fact Sheet on the topic suggests the use of a general term, Idiopathic Environmental Intolerance to Electromagnetic Fields (IEI-EMFs) rather than EHS to avoid introducing assumptions about the etiology of the problem (WHO, 2012).

Nevertheless, concern about EHS has led for public calls to reduce exposure limits to protect EHS individuals. This approach is problematic because of the lack of a demonstrated connection between EMF exposure (of some nature) and the development of EHS symptoms, and lack of any identified exposure level at which such problems would not occur (if in fact they are caused by exposure). There is no doubt that some EHS individuals are seriously affected by their symptoms and need help, but exposure limits are presently not an effective means to address such problems.

12.7.2 Cancer

Numerous epidemiological studies have been conducted on health problems as related to EMF exposure. Of these, the issue of brain cancer as related to long term use of mobile phones has received the most attention, both by scientists and the general public, and the IARC has classified RF energy (mainly from studies related to use of mobile phones) as a "possible" (2B) carcinogen based on "limited evidence in humans for the carcinogenicity of radiofrequency radiation" and "limited evidence in experimental animals for the carcinogenicity of radio frequency radiation" (IARC, 2013).

IARC's use of "possible" reflects a level of suspicion that falls short of that needed to conclude that RF fields "probably" or actually do cause cancer. The European Code Against Cancer (by authors affiliated with IARC but not writing on behalf of that organization) states that "non-ionising types of radiation... including extremely low-frequency electric and magnetic fields as well as radiofrequency electromagnetic fields – are not an established cause of cancer (McColl et al., 2015)".

Three weeks after IARC announced its classification of RF fields as possible carcinogens (2B) based on mobile epidemiology results, WHO EMF Project posted Fact Sheet #193 "Electromagnetic fields and public health: mobile phones" (WHO, 2014). In answering the question "Are there any health effects?" it states: "A large number of studies have been performed over the last two decades to assess whether mobile phones pose a potential health risk. To date, no adverse health effects have been established as being caused by mobile phone use."

While both of these issues (EHS from a broad range of presumed EMF exposures, RF fields and cancer) might (or might not) eventually lead to a revision in RF exposure limits, at present the scientific support for these concerns is an insufficient basis to revise current limits. That does not preclude complementary approaches to addressing public concerns about these issues.

12.8 Precautionary Principle

The BioInitiative Report and other "precautionary" statements refer, explicitly or implicitly, to the PP. Thus, the Wallonia decree cites the Rio Declaration (UNDESA, 1992): "lack of full scientific certainty shall not be used as a reason for postponing cost-effective measures to prevent environmental degradation."

As a statement of principle, most people would consider the Rio Declaration to be unproblematic. The sticking point concerns the term "cost-effective." No environmental or health issue is characterized by "full scientific certainty." The difficult part is to find an appropriate tradeoff between prospective costs and prospective benefits of possible alternative policies to the multiple stakeholders involved in an issue.

The various definitions of the PP vary widely in their implications for environmental and health protection. Wiener and Rogers (2002) and Hammit et al. (2013) identified three "flavors" of the PP:

- *A weak formulation*: Uncertainty does not justify inaction. Thus, the Bergen Declaration (1990) says "[L]ack of full scientific certainty shall not be used as a reason for postponing measures to prevent environmental degradation." The Rio Declaration, a similar formulation, raises the issue of cost effectiveness, and thus opens the door to cost-benefit analysis.

- *A stronger formulation*: Uncertainty justifies or requires action. Thus, the preamble to the Declaration of the Third International Conference on the Protection of the North Sea (Preamble) (1990) says to take action even if there is "no scientific evidence to prove a causal link between emissions [of wastes onto ocean waters] and effects."

- *The strongest formulation*: Uncertainty requires shifting the burden and standard of proof. Thus, Wingspread Statement (1998) says "...the applicant or proponent of an activity or process or chemical needs to demonstrate that the environment and public health will be safe. The proof must shift to the party or entity that will benefit from the activity and that is most likely to have the information" (in Raffensperger and Tickner, 1999).

In its "strongest formulation," the PP proposes that "proponents" of an activity should demonstrate its safety before introducing it to market. Even in countries that do not explicitly recognize the PP, regulatory law may contain similar provisions. For example, the U.S. Food, Drug and Cosmetics Act and its later amendments requires manufacturers to show that a new drug or medical device is "safe and effective" before placing it on the market.

However, "safety" is a human judgment based on social and ethical considerations as well as technical knowledge. One widely used definition of "safety" is "a judgment of the acceptability of risk in a specified situation" (Banta et al., 1978). For example, the U.S. Code of Federal Regulations (C.F.R.) states that a medical device is "safe"

> "...when it can be determined, based upon valid scientific evidence, that the probable benefits to health from use of the device for its intended uses and conditions of use, when accompanied by adequate directions and warnings against unsafe use, outweigh any probable risks." (21 C.F.R. 860.7 (d) (1))

The U.S. Food and Drug Administration (FDA) has many pages of regulations and extensive bureaucratic processes that define the Agency's required standard of proof of safety. Ultimately, the Agency decides about the "safety" of drugs and devices based on scientific data together with cost-benefit considerations.

In the EU, the PP is – by provision of the Treaty on European Union (1992) – the central element in environmental protection in the EU. The Treaty simply states that "Community policy on the environment shall aim at a high level of protection taking into account the diversity of situations in the various regions of the Community. It shall be based on the precautionary principle ..." The Treaty, however, does not define the PP.

In the European context, the meaning of the PP is embodied in several decades of case law in multiple European tribunals. These cases have involved health-related issues such as whether France can exclude genetically modified crops or British beef from its markets or whether Norway and other Scandinavian countries can ban vitamin-enriched corn flakes (Foster, 2017). Some critics have complained that such "precautionary" bans were actually motivated by goals other than health protection. For example, a 2004 report by the World Bank complained that European bans on genetically modified crops were actually motivated by trade protectionism, to protect less competitive European farmers against industrialized agriculture (Anderson et al., 2004).

12.8.1 EC Commentary

To prevent the arbitrary use of the PP, in February 2000 the European Commission (EC, the governing body of the EU) issued an important communication that laid out criteria for applying the PP by EU countries (EC, 2000). This Commentary shaped the development of European law on the issue in the subsequent years. The communication applied to EU nations, but it deserves wider attention as an important attempt by an authoritative source to rationalize the application of the principle.

Two major points emerge in the Opinion about the use of the PP:

1. *"Precautionary" measures must be applied to address identified risks*: For example, the Communication states: "one factor logically and chronologically precedes the decision to act, namely identification of the potentially negative effects of a phenomenon."

2. *"Precautionary" measures must be based on "as best as possible" a review of the scientific evidence*: The Communication states: "A scientific evaluation of the potential adverse effects should be undertaken based on the available data... [t]his requires reliable scientific data and logical reasoning, leading to a conclusion which expresses the possibility of occurrence and the severity of a hazard's impact on the environment, or health of a given population..."

The Commentary outlined a series of requirements for use of the PP (EC Commission, 2000; italics in original):

> Where action is deemed necessary, measures based on the precautionary principle should be, *inter alia*:
>
> - *proportional* to the chosen level of protection,
> - *nondiscriminatory* in their application,
> - *consistent* with similar measures already taken,
> - *based on an examination of the potential benefits and costs* of action or lack of action (including, where appropriate and feasible, an economic cost/benefit analysis),

Radio Frequency Exposure Standards

- *subject to review*, in the light of new scientific data, and
- *capable of assigning responsibility for producing the scientific evidence* necessary for a more comprehensive risk assessment.

The EC communication emphasized that many different "precautionary" responses were possible to a potential risk, ranging from simply "watchful waiting" for further scientific developments, to sponsoring studies to gather more information, to voluntary measures, and to outright bans on a technology.

The Commentary makes it clear that invoking the PP requires an evidentiary basis for harm: public fears about as-yet unproven hazards are not sufficient. It also requires a careful analysis of the scientific record, and commitment to resolve the uncertainties that led to the precautionary policies. Its overall approach is remarkably conservative, that does not differ greatly in approach from the approach taken by the NRC "Red Book."

With a case law extending for nearly three decades, the definition and proper use of the Principle is undoubtedly more settled in Europe than it is elsewhere in the world. As the cornerstone of EU environmental policy according to the Treaty on European Union, there is no dispute about the central role of the PP in the EU. However, even there the Principle remains murky. A 2017 recent legal analysis concluded that "the decision whether or not to apply the precautionary principle [in the EU] appears to be poorly defined, with ambiguities inherent in determining what level of uncertainty and significance of hazard justifies invoking the precautionary principle (Garnett and Parsons, 2017)."

Two paradigm cases illustrate the ends of the spectrum of precautionary versus non-precautionary policies with respect to EMF regulation:

- *Not precautionary*. Construction cranes, when operated in the vicinity of AM radio towers, can build up dangerous RF voltages that can injure a worker if the cranes are not grounded properly. Safe work rules for operating cranes near AM towers address this well-known hazard with little uncertainty surrounding it. This precaution would not properly be considered as an application of the PP.

- *Precautionary*. At least one scientist has called for precautionary measures for MRI imaging based on reports of increases in DNA strand breaks in lymphocytes in patients after imaging, which may possibly increase the risk of cancer later in life (Kaufmann, 2015). Other studies have failed to confirm this effect, including in a recent and apparently well-done study (Critchley et al., 2017), although that study did report subtle effects of MRI examination of undetermined health significance. At best, one can say that some evidence points to possible genotoxic effects of MRI imaging and, if the effect is real, they might have some future health impact to patients.

However, the important question here is whether a patient's outcome is likely to be improved by MRI imaging, given the several known potential (small) risks of the procedure but also potential medical benefits of imaging. Recommending that patients avoid MRI imaging on precautionary grounds because of a speculative small hazard, without considering the prospective benefits of undergoing or the potential risks of foregoing the procedure, is not helpful to patients. As an alternative, "precautionary" measures such as sponsoring more research on the topic, might be warranted if the PP is to be invoked at all (Foster, 2017). But one does not need to invoke the PP to call for further research on the matter.

Science-based exposure limits can coexist consistently with "precautionary" policies. Canada, whose regulatory policies are similar to those of the USA, has in embraced the PP. A 2003 white paper by the Privy Council of Canada (2003) echoes the 2000 EC Commentary but adds: "precautionary measures should be cost-effective, with the goal of generating (i) an overall net benefit for society at least cost, and (ii) efficiency in the choice of measures."

Health Canada states on its website in connection with Safety Code 6:[*]

> Health Canada, as with other federal departments and several regulatory agencies worldwide, applies the precautionary principle as a public policy approach for risk management of possible, but unproven, risks to health. A precautionary approach to decision-making emphasizes the need to take timely and appropriately preventative action, even in the absence of a full scientific demonstration of cause and effect.
>
> The precautionary principle is not a tool for risk assessment. Risk assessments consider all data available in the scientific literature and focus on effects which scientists consider most relevant for human health and based on such an evaluation the Department will take action as required. In the case of electromagnetic fields, there is sufficient evidence supported internationally to show that adherence to the recommended levels of exposure in Safety Code 6 will not cause harm to health.

Later in that document, Health Canada states that it considers that "precaution" has been incorporated in Safety Code 6 through several tiers of "worst case" assumptions in deriving the limits. This characterization has been upheld by courts in other Commonwealth countries with respect to generally similar RF exposure limits in those countries (Telstra, 2006). At least in Commonwealth countries, this interpretation of the PP is legally accepted, to the limited extent that this one court case serves as legal precedent.

In the same sense, both IEEE C95.1-2005 and ICNIRP limits can be described as "precautionary" in their use of safety factors to account for uncertainties in the threshold for identified hazards. IEEE C95.1-2005 states "the safety factor is influenced by the uncertainty in our knowledge of the degree of hazard associated with the hazard exposure threshold and is selected to prevent exceeding the threshold value in human exposure with a sufficiently wide margin." This lines up well with the EC Commentary: the adverse effect has been identified and incorporated a safety factor to account for uncertainty.

Health Canada has, emphatically, adopted science-based limits its approach to setting exposure limits. From Safety Code 6:

> The exposure limits specified in Safety Code 6 have been established based upon a thorough evaluation of the scientific literature related to the thermal and non-thermal health effects of RF fields. Health Canada scientists consider all peer-reviewed scientific studies, on an ongoing basis, and employ a weight-of-evidence approach when evaluating the possible health risks of exposure to RF fields. This approach takes into account the quantity of studies on a particular endpoint (whether adverse or no effect), but more importantly, the quality of those studies. Poorly conducted studies (e.g., those with incomplete dosimetry or inadequate control samples) receive relatively little weight, while properly conducted studies (e.g., all controls included, appropriate statistics, complete dosimetry) receive more weight. The exposure limits in Safety Code 6 are based upon the lowest exposure level at which any scientifically established adverse health effect occurs... It must be stressed that Safety Code 6 is based upon established adverse health effects and should be distinguished from some municipal and/or national guidelines that are based on socio-political considerations.

---

[*] www.canada.ca/en/health-canada/services/environmental-workplace-health/consultations/2015-revisions-safety-code-6-summary-consultation-feedback.html.

Radio Frequency Exposure Standards

In the absence of an authoritative pronouncement for what the PP "means," one can pick and choose among formulations of the PP and argue that the PP "demands" some course of action or other. In fact, the PP does not "demand" any particular action or even any action at all. Like other general prescriptions ("love thy neighbor") the devil is in the details.

12.8.2 Precaution-Based Exposure Limits

A number of countries or local jurisdictions have adopted "precautionary" measures to address public concerns and scientific uncertainty about possible health effects of RF energy, many involving "precautionary" revision to science-based limits. These include adopting precautionary restrictions on the siting of cellular base stations and other transmitting facilities near "sensitive" areas such as schools or hospitals or use of Wi-Fi in schools. Other jurisdictions have revised their RF exposure limits downward for precautionary reasons.

For example, in 1999 Switzerland adopted EMF exposure limits with special reductions for "sensitive" areas "specifically intended to minimise the yet unknown risks" of RF and power-frequency EMFs (Bundesamt, 1999).

Likewise, in 2012, India reduced its exposure limits for RF emission from cellular base stations by a factor of 10 below ICNIRP limits, while retaining ICNIRP limits for transmitters operating outside cellular bands. The country also changed its SAR limits for mobile phones from those of ICNIRP to the older (and somewhat lower) FCC limits currently in place in the USA. A website of the Department of Telecom[*] says, paradoxically, that the "use of mobile services is safe" and at the same time it provides a list of 10 "precautionary guidelines for mobile users" that can reduce the user's exposure to RF energy from handsets.

Many precautionary reductions in RF exposure limits are technology-specific. The Toronto limits apply to cellular base stations (which have generated considerable public controversy in the city) and not to the landmark CN tower in the city center on which communications, radio, and TV broadcast antennas are mounted that collectively transmit more than 1 million watts of power. (These and other broadcast transmitters in the city, however, are "grandfathered" since they were present before the current rules concerning wireless base stations were adopted.) It is inconsistent to reduce exposure limits for RF fields from one technology without taking similar measures against possibly much higher exposures to citizens from RF fields from other technologies as well.

Moreover, the Swiss, Indian, Toronto, Wallonian, Parisian (etc.) limits were not justified (as far as the present authors can determine) by an "as best as possible" scientific review coupled with a commitment to resolve the uncertainties that led to the adoption of the precautionary policies. Rather, in all these cases it seems likely that the "precautionary" limits for RF exposure from cellular base stations (but not other RF transmitting facilities) were political accommodations to a public agitated by the proliferation of cell sites in local communities rather than carefully considered measures against identified hazards.

12.8.3 Other Precautionary Measures

According to the EC Commentary, one can adopt a range of "precautionary" measures, ranging from simply collecting more information to complete bans of a technology. Health agencies around the world have, at times, offered precautionary recommendations

---

[*] www.dot.gov.in/sites/default/files/advertisement_0.pdf.

concerning RF exposure that fall somewhere between these extremes. For a comprehensive review, see Scarfi (2014).

Recommended precautionary measures (as summarized by Scarfi, 2014) include, in increasing level of stringency:

- Calls for more research
- Describing ways in which people *could* reduce RF exposure from use of a cell phone if they so choose (using "hands-free" kits to keep phone away from the head; not using a cell phone where signal levels from the base station are weak, not using a cell phone in enclosed spaces such as elevators)
- Recommending that people *should* reduce their exposure to cell phones (by taking the above steps)
- Discouraging or limiting the use of mobile phones by children
- Banning sales of mobile phones designed for use by children
- Mandatory exposure limits on precautionary grounds.

A full analysis of such recommendations is beyond the scope of this chapter. We note, however, that such advisories are easy for the public to misinterpret and can exacerbate public concerns with no demonstrable potential benefit. Wiedemann and Schütz (2005) noted that "precautionary measures may trigger concerns, amplify EMF-related risk perceptions, and lower trust in public health protection."

For example, Eurobarometer of 2010 reported a survey on "How concerned are you about the potential health risks of mobile phone masts?" (T. N. S. Social and Opinion, 2010). The results varied by country, from 78% of the respondents in Italy, to 6% of respondents in Finland indicating "a large extent" of concern on this issue. More respondents from Italy indicated high concern about this issue than about inadequate housing conditions (72%), exposure to sun (75%) and indoor air quality (72%) – all well established and significant causes of health problems to the population.

The high level of concern by the Italian respondents may have been a result of a long-standing controversy in that country about RF exposures from cellular base stations. Responding to public concerns, different regions of the country adopted low exposure limits for cellular base stations on precautionary grounds while keeping older (ICNIRP) limits for other sources of RF energy. This resulted in a decade-long controversy about possible health hazards from Vatican-owned radio transmitters located outside of Rome, which complied with ICNIRP exposure limits by a large margin but failed to meet the much more stringent "precautionary" limits. The controversy culminated in a health study of the neighboring population near the transmitters, leading to a report in 2010 of an increase in number of cases of childhood leukemia among residents near the transmitters – about the same time that the Eurobarometer survey was conducted. The excess number of cancer cases in the report compared to population incidence rates was very small and the report had little value in demonstrating a hazard from the transmitters, but it was sufficient to raise public concerns even further (Vecchia and Foster, 2002). The Eurobarometer survey concluded:

> asked how the European Union could intervene to support national authorities... the most frequently cited solution, given by nearly half (48%) of EU respondents, is that the European Union should inform the public as to the potential health risks linked to EMFs. The second and third most popular recommendations are setting safety standards for products (39%) and developing guidance for public health protection (36%).

Radio Frequency Exposure Standards 503

A further third (31%) of respondents cite financing research as a possible measure. Similarly strong support is given to setting safety standards for working conditions (27%) and reviewing the status of scientific evidence (23%). The option to harmonise national policies is mentioned by a sixth (16%) of respondents.

All of the measures suggested above could be proposed as "precautionary" measures, but they might also be implemented without formal recourse to the PP (as in fact they have been in many countries that have not adopted the PP in their legal codes).

The present authors believe that arbitrary reduction of RF exposure limits to protect against unknown or unproven hazards is not advisable: it incurs costs while providing no added protection against the hazards for which the limits were designed. Other measures (public education, informing and improving communication with the public, suggesting "precautionary" ways to reduce exposures for people who are concerned about possible hazards, etc.) can be done outside of the framework of setting exposure limits.

The inadvisability of arbitrarily reducing limits on "precautionary" grounds concurs with the recommendation of the WHO Environmental Health Criterion document for ELF Fields (WHO, 2007):

> it is not recommended that the limit values in exposure guidelines be reduced to some arbitrary level in the name of precaution. Such practice undermines the scientific foundation on which the limits are based and is likely to be an expensive and not necessarily effective way of providing protection.

12.9 Future Challenges with RF Standards/Guidelines

Both IEEE C95.1-2005 and ICNIRP (1998) have been under development for decades, without major change in their underlying rationale. Major revisions in ICNIRP and IEEE limits are presently being developed, and are expected to be approved in late 2018 or early 2019. At present, the major changes will most likely be at frequencies above 3–10 GHz, where new communications technologies ("5G" wireless) are beginning to proliferate.[*]

Going forward, the standard-setting process faces major challenges:

- The science-based RF exposure standards (IEEE, ICNIRP) have evolved into highly technical, very lengthy documents (Figure 12.4) that require specialized experience to interpret and implement (or even understand). While this complexity may be required because of the technical complexity of RF dosimetry, it is not desirable from the point of view of transparency.

- The imminent rollout of 5G communications systems, many of which will operate above 3–6 GHz and into the millimeter wave range, will increase the need for reliable standards above the frequency ranges that are chiefly used at present for wireless communications. The short energy penetration depth in tissue above 10 GHz creates technical problems in defining standards and in devising compliance technologies that still need to be addressed. Colombi et al. (2015) pointed out that present exposure standards/guidelines (IEEE, ICNIRP, and FCC) do not provide consistent levels of protection against thermal hazards across the "transition"

---

[*] Readers are advised to consult with the websites of ICNIRP and IEEE ICES for updates to the current standards.

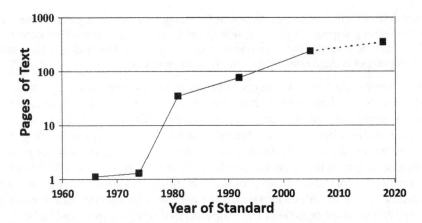

FIGURE 12.4
Increasing length of IEEE C95.1 with edition. Document pages (includes statement of limit and, in later editions, description of rationale and references). The anticipated length of the forthcoming 2018 revision of the standard is indicated also.

frequency in the limits (3 GHz for IEEE C95.1-2005, 10 GHz for ICNIRP (1998)). As a result, the present limits are designed in a way, perhaps inadvertently, that will impose very different limits on the operating power of portable transmitters (used near the body) above and below the limits. One would want the limits to be consistent in level of protection below and above the transition frequency, whatever numerical limits are adopted. These issues are presently being addressed in the most recent, ongoing revisions of both IEEE C95.1-2005 and ICNIRP (1998).

- The scientific literature on biological effects of RF fields is presently growing at a rate of about 300 papers per year (Figure 12.5). Relatively few of these are directly relevant to designing exposure limits. Present work to refine exposure limits above 6–10 GHz is largely based on thermal modeling, but obviously this needs to be better supported by direct experimental data.
- The average quality of the scientific literature in this (and other scientific) fields is declining. This is partly a result of the dramatic rise in the number of online journals, many having questionable standards of peer review. This has resulted in a flood of poor-quality papers.

At the same time, expectations are rising for level of quality in scientific reviews. This has been generally the case in medicine, where the rise of evidence-based medicine has been accompanied by an increasing emphasis on SRs and meta-analysis (as opposed to narrative reviews) for development of practice guidelines. Checklists such as PRISMA, CONSORT, and EQUATOR are becoming the accepted standard for reviews of the medical literature for use in evidence-based medicine, and are fast becoming expected for environmental health reviews (Rooney et al., 2014) and technological risk assessment as well (SCENIHR, 2012).

Reviews done according to these criteria are likely to be more reliable in avoiding bias than simple narrative reviews, but are also far more time consuming to do. If carried out in full detail as outlined in the checklists, a full SR of the entire RF bioeffects literature would be far beyond the capabilities of a volunteer committee – and perhaps for most health agencies as well.

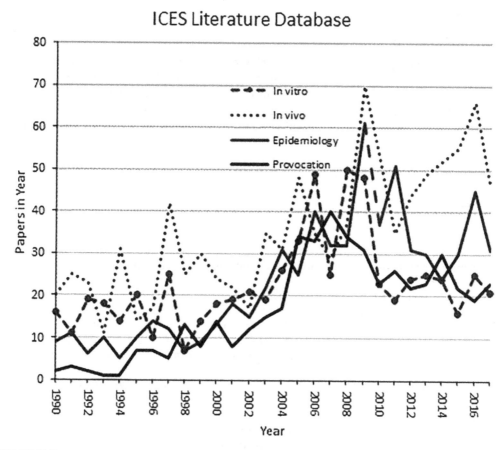

FIGURE 12.5
Growth of RF bioeffects literature (ICES database).

For the hazards for which the ICNIRP and IEEE guidelines/standard are designed to protect against, the scientific issues are relatively well delineated, despite gaps in present knowledge about these issues. But up to date SRs are needed for analysis of potential health risks from long-term exposures to RF fields that remain unproven but nevertheless controversial (e.g., RF fields and cancer, cognitive effects of RF fields and use of wireless technologies). Extensive narrative reviews have already been completed but the literature on these topics is still evolving. Also needed are SRs and meta-analyses related to particular biological endpoints (e.g., genotoxicity, oxidative stress) that might be relevant to potential mechanisms for health effects. SRs of these more limited topics are more feasible (and indeed have been carried out in some cases).

With several thousand related scientific papers, the scientific record about possible health and biological effects of RF energy is among the most extensive of that for any potentially hazardous agent. Health agencies around the world (as well as standards setting bodies in the process of updating their limits) continue to review the RF bioeffects literature. If any major health hazard has presently been overlooked in setting exposure limits, one can assume that the continued reviews of the literature by health agencies will eventually identify it. If that happens, the standards setting process is capable of revising the limits accordingly.

12.10 Conclusion

Exposure to RF energy is an inescapable part of modern life, and it is important to protect public health and safety. Workable and effective exposure limits, together with other protective measures such as product safety standards and safe work practices, are important to protect the population against potential hazards of the useful technologies that utilize RF energy. Developing exposure guidelines is time consuming, but it is an important task.

References

Ågerstrand, M., Beronius, A. 2016. Weight of evidence evaluation and systematic review in EU chemical risk assessment: Foundation is laid but guidance is needed. *Environment International* 92: 590–596.

Anderson, K., Damania, R., Jackson, L. A. 2004. *Trade, standards, and the political economy of genetically modified food*, Vol. 3395. World Bank Publications.

ANSI/IEEE C95.1-1992. 1992. IEEE Standard for Safety Levels with Respect to Human Exposure to RadioFrequency Electromagnetic Fields, 3 kHz to 300 GHz. IEEE, Piscataway NJ.

Arnold, A. W., Itin, P. H. 2010. Laptop computer–induced erythema *ab igne* in a child and review of the literature. *Pediatrics* 126 (5): e1227–e1230.

Banta, H. D., Behney, C. J., Andrulid, D. P. 1978. *Assessing the efficacy and safety of medical technologies.* Office of Technology Assessment, Washington, p. 18.

Betskii, O. V., Devyatkov, N. D., Kislov, V. V. 2000. Low intensity millimeter waves in medicine and biology. *Critical Reviews in Biomedical Engineering* 28 (1&2).

Blackman, C. F., Blank, M., Kundi, M., Sage, C., Carpenter, D. O., Davanipour, Z., Gee D., et al. 2012. The Bioinitiative Report—A Rationale for a Biologically-based Public Exposure Standard for Electromagnetic Fields (ELF and RF). Available on the Internet at: www.bioinitiative.org/report/docs/report.pdf.

Bukhtiyarov, I. V., Rubtsova, N. B., Paltsev, Y. P., Pokhodzey, L. V. 2015. Electromagnetic fields hygienic regulation in Russia. Ways of international harmonization. *Bulgarian Journal of Public Health* 7 (2) Suppl. 1: 130–135.

Bundesamt für Umwelt, Wald und Landschaft, Switzerland, Ordinance of Protection against Nonionising Radiation Explanatory report, 23 Dec. 1999.

Bynum G. D., Pandolf, K. B., Schuette, W. H., Goldman, R. F., et al. 1978. Induced hyperthermia in sedated humans and the concept of critical thermal maximum. *American Journal of Physiology-Regulatory, Integrative and Comparative Physiology* 235 (5): R228–R236.

Cabanac, M. 1983. Face fanning: A possible way to prevent or cure brain hyperthermia. In *Heat stroke and temperature regulation*. Academic Press, Sydney, pp. 213–221.

Carpenter, R. L., Biddle D. K., Van Ummersen, C. A. 1960. Opacities in the lens of the eye experimentally induced by exposure to microwave radiation. *IRE transactions on medical electronics* 3: 152–157.

Chou, C. K. 2015. IEEE EMF exposure and assessment standards activities. *Bulgarian Journal of Public Health* 7 (2) Suppl. 1: 115–120.

Chou, C.-K., Bassen, H., Osepchuk, J., Balzano, Q., Petersen, R. et al. 1996. Radio frequency electromagnetic exposure. *Journal of Bioelectromagnetics* 17: 195–208.

Chou, C.-K., Petersen, R. 2008. Radio frequency exposure and compliance standards for mobile communication devices. In Fujimoto, K., ed., *Mobile antenna systems handbook*. Artech House, pp. 321–342.

Colombi, D., Thors, B., Törnevik, C. 2015. Implications of EMF exposure limits on output power levels for 5G devices above 6 GHz. *IEEE Antennas and Wireless Propagation Letters* 14: 1247–1249.

Colquhoun, D. 2014. An investigation of the false discovery rate and the misinterpretation of p-values. *Royal Society Open Science* 1 (3): 140216.

Commission of the European Communities (EC Commission), Communication on the Precautionary Principle, Brussels 02 February 2000. See http://europa.eu.int/comm/off/com/health_consumer/precaution.htm.

Critchley, W. R., Reid, A., Morris, J., Naish, J. H., et al. 2017. The effect of 1.5 T cardiac magnetic resonance on human circulating leucocytes. *European Heart Journal* 39 (4): 305–312.

D'Andrea, J. A., Gandhi, O. P., Lords, J. L. 1977. Behavioral and thermal effects of microwave radiation at resonant and nonresonant wavelengths. *Radio Science* 12 (6S): 251–256.

Danker-Hopfe, H., Dasenbrock, C., Huss, A., Klaeboe, L., Mjönes, L., et al. 2016. Recent research on EMF and health risk: Eleventh report from SSM's scientific council on electromagnetic fields: including thirteen years of electromagnetic field research monitored by SSM's Scientific Council on EMF and health: How has the evidence changed over time? Available on the Internet at www.stralsakerhetsmyndigheten.se/en/publications/reports/radiation-protection/2016/201615/.

De Lorge, J. O. 1984. Operant behavior and colonic temperature of Macaca mulatta exposed to radio frequency fields at and above resonant frequencies. *Bioelectromagnetics* 5 (2): 233–246.

De Lorge, J. O. 1983. The thermal basis for disruption of operant behavior by microwaves in three animal species. In Adair, E. R., ed., *Microwaves and thermoregulation*. Academic Press, New York, pp. 379–399.

Dewhirst, M. W., Viglianti, B. L., Lora-Michiels, M., Hanson, M., Hoopes, P. J. 2003. Basic principles of thermal dosimetry and thermal thresholds for tissue damage from hyperthermia. *International Journal of Hyperthermia* 19 (3): 267–294.

Dhungel, A., Zmirou-Navier, D., Van Deventer, E. 2014. Risk management policies and practices regarding radio frequency electromagnetic fields: Results from a WHO survey. *Radiation Protection Dosimetry* 164 (1–2): 22–27.

Dimbylow, P. J. 2002. Fine resolution calculations of SAR in the human body for frequencies up to 3 GHz. *Physics in Medicine and Biology* 47 (16): 2835.

Edwards, M. J., Saunders, R. D., Shiota, K. 2003. Effects of heat on embryos and foetuses. *International Journal of Hyperthermia* 19 (3): 295–324.

Eltiti, S., Wallace, D., Ridgewell, A., Zougkou, K. et al. 2007. Does short-term exposure to mobile phone base station signals increase symptoms in individuals who report sensitivity to electromagnetic fields? A double-blind randomized provocation study. *Environmental Health Perspectives* 115 (11): 1603.

European Union (EU). 1999. Council recommendation 1999/519/ on the limitation of exposure of the general public to electromagnetic fields (0 Hz to 300 GHz), Official Journal of the European Union, L 199/59, 30.7.1999. (https://osha.europa.eu/en/legislation/guidelines/council-recommendation-1999-519-ec-on-the-limitation-of-exposure-of-the-general-public-to-electromagnetic-fields-0-hz-to-300-ghz).

European Union (EU). 2013. Directive 2013/35/eu of the European Parliament and of the Council of 26 June 2013 on the minimum health and safety requirements regarding the exposure of workers to the risks arising from physical agents (electromagnetic fields). Official Journal of the European Union L 179/1. Available on the Internet at https://osha.europa.eu/en/legislation/directives/directive-2013-35-eu-electromagnetic-fields.

Federal Communications Commission (FCC). 1996. Telecommunications Act of 1996, Pub. L. No. 104-104, 110 Stat. 56 (1996).

Finnie, J.W., Blumbergs, P. C., Manavis, J., Utteridge, T. D., et al. 2001. Effect of global system for mobile communication (GSM)-like radiofrequency fields on vascular permeability in mouse brain. 2001. *Pathology* 33 (3): 338–340.

Finnie, J. W., Blumbergs, P. C., Manavis, J., Utteridge, T. D. et al. 2002. Effect of long-term mobile communication microwave exposure on vascular permeability in mouse brain. *Pathology* 34 (4): 344–347.

Foster, K. R. 2017. Radiofrequency fields and the precautionary principle. In Wood, A., Karipidis, K., eds., *Non-ionizing radiation protection: Summary of research and policy options*. Wiley, New York, pp. 405–429.

Foster, K. R., Morrissey, J. J. 2011. Thermal aspects of exposure to radiofrequency energy: Report of a workshop. *International Journal of Hyperthermia* 27 (4): 307–319.

Foster, K. R., Moulder, J. E., Budinger, T. F. 2017. Will an MRI examination damage your genes? *Radiation Research* 187 (1): 1–6.

Foster, K. R., Ziskin, M. C., Balzano, Q. 2017. Thermal modeling for the next generation of radiofrequency exposure limits: Commentary. *Health Physics* 113 (1): 41–53.

Foster, K. R., Ziskin, M. C., Balzano, Q., Bit-Bakik, G. 2018. Modeling tissue heating from exposure to radiofrequency energy and its relevance to exposure limits: Heating factor. *Health Physics*. 115(2):295–307.

Gajšek, P., Pakhomov, A. G., Klauenberg, B. J. 2002. Electromagnetic field standards in Central and Eastern European countries: Current state and stipulations for international harmonization. *Health physics* 82 (4): 473–483.

Garnett, K., Parsons, D. J. 2017. Multi-case review of the application of the precautionary principle in european union law and case law. *Risk Analysis* 37 (3): 502–516.

Grigoriev, Y. G. 2017. Methodology of standards development for EMF RF in Russia and by international commissions: Distinctions in approaches. In Markov, M., ed., *Dosimetry in Bioelectromagnetics*. CRC Press.

Guy, A. W., Lin, J. C., Kramar, P. O., Emery, A. F. 1975. Effect of 2450-MHz radiation on the rabbit eye. *IEEE Transactions on Microwave Theory and Techniques* 23 (6): 492–498.

Hammit, J., Rogers, M., Sand, P., Wiener J. B. 2013. *The reality of precaution: Comparing risk regulation in the United States and Europe*. RFF Press, Washington D.C.

Health Canada. 2015. *Limits of exposure to radiofrequency fields at frequencies from 3 kHz to 300 GHz - safety code 6*. Health Canada, Ottawa.

Health Council of the Netherlands, Minister of Housing, Spatial Planning and the Environment (VROM), Critical Review of the BioInitiative Report, Sept 2, 2008. Available on the Internet at https://www.gezondheidsraad.nl/en/task-and-procedure/areas-of-activity/environmental-health/bioinitiative-report.

Hocking, B., Westerman, R. 1999. Radiofrequency electrocution (196 MHz). *Occupational Medicine* 49 (7): 459–461.

IEEE C95.1-1991. 1992. IEEE standard for safety levels with respect to human exposure to radio frequency electromagnetic fields, 3 kHz to 300 GHz. IEEE, Piscataway NJ.

IEEE C95.6-2002, IEEE standard for safety levels with respect to human exposure to electromagnetic fields, 0–3 kHz (2002). IEEE, Piscataway NJ.

IEEE C95.1-2005. 2005. IEEE standard for safety levels with respect to human exposure to radio frequency electromagnetic fields, 3 kHz to 300 GHz. IEEE, Piscataway NJ.

IEEE C95.1a-2010. 2010. IEEE standard for safety levels with respect to human exposure to radio frequency electromagnetic fields-amend 1: Specifies ceiling limits for induced & contact current. IEEE, Piscataway NJ.

International Agency for Research on Cancer (IARC). 2013. Non-ionizing radiation, part 2: Radiofrequency electromagnetic fields. IARC monographs on the evaluation of carcinogenic risks to humans 102 (2013): 1–421. (Available on the Internet at http://monographs.iarc.fr/ENG/Monographs/vol102/.

International Commission on Nonionizing Radiation Protection (ICNIRP). 1998. Guidelines for limiting exposure to time-varying electric, magnetic, and electromagnetic fields (up to 300 GHz). *Health Physics* 74: (4): 494–521.

International Commission on Non-Ionizing Radiation Protection (ICNIRP). 2002. General approach to protection against non-ionizing radiation. *Health Physics* 82 (4): 540–548.

International Commission on Non-Ionizing Radiation Protection. 2006. ICNIRP statement on far infrared radiation exposure. *Health Physics* 91 (6): 630–645.

International Commission on Nonionizing Radiation Protection (ICNIRP). 2009. Exposure to high frequency electromagnetic fields, biological effects and health consequences (100 kHz–300 GHz) - Review of the Scientific Evidence and Health Consequences.

International Commission on Nonionizing Radiation Protection (ICNIRP). 2010. ICNIRP guidelines for limiting exposure to time-varying electric and magnetic fields (1 Hz to 100 kHz). *Health Physics* 99: 818–836.

Johnson, C. C. 1975. LEADER recommendations for specifying EM wave irradiation conditions in bioeffects research. *Journal of Microwave Power* 10 (3): 249–250.

Justesen, D. 1975. Toward a prescriptive grammar for the radiobiology of non-ionising radiations: Quantities, definitions, and units of absorbed electromagnetic energy—an essay. *Journal of Microwave Power* 10 (4): 343–356.

Kaufmann, P. A. 2015. Cardiac magnetic resonance imaging. The case for nonionizing radiation protection and the precautionary principle. *Circ Cardiovasc Imaging* 8: e003885.

Kim, S. Y., Sung, S. A., Ko, G. J., Boo, C. S. et al. 2006. A case of multiple organ failure due to heat stoke following a warm bath. *The Korean Journal of Internal Medicine* 21 (3): 210–212.

Kodera, S., Gomez-Tames, J., Hirata, A. 2018. Temperature elevation in the human brain and skin with thermoregulation during exposure to RF energy. *Biomedical Engineering Online* 17 (1): 1.

Kramár, P., Harris, C., Guy, A. W. 1987. Thermal cataract formation in rabbits. *Bioelectromagnetics* 8 (4): 397–406.

McColl, N., Auvinen, A., Kesminiene, A., Espina, C., et al. 2015. European code against cancer 4th edition: Ionising and non-ionising radiation and cancer. *Cancer Epidemiology* 39: S93–S100.

McRee, D. I. 1979. Review of Soviet/Eastern European research on health aspects of microwave radiation. *Bulletin of the New York Academy of Medicine* 55 (11): 1133.

Merritt, J. H., Chamness, A. F., Allen, S. J. 1978. Studies on blood-brain barrier permeability after microwave-radiation. *Radiation and Environmental Biophysics* 15 (4): 367–377.

Michaelson, S. M. 1971. The Tri-service program-a tribute to George M. Knauf, USAF (MC). *IEEE Transactions on Microwave Theory and Techniques* 16 (2): 131–146.

Moher, D. et al. 2009. Preferred reporting items for systematic reviews and meta-analyses: The PRISMA statement. *Annals of Internal Medicine* 151 (4): 264–269.

National Council on Radiation Protection and Measurements (NCRP). 1981. Radiofrequency electromagnetic fields—properties, quantities and units, biophysical interaction, and measurements. NCRP Report No. 67, NCRP, Bethesda, MD.

National Council on Radiation Protection and Measurements (NCRP). 1986. Report 86, Biological exposure criteria for radiofrequency electromagnetic fields, NCRP, Bethesda, MD.

National Research Council (NRC). 1983. Risk assessment in the federal government: Managing the process. National Academies Press, Washington, DC.

Oizumi, T., Laakso, I., Hirata, A., Fujiwara, O., Watanabe, S., et al. 2013. FDTD analysis of temperature elevation in the lens of human and rabbit models due to near-field and far-field exposures at 2.45 GHz. *Radiation Protection Dosimetry* 155 (3): 284–291.

Osepchuk, J. M., Petersen, R. C. 2003. Historical review of RF exposure standards and the International Committee on Electromagnetic Safety (ICES). *Bioelectromagnetics* 24: S6.

Le Hir, P. 2017. Paris va réduire de 30 % l'exposition aux ondes des antennes-relais, Le Monde 2 March 2017, available on the Internet at www.lemonde.fr/planete/article/2017/03/02/paris-va-reduire-de-30-l-exposition-aux-ondes-des-antennes-relais_5088273_3244.html.

Pakhomov, A. G., Murphy, M. R. 2000. A comprehensive review of the research on biological effects of pulsed radiofrequency radiation in Russia and the former Soviet Union. In Lin J.C. ed., *Advances in Electromagnetic Fields in Living Systems*, vol 3. Springer, Boston, MA 265–290.

Petersen, R. C. 1998. Radiofrequency safety standards-settings in the United States. In Bersani, F., ed., *Electricity and magnetism in biology and medicine*. Plenum Publishing, London, pp. 761–764.

Petersen, R. C. 2009. Radiofrequency/microwave safety standards. In Roach, W. P., ed., *RF dosimetry handbook*, 5th Edition, Available on the Internet at www.dtic.mil/dtic/tr/fulltext/u2/a536009.pdf.

Privy Council of Canada. 2003. A framework for the application of precaution in science-based decision making about risk. Available on the Internet at www.pco-bcp.gc.ca/docs/information/publications/precaution/Precaution-eng.pdf.

Raffensperger, C., Tickner, J. A., eds. 1999. *Protecting public health and the environment: implementing the precautionary principle.* Island Press, pp. 345–346.

Regel, S. J., Negovetic, S., Röösli, M., Berdiñas, V., et al. 2006. UMTS base station-like exposure, well-being, and cognitive performance. *Environmental Health Perspectives* 114 (8): 1270–1275.

Reilly, J. P. 2005. An analysis of differences in the low-frequency electric and magnetic field exposure standards of ICES and ICNIRP. *Health Physics* 89 (1): 71–80.

Repacholi, M. H. 2017. A history of the International Commission on non-ionizing radiation protection. *Health Physics* 113 (4): 282–300.

Repacholi, M., Grigoriev, Y., Buschmann, J., Pioli, C. 2012. Scientific basis for the Soviet and Russian radiofrequency standards for the general public. *Bioelectromagnetics* 33 (8): 623–633.

Rooney, A. A., Boyles, A. L., Wolfe, M. S., Bucher, J. R. and Thayer, K. A. 2014. Systematic review and evidence integration for literature-based environmental health science assessments. *Environmental Health Perspectives* 122 (7): 711.

Röösli, M., Frei, P., Mohler, E., Hug, K. 2010. Systematic review on the health effects of exposure to radiofrequency electromagnetic fields from mobile phone base stations. *Bulletin of the World Health Organization* 88 (12): 887–896.

Rubin, G. J., Nieto-Hernandez, R., Wessely, S. 2010. Idiopathic environmental intolerance attributed to electromagnetic fields (formerly 'electromagnetic hypersensitivity'): An updated systematic review of provocation studies. *Bioelectromagnetics* 31 (1): 1–11.

Scarfi, M. R. 2014. International and national expert group evaluations: Biological/health effects of radiofrequency fields. *International Journal of Environmental Research and Public Health* 11 (9): 9376–9408.

Scientific Committee on Emerging and Newly Identified Health Risks (SCENIHR). 2012. Memorandum on the use of the scientific literature for human health risk assessment purposes – weighing of evidence and expression of uncertainty. Available on the Internet at http://ec.europa.eu/health/scientific_committees/emerging/docs/scenihr_s_001.pdf.

Schulz, K. F., Altman, D. G., Moher, D. 2010. CONSORT 2010 statement: updated guidelines for reporting parallel group randomised trials. *BMC Medicine* 8 (1): 18.

Schwan, H. P. 1992. Early history of bioelectromagnetics. *Bioelectromagnetics* 13 (6): 453–467.

Sharma, H. S., Hoopes, P. J. 2003. Hyperthermia induced pathophysiology of the central nervous system. *International Journal of Hyperthermia* 19 (3): 325–354.

Sienkiewicz, Z., van Rongen, E., Croft, R., Ziegelberger, G., Veyret, B. 2016. A closer look at the thresholds of thermal damage: Workshop report by an ICNIRP task group. *Health Physics* 111 (3): 300.

Simera, I., et al. 2010. A catalogue of reporting guidelines for health research. *European Journal of Clinical Investigation* 40 (1): 35–53. Available on the Internet at www.equator-network.org/.

Staebler, P. 2017. *Human exposure to electromagnetic fields: From extremely low frequency (elf) to radiofrequency.* John Wiley & Sons, New York.

Stam, R. 2011. *Comparison of international policies on electromagnetic fields (power frequency and radiofrequency fields).* National Institute for Public Health and the Environment, The Netherlands.

T. N. S. Opinion and Social. 2010. Eurobarometer 73.3, Electromagnetic Fields, 2010. Available on the Internet at http://ec.europa.eu/public_opinion/archives/ebs/ebs_347_en.pdf.

Tell, R. A., Tell, C. A. 2018. Perspectives on setting safe limits for RF contact currents: A commentary. *BioMedical Engineering Online* 17 (1): 2.

Telstra Corporation Limited v Hornsby Shire Council. 2006. NSW 133, reported in (2006) 146 LGERA 10, Case No. 11097 of 2005 (2006.03.24) (Land and Environment Court of New South Wales) (Judgment).

Tsang, K. S., Swan, M. C., Masood, S. 2011. Full thickness thigh burn caused by a laptop computer: It's hotter than you think. *Burns* 37 (2): e9–e11.

UNDESA. 1992. Rio Declaration on Environment and Development. In Report of the United Nations Conference on Environment and Development, Rio de Janeiro, 3–14 June 1992. Available on the Internet at http://www.un.org/documents/ga/conf151/aconf15126-1annex1.htm.

Ustuner, F. 2012. Practical papers, articles and application notes: interaction of an AM broadcast transmitter with a large crane posing health hazards: A real-world event analysis. *IEEE Electromagnetic Compatibility Magazine* 1 (2): 41–49.

Vecchia P., Scientific Bases of ICNIRP Guidelines, presentation at conference RF fields: Health effects & policy options for protection Melbourne17–18 November 2005.

Vecchia, P., Foster, K. R. 2002. Regulating radio-frequency fields in Italy. *IEEE Technology and Society Magazine* 21 (4): 23–27.

Verschaeve, L. 2012. Evaluations of international expert group reports on the biological effects of radiofrequency fields. In Wireless Communications and Networks-Recent Advances. InTech, 2012. Available on the Internet at www.intechopen.com/books/wireless-communicationsand-networks-recent-advances/evaluations-of-international-expert-group-reports-on-the-biological-effects-of-radiofrequency-fields.

Verschaeve, L., Juutilainen, J., Lagroye, I., Miyakoshi, J., Saunders, R., et al. 2010. In vitro and in vivo genotoxicity of radiofrequency fields. *Mutation Research/Reviews in Mutation Research* 705 (3): 252–268.

Vijayalaxmi, Prihoda, T. J. 2012. Genetic damage in human cells exposed to non-ionizing radiofrequency fields: A meta-analysis of the data from 88 publications (1990–2011). *Mutation Research/ Genetic Toxicology and Environmental Mutagenesis* 749 (1): 1–16.

Wang, H., Wang, B., Normoyle, K. P., Jackson, K., et al. 2014. Brain temperature and its fundamental properties: A review for clinical neuroscientists. *Frontiers in Neuroscience* 8. Article 307, 17 pp. doi: 10.3389/fnins.2014.00307.

Wassermann, E. M. 1996. Risk and safety of repetitive transcranial magnetic stimulation: Report and suggested guidelines from the International Workshop on the Safety of Repetitive Transcranial Magnetic Stimulation, June 5–7, 1996.

Wiedemann, P. M., Schütz, H. 2005. The precautionary principle and risk perception: Experimental studies in the EMF area. *Environmental Health Perspectives* 113 (4): 402.

Wiener, J. B., Rogers, M. D. 2002. Comparing precaution in the United States and Europe. *Journal of Risk Research* 5 (4): 317–349.

Wood, A. W. 2017. Non-ionizing radiation protection: Summary of research and policy options. In Wood, A. W., Karipidis, K., eds., *Non-ionizing radiation protection*. John Wiley & Sons.

World Health Organization (WHO). 2006. Framework for developing health-based EMF standards, WHO Geneva. Available on the Internet at www.who.int/peh-emf/standards/EMF_standards_framework%5b1%5d.pdf?ua=1.

World Health Organization (WHO). 2007. Environmental Health Criteria 238. Extremely low frequency fields. (2007). WHO: Geneva. Available on the Internet at www.who.int/peh-emf/publications/elf_ehc/en/.

World Health Organization (WHO). 2012. Electromagnetic fields and public health: electromagnetic hypersensitivity (factsheet 296). Available on the Internet at www.who.int/peh-emf/publications/facts/fs296/en/.

World Health Organization (WHO). 2014. Electromagnetic fields and public health: Mobile phones. Fact sheet No. 193. Available on the Internet at: www.who.int/mediacentre/factsheets/fs193/en/ (2011).

Wright, G. L. 1976. Critical thermal maximum in mice. *Journal of Applied Physiology* 40 (5): 683–687.

Yarmolenko, P. S., Moon, E. J., Landon, C., Manzoor, A., et al. 2011. Thresholds for thermal damage to normal tissues: An update. *International Journal of Hyperthermia* 27 (4): 320–343.

Zwamborn, A., Vossen, S., van Leersum, S., Ouwens, M. W., Mäkel, W. M. 2003. Effects of global communication system radio-frequency fields on well being and cognitive functions on human beings with and without subjective health complaints. TNO-Report FEL-03-C148.the Hague, Md.: TNO Physics and Electronic Laboratory (2003). Available on the Internet at http://milieugezondheid.be/dossiers/gsm/TNO_rapport_Nederland_sept_2003.pdf.

Index

A

Absorption, in human bodies exposed to far-field of radio frequency sources
  coupling of electromagnetic pulses into human body, 345–348
  head of cell phone users, 348–353
  human body exposed to near-field MRI source, 353–359
  human exposure to field
    produced by coexisting antenna systems, 344–345
    radiated by BTS antennas, 341–344
  specific absorption rate
    in fine resolution anatomical models, 337–341
    induced in cubic cell models, 333–337
AC, see Alternate current (AC)
Accelerated electron, 24
Acetylcholine (ACh) receptors, 190–191
Actin cytoskeleton, 85
Adiabatic boundary condition, 362
ADI formulation, see Alternate-direction implicit (ADI) formulation
Air–tissue boundary, reflection at, 20
α dispersions, 120–121
Alternate current (AC)
  conductor, 34
  electric engines, 44
  fields on cells, nonlinear effects of, 191–203
  power distribution system, 40
  power transmission, 31
Alternate-direction implicit (ADI) formulation, 367–369
Ambient temperature, 373
Amplitude modulated (AM) radio bands, 63
Ampullae of Lorenzini, 266
AM radio bands, see Amplitude modulated (AM) radio bands
Analogical cordless telephones, 62
Anatomically realistic body models
  anatomical family computer models, 324–325
  cubic cell models, 322
  millimeter-resolution model based on MRI scans, 323
  visible human model, 323–324

Anatomically realistic computer models
  absorption in human bodies exposed to far-field of radio frequency sources
    absorption in head of cell phone users, 348–353
    absorption in human body exposed to near-field MRI source, 353–359
    coupling of electromagnetic pulses into human body, 345–348
    human exposure to field radiated by BTS antennas, 341–344
    human exposure to fields produced by coexisting antenna systems, 344–345
    specific absorption rate induced in cubic cell models, 333–337
    specific absorption rate in fine resolution anatomical models, 337–341
  currents induced in human body by low-frequency
    electric blankets, 325–330
    power transmission lines, 330–333
Angular momentum of molecule, 243
Animal navigation models, based on free radicals, 246–247
Anisotropy, 130, 141
  of dielectric and conductive properties of tissue, 189
  of tissue dielectric properties, 129–130
Antenna
  BTS, 341–344
  coexisting systems, 344–345
  dipole, 423
  gain-based formula, 341
  horn, 430
  intermediate/radio frequency, 66
  loop, 424
  military telecommunication transmitters and, 66
  miscellaneous intermediate and radio frequency, 66
  navigational transmitters and, 63–64
  phantom distance, 342
  planar, 351
  telecommunication transmitters and, 64
Anti-ferromagnetism, 144
Artificial depolarization, 83

Artificial direct current fields, in environment
 direct current fields, 31–32
 electrical appliances, 40–42
 exposure in homes, 36–40
 extremely low-frequency
  fields in occupational settings, 45–46
  fields in transportation, 42–45
 high-voltage alternate current power lines,
  32–36
 internal extremely low-frequency induced
  by external and endogenous fields,
  47–50
Artificial hyperpolarization, 83
Assessment standards, 465
Atmospherics, 30
Atomic magnetic moments, 239
Atomic nuclei, 141
Atomic polarization, 104
Automobiles, 43
Average electric field levels, 60, 207

B

Background
 fields, 290
 magnetic field, 175
Base station transmitting antennas, 65
Basic restrictions, 473
β dispersions, 121–122
BHE, see Bio-heat equation (BHE)
Biochemical process, 446
Bioelectrical phenomena, 74
Bioelectric process, 86
Bioelectromagnetics, 436
 experiments with weakly interacting fields,
  264
Bio-heat equation (BHE)
 boundary conditions, 362
 initial conditions, 361
 thermoregulatory responses, 363–364
BioInitiative report, 489–491
Biological amplification, 179–180
"Biological effects" *versus* "health hazards," 494
Biological ionic mobilities atkins, 164
Biological systems, 162–163, 180
Biological transduction mechanisms, 245–246
Biophysical interactions of fields, 22–27
"Biophysical mechanism," 286–287
Biot–Savart's law, 326
Bolometers, 420–421
Boltzmann's constant, 173, 208
Bond energy, 26
Boundary conditions, 8, 15, 119, 318, 320, 362

BTS antennas, human exposure to field
 radiation, 341–344

C

Calorimeters, 420
 Dewar-flask, 428
 twin-well, 427
Calorimetric techniques
 Dewar-flask calorimeter, 428
 twin-well calorimetry, 427
Calorimetry method, 353
Canada, limits in, 485
Cancer, 496
 tissue, 133–134
Canonical model, 313
Carbohydrates, 117
Cell cultures dynamic factors, 444–447
Cell cycle, 77
Cell membrane, 74–75
 electric field on, 185–191
 potential, 75–77
 rectification by, 191–203
Cell surface, effects on
 electromechanical models, 250
 ligand binding, 250
Cellular mobile communication systems, 344
Cellular systems, 436
  CEM43 (thermal dose), 472, 478
Central Limit Theorem, 263, 283
Chemical binding forces, 23
Chemical bonds, 22–27
Chemical noise, 286–290
Chemical reaction rates, changes in
 collision rates, 172–173
 energy, 173–175
 polarization with electric fields, 173
Claussius–Mossoti–Lorentz formulation, 105
Coenzyme B12-dependent reactions, 247
Coexisting antenna systems, human exposure
  to fields production, 344–345
Collinear dipole arrays, 341
Collision rates, changes in, 172–173
Commercial field meters, 403
Competing chemical reactions, 179
Complementary formulation, 341
Complex bioelectromagnetics systems, 448–449
Complex dynamical systems, 245
Complex voltage-sensitive receptors, 91
Computation algorithms
 finite difference time domain methods
  frequency-dependent formulation, 321–322
  traditional method, 319–321

Index

515

finite element method, 318–319
quasi-static impedance method, 315–316
integral equation method of moments
  surface, 317–318
  volume, 316–317
Conduction of electrons in large molecules, 178–179
Conductivity, 411–412
  of tissue at low frequency, 137–138
Contact currents, 475
  safety factors for, 479
"Controlled environments," 473
Conventional blanket, 327
Conventional cars, 43
Conventional electric blanket, 326
Conventional gasoline engines, 43
Cooper pairs, 406–407
Corona discharge, 35
Coulombic force, 90
Coupling of electromagnetic pulses, into human body, 345–348
Crank–Nicolson's scheme, 367
Cryptochromes, in birds, 247
C-type thermocouples, 419
Cubic cell models, 322
Culture container architecture considerations, 438–439
Culture medium dynamic factors, 444
Curers, 59
Current density, 316
Currents induce, in human body by low-frequency
  electric blankets, 325–330
  power transmission lines, 330–333
Cyclotron Resonance, 89
Cylindrical-wave expansion techniques, 342
Cylindrical wave region-closest, 341

D

Debye equation, modeling of tissue properties with, 346–347
δ dispersions, 123
Depolarization, 77
Derived dosimetric quantities, 472
Dewar-flask calorimeter, 428
Diamagnets, 141–142
Diathermy devices, 60
Dictyostelium cells, 84
Dielectric heaters, 59
Dielectric properties
  of biological materials
    carbohydrates, 117

dispersions in tissue, 119–123
electrolytes, 115–116
proteins and other macromolecules, 118–119
water, 113–115
of biological tissue, 411–412
nonlinear, 138–139
permittivity
  of liquids and dense gases, 105–106
  of low pressure gases, 105
quasi-static response, 104
time and frequency dependence of
  nonpolar molecules, 108–109
  permittivity of polar substance—Debye equation, 108–109
  time-dependent polarization – impulse response – Kramers–Krönig relations, 106–108
of tissue
  measurement concepts, 124–125
  review of, 126–137
  uncertainty in measurement of biological materials, 125
Dielectric relaxation, universal law of, 112–113
Dielectric saturation, 24
Dielectric spectroscopy, 137
Dielectric sphere, 317
Dielectrophoresis, 167, 412
Differential power technique, 426
Diode detectors, 413–415
Dipole antenna, 423
Direct current (DC), 10–14
  fields, 31–32
  into tissue, 8–10
  trains operating on, 44–45
Direct detection methods, for free radicals, 245
Direct electromagnetic forces
  cell surface, effects at
    electromechanical models, 250
    ligand binding, 250
  on charges and currents
    electroporation, 252
    ion cyclotron resonance and related ideas, 252–253
    isolated ions and molecules, 252
Dirichelet boundary condition, 362
Discrete time-domain method, 321
Dispersions, dielectric
  α, 120–121
  β, 121–122
  δ, 123
  γ, 122–123
Distribution of relaxation times, 110–112

516 *Index*

Diurnal variations, 30
Domestic ovens, 58
Dosimetric considerations
    derived dosimetric quantities, 472
    primary quantities, 471–472
Dosimetric quantities, induced field and, 301–302
Downstream
    effects, 245
    pathways, 82
Dynamic factors, 447

E

Earth's magnetic field, 30
EAS, see Electronic article surveillance (EAS)
EC Commentary, see European Commission
    (EC) Commentary
ECG, see Electrocardiogram (ECG)
EEG, see Electroencephalogram (EEG)
Einstein's Fluctuation–Dissipation theorem, 269
Electrical appliances, 40–42
Electrical distribution, 36
Electrically powered trains, 44
Electrically stimulated cells, 85
Electrical synapses, 180
Electric blankets, 325–330
Electric cars, 43
Electric field, 47, 316, 408–409
    with biological materials, 162–171
    on cell membranes, 185–191
    dosimetry considerations, 439–444
    measurement, 401–403, 423–424
    polarization with, 173
    sensors, 400
"Electric polarization waves," 26
Electric properties tomography (EPT), 139–140
Electric propulsion systems, 43
Electrified railways/trams, 42–43
Electrocardiogram (ECG), 211
Electrochemical plants, 46
Electrode polarization, 124
Electroencephalogram (EEG), 211
Electrolytes, 115–116
Electromagnetic coupling, 26
Electromagnetic forces
    on charges and currents
        electroporation, 252
        ion cyclotron resonance and related ideas,
          252–253
        isolated ions and molecules, 252
    interacting with other properties
        phase transitions, 254
        water-related effects, 253

Electromagnetic "hypersensitivity," 495–496
Electromagnetic induction, 46
Electromagnetic interference (EMI), 465–466
Electromagnetic theory, 2–4
Electromechanical models, 250
Electronic article surveillance (EAS), 66
Electro-optic meters, 402, 403
Electroporation, 252
Electrostatic field meters, 401–402
Electrosurgical applications, 60
Electrotaxis, 84
ELF, see Extremely low-frequency (ELF)
Elliptical polarization, 34
Embryogenesis, endogenous electric fields
    during early, 77–80
EMI, see Electromagnetic interference (EMI)
Endogenous bioelectrical phenomena, 74
Endogenous electric fields, 251
    during early embryogenesis, 77–80
    migration, 84–85
    nerve sprouting and growth cones, 85–86
    polarization, 83–84
    regeneration, 80–83
    single organs, differentiation of, 80–81
    transporters and ion channels involved in
        bioelectric processes, 86
    wound healing, 81
Endogenous electromagnetic fields, 47–50,
    86–87
Energy
    changes in, 173–175
    effects, 221–222
    fueled membrane transport systems, 75
    impinging on human body, 359
Environmental endogenous electromagnetic
    fields, 87–88
Epithelial folding, 78
E-polarization, 313–314, 411
EPT, see Electric properties tomography (EPT)
E-type thermocouples, 419
European Commission (EC) Commentary,
    498–501
European Union, 484
Exceptions, 222
"Excess noise," 276
Excitation, 22–27
Experimental dosimetry
    dielectric properties of biological tissue,
        411–412
    of static and extremely low-frequency
        electromagnetic fields
        electric field measurement, 401–403
        magnetic field measurement, 403–408

Index 517

Explicit finite difference formulation, 365–366
Exposure limits, precaution-based, 501
Exposure standards, 465
External electric fields, 177, 251
External electric stimulation, 236
External fields, 47–50
External magnetic fields, 48, 251
Extremely low-frequency (ELF), 29, 471
  electric field measurement, 401–403
  magnetic field measurement, 403–408

F

Faraday cage, 75
Faraday coupling, 90–91
Faraday's law, 11, 48
Far field, 56–57, 409–410
  plane waves, 380–383
FDTD methods, see Finite difference time
      domain (FDTD) methods
Federal Communications Commission, U.S.
      (FCC), 373
Feedback
  amplifiers, 180–183
  mechanism, 364
FEM, see Finite element method (FEM)
Ferrimagnetism, 144–145
Ferritin, 147
Ferromagnetism, temperature dependence of,
      145–146
Field zones, 409–410
Filopodia, 86
Finite difference time domain (FDTD)
      methods
  frequency-dependent formulation, 321–322
  traditional method, 319–321
Finite element method (FEM), 318–319
First-order Debye equation, 321
5G communications systems, 503
"Flicker noise," 276
Fluxgate magnetometer, 404–405
FM radio broadcasting, 64
Food heating equipment
  induction cooking stoves, 58
  microwave ovens, 58
Fourier spectrum of noise, 276
Fragmentation of large molecule, 225–228
Free body meters, 402
Freely diffusing radicals, role of, 246
Free radicals
  in biology, 245–248
  mechanism, 244–245
  in solution, 222–225

Free-space
  compliance boundary, 341
  region, 410
Frequency-dependent finite difference time
      domain formulation, 321–322
Full-wave approaches, 342
Fundamental chemical noise, 266
Fundamental interactions
  multiple layers of tissue, 306–310
  spheroidal models, 310–315
  thick tissue layers, 304–306

G

GA, see Golgi apparatus (GA)
Galerkin algorithm, 318
γ dispersions, 122–123
Gastrulation, 78
Gaussian
  elimination, 318
  noise, 283
Geminate correlated radical pair, 238
Generation of radicals, 225–228
Geomagnetic field, 30
Gigahertz range, 29
Globular protein, 118
Glue heaters, 59
Golgi apparatus (GA), 83
Green's functions, 365
Ground-based communication antennas, 64
Ground reference meters, 402, 403
Growth cones, 85–86
Guided waves
  standing waves, 410–411
  waveguide, 411
Gutenberg–Richter power law, 277

H

Hall effect magnetometer, 405–406
Hand-held devices, 64–66
Hand-sets, 65
Harmonic oscillations, 269
Havriliak–Negami relation, 112
HDAC activity, see Histone deacetylase
      (HDAC) activity
Head of cell phone users
  absorption in, 348–353
  temperature increments in, 371–373
Health issues
  cancer, 496
  electromagnetic "hypersensitivity,"
      495–496

Healthy *versus* pathological tissue
    cancerous tissue, 133–134
    ischemic tissue, 134
Heating, 235
Hemoglobin, 147, 228
Hemolytic cleavage of bonds, 225
Heterogeneity, 439
HF band, see High frequency (HF) band
High-energy free electron, 24
Higher-frequency fields, 30
High-field regime, 242
High frequency (HF) band, 63
High-resolution human body model, 339
High-sensitivity meter, 400
High-voltage alternate current power lines, 32–36
Histone deacetylase (HDAC) activity, 80
HMSC, see Human mesenchymal stem cells
        (hMSC)
Hodgkin–Huxley equation, 190
Homogeneity, 103
Hopping activation energy, 178
Horizontal polarization, 317
Horn antenna, 430
Hot-carrier diode, 414
H-polarization, 313–314, 411
Human body
    coupling of electromagnetic pulses into,
        345–348
    exposed to far field of radiating radio
        frequency sources, temperature
        increments in, 369–371
    exposed to near-field MRI source, 353–359
Human exposure
    to field radiated by BTS antennas, 341–344
    to fields produced by coexisting antenna
        systems, 344–345
Human factor, 453–454
Human mesenchymal stem cells (hMSC), 83
Human umbilical vein cells (HUVECs), 229
Hydrophilic regions, 175
Hydrophobic molecules, 75
Hydrophobic regions, 175
Hyperfine
    interaction induced singlet-to-triplet
        conversion, 240–242
    transitions, 3, 243
Hyperthermia devices, 61
Hypothalamic temperature, 363–364

I

IARC, see International Agency for Research on
    Cancer (IARC)

ICNIRP, see International Commission on
    Nonionizing Radiation Protection
    (ICNIRP)
Idealized process of developing science-based
    exposure limits, 465
IF, see Intermediate frequency (IF)
Immunological defense, 246
Incident magnetic field, 221
Incident power density, 471
India, 485
Individual sinusoidal variations, 34
Induced current, 262, 347–348
Induced electric fields, 221, 301–302
Induced voltage, 13
Induction coil magnetometer, 403–404
Induction cooking stoves, 58
Induction heaters, 46, 59–60
Industrial heating
    dielectric heaters, 59
    induction heaters and welders, 59–60
Inhomogeneous complex permittivities, 337
Initial conditions, 361
Initial directional sensing mechanisms, 84
Institute of Electrical and Electronics Engineers
        (IEEE) standard C95.1-2005, 375, 464,
        472–491
Interfacial polarization, 129
Intermediate frequency (IF) electromagnetic
        field sources and exposures
    food heating equipment
        induction cooking stoves, 58
        microwave ovens, 58
    industrial heating
        dielectric heaters, 59
        induction heaters and welders, 59–60
    medical applications
        diathermy devices, 60
        electrosurgical applications, 60
        hyperthermia, 61
        magnetic resonance imaging, 61
    radars, military, 62
    semiconductor manufacturing equipment, 60
    telecommunication transmitters and
        antennas
        FM radio and TV transmission, 64
        military telecommunication transmitters
            and antennas, 66
        miscellaneous intermediate and radio
            frequency antennas, 66
        mobile phone base stations and
            hand-held devices, 64–66
        navigational transmitters and antennas,
            63–64

Index

519

shortwave transmission, 63
Intermediate/radio frequency antennas, 66
Intermolecular interactions, 105
Internal electric fields, 316
Internal extremely low-frequency, 47–50
Internal signaling, 78, 79
Internal temperature regulation mechanism, 363
International Agency for Research on Cancer (IARC), 495
International Commission on Nonionizing Radiation Protection (ICNIRP), 33, 370, 469–470, 472–491
International Electrotechnical Commission (IEC), formulas, 357
International Telecommunications Union (ITU)
    frequency bands for radio spectrum, 62
Intramolecular magnetic fields, 251
In vitro exposure systems
    bioelectromagnetic experimentation, 437–447
    exposure systems
        horn antenna, 430
        radial waveguide, 430
        rectangular waveguide, 429–430
        transverse electromagnetic mode cell, 428–429
    measurements, *in vivo* versus, 128–129
Ion channels, involved in bioelectric processes, 86
Ion cyclotron resonance, 252–253
Ionization, 22–27
Ionospheric processes, 30
Iron
    ferritin, 147
    hemoglobin, 147
    magnetite, 147–148
Irradiated cadaver, 428
Ischemic tissue, 134
Isolated ions/molecules, 252
Isolated magnetite grains, 236
Isotropic system, 244
Iterative method, 318
ITU, see International Telecommunications Union (ITU)

J

J-type thermocouples, 419

K

K-polarization, 313–314, 411
K-type thermocouples, 419

L

Lacking quality assurance can, 454
Lamellipodia, 86
Landé g-factor, 241
Larger biopolymers, 119
Largest stray currents, 37
Larmor precession, 89–90
    changes, 249
    frequency, 222
Lévy distribution, 283
LF, see Low frequency (LF)
LFE, see Low-field effect (LFE)
Ligand binding, 250
Ligand–receptor interaction, 89
Lightning strokes, 24
Linearly polarized plane wave, 304
Lipid bilayer, 75
Local electric field, 40
Local exposure, 475, 484
    safety factors for, 478–479
Local magnetic field, 40
Local specific absorption rate, 355
Lodestone, 266–267
Long conjugated molecules, 178
Long-range attractive forces, 171
Loop antennas, 424
Lorentz
    equation, 2
    power spectrum, 276
Low-field effect (LFE), 242–243
Low-frequency (LF)
    bands, 63
    electric fields, 8–10
    exposures, safety factors for, 477–478
    magnetic fields, 10–14
Low-magnetic-field blanket, 326
Low-water-content materials, 20, 21

M

Macromolecules, 118–119
Magnetic anisotropy, 149
Magnetic dipole moments, 220
Magnetic field, 408
    dosimetry considerations, 439–444
    measurement, 424–425
        fluxgate magnetometer, 404–405
        Hall effect magnetometer, 405–406
        induction coil magnetometer, 403–404
        superconducting quantum interference device magnetometer, 406–408
    sensors, 400

Magnetic flux density, 2, 34, 471
Magnetic permeability, 221
Magnetic properties of matter
    diamagnetic materials, 141–142
    ferromagnetic materials
        anti-ferromagnetism, 144
        ferrimagnetism, 144–145
    paramagnetic materials, 142–143
Magnetic pulses, 219
Magnetic resonance imaging (MRI), 61
    techniques for magnetic susceptibility
        mapping
        magnetic susceptibility in diagnostic
            applications, 150
        QSM *versus* SQUID susceptometry,
            149–150
        quantitative susceptibility mapping, 149
Magnetic susceptibility
    of biological materials, factors affect, 147–149
    mapping, in diagnostic applications, 150
Magnetite, 147–148, 236
Magnetization, 141
Magneto hydrodynamic effect, 11
Magnetometers
    characteristics, 404
    fluxgate, 404–405
    Hall effect, 405–406
    Induction coil, 403–404
    superconducting quantum interference
        device, 406–408
Magnetosensitivity, 266–267
Magnetosomes, 267
Magnetotactic bacterium, 147–148
Man-made fields, 207–212
Maxwell's equations, 2–5, 103, 162, 318, 319, 321,
    400
Mean electric field, 66
Medical applications
    diathermy devices, 60
    electrosurgical applications, 60
    hyperthermia, 61
    magnetic resonance imaging, 61
Medium frequency (MF) bands, 63
Membrane potential, 75–77
Metric specific absorption rate, 301
MF, see Medium frequency (MF) bands
Microenvironmental variables, 448
Microtubule-organizing center (MTOC), 83
Microwave
    frequency, 4
    ovens, 58
    systems, antenna design in, 60
Migration, 84–85

Military radars, 62
Military telecommunication transmitters/
    antennas, 66
Millimeter-resolution model, 323
Minor corona damage, 35
Mobile phone base stations, 64–66
Mobile telecommunication systems, 341
Modern electrical appliances, 40–41
Modern phones, 65
Molecular origin, 141, see *also* Dielectric
    properties
Molecular polarization, 104
MRI, see Magnetic resonance imaging (MRI)
MTOC, see Microtubule-organizing center
    (MTOC)
Multi-diode power sensor, 413
Multiphysics simulation, 450
Multiple-cavity resonances, 207
Multiple layers of tissue, 306–310
Multiple relaxation models, 110–112
Myocardial muscle, 134

N

National Library of Medicine, 323
National limits, 483–488
National Radiological Protection Board (NRPB),
    44
Natural electric fields, 207–212
Naturally occurring fields, 30–31
Navigational transmitters/antennas, 63–64
Near-field, 5–8, 56, 409–410
    radio frequency sources, 374–380
Nernst equation, 447
Nerves/nervous system, 236–237
Nerve sprouting, 85–86
Network analyzer, 422–423
Neural transmitters, 180
1996 database, 126–128
NMR, see Nuclear magnetic resonance (NMR)
Noise, 207–212
    chemical, 286–290
    equilibrium, 265–272
    nonequilibrium, 272–284
    quantum, 284–286
    ratio, signal to, 263–265
Nonequilibrium noise, 272–284
Non-invasive skin impedance spectroscopy,
    137
Nonlinear dielectric properties, 138–139
Nonlinear effects of alternate current fields, on
    cells, 191–203
Nonpolar molecules, 108–109

Index 521

NRPB, see National Radiological Protection Board (NRPB)
Nuclear magnetic resonance (NMR), 61
Numerical methods
  alternate-direction implicit formulation, 367–369
  explicit finite difference formulation, 365–366
  stability criterion, 366–367
Numerical modeling, 448
Nyquist noise, 280

O

Occupational settings, 65
  extremely low-frequency fields in, 45–46
ODC, see Ornithine decarboxylase (ODC)
Open-ended coaxial probes, 125
Optimal meter, 400
Ordered chaos, 87
Organic molecules, 228
Organogenesis, 80
Ornithine decarboxylase (ODC), 197
Oscillating electromagnetic fields, 251
Oscillatory thermal signals, 447
Output power, 65

P

Pacemaker cells, 190
Paging communication system, 66
PAR, see "Project Authorization Request" (PAR)
Parallel polarization, 306
Paramagnetism, 142–143, 222, 228–229
Parametric amplifiers, 183–184
Partial-body specific absorption rate distributions, 355
Pauli Exclusion Principle, 225–226
PEMFs, see Pulsed electromagnetic fields (PEMFs)
Permeability, 411–412
Permittivity, 411–412
  of liquids and dense gases, 105–106
  of low pressure gases, 105
  of polar substance—Debye equation, 108–109
Peroxidase–oxidase system, 245
Personal measurements, 67
Phase transitions, 254
Physical transduction mechanisms, 240
Physics basics, 219–220, 234
Piezoelectric transduction, 24
Planar antennas, 351
"Plane polarization," 34

Plane waves, 333, 409
Polarization, 83–84, 411
  atomic, 104
  with electric fields, changes in, 173
  electrode, 124
  interfacial, 129
  molecular, 104
  plane, 34
  time-dependent, 106–108
Poor project management, 454
Portable systems, 62
Positive temperature coefficient (PTC), 326
  low-magnetic field blanket, 327
Power density, 408–409
Power meters
  calorimeters, 420
  diode detectors, 413–415
  radiofrequency
    thermistors and bolometers, 420–421
    thermocouples, 415–420
Power method, 353
Power sensors, 416–417
Power steering pumps, 43
Power transmission
  coefficient, 304
  lines, 330–333
Precautionary principle, 497–503
Primary quantities, 471–472
"Project Authorization Request" (PAR), 474
Prolonged radio frequency exposures, 383–384
Proteins, 118–119, 175
  reactions, 176–178
Protrusion, 85
PTC, see Positive temperature coefficient (PTC)
Pulsed electromagnetic fields (PEMFs), in therapy, 88–89

Q

Quality assurance, 449–451
Quantitative susceptibility mapping (QSM), 149
Quantized energy, 23
Quantum mechanical formulation, 240
Quantum mechanics, 249
Quantum noise, 284–286
"Quantum tunneling," 285
Quasi-static impedance method, 315–316
Quasi-static response, 104

R

Radars, military, 62
Radial waveguide, 430

Radiation fields, 5–8
Radiative region, 302–303
Radicals, 228–229
  generation of, 225–228
  pair mechanism, 266
Radio frequency (RF)
  absorption metrics
    far field plane waves, 380–383
    near-field radio frequency sources,
      374–380
  dosimetry
    specific absorption rate, 425–426
    specific absorption rate measurements,
      426–428
  electro magnetic field in environments, 67
  experimental dosimetry
    dielectric properties of biological tissue,
      411–412
    fields, 408–411
    measurement, 423–425
    measurement instrumentation, 413–423
  fields, 15–22
  heaters, 59
  identification systems, 66
  sealers, 59
  in vitro exposure systems
    horn antenna, 430
    radial waveguide, 430
    rectangular waveguide, 429–430
    transverse electromagnetic mode cell,
      428–429
Random fluctuations, 207–212
Reactive region, 302
Receptor-ligand binding process, 250
Rectangular waveguide, 429–430
Rectification, of cell membranes, 191–203
"Reference man," 338
Regeneration, 80–83
Regenerative therapy, 83
Resonant transitions, 243–244
Resting potential, 75–77
Resultant magnetic field (RMS), 443
Ritz algorithm, 318
Ritz–Schulten model, 247
RMS, see Resultant magnetic field (RMS)
Rotational angular momentum, 239
Russian federation, 485–487

S

SA, see Spectrum analyzer (SA)
Saline-filled scale model, 335
SAR, see Specific absorption rate (SAR)

Scalar meters, 400
Schottky diode, 414
Schumann resonances, 30
Science-based exposure standards
  ICNIRP (1998) guideline, 469–470
  IEEE C95.1 standard, 467–469
Search-coil magnetometer, 403
Second-order single-pole Lorentz equation, 321
Seebeck
  coefficients, 419
  effect, 415
"Segmented" version, 323
Semiconductor manufacturing equipment, 60
Semiconductor materials, 406
Sensitivity approach, to causality, 453
Sewing machines, 46
Short radio frequency exposures, 383
Shortwave transmission, 63
Shutter-type field mills, 401–402
Signal, 261–262
  to-noise ratio, 263–265
Significant electric fields, 251
Single axis field meters, 443
Single organs, differentiation of, 80–81
Singlet state, 222–223
Six-wire systems, 34
Skin
  depth, 16
  species specific tissue, 134–137
SLE, see Stochastic Liouville equation (SLE)
SMoM, see Surface integral equation method of
      moments (SMoM)
Spatio-temporal considerations, 437–447
Specialized sensory organs, 236
Species specific tissue, skin, 134–137
Specific absorption rate (SAR), 425–426
  in fine resolution anatomical models,
    337–341
  induced in cubic cell models, 333–337
  measurements, 426–428
Specificity, 262–263, 290
Spectrum analyzer (SA), 347–348, 421–422
Spherical-wave expansion techniques, 342
Spheroidal models, 310–315
Spin-correlated radical pair, 238
Spin rephrasing Dg mechanism, 242
Split phase arrangement, 35
SQUID, see Superconducting quantum
      interference device (SQUID)
Stability criterion, 366–367
Standing wave ratio (SWR), 410–411
  specific absorption rate patterns, 310
Static electromagnetic fields, 61

Index

measurements
electric field, 401–403
magnetic field, 403–408
Static signals, 447
Stochasticity, 285
Stochastic Liouville equation (SLE), 240
Stochastic resonance, 184–185
Stratum corneum, 135
Stronger/strongest formulation, 497
Superconducting quantum interference device (SQUID) magnetometer, 406–408
quantitative susceptibility mapping *versus*, 149–150
Surface integral equation method of moments (SMoM), 317–318
Surface treating method, 439
SWR, see Standing wave ratio (SWR)

T

Telecommunication transmitters/antennas
FM radio and TV transmission, 64
military telecommunication transmitters and antennas, 66
miscellaneous intermediate and radio frequency antennas, 66
mobile phone base stations and hand-held devices, 64–66
navigational transmitters and antennas, 63–64
shortwave transmission, 63
TEM cell, see Transverse electromagnetic mode (TEM) cell
Temperature dependence of ferromagnetism, 145–146
Temperature elevations induce
bio-heat equation
boundary conditions, 362
initial conditions, 361
thermoregulatory responses, 363–364
numerical methods for solving thermal problems
alternate-direction implicit formulation, 367–369
explicit finite difference formulation, 365–366
stability criterion, 366–367
in subjects exposed to
temperature increments in head of cell phone users, 371–373
temperature increments in human body exposed to far field of radiating radio frequency sources, 369–371
thermoregulatory responses, 363–364

Temperature increments
in head of cell phone users, 371–373
in human body exposed to far field of radiating radio frequency sources, 369–371
Temperature rise, see *also* Radio frequency absorption metrics
TEP, see Transepithelial potential (TEP)
Thermal analysis, 360
Thermal dose CEM43, 472, 478
Thermal effects, 203–207, 476
Thermal energy, 26
Thermally insulated surface, 362
"Thermal" standards, 488–489
Thermistors, 420–421
Thermocouples, 415–420, 448
Thermodynamic equilibrium, 208
Thermolysis, 225
Thermoregulation, 18
Thermoregulatory responses, 363–364
Thick tissue layers, 304–306
Three orthogonal sensors, 400
Three-phase systems, 36
Three-wire systems, 34
Time and frequency dependence of dielectric response
nonpolar molecules, 108–109
permittivity of polar substance—Debye equation, 108–109
time-dependent polarization – impulse response – Kramers–Krönig relations, 106–108
Time-dependent Maxwell's curl equations, 319, 321
Time-dependent polarization – impulse response – Kramers–Krönig relations, 106–108
Time-varying magnetic fields, 221, 243–244
Tissue
conductivity, 326
dielectric dispersions in, 119–123
folding process, 74
structure of, 149
Toroidal device, 262
Traditional finite difference time domain method, 319–321
Transepithelial potential (TEP), 77
Transient
radiations, 345–346
signals, 447
Transmitters, 62
characteristics of, 63
Transportation, extremely low-frequency fields in, 42–45

524   *Index*

Transporters, involved in bioelectric processes, 86

Transverse electromagnetic mode (TEM) cell, 428–429

Triangular expansion, 317

Triplet state, 222–223, 241

Tri-Service research program, 469

T-type thermocouples, 419

TV transmission, 64

Twin-well calorimetry, 427

U

Ultra-high frequency (UHF) bands, 64

Uncertainty, 449–451

Uniform theory of diffraction (UTD), 344

Universal law of dielectric relaxation, 112–113

V

Validation, 449–451

VAR, see Volumetric absorption rate (VAR)

Variation, 449–451
    of dielectric properties with age, 130–132

Vertical polarization, 317

Very-high frequency (VHF) band, 64

Very low-frequency (VLF), 30

Vibration detection, 237

Visible human (VH) model, 323–324, 338

Voltage-sensitive phosphatases (VSP), 91

Voltage-sensitive receptors, 91

Volume integral equation method of moments (VMoM), 316–317

Volumetric absorption rate (VAR), 375

VSP, see Voltage-sensitive phosphatases (VSP)

W

Water, 113–115, 175
    related effects, 253

Waveguide, 411
    rectangular, 429–430
    radial, 430

Weak external magnetic fields, 239

Weak formulation, 497

Welders, 46, 59–60

Whole-body exposure, 475
    safety factors for, 476–477

World Health Organization (WHO), 464

Wound healing, 80

Z

Zeeman
    effect, 11, 222
    splitting, 175